Food Hypersensitivity and Adverse Reactions

CLINICAL ALLERGY AND IMMUNOLOGY

Series Editor

MICHAEL A. KALINER, M.D.

Medical Director
Institute for Asthma and Allergy
Washington, D.C.

Food Hypersensitivity and Adverse Reactions

A Practical Guide for Diagnosis and Management

edited by

Marianne Frieri
Nassau County Medical Center, East Meadow,
and State University of New York at Stony Brook
Stony Brook, New York

Brett Kettelhut
Children's Hospital Medical Center
and Cincinnati Allergy and Asthma Center
Cincinnati, Ohio

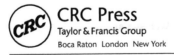

CRC Press
Taylor & Francis Group
Boca Raton   London   New York

CRC Press is an imprint of the
Taylor & Francis Group, an **informa** business

First published 1999 by Marcel Dekker, Inc.

Published 2018 by CRC Press
Taylor & Francis Group
6000 Broken Sound Parkway NW, Suite 300
Boca Raton, FL 33487-2742

© 1999 by Taylor & Francis Group, LLC
CRC Press is an imprint of Taylor & Francis Group, an Informa business

First issued in paperback 2019

No claim to original U.S. Government works

ISBN 13: 978-0-367-45563-7 (pbk)
ISBN 13: 978-0-8247-9903-8 (hbk)

Visit the Taylor & Francis Web site at
http://www.taylorandfrancis.com

and the CRC Press Web site at
http://www.crcpress.com

Preface

Our objective in preparing this book was to provide a resource offering up-to-date basic science and relevant clinical expertise in the area of food hypersensitivity. The contributors are highly qualified experts in the many aspects of this field, authors able to present state-of-the-art and practical information.

The text is divided into five parts. The basic science section (Parts I and II) reviews the allergic and immunologic basis for food hypersensitivity. The clinical section (Parts III and IV) discusses in detail clinical manifestations, including prevalence, unusual presentations, diagnosis, prevention, and treatment. Part V contains chapters on the management of the hospitalized patient with food hypersensitivity, diets, and hypoallergenic formulas, as well as a list of patient resources. In order to achieve completeness in each of the five parts, some of the presented areas overlap.

Several chapters contain detailed information on immunologic mechanisms including food allergen characterization, food contaminants, and "hidden foods." Other chapters discuss non-IgE-mediated topics and atypical cutaneous manifestations. The presentation of neurologic, autoimmune, and psychological topics provides information for an integrated team approach in evaluating the food-allergic patient.

The book will be of great interest to and will provide an important scientific and clinical reference for internists, pediatricians, family practitioners, allergists-immunologists, gastroenterologists, dermatologists, psychologists, psychiatrists, food scientists, dieticians, medical students, students in nutrition programs, teachers of nutritional science, and executives in the food industry.

Marianne Frieri
Brett Kettelhut

Contents

Contributors

Daryl R. Altman, M.D.   Little Neck, New York

Amal Halim Assa'ad, M.D.   Division of Pulmonary Medicine, Allergy, and Immunology, Children's Hospital Medical Center, Cincinnati, Ohio

Sami L. Bahna, M.D., D.P.H.   Division of Allergy/Immunology, University of South Florida, All Children's Hospital, St. Petersburg, Florida

Clifford W. Bassett, M.D.   Little Neck, New York

Vincent S. Beltrani, M.D.   Department of Dermatology, College of Physicians and Surgeons, Columbia University, New York, New York

Lawrence T. Chiaramonte, M.D.   Little Neck, New York

John J. Condemi, M.D., F.A.C.P.   Department of Medicine, University of Rochester, Rochester, New York

John Joseph Costa, M.D.   Beth Israel Deaconess Medical Center and Harvard Medical School, Boston, Massachusetts

Michael K. Farrell, M.D.   University of Cincinnati College of Medicine, Children's Hospital Medical Center, Cincinnati, Ohio

Ira Finegold, M.D., M.S. Allergy and Infectious Disease Section, St. Luke's–Roosevelt Medical Center, New York, New York

Marianne Frieri, M.D., Ph.D. Division of Allergy-Immunology, Nassau County Medical Center, East Meadow, and State University of New York at Stony Brook, Stony Brook, New York

Stephen J. Galli, M.D. Beth Israel Deaconess Medical Center and Harvard Medical School, Boston, Massachusetts

Susan L. Hefle, M.D. Food Allergy Research and Resource Program, University of Nebraska, Lincoln, Nebraska

David J. Hill, M.D. Royal Children's Hospital, Melbourne, Australia

Clifford S. Hosking, M.D. Royal Children's Hospital, Melbourne, Australia

Arne Høst, M.D., D.Sc. Department of Pediatrics, Odense University Hospital, Odense, Denmark

Michael A. Kaliner, M.D. Department of Medicine, Institute for Asthma and Allergy, George Washington University School of Medicine, Washington, D.C.

William T. Kniker, M.D. Department of Pediatrics, University of Texas Health Science Center at San Antonio

Samuel B. Lehrer, Ph.D. Department of Medicine and Clinical Immunology, Tulane University Medical Center, New Orleans, Louisiana

Lyndon E. Mansfield, M.D. El Paso Institute for Medical Research and Development and University of Texas at El Paso, El Paso, Texas

Anne Muñoz-Furlong The Food Allergy Network, Fairfax, Virginia

Mandakolathur R. Murali, M.D. Williston Park, New York

Gerald Reese, M.D. Department of Medicine and Clinical Immunology, Tulane University Medical Center, New Orleans, Louisiana

John C. Selner, M.D. Department of Pediatrics, University of Colorado Health Sciences Center, Denver, Colorado

Herman Staudenmayer, Ph.D. Behavioral Medicine & Biofeedback Clinic of Denver, Denver, Colorado

Susan C. Sturgess, M.S., R.D., C.N.S.D.   Division of Gastroenterology, Hepatology, and Nutrition, Winthrop-University Hospital, Mineola, New York

Steve L. Taylor, Ph.D.   Department of Food Science and Technology, University of Nebraska, Lincoln, Nebraska

Saul Teichberg, Ph.D.   Department of Pediatrics and Laboratories, North Shore University Hospital, Manhasset, New York

Abba I. Terr, M.D.   Stanford University School of Medicine, Stanford, California

Jaya M. Therattil, M.D.   Division of Allergy and Immunology, Nassau County Medical Center, East Meadow, New York

Stephanie Torrens, M.S., R.D.   Massapequa Park, New York

Barry K. Wershil, M.D.   Children's Hospital and Harvard Medical School, Boston, Massachusetts

1

Mast Cells and Basophils: Basic Biology and Roles in Gastrointestinal Diseases

JOHN JOSEPH COSTA AND STEPHEN J. GALLI

Beth Israel Deaconess Medical Center and Harvard Medical School, Boston, Massachusetts

BARRY K. WERSHIL

Children's Hospital and Harvard Medical School, Boston, Massachusetts

Mast cells and basophils are thought to be critical effector cells in immunoglobulin E– (IgE)-dependent host responses to parasites and allergic diseases. These cells may also have important functions in a variety of other immunological, pathological, and perhaps physiological processes, involving the gastrointestinal tract and other anatomic sites. However, the difficult issue is not to determine what mast cells and basophils *might* do in these responses but what they *actually* do and *how* they do it, and, beyond that, to ascertain the *relative importance* of these cells as compared to other cell types that may express similar or overlapping functions. Unfortunately, despite decades of intensive study and the revelation of many interesting and potentially important findings, our understanding of the roles played by mast cells and basophils in health and disease is still incomplete.

1

TABLE 1 Comparison of Human Mast Cells and Basophils

Characteristic	Basophils	Mast Cells
Natural History		
Origin of precursor cells	Bone marrow	Bone marrow
Site of maturation	Bone marrow	Connective tissues (a few in the bone marrow)
Mature cells in the circulation	Yes (usually <1% of blood leukocytes)	No
Mature cells recruited into tissues from circulation	Yes (during immunologic, inflammatory response)	No
Mature cells normally residing in connective tissues	No (not detectable by microscopy)	Yes
Proliferative ability of morphologically mature cells	None reported	Yes (under certain circumstances)
Life span	Days (like other granulocytes)	Weeks to months (based on studies in rodents)
Mediators		
Major mediators stored preformed in cytoplasmic granules	Histamine, chondroitin sulfates, neutral protease with bradykinin-generating activity, β-glucoronidase, elastase, cathepsin G–like enzyme, major basic protein, Charcot-Leyden crystal protein	Histamine, heparin, and/or chondroitin sulfates; neutral proteases (chymase and/or tryptase), many acid hydrolases, cathepsin G, carboxypeptidase
Major lipid mediators produced upon appropriate activation	LTC_4	Prostaglandin D_2, LTC_4, platelet-activating factor
Cytokines released upon appropriate activation	IL-4, IL-13, MIP-1α	TNF-α, IL-4, IL-5, IL-6, IL-8, IL-13, β-FGF (mouse mast cells produce many more)
Surface structures		
Ig receptors	FcεRI, FcγRII(CDw32)	FcεRI
Cytokine/growth factor receptors	IL-2(CD25), IL-3, IL-4, IL-5, IL-8, SCF (some basophils express low numbers of c-kit receptors	SCF (c-kit receptor)
Cell adhesion structures	LFA-1 α chain (CD11a), C43bi receptor (CD11b) gp 150/95 (CD11c), LFA-1 β chain (CD18), ICAM-1 (CD54), and CD44	ICAM-1 (CD54), CD44

IL, interleukin; SCF, stem cell factor; LFA, lymphocyte function-associated antigen; ICAM, intercellular adhesion molecule; Ig, immunoglobulin; LTC_4, leukotriene C_4; MIP, macrophage inflammatory protein; TNF, tumor necrosis factor; β-FGF, LFA,
Source: Ref. 80.

As detailed in Table 1, mast cells and basophils share several notable features besides their distinctive metachromatic staining properties. Both cell types are derived from bone marrow progenitor cells, and both mast cells and basophils are major sources of histamine and other potent chemical mediators implicated in a wide variety of inflammatory and immunologic processes, including allergic disorders with components of immediate hypersensitivity [1–4]. In all mammalian species yet analyzed, both mast cells and basophils express plasma membrane receptors (Fc$_e$RI) that specifically bind with high affinity the Fc portion of IgE antibodies [5,6].

Although it once was believed that basophils might be circulating precursors of mast cells or that mast cells were tissue basophils, current evidence indicates that mature basophils are terminally differentiated circulating granulocytes that can infiltrate tissues or appear in exudates during a variety of inflammatory or immunologic processes. By contrast, morphologically identifiable mast cells do not normally circulate but reside in virtually all normal vascularized tissues.

After sensitization with IgE, exposure to specific multivalent antigen triggers both cell types to undergo an integrated, noncytolytic series of biochemical [5–7] and ultrastructural [8] alterations, often called anaphylactic degranulation or exocytosis, that results in the exposure of the matrices of the cytoplasmic granules to the external medium. These events are associated with the release of the cells' preformed mediators, which are stored in the cytoplasmic granules (such as histamine, heparin or other sulfated proteoglycans, and certain proteases); the de novo synthesis and release of lipid mediators (such as prostaglandin D$_2$ and/or leukotriene C$_4$); and the release of multifunctional cytokines. In addition, a number of stimuli other than IgE and antigen can induce mediator release from mast cells and basophils, providing an alternative mechanism by which these cells might participate in inflammatory reactions in which IgE has no demonstrable role [1–4]. These and many other lines of evidence strongly suggest that mast cells and basophils can serve as biologically significant sources of proinflammatory and immunoregulatory mediators that contribute importantly to the development of many of the clinically relevant features and consequences of allergic diseases and other immunologic disorders.

DEVELOPMENT AND DISTRIBUTION

Mast Cell Distribution

Mast cells are distributed throughout normal connective tissues, where they often lie adjacent to blood and lymphatic vessels, near or within nerves, and beneath epithelial surfaces, that are exposed to the external environment, such as those of the respiratory and gastrointestinal systems and the skin [2,4,9]. Mast cells are also a normal if numerically minor component of the bone marrow and lymphoid tissues. However, unlike mature basophils, mature mast cells do not circulate in the blood.

The abundance of mast cells in normal gastrointestinal (GI) tissues and the ability of mast cells and basophils to release inflammatory mediators in response to multiple immunologic and nonimmunologic stimuli have fueled speculation that these cells may play an important role in gastrointestinal pathophysiological processes [10,11]. Mast cells are ordinarily distributed throughout the entire length of the normal gastrointestinal tract, and in humans, mast cells are particularly prominent in the stomach and small intestine [12]. Mast cells within the GI tract can be seen in the epithelium, mucosa, submucosa, muscle layers, and serosa of the bowel. The close proximity of the mast cells to these different elements of the GI tract may have important functional significance. For example, Stead et al. [13,14] have shown that mast cells in the GI tract of rodent species and humans lie in close anatomical proximity to peptidergic containing nerve cells, and in particular, substance P–containing nerves [13]. At the present time, it is not clear whether the anatomical relationship between mast cells and peptidergic nerves is the result of random association or directed interactions [15].

In humans and many other mammalian species, mast cell numbers in normal tissues exhibit considerable variation according to anatomic sites [4,9] and in association with certain inflammatory or immunological reactions [16]. The numbers of mast cells at sites of chronic inflammation due to a variety of different causes may well be many times higher than in the corresponding normal tissues [16,17]. Such findings as changes in the number of mast cells at various anatomical sites and/or evidence of activation of the cells for mediator release have been observed in a wide spectrum of adaptive or pathological immune or inflammatory responses in the GI tract (Table 2).

TABLE 2 Human Disorders with Evidence Supporting a Role for Mast Cells and/or Basophils in the Pathogenesis of the Inflammatory Response

Food-induced hypersensitivity reactions
Parasitic infections
Inflammatory bowel disease: Crohn's disease
                             ulcerative colitis
Celiac disease (gluten-sensitive enteropathy)
Helicobacter pylori–induced gastritis/ulcer
Pseudomembranous enterocolitis (*Clostridium difficile*–induced enterocolitis)
Eosinophilic gastroenteritis
GI involvement in systemic connective tissue diseases
Ethanol-induced gastritis/ulcer

Mast Cell Heterogeneity

The concept of mast cell heterogeneity is based on evidence derived from studies in humans and experimental animals indicating that mast cells can vary in several aspects of phenotype, including morphological characteristics histochemical features, mediator content, and response to drugs and stimuli of activation [4,9,18–21]. Human mast cells in several anatomical sites can be classified on the basis of their protease content. Mast cells that express immunoreactivity for tryptase (localized predominantly to scroll-containing cytoplasmic granules), but no detectable chymase (less than 0.04 pg per cell) are denoted as MC_T. Other mast cells, termed MC_{TC}, contain immunoreactivity for *both* tryptase and chymase (predominantly localized to crystal-containing cytoplasmic granules) [4,22]. MC_T predominates in the lung, nasal mucosa, and small intestinal mucosa. MC_{TC} predominates in the skin and small intestinal submucosa [4,22]. Although the functional significance of mast cell heterogeneity remains uncertain, experimental data from rodents have confirmed the ability of microenvironmental factors, such as cytokines, to influence the development of mast cell phenotypic variation and have also shown that certain phenotypic changes within mast cell populations can be reversible [9].

Stem Cell Factor and c-*kit*

The study of mast cell development and function has been aided by the identification of mutant mice that exhibit a profound deficiency in tissue mast cells [9,19,23,24]. The mast cell deficiency and other phenotypic abnormalities expressed by $WBB6F_1$–Kit^W/Kit^W–v or $WCB6F_1$–Mgf^{Sl}/Mgf^{Sl}–d mice reflect the consequences of these mutations on the production and/or function of the stem cell factor receptor (SCFR; CD117), which is encoded at the *W* locus in the mouse by the c-*kit* protooncogene, or on the production or function of SCF, the ligand for this receptor, which is encoded at the *Sl* locus in the mouse [24–26]. Specifically, the W^v mutation results in an amino acid substitution in the kinase domain, which dramatically reduces the kinase activity, and *W* is an exon skip mutation of c-*kit* that results in no cell surface expression of the receptor [24–26]. The *Sl* mutation is a deletion of all SCF coding sequences, and the Sl^d allele encodes an SCF transcript that lacks sequences for the intracytoplasmic and transmembrane domains of the molecule [24–26].

The effects of SCF on mast cell development are notable for both their diversity and their importance in the natural history of this particular hematopoietic lineage. SCF has been shown to influence the recruitment, retention, and/or survival of mast cell precursors as well as to promote the proliferation and maturation of these cells [27,28]. SCF is the only cytokine that can induce significant proliferation of either immature mouse mast cells or mature mouse connective tissue mast cells (CTMCs) [27–29]. Repeated injection of recombinant rat SCF into the skin of Sl/Sl^d mice resulted in the local development of a large number of mast cells with phenotypic characteristics of CTMCs, and many of the mast cells in these sites were undergoing proliferation [22,28]. The effect of SCF on mast cell survival is most likely mediated via suppression of mast cell apoptosis, which has been demonstrated both in vitro and in vivo [30,31]. In vivo experiments have demonstrated that an impressive SCF-induced mast cell hyperplasia occurs both in rodents and in nonhuman primates injected with this cytokine. In cynomolgus monkeys treated with recombinant human SCF (rhSCF) at 6 mg/kg per day for 21 days increased numbers of mast cells developed at all sites examined except the central nervous system (CNS), with increases ranging from 3-fold in the heart to 1500-fold in the spleen [32]. Remarkably, mast cell numbers in most sites declined to the baseline numbers observed in vehicle-treated control monkeys by 15 days after cessation of rhSCF administration. Moreover, the rhSCF-treated monkeys appeared to be clinically well, not only throughout the course of treatment, but also during the period when mast cell populations were declining precipitously to normal levels.

Mast Cell and Basophil Development in Humans

Culture of human bone marrow cells or umbilical cord blood cells in suspension in the presence of interleukin 3 (IL-3) generates populations highly enriched in basophils (25% or more), with the remaining cells consisting of neutrophils, eosinophils, monocytes, and rare mast cells [33–35]. Moreover, high-affinity binding sites for IL-3 have been identified on the human basophil surface [36], and basophil numbers are slightly increased in the blood of patients who are treated with rhIL-3 [37]. Although these findings indicate that IL-3 is an important growth factor for human basophils, other cytokines can also contribute to the development of this lineage [38,39]. Granulocyte macrophage colony-stimulating factor (GM-CSF), but not granulocyte CSF (G-CSF) or macrophage CSF (M-CSF), can enhance the growth of basophils from peripheral blood. IL-5 and nerve growth factor (NGF) may also synergize with other growth factors to enhance basophil development in vitro [40]. Although basophils also express receptors for several other cytokines, including IL-2, IL-4, and IL-8, neither these cytokines, IL-1, nor IL-6 appears to promote significant basophil differentiation [38,39].

Like other granulocytes, basophils differentiate and mature in the bone marrow and then circulate in the blood. In humans, the basophil is the least common blood granulocyte, with a prevalence of approximately 0.5% of total leukocytes and approximately 0.3% of nucleated marrow cells [41]. Both cytogenetic evidence and in vitro studies [41] indicate that basophils share a precursor with other granulocytes and monocytes. Specifically, human basophils are derived from pluripotent CD34[+] hematopoietic progenitor cells [42]. Human basophils appear to exhibit kinetics of production and peripheral circulation similar to that of eosinophils [41]. However, unlike the eosinophil, the basophil ordinarily does not occur in peripheral tissues in significant numbers. Basophils can infiltrate sites of many immunological or inflammatory processes, often in association with eosinophils, and participate in the reactions to some tumors [43]. In such cases, basophils are readily distinguishable from mast cells residing in the same tissues [44].

Experiments employing immunomagnetic selection approaches show that the bone marrow progenitor for human mast cells also resides in the CD34[+] population of hematopoietic progenitor cells [42]. Mast cells that express phenotypic characteristics of mature human mast cells can be derived by culturing appropriate progenitor cells together with mouse 3T3 fibroblasts [45]. These mast cells coexpress cell surface IgE receptors and cytoplasmic granules that contain tryptase. In addition, they express a variety of cytoplasmic granule morphological characteristics, including the scroll, mixed, reticular, dense-core, and homogeneous patterns found in the mature human mast cells that occur in normal tissues [46].

In vitro studies have demonstrated that culture of human bone marrow or peripheral blood mononuclear cells, human umbilical cord blood mononuclear cells, and human fetal liver cells with rhSCF used as the only exogenous cytokine results in the development of mast cells [47–50]. However, the human mast cells that develop in cultures supplemented with soluble rhSCF appear to be only a subset of the human mast cell phenotypes observed in vivo. For example, these rhSCF-derived human mast cells express little or no cytoplasmic granule–associated chymase [48,50]. Recently, Costa et al. [51] quantified mast cell numbers in skin biopsy samples obtained from patients enrolled in phase I study of rhSCF. Treatment of these subjects with rhSCF at 5 to 50 µg/kg per day for 14 days resulted in about a 60% increase in the number of dermal mast cells in skin distant from the SCF injection sites. These data indicate that rhSCF can induce mast cell hyperplasia in vivo in humans.

The systemic expansion of mast cell numbers in mice, rats, monkeys, or humans receiving exogenous SCF suggests that changes in the level of expression of endogenous SCF may explain at least in part some of the striking alterations in mast cell numbers noted in association with a variety of repairative responses, immunological reactions, and disease processes [24]. Moreover, it is likely that the wide variation in the numbers of mast cells ordinarily present in different normal tissues may reflect differences in the levels of endogenous SCF bioactivity expressed at the various anatomical sites.

MEDIATORS

Basophils and mast cells contain, or elaborate on appropriate stimulation, a diverse array of potent biologically active mediators [1–4]. Some of these products are stored preformed in the cells' cytoplasmic granules (e.g., proteoglycans, proteases, histamine); others are synthesized upon activation of the cell by IgE and antigen or other stimuli (e.g., products of arachidonic acid oxidation through the cyclooxygenase or lipoxygenase pathways and, in some cells, platelet activating factor [PAF]. Cytokines are the most recently identified group of mast cell and basophil mediators, at least one of which, tumor necrosis factor α (TNF-α), can be both performed and stored as well as newly synthesized by activated cells [52,53]. These agents can mediate a diverse array of effects in inflammation, immunity, and tissue remodeling and can influence the clotting, fibrinolytic, complement, and kinin systems.

Preformed Mediators

Mediators stored preformed in the cytoplasmic granules include histamine, proteoglycans, serine proteases, carboxypeptidase A, and small amounts of sulfatases and exoglycosidases. Mast cells and basophils form histamine by the decarboxylation of histidine and store histamine as an ionic complex with the highly charged carboxyl and/or sulfate groups of the glycosaminoglycan side chains of the proteoglycans. Mast cells isolated from human lung, skin, lymphoid tissue, or small intestine contain about 3 to 8 pg of histamine per cell, and human basophils contain about 1 to 2 pg per cell [2–4]. Studies in genetically mast cell–deficient and congenic normal mice indicate that mast cells account for nearly all of the histamine stored in normal tissues, with the exception of the glandular stomach and the CNS [54]. Basophils are the source of most of the histamine in normal human blood [55].

Human mast cell populations contain variable mixtures of heparin (about 60 kDa) and chondroitin sulfate proteoglycans [56,57]. Although the sulfated glycosaminoglycans of normal human blood basophils have not been characterized, chondroitin sulfates account for the majority of the proteoglycans in the basophils of patients with myelogenous leukemia [58]. Proteoglycans are composed of a central protein core with extended unbranched carbohydrate side chains (glycosaminoglycans) of repeating disaccharide subunits [59]. The central protein core of heparin has numerous serine-glycine repeating residues that, besides conferring protease resistance to the proteoglycan, form the attachment points for glycosaminoglycans. Each disaccharide of the glycosaminoglycans has between zero, and in the case of heparin, three sulfate groups, whose high charge contributes to many of the characteristic physicochemical properties of these molecules [4,59].

Mast cell and basophil proteoglycans probably have several biological functions both within and outside the cells. By ionic interactions they bind histamine, neutral proteases, and carboxypeptidases, and they may contribute to the packaging and storage of these molecules within the secretory granules. When the granule matrices are exposed to physiological conditions of pH and ionic strength during degranulation, the various mediators associated with the proteoglycans dissociate at different rates, histamine very rapidly but tryptase and chymase much more slowly [4]. In addition to regulating the kinetics of release of mediators from the granule matrices, proteoglycans can regulate the activity of some of the associated mediators. For example, heparin stabilizes tryptase in a configuration required for its normal enzymatic activity [4,60].

Neutral proteases are the major protein component of mast cell secretory granules. Both basophils and mast cells contain enzymes with TAME-esterase activity, which can be used as a marker of mast cell or basophil activation in vivo. By weight, tryptase is the major enzyme stored in the cytoplasmic granules of human mast cells, and this neutral protease has been detected in most, if not all, human mast cell populations that have been examined [4]. At least two tryptase genes occur in the human genome, encoding α-tryptase and β-tryptase (approximately 93% homology). Current evidence suggests that β-tryptase is released primarily in association with extensive, systemic anaphylactic-type mast cell degranulation [61]. β-Tryptase is not detectable (< 1–2 ng/ml) in serum obtained from healthy subjects but has been detected at high concentrations in cases of allergen-induced anaphylaxis or systemic mastocytosis. Human mast cell tryptase is a serine endopeptidase that exists in the granule in active form as a tetramer of 134 kDa containing subunits of 31 to 35 kDa, each of which contains an active site [4]. Negligible amounts of tryptase have been identified in normal human basophils by immunoassay [22]. Because this enzyme appears to be unique to the human mast cell, measurements of mast cell tryptase in biological fluids such as plasma, serum, and inflammatory exudates have been used to assess mast cell activation in these settings [62]. Tryptase is stored in the cytoplasmic granules in the active tetrameric form as a complex that is stabilized by its association with heparin and perhaps other proteoglycans within the mast cell granule [60]. The function of mast cell tryptase in vivo is unknown. Mast cell chymase is also a serine protease that is stored in active form in the mast cell granule, but as a monomer with a molecular weight of 30 kDa [63,64]. Human basophils, like eosinophils, can form Charcot-Leyden crystls and contain Charcot-Leyden crystal protein (lysophospholipase) in quantities similar to that of eosinophils [65]. This protein has been localized ultrastructurally to the major cytoplasmic granule population of basophils [66].

Newly Synthesized Lipid Mediators

The activation of mast cells with appropriate stimuli not only causes the secretion of preformed granule-associated mediators but also can initiate the de novo synthesis of certain lipid-derived substances. Of particular importance are the cyclooxygenase and lipoxygenase metabolites of arachidonic acid, which have potent inflammatory activities and which may also play a role in modulating the release process itself [67]. The major cyclooxygenase product of mast cells is prostaglandin D_2 (PGD_2), and the major lipoxygenase products derived from mast cells and basophils are the sulfidopeptide leukotrienes (LTs): LTC_4, LTD_4, and LTE_4 [67]. Human mast cells, but not human basophils, also can produce LTB_4, albeit in much smaller quantities than PGD_2 or the sulfidopeptide leukotrienes [67].

There are three patterns of release of products of arachidonic acid metabolism by human mast cells and basophils: (a) Gut or lung mast cells produce similar amounts of LTC_4 and PGD_2, (b) skin mast cells chiefly produce PGD_2, (c) basophils generate only LTC_4.

Cytokines

Many cytokine-dependent processes are implicated in allergic inflammation, including the upregulation of the IgE response itself (e.g., IL-4, IL-5, IL-6, IL-13), the enhancement or induction of basophil recruitment (e.g., tumor necrosis factor α [TNF-α], IL-4), or mediator production (e.g., IL-3, IL-4, macrophage inflammatory protein 1α [MIP-1 α]), the promotion of eosinophil development/survival (e.g., IL-5, IL-3, granulocyte/macrophage colony-stimulating factor [GM-CSF]), and recruitment (e.g., IL-3, IL-5, GM-CSF, lymphocyte chemotactic factor [LCF], regulated an activation, normal T cell expressed and secreted [RANTES], MIP-1 α), and the recruitment of moncytes and T cells (e.g., MIP-1 α, RANTES) [1,68–75]. Much of the ability of certain cytokines (i.e., IL-1 and TNF-α) to promote allergic inflammation is thought to reflect the capacity of these agents to enhance the recruitment of leukocytes by inducing the increased expression of adhesion molecules, such as P- and E-selectin, vascular cell adhesion molecule (VCAM-1), and intercellular adhesion molecule (ICAM-1), on vascular endothelial cells [76–79]. However, cytokines may critically influence many other stages in the development of allergic inflammation, as well as regulate some of the local consequences of these responses.

In addition to the effects attributed to the "traditional" mast cell– and basophil-derived mediators already described, it is now clear that mast cells and basophils can influence many important aspects of the pathogenesis of allergic inflammation in asthma and other allergic disorders via the elaboration of multifunctional cytokines [52,53]. Indeed, we have hypothesized that the production of cytokines represents one of the critical links among IgE-dependent mast cell activation that occurs immediately after allergen challenge in atopic subjects, the inflammation that develops during the subsequent late-phase reactions to such provocation, and the persistent inflammation and associated tissue changes that are characteristic of chronic allergic disorders [80].

Studies in mast cell–reconstituted genetically mast cell–deficient mice have demonstrated that mast cells are required for essentially all of the leukocyte infiltration observed in the skin [81] or stomach wall [82] after challenge with IgE and specific antigen. A similar approach was used to show that mast cells importantly contribute to the eosinophil infiltration elicited in the lungs in response to aerosol allergen challenge in sensitized mice [83]. In the skin, approximately 50% of such IgE-and mast cell–dependent leukocyte infiltration can be inhibited by using an antibody to recombinant mouse TNF-α [81]. Moreover, mast cells accounted for virtually all of the upregulated expression of TNF-α ribonucleic acid (mRNA) observed within 60–90 min of antigen challenge at cutaneous sites that had been injected with IgE [84].

In IgE-dependent reactions, mast cells are likely to represent the critical initial source of TNF-α, since other cellular elements of allergic inflammation that also can produce this cytokine, such as macrophages, T cells, and B cells, apparently contain little or no preformed TNF-α bioactivity, whereas certain mature, "resting" (nonactivated) mouse mast cells contain preformed stores of TNF-α available for immediate release upon appropriate stimulation of the cells.

However, mast cells represent a potential source of many cytokines, in addition to TNF-α, that might influence allergic inflammation, and the synthesis and release of these products can be induced via IgE-dependent mechanisms. IL-3-dependent in vitro–derived mouse mast cells or mast cell lines activated via the Fc$_\varepsilon$RI contain increased levels of mRNA for many cytokines (IL-1α, IL-3, IL-4, IL-5, IL-6, and GM-CSF and the chemokines MIP-1 α, MIP-1β, MCAF [monocyte chemotactic protein 1 (MCP-1)] (MCP-1), and I-309) and secrete substances with the corresponding bioactivities (IL-1, IL-3, IL-4, IL-6, GM-CSF) [85–87]. Certain mouse mast cell populations can also generate the C-C chemokine, MARC [88], as well as IL-9 and IL-13 [89].

Studies of human mast cell cytokine production have been slower to emerge, in part because of the difficulty of obtaining highly purified preparations of human mast cells. Recent advances in technology that now permit isolation of significant numbers of mast cells from human tissues along with techniques to colocalize mast cell–specific markers and various cytokines in human biopsy specimens clearly have greatly extended our knowledge of human mast cell cytokine production.

Such studies have shown that *human* mast cells can represent a potential source of many cytokines, including TNF-α, bFGF, IL-4, IL-5, IL-6, IL-8, and IL-13 [90,91].

Several groups have demonstrated either de novo or enhanced cytokine production by mast cells in response to IgE-dependent activation, an observation with obvious relevance to pathogenesis of allergic inflammation. Benyon et al. [92] demonstrated that stimulation of purified human skin mast cells with anti-IgE induced these cells to release TNF-α bioactivity, and Gordon et al. [93] showed that, upon challenge with anti-IgE, highly purified human lung mast cells released TNF-α bioactivity and exhibited increased steady-state levels of TNF-α mRNA. Ohkawara et al. [94] showed that challenge of human lung fragments with anti-IgE antibodies in vitro caused three resident cell populations in human lung fragments to express TNF-α immunohistochemically 4 hr after anti-IgE challenge in vitro—mast cells, tissue and alveolar macrophages, and bronchial epithelial cells—whereas no cells exhibited TNF-α immunoreactivity in specimens incubated with medium alone. Finally, Okayama and colleagues [95], using reverse transcription polymerase chain reaction (RT-PCR) and enzyme-linked immunosorbent assay (ELISA) to study human lung mast cell preparations of greater than 94%–99% purity, provided evidence that the c-*kit* ligand, stem cell factor (SCF), and anti-IgE can induce lung mast cells to produce TNF-α, with up to 150 pg TNF-α/10^6 mast cells being generated into the supernatant within 4 hr.

In vitro studies also have confirmed human mast cells as a potentially significant source of IL-5. Okayama and colleagues used RT-PCR and (ISH) in highly purified (>93%) human lung mast cells to demonstrate highly consistent IgE-dependent expression of IL-5 mRNA, which persisted from 24 through 48 approx to 72 hr after activation [96]. In addition, the strength of the IL-5 mRNA signal was positively correlated with the anti-IgE concentration used to activate the cells and immunoreactive IL-5 could be detected by 8 hr after challenge in the culture supernatants [96]. Schulman and coworkers [97] also have demonstrated induction of IL-5 mRNA by both PCR and ISH in both human lung explants and preparations of highly purified human lung mast cells stimulated with anti-IgE antibodies. although secretion of IL-5 protein required costimulation with phorbol ester.

Other investigators have documented enhanced mast cell cytokine expression in nasal or lung tissue from symptomatic atopic individuals as compared to nonallergic control subjects. Bradding et al. [98] used IHC to assess the distribution and identity of cells that expressed IL-4, IL-5, IL-6, and TNF-α in the airways of normal individuals and subjects with mildly symptomatic atopic asthma. In biopsy samples of both the normal and asthmatic airways, many cells stained for each of the four cytokines, and most of these cells were identified as mast cells according to their tryptase content. In addition, there was a highly significant sevenfold mean increase in the number of cells staining for TNF-α in the biopsy specimens of asthmatic as opposed to normal subjects. Also, approximately twice as many mast cells had positive findings for TNF-α by IHC in the biopsy specimens of subjects with asthma as in the specimens of normal subjects. Moreover, most of the TNF-α cells in the biopsy samples were mast cells, both in the airways of normal subjects (range = 50%–100%) and in the airways of subjects with asthma (range = 75%–100%). Immunohistochemical analysis also has revealed that some mast cells in nasal turbinate specimens from patients with allergic rhinitis or from nonatopic subjects display immunoreactivity for IL-4, IL-5, and IL-6 [99].

Sun Ying et al. used a combination of ISH and IHC to examine bronchial biopsy specimens and cytospins of bronchoalveolar lavage (BAL) fluid from mildly atopic asthmatic patients and nonatopic controls [100]. In both the BAL fluid and the biopsy samples, approximately 15% of the IL-4 and IL-5-positive cells were identified as tryptase-positive mast cells [100]. Furthermore, biopsy results from the atopic asthmatics showed significantly increased percentages of tryptase-positive mast cells coexpressing IL-4 and IL-5 mRNA, but not IL-2 or interferon γ(IFN-γ) as compared to those of the nonatopic controls [100].

Glucocorticoids can inhibit cytokine production in many cell types, as can cyclosporin A (CsA), and these effects have been proposed to be among the important mechanisms of action of these agents in patients with asthma [101–104]. Using an in vivo mouse model of IgE- and mast cell–dependent passive cutaneous anaphylaxis. Wershil and coworkers demonstrated that both dexamethasone and CsA could significantly suppress the tissue swelling and leukocyte infiltration associated with IgE-, mast cell–, and TNF—induced inflammation [105]. In the same study, it was shown that either dexamethasone or CsA markedly suppressed TNF-α secretion by mouse mast cells challenged with IgE and antigen in vitro [105]. This work raises the possibility that *one* of the ways glucocorticoids (or CsA) can suppress inflammatory responses is through effects on mast cell cytokine production.

The ability of basophils to serve as a source of multifunctional cytokines has been less extensively studied. However, several reports have demonstrated that mature human basophils isolated from peripheral blood can release IL-4 in response to Fc$_\epsilon$RI-dependent activation, and such release can be enhanced in basophils exposed to IL-3 but not to IL-5, GM-CSF, or nerve growth factor (NGF) [106–109]. Stimulation of human basophils via Fc$_\epsilon$RI crosslinking also yields release of IL-13, and basophil IL-13 synthesis also can be increased by preincubation with IL-3 [110]. IL-4 derived from mast cells or basophils at sites of allergic inflammation may play a role in T cell differentiation toward a TH2 phenotype. Since both human basophils and mast cells can express the CD40 ligand, it is possible these cell types may be able to contribute to IgE production by promoting immunoglobulin class switching [111]. Recent studies of human basophils have also demonstrated synthesis and secretion of MIP-1 α, raising the possibility of autocrine augmentation of mediator release [112].

MECHANISMS OF ACTIVATION

Fc$_\varepsilon$RI-Mediated Activation

The best understood cellular event that underlies expression of basophil or mast cell function is degranulation, a stereotyped constellation of stimulus-activated biochemical and morphological events that result in the fusion of the cytoplasmic granule membranes with the plasma membrane (with external release of granule-associated mediators). Although a variety of agents can initiate basophil or mast cell degranulation, the best-studied pathway of stimulation is transduced through Fc$_\varepsilon$RI expressed on the basophil or mast cell surface [5–7]. The Fc$_\varepsilon$RI consists of one α, one β, and two identical disulfide-linked γ chains, all components of which have been cloned and sequenced [5,6]. When adjacent Fc$_\varepsilon$RIs are bridged, by either bivalent or multivalent antigen interaction with receptor-bound IgE or by antibodies directed against either receptor-bound IgE or the receptor itself, the cells are rapidly activated for the release of stored and newly generated mediators. This process is energy- and temperature-dependent; requires the mobilization of calcium, which results in increased levels of free calcium in the cytosol; and occurs without evidence of toxicity to the responding cell. It has been shown that the bridging of only a few hundred pairs of IgE molecules is sufficient to trigger human basophil histamine release [113].

Because so little of a basophil's or mast cell's Fc$_\varepsilon$RI must be bridged to initiate the degranulation response, these cells may be sensitized simultaneously with IgE antibodies of many different specificities and therefore can react to stimulation by many different antigens. IgE- and antigen-dependent activation is the basis for the immunologically specific expression of mast and basophil function in IgE-dependent immune responses and allergic disorders. For many years, mast cells and basophils were thought to be unique in their expression of the high-affinity receptor (Fc$_\varepsilon$RI) that specifically binds IgE antibodies. However, it is now known that dermal Langerhans' cells and, under certain circumstances, other cell types such as monocytes and eosinophils can also express high-affinity Fc$_\varepsilon$RI [114–117].

Regulation of IgE Receptor Expression

Mast cells and basophils must display high-affinity IgE receptors (Fc$_\varepsilon$RI) on their surface in order to express significant IgE- and antigen-specific effector function. Yet the factors that regulate that Fc$_\varepsilon$RI expression on the surface of these effector cells are incompletely understood [5,6,118]. Two groups demonstrated independently that the level of Fc$_\varepsilon$RI expression on circulating human basophils can exhibit a positive correlation with the serum concentration of IgE [119–121]. However, the basis for this association was not determined. Other studies have demonstrated that short-term incubation of the rat basophilic leukemia cell line (RBL-2H3), a long-term malignant cell line with characteristics most similar to those of mast cells [122], with IgE in vitro can result in roughly a doubling of the cells' surface expression of $Fc_\varepsilon RI$ [123,124]. These studies also showed that this effect, which was insensitive to inhibition by cycloheximide, probably largely reflected IgE-dependent suppression of the elimination of $Fc_\varepsilon RI$ from the cell surface. However, the relevance of these observations to normal mast cells was not clear. More importantly, it was not established whether IgE-induced increases in $Fc_\varepsilon RI$ expression resulted in enhanced responsiveness to IgE-dependent release of proinflammatory mediators.

Yamaguchi et al. have recently reported that exposure to IgE results in a striking (up to 32-fold) upregulation of surface expression of $Fc_\varepsilon RI$ on mouse mast cells in vitro or in vivo [125]. In addition, baseline levels of $Fc_\varepsilon RI$ expression on peritoneal mast cells from genetically IgE-deficient (IgE –/–) mice were dramatically reduced (by ~83%) compared to those on cells from corresponding normal mice. In vitro studies indicated that the IgE-dependent upregulation of mouse mast cell $Fc_\varepsilon RI$ expression has two components: an early cycloheximide-insensitive phase followed by a later and more sustained component that is highly sensitive to inhibition by cycloheximide. IgE-dependent upregulation of $Fc_\varepsilon RI$ expression in turn significantly enhanced the ability of mouse mast cells to release serotonin, IL-6, and IL-4 in response to challenge with IgE and specific antigen.

In a related study [126], Lantz and coworkers demonstrated that the level of $Fc_\varepsilon RI$ expression on bone marrow basophils in mice infected with the nematode *Strongyloides venezuelensis* exhibits a strong positive correlation with the serum concentration of IgE, as was previously reported for human blood basophils. Moreover, the administration of IgE in vivo can significantly upregulate $Fc_\varepsilon RI$ expression on mouse basophils, and genetically IgE-deficient (IgE –/–) mice exhibit a dramatic (~81%) reduction of basophil $Fc_\varepsilon RI$ expression compared to the corresponding normal (IgE +/+) mice.

The finding that IgE can be a major regulator of mouse mast cell and basophil $Fc_\varepsilon RI$ expression in vivo and that IgE-dependent enhancement of mast cell $Fc_\varepsilon RI$ expression permits mast cells to respond to antigen challenge with increased production of proinflammatory and immunoregulatory mediators identifies a potentially important mechanism for enhancing the expression of effector cell function in IgE-dependent allergic reactions or immunological responses to parasites.

Nonimmunologic Direct Activation

In addition to IgE and specific antigen, a variety of biological substances, including products of complement activation and certain cytokines, chemical agents, and physical stimuli, can elicit release of basophil or mast cell mediators. However, the responsiveness of human basophils and different populations of human mast cells to individual stimuli varies. For example, cutaneous mast cells appear to be much more sensitive to stimulation by neuropeptides than are pulmonary mast cells [2,3,127]. Moreover, these stimuli can induce a pattern of mediator release that differs from the one associated with $Fc_\varepsilon RI$-dependent mast cell activation.

Morphine and other narcotics are among the pharmacological agents that can induce mast cell mediator release, but these agents preferentially activate certain populations of mast cells, such as skin mast cells [127]. In this respect the agents are similar to neuropeptides, which can trigger mediator release from human skin mast cells but not significantly from human basophils or gut or lung mast cells.

A considerable body of evidence indicates that cytokines can directly release and/or augment IgE-stimulated mediator release in mast cells and basophils, but often with markedly different responses in each cell type. Members of both the C-C branch of the chemokine cytokine superfamily [128] as well as the C-X-C branch of this group are potent basophil secretogogues [129–135]. MCAF, MIP-1α, CTAP-III, and NAP-2 all cause direct dose-dependent histamine release from basophils [129–135], and some of them also enhance anti-IgE-induced basophil mediator release. Interestingly, another member of the C-X-C group, IL-8, can inhibit the release of histamine from basophils in response to certain stimuli [136]. IL-1, IL-3, IL-5, and GM-CSF also have been shown to cause basophil histamine release directly, or to enhance the basophil histamine release observed in response to other stimuli.

Under certain circumstances SCF can directly induce mouse mast cell degranulation and mediator release and can enhance the mast cell mediator release that is observed upon IgE-dependent activation of these cells [137,138]. SCF can also augment IgE-dependent mediator release from human mast cells [139,140]. At high concentrations it can directly promote mediator release from human basophils in vitro [139] and can induce anaphylactic-type degranulation from human cutaneous mast cells in vivo [51]. In phase I trials, daily subcutaneous administration of rhSCF 5 to 50 µg/kg per day for 14 days resulted in wheal and flare reactions at the rhSCF injection sites. Electron microscopic evaluation revealed extensive anaphylactic degranulation of cutaneous mast cells at these sites [51]. These subjects also developed increased serum levels of mast cell α-tryptase and increased urinary levels of the major histamine metabolite, methyl-histamine. Some of the patients receiving rhSCF experienced other adverse events suggestive of mast cell activation and mediator release, including upper airway symptoms such as cough, hoarseness, and laryngeal spasm and in one patient, transient hypotension [51].

In contrast, the long-term administration of SCF to mice in vivo can *di-*

minish the mast cell's responsiveness to stimulation by IgE and antigen and can *decrease* the severity of IgE-dependent passive anaphylaxis [141]. Although the explanation for these in vivo findings remains to be determined, the results certainly indicate that the effects of SCF on mast cell function may be quite complex.

FUNCTIONAL ROLES IN HEALTH AND DISEASE

Immediate Hypersensitivity

The immediate hypersensitivity reaction is the pathophysiological hallmark of allergic rhinitis, allergic asthma, and anaphylaxis, and the central role of the mast cell in the pathogenesis of these disorders is widely accepted [1–4]. An immediate hypersensitivity reaction is initiated by the interaction of antigen-specific IgE molecules on the surface of mast cells and/or basophils with the relevant multivalent antigen. The physiological effects are due to the biological responses of target cells (vascular endothelial cells, smooth muscle, glands, leukocytes, and so on) to mediators released by activated mast cells and/or basophils.

Immediate allergic reactions are usually accompanied by an increase in local levels of LTC_4 and PGD_2 and by the liberation of histamine and tryptase [2–4]. Although there are several possible cellular sources for some of these mediators, tryptase is thought to be strictly mast cell–derived, providing the strongest biochemical evidence implicating mast cells in these responses in humans.

Studies utilizing mast cell–deficient mice have shown that essentially all of the augmented vascular permeability, tissue swelling, and deposition of cross-linked ^{125}I-fibrin associated with IgE-dependent passive cutaneous anaphylaxis reactions and with IgE-dependent reactions in the stomach wall is mast cell–dependent [142,143]. In humans, mast cell participation in the immediate phase of type I reactions in several anatomical sites has been clearly established by several lines of evidence, including studies demonstrating release of both histamine and tryptase, with a strong correlation between levels of these two mediators, in the nasal secretions or skin blister fluids induced by exposure to allergen [144].

Late-Phase Responses

In many allergic patients the immediate reaction to cutaneous antigenic challenge is followed 4 to 8 hr later by persistent swelling and leukocyte infiltration, termed the late-phase reaction (LPR) [145]. LPRs may follow IgE-dependent reactions in the respiratory tract, nose, and other anatomical locations as well as in the skin. Moreover, many of the clinically significant consequences of IgE-dependent reactions, both in the respiratory tract and in the skin, are now thought to reflect the actions of the leukocytes recruited to these sites during LPR rather than the direct effects of the mediators released by mast cells at early intervals after antigen challenge [80,145]. Several lines of evidence derived from both clinical and animal studies suggest that the leukocyte infiltration associated with LPR is a result of mast cell degranulation. Thus, studies in mast cell–reconstituted mice have demonstrated that the influx of leukocytes at sites of IgE-dependent cutaneous reactions, which reaches maximal levels 6 to 12 hr after antigen challenge, is entirely mast cell–dependent [81]. Furthermore, the injection of anti-TNF-α antiserum at sites of IgE-dependent cutaneous mast cell activation diminishes the leukocyte infiltration observed at the reactions by about 50% [81].

In humans, the leukocytes recruited to sites of LPR include basophils, eosinophils, neutrophils, and macrophages; all of these cells may influence the reactions by providing additional proinflammatory mediators and cytokines. The recruitment and activation of basophils at LPR sites are supported by analyses of nasal lavage or bronchoalveolar lavage fluids obtained several hours after antigen challenge that demonstrate elevations in histamine level, TAME-esterase activity, and LTC_4 but not PGD_2 or tryptase level [146–148].

Mast Cell–Leukocyte Cytokine Cascades

Galli et al. have formulated the hypothesis that a "mast cell–leukocyte cytokine cascade" critically contributes to the initiation and perpetuation of IgE-dependent allergic inflammation in the airways and other sites [80,90]. Specifically, it is proposed that the activation of mast cells through the $Fc_\varepsilon RI$ initiates the response, in part through the release of TNF-α and other cytokines that can influence the recruitment and function of additional effector cells (Fig. 1). These recruited cells then can influence the further progression of the inflammatory response by providing additional sources of certain cytokines (that can also be produced by mast cells stimulated by ongoing exposure to allergen), as well as new sources of cytokines and other mediators that may not be produced by mast cells. Finally, mast cell activation may directly or indirectly promote the release of cytokines from certain resident cells in the respiratory tract, such as alveolar macrophages and bronchial epithelial cells.

Thus, within the local microenvironment in which an allergic response has been elicited, cytokines from mast cells and other resident cells, along with those from recruited leukocyte sources, exert complex effects on other resident cells such as vascular endothelial cells, fibroblasts, epithelial cells, nerves, and mast cells. These contribute to the vascular and epithelial changes and to the tissue remodeling, angiogenesis, and fibrosis that are so prominent in many disorders associated with mast cell activation and leukocyte infiltration. At certain points in the natural history of these processes, mast cell–or eosinophil-derived cytokines may also contribute to the downregulation of the response.

The mast cell–leukocyte cytokine cascade hypothesis thus proposes that mast cell–derived cytokines have a critical role in the initiation of the effector limb of IgE-dependent allergic inflammation and importantly contribute to the perpetuation of the response, but that the manifestations of allergic inflammation, once the response is established, reflect the contributions of the mast cell and many other resident or recruited cell types, including cells that may be recruited by mast cell–dependent mechanisms..

Parasitic Diseases

Several lines of evidence indicate that mast cells or basophils may have similar, overlapping, or complementary functions in immune responses to ectoparasites, worms, and perhaps other parasites, with the relative contributions of each cell type varying according to the type of parasite, species of host animal, and other factors.

Infection with helminthic parasites is associated with increased levels of parasite-specific and nonspecific IgE and with mast cell hyperplasia [149,150]. Moreover, the ability of worm antigens to cause degranulation of mast cells obtained from parasite-infected animals and the toxic properties of some mast cell mediators on these parasites are well documented [149,150]. Finally, some mast cell– or basophil-derived mediators, including histamine and serotonin, have physiological effects on vascular permeability, intestinal ion and mucus secretion, and/or gut motility that may enhance local expressions of host defense against parasites [149,150]. Accordingly, it has been hypothesized that mast cell and basophil sensitization by parasite-specific IgE followed by mast cell and basophil degranulation in response to exposure to parasite antigens promotes the expulsion of the parasites.

In accord with this hypothesis, studies of *Trichinella spiralis* and *Strongyloides ratti* infections and some experiments with the roundworm *Nippostrongylus brasiliensis* showed that the duration of these experimental parasite infections was longer in mast cell–deficient mice than in normal animals [151]. However, the impairment of immunity in mast cell–deficient mice was never as severe as that in athymic nude mice, and in each instance the mast cell–deficient mice eventually were able to resolve the infection. Moreover, the successful elimination of parasites in the absence or virtual absence of a specific IgE response has also been reported [152,153]. Thus, several lines of evidence indicate that mucosal mast cell hyperplasia and activation may contribute to host defense against certain helminthic infections, but in most cases mast cells may not represent an essential component of these immune responses.

The most compelling evidence for a role for mast cells or basophils in

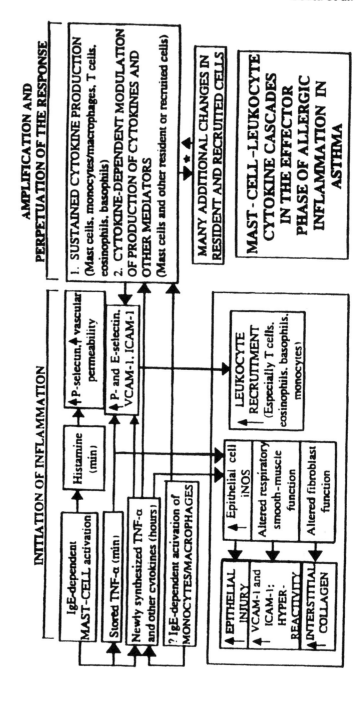

FIGURE 1 A greatly simplified diagram of the pathogenesis of allergic inflammation in asthma and some of its consequences. The diagram is limited to the effector phase of allergic inflammation and focuses primarily on the roles of IgE, mast cells, and cytokines, especially TNF-α. In sensitized subjects, allergic inflammation is insulated by the responses of mast cells, monocytes/macrophages, and perhaps other resident cells (e.g., T cells) to a specific allergen and can then be amplified and sustained, especially in response to persistent or repeated allergen exposure, by the actions of both resident and recruited cells. TNF-α has effects on both resident cells (e.g., vascular endothelial cells, epithelial cells, smooth-muscle cells, and fibroblasts) and recruited leukocytes which can contribute to several of the clinical and pathologic features of asthma. Mast cells and resident monocytes/macrophages may represent the most important initial sources of TNF-α after allergen exposure, but many other effector cells, including T cells, eosinophils, and neutrophils, may provide additional sources of TNF-α during later phases of the inflammatory response. The cytokine production associated with allergic inflammation in asthma can result in many changes in the phenotype, function, and, in some cases, numbers of resident cells, and some of these changes in turn can influence cytokine production by mast cells and other effector cells at these sites. Moreover, many mediators other than cytokines, such as histamine (derived from mast cells or basophils), mast-cell tryptase, and lipid mediators (from many cell types) can have actions that overlap and/or modulate certain cytokine-dependent effects. Note that mast cells (and mast-cell-derived cytokines) have also been implicated in the *afferent limb* of allergic responses and even in the *resolution* of allergic inflammation (see text). *Source:* Ref. 90.

defense against parasites is in immune responses to ectoparasites such as ticks. However, the relative importance of basophils and mast cells in these reactions to ticks may vary according to the species of host and the tick. Studies of genetically mast cell–deficient mice adoptively reconstituted with mast cells have demonstrated that IgE and mast cells are essential for the expression of immune resistance to the cutaneous feeding of larval *Haemaphysalis longicornis* ticks [154]. In contrast, basophils may be more important than mast cells in immune resistance to the feeding of a different tick species, *Dermacentor variabilis*, in mice [155], and both basophils and eosinophils appear to be required for immune resistance to the feeding of larval *Amblyomma americanum* ticks in guinea pigs [156].

Immediate-Type Hypersensitivity Reactions in the Gastrointestinal Tract

Adverse reactions to food may be mediated by a number of different mechanisms [157–159]. For example, immediate-type hypersensitivity responses can be observed in patients with elevated circulating levels of IgE antibodies against specific food antigens. Upon ingestion of the offending antigen, a variety of clinical symptoms can result; these may vary in severity from mild complaints, such as nausea and bloating, to more severe reactions, such as systemic anaphylaxis [157–160]. In most cases, the reaction occurs rapidly after the exposure to antigen (10–30 min) and then wanes.

Reimann et al. [161,162] reported that the direct challenge of the gastric mucosa of allergic individuals with specific antigen produced a reaction characterized endoscopically by edema, erythema, and petechial hemorrhages. In other studies, intestinal segments from experimental animals sensitized to either certain intestinal parasites or specific food antigens, and then challenged with the appropriate antigen, have been shown to develop electrophysiological changes indicative of fluid and electrolyte secretion by the epithelium [163–165]. The secretory response evoked as a result of either parasite antigens or food antigens could be divided into two phases—a rapid phase I response and a later, more prolonged phase II response—and several lines of evidence implicated mast cells in the development of these antigen-driven responses. Mast cell–derived mediators, such as histamine or serotonin (in rodent species), were released after antigen challenge in either parasite- [163] or food antigen–induced [166] hypersensitivity reactions and could recapitulate the phase I response. The phase II response was mimicked by stimulation of the epithelium with prostaglandin E_2 [163], but since mucosal mast cells predominantly generate mediators of the lipooxygenase pathway of arachidonic acid metabolism [2–4], a source for PGE_2 production could not be identified at that time.

Enteric nerves may also play a role in these hypersensitivity responses. The close anatomic relationship that exists between mast cells and nerves in the GI tract may allow relatively high concentrations of mast cell–activating neuropeptides, such as substance P, to be delivered directly to the mast cell. This speculation is supported by several functional studies. For example, direct neural stimulation of rat ileum results in mast cell degranulation [167]. Furthermore, Perdue et al. have shown that mast cells significantly contribute to ion secretion driven by electrical transmural stimulation of mouse small intestine [168], providing evidence of functional communication among nerves, mast cells, and intestinal epithelial cells.

Recent studies have examined whether IgE-dependent late-phase responses can be elicited in the stomach wall of mice and have investigated the role of mast cells in this reaction [82]. IgE-dependent gastric inflammation was elicited in genetically mast cell–deficient Kit^{W}/Kit^{W-v} mice, the congenic normal (+/+) mice, and mast cell–deficient Kit^{W}/Kit^{W-v} mice that had undergone local and selective reconstitution of gastric mast cell populations. IgE-dependent gastric reactions were associated with mast cell degranulation and the infiltration of both neutrophils and mononuclear cells in normal mice [82]. In contrast, no significant leukocyte infiltration was observed in mast cell–deficient $Kit^{W}/Kit^{W}-v$ mice. However, in mast cell–reconstituted $Kit^{W}/Kit^{W}-v$ mice, IgE-dependent reactions were associated with the infiltration of neutrophils and mononuclear cells [82]. These results show that late-phase reactions can occur during IgE-dependent gastric inflammation in the mouse and that the infiltration of both neutrophils and mononuclear cells that is observed during this reaction is mast cell–dependent.

Inflammatory Bowel Disease

Crohn's disease and ulcerative colitis are chronic diseases of the GI tract of unknown cause. However, mucosal immune responses are thought to play a central role in the pathogenesis of both conditions [169]. Although Crohn's disease and ulcerative colitis together constitute inflammatory bowel disease (IBD), these two disease processes have distinct clinical and pathological characteristics. Crohn's disease is characterized by granulomatous inflammation that can involve any portion of the GI tract (from mouth to anus) and typically occurs in a discontinuous anatomical distribution. Moreover, the inflammation in Crohn's disease is typically transmural: i.e., it may occur throughout the entire thickness of the bowel wall from epithelium to serosa. By contrast, the inflammation seen in ulcerative colitis is predominantly mucosal, occurs only in the colon, and is typically anatomically continuous, generally occurring from the distal colon to more proximal colon.

There is extensive morphologic evidence that mast cells and basophils participate in the inflammatory response seen in IBD. Ultrastructural analysis of Crohn's disease specimens has shown a marked increase in the number of mast cells present in inflamed tissue in the mucosa, submucosa, and muscle layers of the gut [170–172]. Mast cells have also been identified as a component of the granuloma that is the pathological hallmark of Crohn's disease [173]. Basophils are also present in the lamina propria of the gut involved by Crohn's disease, but in relatively small numbers [170,174]. However, both mast cells and basophils in the lesions of Crohn's disease exhibited morphological evidence of noncytolytic degranulation [170,175].

In ulcerative colitis, the number of mast cells can also be increased [174–176], and many investigators consider mast cell involvement in IBD to promote the inflammatory response. However, in some patients, an unusual distribution of mast cells has been found along the line of demarcation between inflamed tissue and histologically normal tissue [176]. Although the significance of this finding is not known, it has been suggested that mast cells may act to limit inflammation at the margins of the disease [176].

In addition to increased numbers of mast cells, there is evidence of altered mast cell function in IBD. Mast cells isolated from involved areas of ulcerative colitis are more responsive to stimulation through the $Fc_\varepsilon RI$ than are mast cells from uninvolved segments or control specimens [177]. The significance of this finding is not clear, particularly in light of the fact that IgE levels are not typically elevated in IBD. Furthermore, although anaphylactic degranulation of mast cells and basophils in the GI tract in IBD has been described, it is rare, and another mechanism of mast cell and basophil degranulation, termed piecemeal degranulation, has been identified more frequently. Piecemeal degranulation, characterized by variable losses of cytoplasmic granule contents resulting in nonfused, empty granule containers in undamaged mast cells or basophils [8], has also been identified as a mechanism of mast cell mediator release at sites of cutaneous inflammation in IL-4 transgenic mice [178]. It is possible that such nonanaphylactic activation of mast cells and basophils may result in the prolonged secretion of mediators and/or cytokines at sites of active IBD, or in other types of inflammatory responses in the GI tract.

Since the neuropeptide substance P can induce mast cell degranulation, the demonstration that there is a significant increase in the expression of the high-affinity receptor for substance P in areas of active IBD has suggested a role for substance P in IBD [179]. Substance P has been shown to cause the release of TNF-α from a cloned murine mast cell line [180], and, in foreskin explants, substance P elicits mast cell degranulation and induces the expression of the leukocyte adhesion molecule, endothelial-leukocyte adhesion molecule 1 (ELAM-1) [181]. Taken together, these findings support the possibility that substance P/mast cell interactions may promote the inflammatory response in IBD.

Other GI Diseases

In addition to IBD, mast cells and basophils have been implicated in many other inflammatory conditions involving the GI tract (Table 2). Celiac disease or gluten-sensitive enteropathy is a malabsorptive disorder caused by the ingestion of gluten and is characterized by small intestinal villus atrophy, crypt hyperplasia, and the infiltration of inflammatory cells into the mucosa and lamina propria. Several studies have demonstrated an increase in the number of mast cells and basophils at sites of active disease [182,183]. Lavo et al. [184] reported that a provocative challenge with gliadin resulted in a rise in jejunal histamine content, suggesting that gliadin may directly or indirectly activate mast cell and/or basophils in this condition.

It has also been suggested that mast cells participate in the inflammatory reaction elicited by *Helicobacter pylori*, an etiological agent associated with the development of gastric and duodenal ulcer disease. For example, rat mesenteric venules superfused with an extract of *H. pylori* developed a rapid increase in microvascular albumin leakage in association with mast cell degranulation [185]. Extracts prepared from *H. pylori* potentiated the release of histamine stimulated by either bile acids [186] or calcium ionophores [187]. Although such studies do indicate direct action of *H. pylori* on the mast cell, Aceti et al. [188] reported that 84% of the patients they examined with *H. pylori*–associated gastritis had evidence of the production of specific IgE antibodies directed against *H. pylori*. If this observation is confirmed, then this work may have identified an immunological mechanism for mast cell and/or basophil activation in this disease.

Other GI diseases in which mast cells are thought to be involved include eosinophilic gastroenteritis [189], collagenous colitis [190,191], *Clostridium difficile* toxin A–induced enterocolitis [192,193], and certain GI manifestations of systemic connective tissue disease [194]. However, the precise role of mast cells in these diseases is not known. Indeed, with the exception of IgE-dependent reactions in the gut (e.g., certain food allergies), the roles of mast cells or basophils in all of the GI disorders in which these cells have been implicated remain to be determined.

REFERENCES

1. Costa JJ, Galli SJ. Mast cells and basophils. In: Rich R, Fleisher TA, Schwartz BD, Shearer WT, Strober W, eds. Clinical Immunology: Principles and Practice. St. Louis: Mosby, 1996, pp 408–430.
2. Galli SJ, Lichtenstein LM. Biology of mast cells and basophils. In: Middleton E, Reed CE, Ellis EF, Adkinson NF, Yunginger JW, eds. Allergy: Principles and Practice. St. Louis: Mosby, 1988, pp 106–134.

3. Holgate ST, Robinson C, Church MK. Mediators of immediate hypersensitivity. In: Middleton EJ, Reed CE, Ellis EF, Adkinson NF, Yunginger JW, Busse WW, eds. Allergy: Principles and Practice. St. Louis: Mosby, 1993, pp 267–301.
4. Schwartz L, Huff T. Biology of mast cells and basophils. In: Middleton E, Reed CE, Ellis EF, Adkinson NF, Yunginger JW, Busse WW, eds. Allergy: Principles and Practice. St. Louis: Mosby, 1993, pp 135–168.
5. Beaven MA, Metzger H. Signal transduction by Fc receptors: the $Fc_\varepsilon RI$ case. Immunol Today 1993; 14:222–226.
6. Kinet JP. The high-affinity receptor for IgE. Curr Opin Immunol 1989; 2:499–505.
7. Benhamou M, Siraganian RP. Protein-tyrosine phosphorylation: an essential component of FcεRI signaling. Immunol Today 1992; 13:195–197.
8. Dvorak AM. Basophil and mast cell degranulation and recovery. In: Harris JR, ed. Blood Cell Biochemistry. Vol. 4. New York: Plenum Press, 1991.
9. Galli SJ. New insights into "the riddle of the mast cells": microenvironmental regulation of mast cell development and phenotypic heterogeneity. Lab Invest 1990; 62:5–33.
10. Wershil BK, Galli SJ. Gastrointestinal mast cells: new approaches for analyzing their function in vivo. Gastroenterol Clin North Am 1991; 20:613–627.
11. Marshall JS, Bienenstock J. The role of mast cells in inflammatory reactions of the airways, skin and intestine. Curr Opin Immunol 1994; 6:853–859.
12. Norris HT, Zamcheck N, Gottlieb LS. The presence and distribution of mast cells in the human gastrointestinal tract. Gastroenterology 1963; 44:448–454.
13. Stead RH, Tomioka M, Quinonez G, Simon GT, Felten SY, Bienenstock J. Intestinal mucosal mast cells in normal and nematode-infected rat intestines are in intimate contact with peptidergic nerves. Proc Natl Acad Sci USA 1987; 84:2975–2979.
14. Stead RH, Dixon MF, Bramwell NH, Riddell RH, Bienenstock J. Mast cells are closely apposed to nerves in the human gastrointestinal mucosa. Gastroenterology 1989; 97:575–585.
15. Arizono N, Matsuda S, Hattori T, Kojima Y, Maeda T, Galli SJ. Anatomical variation in mast cell nerve associations in the rat small intestine, heart, lung, and skin: similarities of distances between neural processes and mast cells, eosinophils, or plasma cells in the jejunal lamina propria. Lab Invest 1990; 62:626–634.
16. Enerback L, Pipkom U, Aldenborg F, Wingren U. Mast cell heterogeneity in man: properties and function of human mucosal mast cells. In: Galli SJ, Austen KF, eds. Mast Cell and Basophil Differentiation and Function in Health and Disease. New York: Raven Press, 1989.
17. Bienenstock J, Blennerhassett M, Kakuta Y, et al. Evidence for central and peripheral nervous system interaction with mast cells. In: Galli SJ, Austen KF, eds. Mast Cell and Basophil Differentiation and Function in Health and Disease. New York: Raven Press, 1989.
18. Enerback L. Mast cell heterogeneity: the evolution of the concept of a specific mucosal mast cell. In: Befus AD, Bienenstock J, Denburg JA, eds. Mast Cell Differentiation and Heterogeneity. New York: Raven Press, 1986.
19. Kitamura Y. Heterogeneity of mast cells and phenotypic changes between subpopulations. Annu Rev Immunol 1989; 7:59–76.

20. Miller HRP, Huntley JF, Newlands GFJ, et al. Mast cell granule proteases in mouse and rat: a guide to mast cell heterogeneity and activation in the gastrointestinal tract. In: Galli SJ, Austen KF, eds. Mast Cell and Basophil Differentiation and Function in Health and Disease. New York: Raven Press, 1989.

21. Bienenstock J, Befus AD, Denburg JA. Mast cell heterogeneity: basic questions and clinical implications. In: Befus AD, Bienenstock J, Denburg JA, eds. Mast Cell Differentiation and Heterogeneity. New York: Raven Press, 1986.

22. Irani AA, Schechter NM, Craig SS, DeBlois G, Schwartz LB. Two types of human mast cells that have distinct neutral protease compositions. Proc Natl Acad Sci USA 1986; 83:4464–4468.

23. Galli SJ, Kitamura Y. Animal model of human disease: genetically mast cell-deficient W/Wᵛ and S/S1ᵈ mice: their value for the analysis of the roles of mast cells in biological responses in vivo. Am J Pathol 1987; 127:191–198.

24. Galli SJ, Zsebo KM, Geissler EN. The kit ligand, stem cell factor. Adv Immunol 1994; 55:1–96.

25. Williams DE, de Vries P, Namen AE, Widmer MB, Lyman SD. The Steel factor. Dev Biol 1992; 151:368–376.

26. Besmer P. The *kit* ligand encoded at the murine *Steel* locus: a pleiotropic growth and differentiation factor. Curr Opin Cell Biol 1991; 3:939–946.

27. Tsai M, Shih LS, Newlands GF, Takeishi T, Langley KE, Zsebo KM, Miller HR, Geissler EN, Galli SJ. The rat c-kit ligand, stem cell factor, induces the development of connective tissue-type and mucosal mast cells in vivo: Analysis by anatomical distribution, histochemistry, and protease phenotype. J Exp Med 1991; 174:125–131.

28. Zsebo KM, Williams DA, Geissler EN, Broudy VC, Martin FH, Atkins HL, Hsu RY, Birkett NC, Okino KH, Murdock DC, Jacobsen FW, Langley KE, Smith KA, Takeishi T, Cattanach BM, Galli SJ, Suggs SV. Stem cell factor (SCF) is encoded at the S1 locus of the mouse and is the ligand for the c-kit tyrosine kinase receptor. Cell 1990; 63:213–224.

29. Tsai M, Takeishi T, Thompson H, Langley KE, Zsebo KM, Metcalfe DD, Geissler EN, Galli SJ. Induction of mast cell proliferation, maturation, and heparin synthesis by the rat c-kit ligand, stem cell factor. Proc Natl Acad Sci USA 1991; 88:6382–6386.

30. Mekori YA, Oh CK, Metcalfe DD. IL-3-dependent murine mast cells undergo apoptosis on removal of IL-3: prevention of apoptosis by c-kit ligand. J Immunol 1993; 151:3775–3784.

31. Iemura A, Tsai M, Ando A, Wershil BK, Galli SJ. The c-kit ligand, stem cell factor, promotes mast cell survival by suppressing apoptosis. Am J Pathol 1994; 144:321–328.

32. Galli SJ, Iemura A, Garlick DS, Gamba-Vitalo C, Zsebo KM, Andrews RG. Reversible expansion of primate mast cell populations in vivo by stem cell factor. J Clin Invest 1993; 91:148–152.

33. Kirshenbaum AS, Goff JP, Dreskin SA. Interleukin-3-dependent growth of basophil-like and mast-like cells from human bone marrow. J Immunol 1989; 42:2424–2429.

34. Aglietta M, Camussi G, Piacibello W. Detection of basophils growing in semisolid agar culture. Exp Hematol 1981; 9:95–100.

35. Valent P, Schmidt G, Besemer J, Mayer P, Zenke G, Liehl E, Hinterberger W, Lechner K, Maurer D, Bettelheim P. Interleukin-3 is a differentiation factor for human basophils. Blood 1989; 73:1763–1769.

36. Valent P, Besemer J, Muhm M, Majdic O, Lechner K, Bettelheim P. Interleukin-3 activates human blood basophils via high affinity binding sites. Proc Natl Acad Sci USA 1989; 86:5542–5546.

37. Ganser A, Lindemann A, Seipelt G, Ottman OG, Herrmann F, Eder M, Frisch J, Schulz G, Mertelsmann R, Hoelzer D. Effects of recombinant human interleukin-3 patients with normal hematopoiesis and in patients with bone marrow failure. Blood 1990; 76:666–676.

38. Denburg JA. Cytokine-induced human basophil/mast cell growth and differentiation in vitro. Springer Semin Immunopathol 1990; 12:401–414.

39. Valent P, Bettelheim P. The human basophil. Crit Rev Oncol Hematol 1990; 10:327–352.

40. Tsuda T, Wong DA, Dolovich J, Bienenstock J, Marshall J, Denburg JA. Synergistic effects of nerve growth factor and granulocyte-macrophage colony-stimulating factor on human basophilic cell differentiation. Blood 1991; 77:971–979.

41. Galli SJ, Dvorak AM. Production, biochemistry, and function of basophils and mast cells. In: Beutler E, Lichtman MA, Coller BS, Kipps TJ, eds. Williams Hematology. New York: McGraw-Hill, 1995, pp 805–810.

42. Kirshenbaum AS, Kessler SW, Goff JP, Metcalfe DD. Demonstration of the origin of human mast cells from CD34+ bone marrow progenitor cells. J Immunol 1991; 146:1410–1415.

43. Galli SJ, Dvorak AM, Dvorak HF. Basophils and mast cells: morphologic insights into their biology, secretory patterns and function. Prog Allergy 1984; 34:1–141.

44. Dvorak AM, Dvorak HF, Galli SJ. Ultrastructural criteria for identification of mast cells and basophils in humans, guinea pigs, and mice. Am Rev Respir Dis 1983; 128:S49–S52.

45. Furitsu T, Saito H, Dvorak AM, Schwartz LB, Irani AM, Burdick JF, Ishizaka K, Ishizaka T. Development of human mast cells in vitro. Proc Natl Acad Sci USA 1989; 86:10039–10043.

46. Dvorak AM, Furitsu T, Ishizaka T. Ultrastructural morphology of human mast cell progenitors in sequential cocultures of cord blood cells and fibroblasts. Int Arch Allergy Immunol 1993; 100:219–229.

47. Kirshenbaum AS, Goff JP, Kessler SW, Mican JM, Zsebo KM, Metcalfe DD. Effect of IL-3 and stem cell factor on the appearance of human basophil and mast cells from CD34+ pluripotent progenitor cells. J Immunol 1992; 148:772–777.

48. Mitsui H, Furitsu T, Dvorak AM, Irani A-MA, Schwartz LB, Inagaki N, Takei M, Ishizaka K, Zsebo KM, Gillis S, Ishizaka T. Development of human mast cells from umbilical cord blood cells by recombinant human and murine c-*kit* ligand. Proc Natl Acad Sci USA 1993; 90:735–739.

49. Valent P, Spanblochl E, Sperr WR, Sillaber C, Zsebo KM, Agis H, Strobl H, Geissler K, Bettelheim P, Lechner K. Induction of differentiation of human mast

cells from bone marrow and peripheral blood mononuclear cells by recombinant human stem cell factor/kit-ligand in long-term culture. Blood 1992; 80:2237–2245.

50. Irani A-MA, Nilsson G, Mettinen U, Craig SS, Ashman LK, Ishizaka T, Zsebo KM, Schwartz LB. Recombinant human stem cell factor stimulates differentiation of mast cells from dispersed fetal liver cells. Blood 1992; 80:3009–3021.

51. Costa JJ, Demetri GD, Harrist TJ, Dvorak AM, D.F. H, Merica EA, Menchaca DM, Gringeri AJ, Schwartz LB, Galli SJ. Recombinant human stem cell factor (c-kit ligand) promotes human mast cell and melanocyte hyperplasia and functional activation in vivo. J Exp Med 1996; 183:2681–2686.

52. Gordon JR, Burd PR, Galli SJ. Mast cells as a source of multifunctional cytokines. Immunol Today 1990; 11:458–464.

53. Costa JJ, Burd PR, Metcalfe DD. Mast cell cytokines. In: Kaliner MA, Metcalfe DD, eds. The Role of the Mast Cell in Health and Disease. New York: Marcel Dekker, 1992.

54. Yamatodani A, Maeyama K, Watanabe T, Wada H, Kitamura Y. Tissue distribution of histamine in a mutant mouse deficient in mast cells: clear evidence for the presence of non-mast cell histamine. Biochem Pharmacol 1982; 31:305–309.

55. Porter JF, Mitchell RGL. Distribution of histamine in human blood. Physiol Rev 1972; 52:361–381.

56. Stevens RL, Fox CC, Lichtenstein LM, Austen KF. Identification of chondroitin sulfate E proteoglycans and heparin proteoglycans in the secretory granules of human lung mast cells. Proc Natl Acad Sci USA 1988; 85:2284–2287.

57. Thompson HL, Schulman ES, Metcalfe DD. Identification of chondroitin sulfate E in human lung mast cells. J Immunol 1988; 140:2708–2713.

58. Metcalfe DD, Bland CE, Wasserman SI. Biochemical and functional characterization of proteoglycans isolated from basophils of patients with chronic myelogenous leukemia. J Immunol 1984; 132:1943–1950.

59. Kjellen L, Lindahl U. Proteoglycans: structures and interactions. Annu Rev Biochem 1991; 60:443–475.

60. Schwartz LB, Bradford TR. Regulation of tryptase from human lung mast cells by heparin stabilization of the active tetramer. J Biol Chem 1986; 261:7372–7379.

61. Schwartz LB, Sakai K, Bradford TR, Ren S, Zweiman B, Worobec AB, Metcalfe DD. The alpha form of human tryptase is the predominant type present in blood at baseline in normal subjects and is elevated in those with systemic mastocytosis. J Clin Invest 1995; 96:2702–2710.

62. Schwartz LB, Metcalfe DD, Miller JS, Earl H, Sullivan T. Tryptase levels as an indicator of mast cell activation in systemic anaphylaxis and mastocytosis. N Engl J Med 1987; 316:1622–1626.

63. Schechter NM, Franki JE, Geesin JC, Lazarus GS. Human skin chymotryptic proteinase. 1. Isolation and relation to cathepsin G and rat mast cell protease. J Biol Chem 1983; 258:2973–2978.

64. Johnson LA, Moon KE, Eisenberg M. Purification to homogeneity of the human skin chymotryptic proteinase "chymase." Anal Biochem 1986; 155:358–364.

65. Ackerman SJ, Corrette SE, Rosenberg HJ, Bennett JC, Mastrianni DM, Nicholson-

Weller A, Weller PF, Chin DT, Tenen DG. Molecular cloning and characterization of human eosinophil Charcot-Leyden crystal protein (lysophospholipase): similarities to IgE binding proteins and the S-type animal lectin superfamily. J Immunol 1993; 150:456–468.

66. Dvorak AM, Ackerman SJ. Ultrastructural localization of the Charcot-Leyden crystal protein (lysophospholipase) to granules and intragranular crystals in mature human basophils. Lab Invest 1989; 60:557–567.

67. Valone FH, Boggs JM, Goetzl EJ. Lipid mediators of hypersensitivity and inflammation. In: Middleton E, Reed CE, Ellis EF, Adkinson NF, Busse WW, eds. Allergy: Principles and Practice. St. Louis: Mosby, 1993:302–319.

68. Vercelli D, Geha RS. Control of IgE synthesis. In: Middleton E, Reed CE, Ellis EF, Adkinson NF, Yunginger JW, Busse WW, eds. Allergy: Principles and Practice. St. Louis: Mosby, 1993, pp 93–104.

69. Sutton BJ, Gould HJ. The human IgE network. Nature 1993; 366:421–428.

70. Romagnani S. Human TH1 and TH2 subsets: doubt no more. Immunol Today 1992; 12:256–257.

71. Weller PF. The immunobiology of eosinophils. N Engl J Med 1991; 324:1110–1118.

72. Punnonen J, Aversa G, Cocks BG, De Vries JE. Role of interleukin-4 and interleukin-13 in synthesis of IgE and expression of CD23 by human B cells. Allergy 1994; 49:576–586.

73. Taub DD, Lloyd AR, Wang J-M, Oppenheim JJ, Kelvin DJ. The effects of human recombinant MIP-1α, MIP-1β, and RANTES on the chemotaxis and adhesion of T cell subsets. In: Lindley IJD, Westwick J, Kunkel S, eds. The Chemokines: Biology of the Inflammatory Peptide Supergene Family II. New York: Plenum Press, 1993, pp 139–146.

74. Rot A, Krieger M, Brunner T, Bischoff SC, Schall TJ, Dahinden CA. RANTES and macrophage inflammatory protein 1 alpha induce the migration and activation of normal human eosinophil granulocytes. J Exp Med 1992; 176:1489–1495.

75. Kaplan AP, Kuna P, Reddigari SR. Chemokines as allergic mediators: relationship to histamine releasing factors. Allergy 1994; 49:495–501.

76. Wardlaw AJ, Walsh GM, Symon FA. Mechanisms of eosinophil and basophil migration. Allergy 1994; 49:797–807.

77. Bochner BS, Schleimer RP. The role of adhesion molecules in human eosinophil and basophil recruitment. J Allergy Clin Immunol 1994; 94:427–438.

78. Bevilacqua MP. Endothelial-leukocyte adhesion molecules. Annu Rev Immunol 1993; 11:767–804.

79. Springer TA. Traffic signals for lymphocyte recirculation and leukocyte emigration: the multistep paradigm. Cell 1994; 76:301–314.

80. Galli SJ. New concepts about the mast cell. N Engl J Med 1993; 328:257–265.

81. Wershil BK, Wang ZS, Gordon JR, Galli SJ. Recruitment of neutrophils during IgE-dependent cutaneous late phase reactions in the mouse is mast cell-dependent: partial inhibition of the reaction with antiserum against tumor necrosis factor-alpha. J Clin Invest 1991; 87:446–453.

82. Wershil BK, Furuta GT, Wang Z-S, Galli SJ. Mast-cell dependent neutrophil and

mononuclear cell recruitment in immunoglobulin E-induced gastric reactions in mice. Gastroenterology 1996; 110:1482–1490.

83. Kung TT, Stelts D, Zurcher JA, Jones H, Umland SP, Kreutner W, Egan RW, Chapman RW. Mast cells modulate allergic pulmonary eosinophilia in mice. Am J Respir Cell Mol Biol 1995; 12:404–409.

84. Gordon JR, Galli SJ. Release of both preformed and newly synthesized tumor necrosis factor a (TNF-α)/cachectin by mouse mast cells stimulated by the FcεRI: a mechanism for the sustained action of mast cell-derived TNF-α during IgE-dependent biological responses. J Exp Med 1991; 174:103–107.

85. Plaut M, Pierce JH, Watson CJ, Hanley-Hyde J, Nordan RP, Paul WE. Mast cell lines produce lymphokines in response to cross-linkage of Fc$_ε$RI or to calcium ionophores. Nature 1989; 339:64–67.

86. Wodnar-Filipowicz A, Heusser CH, Moroni C. Production of the haemopoietic growth factors GM-CSF and interleukin-3 by mast cells in response to IgE receptor-mediated activation. Nature 1989; 339:150–152.

87. Burd PR, Rogers HW, Gordon JR, Martin CA, Jayaraman S, Wilson SD, Dvorak AM, Galli SJ, Dorf ME. Interleukin 3-dependent and -independent mast cells stimulated with IgE and antigen express multiple cytokines. J Exp Med 1989; 170:245–257.

88. Kulmburg PA, Huber NE, Scheer BJ, Wrann M, Baumruker T. Immunoglobulin E plus antigen challenge induces a novel intercrine/chemokine in mouse mast cells. J Exp Med 1992; 176:1773–1778.

89. Hultner L, Huls C, Kremer J-P, Kaspers U, Broszeit H, Schmitt E. IL-1 upregulates expression of IL-2 and IL-3 as well as TH2-type cytokines (IL-5, IL-6, IL-9, IL-13) in activated mouse bone marrow-derived mast cells (Abstr 19). J Invest Dermatol 1994; 103:620

90. Galli SJ, Costa JJ. Mast cell-leukocyte cytokine cascades in allergic inflammation. Allergy 1995; 50:851–862.

91. Costa JJ, Church MK, Galli SJ. Mast cell cytokines in allergic inflammation. In: Holgate ST, Busse W, eds. Inflammatory Mechanisms in Asthma. New York: Marcel Dekker, 1997.

92. Benyon RC, Bissonnette EY, Befus AD. Tumor necrosis factor-alpha dependent cytotoxicity of human skin mast cells is enhanced by anti-IgE antibodies. J Immunol 1991; 147:2253–2258.

93. Gordon JR, Post T, Schulman ES, Galli SJ. Characterization of mouse mast cell TNF-α induction in vitro and in vivo, and demonstration that purified human lung mast cells contain TNF-α. FASEB J 1991; 5:A1009.

94. Ohkawara Y, Yamauchi K, Tanno Y, Tamura G, Ohtani H, Nagura H, Ohkuda K, Takishima T. Human lung mast cells and pulmonary macrophages produce tumor necrosis factor-alpha in sensitized lung tissue after IgE receptor triggering. Am J Respir Cell Mol Biol 1992; 7:385–392.

95. Okayama Y, Lau LCK, Church MK. TNF-α production by human lung mast cells in response to stimulation by stem cell factor and Fc$_ε$RI cross-linkage.

96. Okayama Y, Petit-Frere C, Kassel O, Semper A, Quint D, Tunon-de-Lara MJ, Bradding P, Holgate ST, Church MK. IgE-dependent expression of mRNA for IL-4 and IL-5 in human lung mast cells. J Immunol 1995; 155:1796–1808.

97. Jaffe JS, Glaum MC, Raible DG, Post TJ, Dimitry E, Govindarao D, Wang Y, Schulman ES. Human lung mast cell IL-5 gene and protein expression: temporal analysis of upregulation following IgE-mediated activation. Am J Respir Cell Mol Biol 1995; 13:665–675.

98. Bradding P, Roberts JA, Britten KM, Montefort S, Djukanovic R, Mueller R, Heusser CH, Howarth PH, Holgate ST. Interleukin-4, -5, and -6 and tumor necrosis factor-alpha in normal and asthmatic airways: evidence for the human mast cell as a source of these cytokines. Am J Respir Cell Mol Biol 1994; 10:471–480.

99. Bradding P, Feather IH, Wilson S, Bardin PG, Heusser CH, Holgate ST, Howarth PH. Immunolocalization of cytokines in the nasal mucosa of normal and perennial rhinitic subjects: the mast cell as a source of IL-4, IL-5, and IL-6 in human allergic mucosal inflammation. J Immunol 1993; 151:3853–3865.

100. Ying S, Durham SR, Corrigan CJ, Hamid Q, Kay AB. Phenotype of cells expressing mRNA for TH2-type (interleukin 4 and interleukin 5) and TH1-type (interleukin 2 and interferon gamma) cytokines in bronchoalveolar lavage and bronchial biopsies from atopic asthmatic and normal control subjects. Am J Respir Cell Mol Biol 1995; 12:477–487.

101. Robinson DS, Durham SR, Kay AB. Cytokines. III. Cytokines in asthma. Thorax 1993; 148:401–406.

102. Schleimer RP. Glucocorticosteroids. Their mechanisms of action and use in allergic diseases. In: Middleton EJ, Ellis EF, Adkinson NFJ, Yunginger JW, Busse WW, eds. Allergy: Principles and Practice. St. Louis: Mosby, 1993, pp 893–925.

103. Robinson D, Hamid Q, Ying S, Bentley A, Assoufi B, Durham S, Kay AB. Prednisolone treatment in asthma is associated with modulation of bronchoalveolar lavage cell interleukin-4, interleukin-5, and interferon-γ cytokine gene expression. Am Rev Respir Dis 1993; 148:401–406.

104. Alexander AG, Barnes NC, Kay AB. Trial of cyclosporin in corticosteroid-dependent chronic severe asthma. Lancet 1992; 339:324–328.

105. Wershil BK, Furuta GT, Lavigne JA, Roy Choudhury A, Wang Z-S, Galli SJ. Dexamethasone or cyclosporin A suppresses mast cell-leukocyte cytokine cascades: multiple mechanisms of inhibition of IgE- and mast cell-dependent cutaneous inflammation in the mouse. J Immunol 1995; 154:1391–1398.

106. Brunner T, Heusser CH, Dahinden CA. Human peripheral blood basophils primed by interleukin 3 (IL-3) produce IL-4 in response to immunoglobulin E receptor stimulation. J Exp Med 1993; 177:605–611.

107. Arock M, Merle-Beral H, Dugas B, Ouaaz F, Le Goff L, Vouldoukis I, Mencia-Huerta J-M, Schmitt C, Leblond-Missenard V, Debre P, Mossalayi MD. IL-4 release by human leukemic and activated normal basophils. J Immunol 1993; 151:1441–1447.

108. MacGlashan D, Jr., White JM, Huang SK, Ono SJ, Schroeder JT, Lichtenstein LM. Secretion of IL-4 from human basophils: the relationship between IL-4 mRNA and protein in resting and stimulated basophils. J Immunol 1994; 152:3006–3016.

109. Schroeder JT, MacGlashan DM, Kagey-Sobotka A, White JM, Lichtenstein LM. IgE-dependent IL-4 secretion by human basophils: the relationship between cytokine production and histamine release in mixed leukocyte cultures. J Immunol 1994; 153:1818–1817.

110. Li H, Sim TC, Alam R. IL-13 released by and localized in human basophils. J Immunol 1996; 156:4833–4838.

111. Gauchat J-F, Henchoz S, Mazzei G, Aubry J-P, Brunner T, Blasey H, Life P, Talabot D, Flores-Romo L, Thompson J, Kishi K, Butterfield J, Dahinden C, Bonnefoy J-Y. Induction of human IgE synthesis in B cells by mast cells and basophils. Nature 1993; 365:340–343.

112. Li H, Sim TC, Grant JA, Alam R. The production of macrophage inflammatory protein-1 alpha by human basophils. J Immunol 1996; 157:1207–1212.

113. Dembo M, Goldstein B, Sobotka AK, Lichtenstein LM. Degranulation of human basophils: quantitative analysis of histamine release and desensitization due to a bivalent penicilloyl hapten. J Immunol 1979; 123:1864–1872.

114. Wang B, Rieger A, Kilgus O, Ochiai K, Maurer D, Fodinger D, Kinet J-P, Stingl G. Epidermal Langerhans cells from normal human skin bind monomeric IgE via Fc$_\epsilon$RI. J Exp Med 1992; 175:1353–1365.

115. Bieber T, de la Salle H, Wollenberg A, Hakimi J, Chizzonite R, Ring J, Hanau D, de la Salle C. Human epidermal Langerhans cells express the high-affinity receptor for immunoglobulin E (Fc$_\epsilon$RI). J Exp Med 1992; 175:1285–1290.

116. Gounni AS, Lamkhioued B, Ochiai K, Tanaka Y, Delaporte E, Capron A, Kinet JP, Capron M. High-affinity IgE receptor on eosinophils is involved in defense against parasites. Nature 1994; 367:183–186.

117. Maurer D, Fiebiger E, Reininger B, Wolff-Winiski B, Jouvin M-H, Kilgus O, Kinet J-P, Stingl G. Expression of functional high affinity IgE receptors (Fc$_\epsilon$RI) on monocytes of atopic individuals. J Exp Med 1994; 179:745–750.

118. Ravetch JV, Kinet J-P. Fc receptors. Annu Rev Immunol 1991; 9:457–492.

119. Conroy MC, Adkinson NF, Jr., Lichtenstein LM. Measurement of IgE on human basophils: relation to serum IgE and anti-IgE-induced histamine release. J Immunol 1977; 118:1317–1321.

120. Stallman PJ, Aalberse RC, Bruhl PC, van Elven EH. Experiments on the passive sensitization of human basophils, using quantitative immunofluorescence microscopy. Int Arch Allergy Appl Immunol 1977; 54:364–373.

121. Malveaux FJ, Conroy MC, Adkinson NF, Jr., Lichtenstein LM. IgE receptors on human basophils: relationship to serum IgE concentration. J Clin Invest 1978; 62:176–181.

122. Seldin DC, Adelman S, Austen KF, Stevens RL, Hein A, Caulfield JP, Woodbury RG. Homology of the rat basophilic leukemia cell and the rat mucosal mast cell. Proc Natl Acad Sci USA 1985; 82:3871–3875.

123. Furuichi K, Rivera J, Isersky C. The receptor for immunoglobulin E on rat basophilic leukemia cells: effect of ligand binding on receptor expression. Proc Natl Acad Sci USA 1985; 82:1522–1525.

124. Quarto R, Kinet J-P, Metzger H. Coordinate synthesis and degradation of the α, β and γ subunits of the receptor for immunoglobulin E. Mol Immunol 1985; 22:1045–1051.

125. Yamaguchi M, Lantz CS, Oettgen HC, Katona IM, Fleming T, Miyajima I, Kinet J-P, Galli SJ. IgE enhances mouse mast cell Fc$_\epsilon$RI expression in vitro and in vivo: evidence for a novel amplification mechanism in IgE-dependent reactions. J Exp Med 1997; 185:663–672.

126. Lantz CS, Yamaguchi M, Oettgen HC, Katona IM, Miyajima I, Kinet J-P, Galli SJ. IgE regulates mouse basophil $Fc_\epsilon RI$ expression in vivo. J Immunol 1997; 158:2517–2521.

127. Church MK, Benyon RC, Rees PH, et al. Functional heterogeneity of human mast cells. In: Galli SJ, Austen KF, eds. Mast Cell and Basophil Differentiation and Function in Health and Disease. New York: Raven Press, 1989.

128. Oppenheim JJ, Zachariae CO, Mukaida N, Matsushima K. Properties of the novel proinflammatory supergene "intercrine" cytokine family. Annu Rev Immunol 1991; 9:617–648.

129. Dahinden CA, Kurimoto Y, De Weck AL, Lindley I, Dewald B, Baggiolini M. The neutrophil-activating peptide NAF/NAP-1 induces histamine and leukotriene release by interleukin 3-primed basophils. J Exp Med 1989; 170:1787–1792.

130. Reddigari SR, Kuna P, Miragliotta GF, Kornfeld D, Baeza ML, Castor CW, Kaplan AP. Connective tissue-activating peptide-III and its derivative, neutrophil-activating peptide-2, release histamine from human basophils. J Allergy Clin Immunol 1992; 89:666–672.

131. Kuna P, Reddigari SR, Rucinski D, Oppenheim JJ, Kaplan AP. Monocyte chemotactic and activating factor is a potent histamine-releasing factor for human basophils. J Exp Med 1992; 175:489–493.

132. Bischoff SC, Krieger M, Brunner T, Dahinden CA. Monocyte chemotactic protein 1 is a potent activator of human basophils. J Exp Med 1992; 175:1271–1275.

133. Alam R, Lett-Brown MA, Forsythe PA, Anderson-Walters DJ, Kenamore C, Kormos C, Grant JA. Monocyte chemotactic and activating factor is a potent histamine-releasing factor for basophils. J Clin Invest 1992; 89:723–728.

134. Alam R, Forsythe PA, Stafford S, Lett-Brown MA, Grant JA. Macrophage inflammatory protein-1 alpha activates basophils and mast cells. J Exp Med 1992; 176:781–786.

135. Kuna P, Reddigari SR, Schall TJ, Rucinski D, Sadick M, Kaplan AP. Characterization of the human basophil response to cytokines, growth factors, and histamine releasing factors of the intercrine/chemokine family. J Immunol 1993; 150:1932–1943.

136. Kuna P, Reddigari SR, Kornfeld D, Kaplan AP. IL-8 inhibits histamine release from human basophils induced by histamine-releasing factors, connective tissue activating peptide III, and IL-3. J Immunol 1991; 147:1920–1924.

137. Wershil BK, Tsai M, Geissler EN, Zsebo KM, Galli SJ. The rat c-kit ligand, stem cell factor, induces c-kit receptor-dependent mouse mast cell activation in vivo: evidence that signaling through the c-kit receptor can induce expression of cellular function. J Exp Med 1992; 175:245–255.

138. Coleman JW, Holliday MR, Kimber I, Zsebo KM, Galli SJ. Regulation of mouse peritoneal mast cell secretory function by stem cell factor, IL-3 or IL-4. J Immunol 1993; 150:556–562.

139. Columbo M, Horowitz EM, Botana LM, MacGlashan DW, Jr., Bochner BS, Gillis S, Zsebo KM, Galli SJ, Lichtenstein LM. The human recombinant c-kit receptor ligand, rhSCF, induces mediator release from human cutaneous mast cells and enhances IgE-dependent mediator release from both skin mast cells and peripheral blood basophils. J Immunol 1992; 149:599–608.

140. Bischoff SC, Dahinden CA. c-kit ligand: a unique potentiator of mediator release by human lung mast cells. J Exp Med 1992; 175:237–244.

141. Ando A, Martin TR, Galli SJ. Effects of chronic treatment with the c-kit ligand, stem cell factor, on immunoglobulin E-dependent anaphylaxis in mice: genetically mast cell-deficient Sl/Sl^d mice acquire anaphylactic responsiveness, but the congenic normal mice do not exhibit augmented responses. J Clin Invest 1993; 92:1639–1649.

142. Wershil BK, Mekori YA, Murakami T, Galli SJ. ^{125}I-fibrin deposition in IgE-dependent immediate hypersensitivity reactions in mouse skin: demonstration of the role of mast cells using genetically mast cell-deficient mice locally reconstituted with cultured mast cells. J Immunol 1987; 139:2605–2614.

143. Wershil BK, Galli SJ. ^{125}I-fibrin deposition in IgE-dependent gastric reactions in the mouse: the role of mast cells (MCs). FASEB J 1989; 3:A789.

144. Alter SC, Schwartz LB. Tryptase: an indicator of mast cell-mediated allergic reactions. Provocative Challenge Proc 1989; 167.

145. Lemanske RFJ, Kaliner MA. Late phase allergic reactions. In: Middleton EJ, Reed CE, Ellis EF, Adkinson NF, Yunginger JW, Busse WW, eds. Allergy: Principles and Practice. St. Louis: Mosby, 1993, pp 320–361.

146. Bascom R, Wachs M, Naclerio RM, Pipkorn U, Galli SJ, Lichtenstein LM. Basophil influx occurs after nasal antigen challenge: effects of topical corticosteroid pretreatment. J Allergy Clin Immunol 1988; 81:580–589.

147. Liu MC, Hubbard WC, Proud D, Stealey BA, Galli SJ, Kagey-Sobotka A, Bleecker ER, Lichtenstein LM. Immediate and late inflammatory responses to ragweed antigen challenge of the peripheral airways in allergic asthmatics: cellular, mediator, and permeability changes. Am Rev Respir Dis 1991; 144:51–58.

148. Guo C-B, Liu MC, Galli SJ, et al. Identification of IgE bearing cells in the late phase response to antigen in the lung as basophils. Am J Resp Cell Mol Biol 1994; 10:384–390.

149. Jarrett EEE, Miller HRP. Production and activities of IgE in helminth infection. Prog Allergy 1982; 31:178–233.

150. Askenase PW. Immunopathology of parasitic diseases: involvement of basophils and mast cells. Springer Semin Immunopathol 1980; 2:417.

151. Reed ND. In: Galli SJ, Austen KF, eds. Mast Cell and Basophil Differentiation and Function in Health and Disease. New York: Raven Press, 1989.

152. Jacobson RH, Reed ND, Manning DD. Expulsion of *Nippostrongylus brasiliensis* from mice lacking antibody production potential. Immunology 1977; 32:867–874.

153. Watanabe N, Katakura K, Kobayashi A, Okumura K, Ovary Z. Protective immunity and eosinophilia in IgE-deficient SJA/9 mice infected with *Nippostrongylus brasiliensis* and *Trichinella spiralis*. Proc Natl Acad Sci USA 1988; 85:4460–4462.

154. Matsuda H, Watanabe N, Kiso Y, Hirota S, Ushio H, Kannan Y, Azuma M, Koyama H, Kitamura Y. Necessity of IgE antibodies and mast cells for manifestation of resistance against larval *Haemaphysalis longicornis* ticks in mice. J Immunol 1990; 144:259–262.

155. Steeves EB, Allen JR. Basophils in skin reactions of mast cell-deficient mice infested with *Dermacentor variabilis*. Int J Parasitol 1990; 20:655–667.

156. Brown SJ, Galli SJ, Gleich GJ, Askenase PW. Ablation of immunity to *Amblyomma americanum* by anti-basophil serum: cooperation between basophils and eosinophils in expression of immunity to ectoparasites (ticks) in guinea pigs. J Immunol 1982; 129:790–796.

157. Barrett KE, Metcalfe DD. The mucosal mast cell and its role in gastrointestinal allergic diseases. Clin Rev Allergy 1984; 2:39–53.

158. Sampson HA, Metcalfe DD. Immediate reactions to foods. In: Metcalfe DD, Sampson HA, Simon RA, eds. Food Allergy: Adverse Reactions to Foods and Food Additives. Cambridge: Blackwell, 1991, pp 99–112.

159. Gall DG. Gastrointestinal anaphylaxis: effect on gastric and intestinal function: immunophysiology of the gut. Bristol-Myers Squibb/Mead Johnson Nutrition Symposia, San Diego.

160. Bochner BS, Lichtenstein LM. Anaphylaxis. N Engl J Med 1991; 324:1785–1790.

161. Reimann HJ, Ring J, Ultsch B, Wendt P. Intragastral provocation under endoscopic control (IPEC) in food allergy: mast cell and histamine changes in gastric mucosa. Clin Allergy 1985; 15:195–202.

162. Reimann HJ, Lewin J. Gastric mucosal reactions in patients with food allergy. Am J Gastroenterol 1988; 83:1212–1219.

163. Castro GA, Harari Y, Russell D. Mediators of anaphylaxis-induced ion transport in small intestine. Am J Physiol 1987; 253:G540–G548.

164. Perdue MH, Gall DG. Intestinal anaphylaxis in the rat: jejunal response to in vitro antigen exposure. Am J Physiol 1986; 250:G427–G431.

165. Perdue MH, Marshall J, Masson S. Ion transport abnormalities in inflamed rat jejunum: involvement of mast cells and nerves. Gastroenterology 1990; 98:561–567.

166. Perdue MH, Chung M, Gall DG. Effect of intestinal anaphylaxis on gut function in the rat. Gastroenterology 1984; 86:391–397.

167. Bani-Sacchi T, Barattini M, Bianchi S, Blandina P, Brunelleschi S, Fantozzi R, Mannaioni PF, Masini E. The release of histamine by parasympathetic stimulation in guinea-pig auricle and rat ileum. J Physiol 1986; 371:29–43.

168. Perdue MH, Masson S, Wershil BK, Galli SJ. Role of mast cells in ion transport abnormalities associated with intestinal anaphylaxis: correction of the diminished secretory response in genetically mast cell-deficient W/W^v mice by bone marrow transplantation. J Clin Invest 1991; 87:687–693.

169. Schreiber S, Raedler A, Stenson WF, MacDermott RP. The role of the mucosal immune system in inflammatory bowel disease. Gastroenterol Clin North Am 1992; 21:421–502.

170. Dvorak AM, Monahan RA, Osage JE, Dickersin GR. Crohn's disease: transmission electron microscopic studies. II. Immunologic inflammatory response: alterations of mast cells, basophils, eosinophils, and the microvasculature. Hum Pathol 1980; 11:606–619.

171. Dvorak AM, Monahan RA. Crohn's disease: mast cell quantitation using one micron plastic sections for light microscopic study. Pathol Annu 1983; 1:181–190.

172. Ranlov P, Nielsen MH, Wanstrup J. Ultrastructure of the ileum in Crohn's disease: immune lesions and mastocytosis. Scand J Gastroenterol 1972; 7:471–476.

173. Rao SN. Mast cells as a component of the granuloma in Crohn's disease. J Pathol 1973; 109:79–82.
174. Dvorak AM, McLeod RS, Onderdonk A, Monahan-Earley RA, Cullen JB, Antonioli DA, Morgan E, Blair JE, Estrella P, Cisneros RL, Cohen Z, Silen W. Human gut mucosal mast cells: ultrastructural observations and anatomic variation in mast cell–nerve associations in vivo. Int Arch Allergy Immunol 1992; 99:158–168.
175. Dvorak AM, McLeod RS, Onderdonk A, Monahan-Earley RA, Cullen JB, Antonioli DA, Morgan E, Blair JE, Estrella P, Cisneros RL, Silen W, Cohen Z. Ultrastructural evidence for piecemeal and anaphylactic degranulation of human gut mucosal mast cells in vivo. Int Arch Allergy Immunol 1992; 99:74–83.
176. King T, Biddle W, Bhatia P, Moore J, Miner P, Jr. Colonic mucosal mast cell distribution at line of demarcation of active ulcerative colitis. Dig Dis Sci 1992; 37:490–495.
177. Fox CC, Lazenby AJ, Moore WC, Yardley JH, Bayless TM, Lichtenstein LM. Enhancement of human intestinal mast cell mediator release in active ulcerative colitis. Gastroenterology 1990; 99:119–124.
178. Dvorak AM, Tepper RI, Weller PF, Morgan ES, Estrella P, Monahan-Earley RA, Galli SJ. Piecemeal degranulation of mast cells in the inflammatory eyelid lesions of interleukin-4 transgenic mice: evidence of mast cell histamine release in vivo by diamine oxidase-gold enzyme-affinity ultrastructural cytochemistry. Blood 1994; 83:3600–3612.
179. Mantyh CR, Gates TS, Zimmerman RP, Welton ML, Passaro E, Jr., Vigna SR, Maggio JE, Kruger L, Mantyh PW. Receptor binding sites for substance P, but not substance K or neuromedin K, are expressed in high concentrations by arterioles, venules, and lymph nodules in surgical specimens obtained from patients with ulcerative colitis and Crohn disease. Proc Natl Acad Sci USA 1988; 85:3235–3239.
180. Ansel JC, Brown JR, Payan DG, Brown MA. Substance P selectively activates TNF-α gene expression in murine mast cells. J Immunol 1993; 150:4478–4485.
181. Matis WL, Lavker RM, Murphy GF. Substance P induces the expression of an endothelial-leukocyte adhesion molecule by microvascular endothelium. J Invest Dermatol 1990; 94:492–495.
182. Marsh MN, Hinde J. Inflammatory component of celiac sprue mucosa. I. Mast cells, basophils, and eosinophils. Gastroenterology 1985; 89:92–101.
183. Wingren U, Hallert C, Norrby K, Enerback L. Histamine and mucosal mast cells in gluten enteropathy. Agents Actions 1986; 18:266–268.
184. Lavo B, Knutson L, Loof L, Odlind B, Venge P, Hallgren R. Challenge with gliadin induces eosinophil and mast cell activation in the jejunum of patients with celiac disease. Am J Med 1989; 87:655–660.
185. Kurose I, Granger DN, Evans D, Jr., Evans DG, Graham DY, Miyasaka M, Anderson DC, Wolf RE, Cepinskas G, Kvietys PR. *Helicobacter pylori*–induced microvascular protein leakage in rats: role of neutrophils, mast cells, and platelets. Gastroenterology 1994; 107:70–79.
186. Masini E, Bechi P, Dei R, Di Bello MG, Sacchi TB. *Helicobacter pylori* potentiates histamine release from rat serosal mast cells induced by bile acids. Dig Dis Sci 1994; 39:1493–1500.

187. Bechi P, Dei R, Di Bello MG, Masini E. *Helicobacter pylori* potentiates histamine release from serosal rat mast cells in vitro. Dig Dis Sci 1993; 38:944–949.

188. Aceti A, Celestino D, Caferro M, Casale V, Citarda F, Conti EM, Grassi A, Grilli A, Pennica A, Sciarretta F, Basophil-bound and serum immunoglobulin E directed against *Helicobacter pylori* in patients with chronic gastritis. Gastroenterology 1991; 101:131–137.

189. Lemanske R, Jr., Atkins FM, Metcalfe DD. Gastrointestinal mast cells in health and disease. Part II. J Pediatr 1983; 103:343–351.

190. Flejou JF, Grimaud JA, Molas G, Baviera E, Potet F. Collagenous colitis: ultra-structural study and collagen immunotyping of four cases. Arch Pathol Lab Med 1984; 108:977–982.

191. Baum CA, Bhatia P, Miner P. Increased colonic mucosal mast cells associated with severe watery diarrhea and microscopic colitis. Dig Dis Sci 1989; 34:1462–1465.

192. Pothoulakis C, Karmeli F, Kelly CP, Eliakim R, Joshi MA, O'Keane CJ, Castagli-uolo I, LaMont JT, Rachmilewitz D. Ketotifen inhibits *Clostridium difficile* toxin A–induced enteritis in rat ileum. Gastroenterology 1993; 105:701–707.

193. Pothoulakis C, Castagliuolo I, LaMont JT, Jaffer A, O'Keane JC, Snider RM, Leemah SE. CP-96, 345, a substance P antagonist, inhibits rat intestinal responses to *Clostridium difficile* toxin A but not cholera toxin. Proc Natl Acad Sci USA 1994; 91:947–951.

194. DeSchryver-Kecskemeti K, Clouse RE. Perineural and intraneural inflammatory infiltrates in the intestines of patients with systemic connective-tissue disease. Arch Pathol Lab Med 1989; 113:394–398.

2

Humoral and Cellular Immunity

MARIANNE FRIERI
Nassau County Medical Center, East Meadow, and State University of New York at Stony Brook, Stony Brook, New York

THE MUCOSAL IMMUNE SYSTEM

The intestinal processing of antigen absorption and handling and the local secretory immune reaction, including nonimmunological factors, are important components that influence the mucosal barrier of the gastrointestinal tract [1]. The mucosal immune system is a significant regulator of the homeostatic balance in the gastrointestinal tract. Antigen or food protein uptake by specialized epithelial or microfold (M) cells can react with intraepithelial lymphocytes within Peyer's patches [1,2]. Lymphoid nodules in this environment also contain mast cells, which, upon degranulation, can cause local immunosuppression of lymphocyte function [3] (Fig. 1).

HUMORAL IMMUNITY

Immunoglobulin Production

The humoral immune system plays a major role in mucosal immunity via immunoglobulin E (IgE) and IgA bearing cells in lymphoid tissue [2]. Peyer's

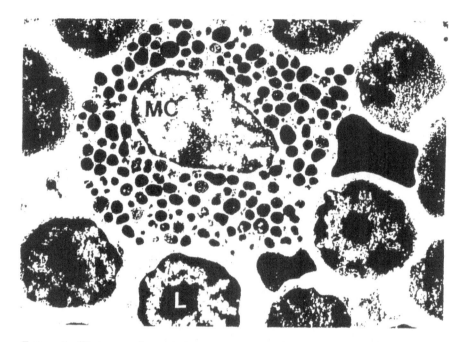

FIGURE 1 Electron micrograph of a lymph node with intranodal mast cells (MC) located among macrophages, reticular fibers, and lymphocytes (L) in the medullary lymphatic sinuses. (Courtesy of Dr. Arthur O. Anderson, Assistant Professor of Pathology and Biology, University of Pennsylvania, Philadelphia, Pennsylvania.)

patches are enriched for IgA precursor, which migrates via the lymphatics to the mesentery lymph node, thoracic duct, and other secretory tissue within the lacrimal, salivary, mammary gland, respiratory, and genitourinary systems [4]. Increased levels of IgE and IgD have been reported with milk protein sensitivity and milk-protein-induced respiratory disease [5]. Increased IgD levels have also been associated with the hyper-IgE syndrome [6], endocrine disorders, immunodeficiencies associated with IgA deficiency, malignancy, and human immunodeficiency virus (HIV) infection [7].

Connective tissue skin mast cells are degranulated primarily via IgE, and T cell–dependent mucosal mast cells may preferentially respond to IgG_4 antibodies that we and others have demonstrated in IgE-negative food-hypersensitive patients [8,9]. In a preliminary study on humoral immune responses to selected food proteins in patients with Crohn's disease, an IgG_4 response may indicate a reaction to gastrointestinal immunization or antigenic leakage [10].

A more recent animal study that examined intestinal inflammation induced during cow's milk protein sensitization revealed a larger degree of sensitization via specific IgE and IgG antibodies [11]. Thus, intestinal inflammation increasing gut permeability enhances the sensitization process.

The involvement of interleukin 4 (IL-4), which can enhance the production of IgG_4 from purified human B cells, has been demonstrated in spontaneous in vitro IgE synthesis in patients with atopic dermatitis [12]. In preliminary studies in several patients with atopic dermatitis and a history of food hypersensitivity to milk antigen, we demonstrated B cell growth factor in peripheral blood mononuclear cells stimulated with milk protein [13].

The Role of Immune Complexes

Intact antigenic macromolecules from food protein can traverse the epithelium of the gastrointestinal tract, generating active secretion of IgA with immune complex formation [2]. (Fig. 2) IgA production appears to be increased when immunization is induced by the oral route. However, IgG appears preferentially after parenteral injection [14]. In animal studies, formation of β-lactoglobu-

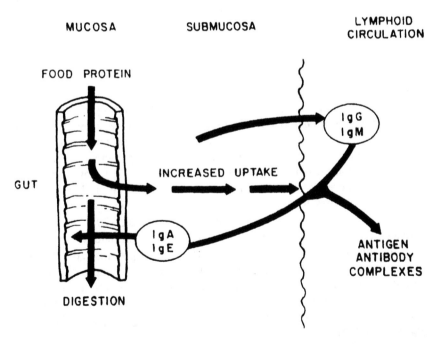

Figure 2 Immunoglobulin (Ig) production with food protein traversing intestinal mucosal barriers. Food antigen–antibody complexes can develop in the systemic circulation but are normally removed by the reticuloendothelial system.

lin–mucosal IgA immune complexes escaping the mucosal IgA trap and then binding with specific IgG and IgE has been suggested [11]. Gut-associated lymphoid tissue is a rich source of IgA precursor cells. Newborns have a decreased concentration of IgA in saliva, stool, and serum which may contribute to the increased incidence of intestinal allergy in infants [1].

When oral immunization is performed, large and/or long-term consecutive doses of antigens are required for induction of IgA antibody against food antigens [15]. Konishi et al. studied the biliary immune response to orally presented food antigen, ovomucoid, and its potentiation by cholera toxin B in mice [15]. The relationship between serum and biliary IgA and IgG antibodies suggested that immunization with cholera toxin B subunit, which can induce a gut immune response against nonrelated antigens, potentiates biliary antiovomucoid responses by increasing antibody levels and also by modulating the process specific to mucosal presentation of antigen [15].

Of interest, IgA has been shown to be an activator of eosinophil cytokine production, which may play a role in eosinophilic gastroenteritis [16]. In a Finnish study, jejunal biopsy specimens studied from 25 patients with IgA deficiency revealed a significant increase of intraepithelial CD25$^+$ cells, supporting the theory that enhanced T cell activation is present in the intestine of these patients as a result of ineffective antigen elimination or chronic infection [17]. Peyer's patch B cells have also been shown to produce increased amounts of IgA in response to substance P, which is a late-acting cofactor supporting IL-6-mediated IgA production [18].

Immune complexes can activate complement, resulting in either activation of mast cells or chemotaxis of polymorphonuclear leukocytes with release of mast cell mediators or proteolytic enzyme release. Cow's milk and egg protein immune complexes with specific IgA may develop, increasing the potential for immune-mediated reactions in the newborn [19]. IgG$_1$ antibodies appear to be more effective in activating complement. The production of IgG and IgG$_1$ antibodies to cytoskeletal protein tropomyosin by lamina propria cells was demonstrated in patients with ulcerative colitis [20]. The degree of activated complement deposition has been shown to correlate with inflammation; this finding may explain autoimmunity in these patients [20]. Bonnefay and coworkers have found a subset of anti-CD21 monoclonal antibodies that stimulate IgE production, providing a potential mechanism for how soluble Fc ε RII (sFc$_ε$RII) modulates human IgE production [21,22]. Human basophils and mast cells also express the CD40 ligand, leading to IgE production by class switch [23].

The pathogenetic mechanisms in food-induced allergic diseases via the gut-associated tissue involving humoral immunity, antigen-antibody complexes, and Th1 of Th2 cells has recently been reviewed in relation to oral tolerance [24].

CELLULAR IMMUNITY

Proliferative Studies

Cell-mediated or delayed hypersensitivity reactions develop over 24–48 hr when actively sensitized lymphocytes of the Th_1 subtype release various cytokines such as interleukin 2 (IL-2) and gamma interferon (γ-IFN) interacts with specific antigen. In one study, the combination of cord blood IgE and the proliferative response of cord blood lymphocytes to food antigens appeared to be useful for the prediction of allergic disorders [25]. IL-2 production of cord blood lymphocytes stimulated with food antigens in 24 newborn infants correlated well with proliferative response to ovalbumin or bovine serum albumin [25].

In earlier studies Kondo et al. and Pene et al. evaluated lymphocyte responses to food antigens in patients with atopic dermatitis sensitive to foods and IgE production by normal human lymphocytes induced by IL-4 and suppressed by IFN and prostaglandin E_2 [26,27].

In a more recent study of 194 food-sensitive children with atopic dermatitis, lymphocyte proliferation in response to food antigens and specific IgE antibodies was evaluated with respect to age [28]. Proliferative responses to peripheral blood mononuclear cells to food antigens decreased rapidly after patients were placed on elimination diets [19]. The authors proposed that such diets may trigger a reduction in the responsiveness of food-sensitive CD4+ cells, possibly with oral tolerance or the development of absorptive functions, inducing these immunologic changes [27]. Kondo et al. determined that by combining the sensitivity and specificity values, a stimulation index >2.0 served as a convenient method to mark a specific offending food in food-sensitive atopic dermatitis [29]. Proliferative responses of peripheral blood mononuclear cells to food antigens may be more useful than RAST scores for detection of offending foods in food-sensitive atopic dermatitis [29].

The Role of Cytokines

Cytokines and their role in the pathogenesis of severe food hypersensitivity reactions were evaluated by Jaffe and Metcalfe [30]. Cytokine production from peripheral T cells was found to be abnormal after mitogenic stimulation, which may contribute to elevated IgE level and eosinophilia [30].

CD4-positive T helper cells can be functionally divided on the basis of their cytokine secretion pattern after activation [24]. Th1 effector cells predominantly secrete IFN-γ and interleukin 2 (IL-2), which trigger delayed hypersensitivity responses.

The basic regulatory mechanisms of oral tolerance have been shown to involve suppressive cytokines such as transforming growth factor β (TGF-β) secreting CD8$^+$ cells, which can then act on other immune cells, which are naive to the antigen and suppress their reactivity [31].

After passage through the mucosa and processing by antigen presenting cells, the antigen is presented to lymphocytes for subsequent reactions. Selected presentation in association with class I antigens may lead to specific CD8$^+$ T suppressor cell activation, whereas class II antigens activate CD4$^+$ T cells and lead to memory induction. Thus, a regulatory interaction between CD4$^+$ and CD8$^+$ T cells is possible [31]. Activated CD8$^+$ T cells can also provide a negative signal to autoreactive cells in affected target organs provided by TGF-β. In the absence of a costimulatory signal (e.g., via CD28-CD8$^+$ [B7 family]), T-cell anergy or tolerance could be induced [31].

In a preliminary study in our division, in several atopic patients with allergic rhinitis, asthma, atopic dermatitis, or urticaria and a history of food hypersensitivity and milk or egg protein positivity via skin test or specific IgE, milk-or egg-specific IL-2-triggered T-cell proliferation was demonstrated [32].

Induction of IL-2 responsiveness is necessary for antigen-activated T cells to induce cell-mediated immunity. Noma et al. evaluated antigen-specific induction of IL-2 responsiveness to ovalbumin-stimulated lymphocytes from patients with egg-white allergy [33]. These authors further investigated IL-2 responsiveness and class II major histocompatibility complex (MHC) involvement with ovalbumin antigen by adhering cells and T-cell activation in patients with hen egg allergy [34]. The IL-2 responding cells were shown to consist mainly of CD3$^+$, CD2$^+$, CD4$^+$, CD8$^-$, CD45 RA$^+$ cells, which could act as helper cells for IgE production or effector cells for delayed-type hypersensitivity. The DQ-bearing and/or DP-bearing adhering cells appeared to have a key function in presenting ovalbumin antigen to allergen-specific responder CD4$^+$ T cells [34]. In studies in our division, we were also able to demonstrate antigen-specific IL-2 and IL-6 production in mononuclear cells from patients with autoimmune disease [35,36].

We further investigated the role of cellular and serum IFN, serum IL-4, and IgE levels in seven patients with atopic dermatitis [37]. Mitogen- or antigen-stimulated cellular IL-4 levels were detected in three patients, but less cellular IFN was noted than in normal control subjects. Thus, cellular and humoral IL-4 and γ-IFN production can be dysregulated in certain patients with atopic dermatitis [37]. IL-4, a T cell–derived glycoprotein produced by activated T lymphocytes, can increase the growth of mast cells and IgE production and stimulate deoxyribonucleic acid (DNA) synthesis by B cells [38].

In a study of serum IL-4 detection in our division, 15 atopic pediatric and adult patients evaluated for food hypersensitivity, dietary modification improved cutaneous and gastrointestinal symptoms in 11 patients, and all had decreased IL-4 levels after dietary elimination of the incriminated foods [32]. The mean percentage of serum IL-4 also decreased in 67%, correlating with clinical scores and lymphocyte proliferative cytokine responses to food antigens, and postdietary elimination was inhibited by anti-IL-4 [32]. In a later open-challenge study in food-hypersensitive patients, we were able to demonstrate serum and food antigen-stimulated IL-4 decline after dietary restriction [39]. IL-4- and IL-2-induced lymphocyte proliferation to egg and milk protein also declined in several patients after dietary modification. Elimination diets could reduce the proliferative responses of peripheral blood mononuclear cells to food antigens in vitro or enhance mucosal antibody responses [40,41].

Recently, a specific T cell–mediated immune response to casein was found in the blood of adolescent and adult patients with milk-related exacerbation of atopic dermatitis [42]. In contrast to house dust mite–specific T cells, casein-specific T cells of adult patients who respond to cow's milk with worsening of atopic dermatitis produce little or no IL-4 [42]. Thus, in older patch test lesions and in chronic lesions of atopic dermatitis, type 2 cytokines such as IL-4 are downmodulated and type 1 cytokines such as IFN-γ may be predominant [43]. Beyer et al. in evaluating peripheral blood mononuclear cells from children with atopic dermatitis after stimulation with cow's milk or egg allergen noted the combined assessment of CD4$^+$CD45 RO$^+$ and CD4 L-selectin expression on T cells by flow cytometry may predict the development of severe allergic reactions [44].

Benlounes et al. demonstrated that intact rather than intestinally processed protein stimulates peripheral blood mononuclear cells to release tumor necrosis factor α and alter intestinal barrier capacity [45]. The threshold for peripheral blood mononuclear cell reactivity to milk antigens was also shown to decrease considerably during active cow's milk allergy with intestinal symptoms, suggesting TNF-α may be a good marker of immune reactivity to milk antigens [45].

Shinbara et al. reported on IL-4 and γ-IFN production from ovalbumin-stimulated lymphocytes in egg-sensitive children [46]. Levels of IFN production from IL-2 [stimulated or both ovalbumin-stimulated] and peripheral blood mononuclear cells from egg-sensitive patients with atopic dermatitis was significantly higher than that of healthy children and those with immediate allergic symptoms [43].

A study using lymphocyte transformation tests was performed in healthy adults to determine the mitogen-induced lymphocyte proliferative responses to bovine caseins hydrolyzed with pepsin and trypsin and bovine caseins hydrolyzed with enzymes derived from *Lactobacillus casei* [47]. Lymphocyte proliferation was only stimulated with K-casein hydrolyzed with pepsin and trypsin with 10 μg/ml of PHA; however, suppression of lymphocyte proliferation was noted with the bacterial hydrolyzed caseins [47]. This study established that degradation of food antigens with *L. casei*–derived enzymes modifies their immunomodulatory activity and leads to suppression of peripheral blood mononuclear cells in health. Such suppression of cell-mediated immunity with simultaneous preservation of IgG production and γ-IFN producing T cell reactivity evolves after a phase of T cell–mediated regulation as a result of continuous allergen exposure [48]. In a similar fashion, we showed that mast cell mediators such as heparin proteoglycan can be suppressive on mitogen-induced lymphocyte responsiveness [3].

The Role of Mast Cell Mediators

There are a variety of forms of arthritis that appear causally related to a primary process in the gastrointestinal tract [49]. Mast cells that occur in both the synovium and gastrointestinal tract which can, upon degranulation, release numerous mediators of inflammation, resulting in pain, synovial, mucosal edema, and mucus production. The function of MHC class II antigens and presentation to CD4+ T helper cells support the possibility that external antigens influence rheumatoid arthritis [50]. Some foods or components might influence subgroups of rheumatoid arthritis patients, although this theory is unproved [50].

In a study in our division, increased IL-4 production in response to mast cell mediators and human type I collagen was demonstrated in mononuclear cells from 21 patients with rheumatoid arthritis [51]. When cells from all patients were divided into atopic and nonatopic groups, decreased lymphocyte proliferation with all stimuli occurred in 90% of mononuclear cell cultures from atopic patients compared to nonatopic patients [51]. Increased lymphocyte proliferation in all nonatopic patients paralleled decreased allergic scores. Thus, a possible feedback mechanism in atopic individuals due to IL-4 might occur with decreased T-cell proliferation in the presence of mast cell mediators.

Perhaps a similar mechanism to that which occurs in patients with atopic dermatitis with transient suppression of cell-mediated immune responses is an explanation for these findings [51].

Recent additional topics addressing humoral and cellular immune reactions related to food hypersensitivity have been summarized in another article by the author [52].

REFERENCES

1. Wershil BK, Walker WA. The mucosal barrier, IgE-mediated gastrointestinal events and eosinophilic gastroenteritis. Gastroenterol Clin North Am 1992; 21:387–404.
2. Frieri M. IgE/IgA bearing cells in gut lymphoid tissue with special emphasis on food allergy. In: Chiaramonte L, Schneider A, Lifshitz F, eds. Food Allergy: A Practical Approach to Diagnosis and Management. New York: Marcel Dekker, 1988, pp 45–70.
3. Frieri M, Metcalfe, DD. Analysis of the effect of mast cell granules in lymphocyte

blastogenesis: identification of heparin as a granule associated suppressor factor. J Immunol 1983; 131: 1942–1949.

4. Brandtzaeg P. Transport models for secretory IgA and secretory IgM. Clin Exp Immunol 1981; 44:221.

5. Galaint S, Nussbaum E, Wittner R et al. Increased IgD milk antibody responses in a patient with Down's syndrome, pulmonary hemosiderosis and cor pulmonale. Ann Allergy 1983; 51:446.

6. Joseph SH, Buckley RH. Serum IgD concentrations in normal infants, children and adults and in patients with elevated IgE. J Pediatr 1980; 96:417.

7. Papadoupolos NM, Frieri M. The presence of immunoglobulin D in endocrine disorders and diseases of immunoregulation, including the acquired immunodeficiency syndrome. J Clin Immunol Immunopathol 1984; 32:248.

8. Nakagawa T, Mukoyama T, Baba M et al. Egg white–specific IgE and IgG_4 antibodies in atopic children. Ann Allergy 1986; 57:359–362.

9. Frieri M, Bhat B, Zitt M et al. Specific immunoglobulin G_4 and E levels in food-sensitive patients. Immunol Allergy Pract 1988; 10:9–16.

10. Frieri M, Claus M, Boris M et al. Preliminary investigation on humoral and cellular immune responses to selected food proteins in patients with Crohn's disease. Ann Allergy 1990; 64:345–351.

11. Fargeas MJ, Theodorou V, Mare J et al. Boosted systemic immune and local responsiveness after intestinal inflammation in orally sensitized guinea pigs. Gastroenterology 1995; 109:53–62.

12. Vollenweider S, Saurat JH, Rochen M, Hauser C. Evidence suggesting involvement of interleukin 4 production in spontaneous in vitro IgE synthesis in patients with atopic dermatitis. J Allergy Clin Immunol 1991; 87:1088–1095.

13. Frieri M. Preliminary investigation of interleukin-4 for food hypersensitivity in atopic patients. Clin Res 1990; 38:486a.

14. Kleinman RE, Walker WA. Antigen processing and uptake from the intestinal tract. Clin Rev Allergy 1984; 2:25–37.

15. Konishi YS, Kumagai S. Biliary immune response to orally presented food antigen, ovomucoid and its potentiation by cholera toxin B subunit. Scand J Immunol 1992; 35:597–602.

16. Dubucquoi S, Desreumaux P, Tanin A et al. Interleukin 5 synthesis of eosinophils: association with granules and immunoglobulin-dependent secretion. J Exp Med 1994; 179:703–708.

17. Klemola T, Savilahti E, Arato A. Immunohistochemical findings in jejunal specimens from patients with IgA deficiency. Gut 1995; 37:519–523.

18. Bost KL, Pascual DW. Substance P: a late-acting lymphocyte differentiation cofactor. Am J Physiol 1992; 262:537–545.

19. Soothill JF. Food allergy. In: Pepys J, Edward AM, eds. The Mast Cell, Its Role in Health and Disease. New York: Focal Press, 1979.

20. Biancone L, Mandal A, Yang H et al. Production of IgG, IgG1 antibodies to cytoskeletal protein by lamina propria cells in cells in ulcerative colitis Gastroenterology 1995; 109:3–12.

21. Henchoz S, Gauchat JF, Aubry JP, Graber P, Pochon S, Bonnefoy JY. Stimulation of human IgE production by a subset of anti-CD21 monoclonal antibodies: requirement of a co-signal to modulate gene transcripts. Immunology 1994; 81:285–290.

22. Bonnefay JY, Pachon S, Aubry JP et al. A new pair of surface molecules involved in human IgE regulation. Immunol Today 1993; 14:1–2.

23. Gauchat JF, Henchoz S, Mazzel G, Aubry JP, Brannert T, Blasey H, Life P, Talabot D, Fiores-Romo L, Thompson J, et al. Induction of human IgE synthesis in B cells by mast cells and basophils. Nature 1993; 365:340–343.

24. Strobel S. Oral tolerance: immune responses to food antigens. In: Metcalfe DD, Sampson HA, Simon RA, eds. Food Allergy: Adverse Reactions to Foods and Food Additives, 2nd ed. Cambridge, MA: Blackwell Science, 1997.

25. Kobayashi Y, Konda N, Shinoda S, Kasahara KK, Iwagas, O et al. Predictive values of cord blood IgE and cord blood lymphocyte responses to food antigens in allergic disorders during infancy. J Allergy Clin Immunol 1994; 94:907–916.

26. Kondo N, Agata H, Fukotomi O, Motoyoshyi F, Orii T et al. Lymphocyte responses to food antigens in patient with atopic dermatitis who are sensitive to foods. J Allergy Clin Immunol 1990; 86:253–260.

27. Pene J, Rousset F, Briere F, Chietien I, Bonnefoy JY, Spits H, Yolota T, Arai N, Araik, I, Banchereau J, Voies J et al. IgE production by normal human lymphocytes is induced by interleukin 4 and suppressed by interferons γ and g and interleukin-4 production of ovalbumin-stimulated lymphocytes in egg-sensitive children. Ann Allergy Asthma Immunol 1996; 77:60–66.

28. Iida S, Kondo N, Agata H, Shinoda S, Shimbara M, Nishida T, Fukotumi O, Orii, T et al. Differences in lymphocyte proliferative responses to food antigens and specific IgE antibodies to foods with age among food-sensitive patients with atopic dermatitis. Ann Allergy Asthma Immunol 1995; 74:334–340.

29. Kondo N, Kaneko H, Fukao T et al. High sensitivity and specificity of proliferative responses of lymphocytes to food antigens for detection of the offending food in patients with food-sensitive atopic dermatitis. Pediatr Asthma Allergy Immunol 1996; 10:175–180.

30. Jaffe TS, Metcalfe DD. Cytokines and their role in the pathogenesis of severe food hypersensitivity reactions. Ann Allergy 1993; 71:362–364.

31. Miller A, Lider O, Weiner HL. Antigen-driven bystander suppression after oral administration of antigens. J Exp Med 1981; 174:791–7981.

32. Frieri M, Martinez S, Agarwal K, Trotta P et al. A preliminary study of interleukin 4 detection in atopic pediatric and adult patients: effect of dietary modification. Pediatr Asthma Allergy Immunol 1993; 7:27–35.

33. Noma T, Kawano Y, Yoshizawa I, Itoh M, Mukouyama T, Baba M, Yata J et al. Antigen specific induction of IL-2 responsiveness of ovalbumin (OVA)-stimulated lymphocytes from patients with egg-white allergy and their regulation by the supernatant of normal lymphocytes. Ann Allergy 1990; 64:33–41.

34. Noma T, Yoshizawa I, Maeda K, Baba M, Yata J et al. Initial events and T cell activation in lymphokine-mediated allergic responses in patients with hen egg allergy. Ann Allergy 1994; 73:76–84.

35. Hawryklo E, Spertus A, Mele C, Oster N, Frieri M. Increased interleukin-2 in response to human type I collagen in patients with systemic sclerosis. Arthritis Rheum 1991; 34:530–587.
36. Gurram M, Pahwa S, Frieri M. Interleukin 6 production in response to type I human collagen in patients with systemic sclerosis. Ann Allergy 1995; 73:493–496.
37. Knapik M, Frieri M. Altered cytokine production in atopic dermatitis: a preliminary study. Pediatr Asthma Allergy Immunol 1993; 7:127–133.
38. Paul WE, Ohara J. B cell stimulatory factor/interleukin-4. Annu Rev Immunol 1987; 5:429.
39. Chavarria V, Frieri M, Young R, Zitt M, Karnik A, Kurpad C, Fitzgerald D. Interleukin-4 and plasma histamine levels in challenged food hypersensitive patients. Ann Allergy 1994; 72:57a.
40. Isolauri E, Suomalaineu H, Kaila M, Jalonen T, Soppi E, Virtanen E, Arvilommi H et al. Local immune responses in patients with cow milk allergy: follow-up of patients retaining allergy or becoming tolerant. J Pediatr 1992; 120:9–15.
41. Agata H, Kondo N, Fukutomi O, Shinoda S, Orii T et al. Effect of elimination diets on food specific IgE antibodies and lymphocyte proliferative responses to food antigens in atopic dermatitis patients exhibiting sensitivity to food allergens. J Allergy Clin Immunol 1993; 91:668–679.
42. Werfel T, Ahlers G, Schmidt P, Boeker M, Kapp A, Neumann C. Milk-responsive atopic dermatitis is associated with a casein-specific lymphocyte response in adolescent and adult patients. J Allergy Clin Immunol 1997; 99:124–133.
43. Greive M. Walther S, Gyufka K, Czech W, Schopf E, Krutmann J. Analysis of the cytokine pattern expressed in situ in inhalent allergen patch test reactions of atopic dermatitis patients. J Invest Dermatol 1995; 105:407–10.
44. Beyer K, Niggemann B, Nasert S, Renz H, Wahn U et al. Severe allergic reactions to foods are predicted by increased of CD45 RO⁺ T cells and loss of L-selection expression. J Allergy Clin Immunol 1997; 99:522–529.
45. Benlounes N, Dupont C, Candalh C, Agnes Blaton M, Darmon N, Resjeux JF, Heyman M et al. The threshold for immune cell reactivity to milk antigens decreases in cow's milk allergy with intestinal symptoms. J Allergy Clin Immunol 1996; 98:781.
46. Shinbara M, Kondo N, Agata H, Fukutomi O, Kuwabara N, Kobayashi Y, Miura M, Orii T et al. Interferon-γ and interleukin-4 production of ovalbumin-stimulated lymphocytes in egg-sensitive children. Ann Allergy Asthma Immunol 1996; 77:60–66.
47. Sutas Y, Soppi E, Karhonen H, Liisa-Syväoja E, Saxelin M, Rokka T, Isolauri E et al. Suppression of lymphocyte proliferation in vitro by bovine caseins hydrolyzed with *Lactobacillus casei* GG-derived enzymes. J Allergy Clin Immunol 1996; 98:216–224.
48. McMenamin C, Holt PG. The natural immune response to inhaled soluble protein antigens involves major histocompatibility complex (MHC) class I-restricted CD8⁺ T cell-mediated, but MHC class II-restricted CD4⁺ T cell-dependent immune deviation resulting in selective suppression of immunoglobulin E production. J Exp Med 1993; 178:889–899.

49. Inman RD. Antigens, the gastrointestinal tract and arthritis. Rheum Dis Clin North Am 1991; 17(2):309–321.

50. Van de Laar MA, van der Korst JK. Rheumatoid arthritis, food and allergy. Semin Arthritis Rheum 1991; 21(1):12–23.

51. Frieri M, Agarwal K, Datar A, Trotta P et al. Increased interleukin-4 production in response to mast cell mediators and human type collagen in patients with rheumatoid arthritis. Ann Allergy 1994; 72:360–367.

52. Frieri M. Food Allergy. In: Kaliner M, ed. Current Review of Allergic Diseases, Current Medicine, 1999, pp 173–182, Blackwell Science.

3

Antigen Absorption and the Gut Barrier

SAUL TEICHBERG
North Shore University Hospital, Manhasset, New York

INTRODUCTION

The apical surface of the intestinal mucosa faces a luminal external milieu with remarkably diverse and changeable ecological conditions. This includes variable pH, electrolytes, nutrients, digestive enzymes, bile salts, and their micelles; transient alterations in luminal osmotic pressure; beneficial and pathogenic microbes and their metabolites; as well as toxigenic or potentially antigenic molecules [68,82]. Consequently, one of the central functions of the intestinal epithelium, intraepithelial lymphocytes, and lamina propria lymphoid and effector cells is to provide a barrier, protecting the internal environment from noxious or damaging elements of the external mileu of the intestine. A key component of this gut barrier concerns the mechanisms that exclude foreign antigens and toxigenic macromolecules from the mucosa and internal environment [34,51,61,68,82]. In addition to its protective role in excluding antigens, the gut barrier permits some macromolecules that may be of benefit to the host to cross the epithelium. This includes orally derived antigen induction of systemic immune tolerance and absorption of potential trophic factors.

COMPONENTS OF THE GUT BARRIER

Physiological Factors

The mature mammalian gut barrier is composed of several physiological, immunological, and structural components that play a role in the exclusion of foreign antigens and toxigenic macromolecules from the internal environment. Physiological barrier components include normal peristalsis and gut motility, gastrointestinal digestive processes, and mucus release. Peristalsis decreases the potential for antigen absorption by limiting contact time between luminal contents and the apical surface of the intestinal mucosa. Peristalsis also helps to prevent colonization of the upper small intestinal lumen with bacterial flora; the latter may secrete damaging metabolic products such as deconjugated bile salts and alcohols that can alter the integrity of the gut barrier [68,72,82,88]. Low gastric pH, gastric protease activity, pancreatic digestive enzymes, and brush border peptidases all participate in the process of hydrolyzing potential antigens in the gut lumen [61,77]. The end products of this digestion are di- and tripeptides and amino acids, substrates for normal intestinal absorption. Some fragmented oligopeptides are also produced during luminal digestion. Even if they are absorbed into the gut epithelium and across the mucosa, the evidence suggests that these partially digested peptides display reduced ability to elicit immunological responses [23,45,52]. Mucus, which contains numerous glycoproteins and is released by goblet cells, also acts as a barrier to antigen or toxin penetration across the intestinal mucosa. Binding to secreted mucus may prevent access of potential antigens onto the cell surface. Mucus may also act as a barrier by "washing" off antigen or antigen–antibody complexes adherent to the brush border [78,82].

Immunological Mechanisms

In adult mammals there are important gut immune antigen excluding protective mechanisms, generally mediated by mucosal secretory antibody (secretory immunoglobulin A [S-IgA]) a part of the gut associated lymphoid system (GALT). This topic has been extensively reviewed [31,34,61,65]. In response to penetration of luminal antigen across some portion of the intestinal mucosa, there are sampling and processing of macromolecules by lymphocytes and antigen presenting cells. These include macrophages and dendritic cells. After interaction with T lymphocytes, S-IgA is synthesized by lamina propria plasma cells. The S-IgA then binds to secretory component (SC), a glycoprotein receptor at the basolateral epithelial surface. The complex of S-IgA and SC is endocytosed and transported within vesicles, from the basal to the apical surface of the epithelium, and then released into the gut lumen by exocytosis. S-IgA is generally directed against antigens and toxigenic organisms, such as *Vibrio cholerae,* to which the intestine has been exposed [16,34,47,61,65]. Some data suggest that binding and immobilization of luminal antigens to S-IgA may promote more efficient digestion by luminal pancreatic proteases [77].

In neonatal mammals immune exclusion mechanisms may be quite complex, involving lymphocyte trafficking and immunoglobulin transport from mother to young via breast milk, particularly colostrum [25,34,51,57,65]. Maternal B lymphocytes, capable of producing S-IgA against antigens that they have sampled in the intestine of the mother, can migrate to the breast, where they release immunoglobulin in maternal milk. Some maternal lymphocytes may also be transferred into the milk [34]. Thereby, the neonate acquires secretory immunity against dietary or other antigens to which the mother has been exposed. In the neonatal period of many mammals, including humans, the secretory immune system is immature. Therefore, this lymphocyte trafficking and secretory immunoglobulin production on the gut to breast to neonatal intestine axis may be of great physiological importance. The maternal lymphocytes and S-IgA survive in the gastrointesinal environment of the neonate in part because of the relative gastric achlorhydria.

Structural Mechanisms: Zonula Occludens

In addition to physiological and immune mechanisms, there is a formidable gut epithelial structural barrier to the absorption of antigens. This barrier includes the tight junction or zonula occludens (ZO). The ZO is a specialized cell–cell junctional structure, joining the lateral plasma membranes of adjacent epithelial cells at their most apical region, beneath the microvillus brush border (Figs. 1 and 2). Structurally, ZOs joining intestinal absorptive epithelial cells are composed of a meshlike network of intramembranous particles that form strands and are embedded within the adjacent lateral plasma membranes (Fig. 1) [30,39,40,43,46]. The ZO normally presents a physical barrier to paracellular (between the cells) diffusion of even small macromolecules, between the gut lumen and the basolateral intercellular spaces of the epithelium. Normally, only water and some electrolytes, principally cations, traverse the ZO [14,30,41,55].

Many studies have revealed an inherent variability in the structural organization found in the ZOs of the intestinal mucosa. Because of the meshlike quality of the gut ZO, there is considerable variation in the number of strands a molecule is required to traverse in order to cross the ZO at different loci, within the same cell or a given cell type (Fig. 1). Intestinal epithelial ZO variability is also a result of differences in the mean number of ZO strands and organization among the several epithelial cell types of the intestine For example, ZOs involv-

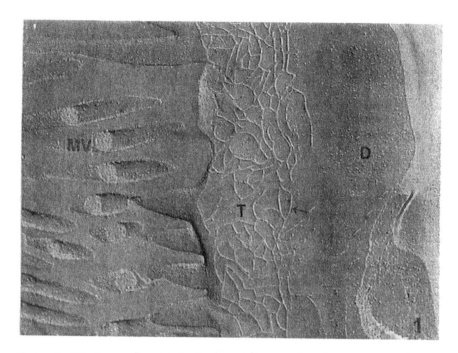

FIGURE 1 Electron micrograph of a freeze fractured replica of an absorptive cell junction from the rabbit ileum. The tight junction (T) shows the characteristic meshlike network of intramembranous strands (arrow). This meshlike property results in an inherent variability in the number of strands within the junction at any given point, as illustrated in the micrograph. A desmosome is at D and the apical microvillus surface at MV. x57,000.

ing goblet cells are less well organized and have fewer strands than junctions between absorptive cells. ZOs involving cup cells show a more organized parallel array of junctional strands [43,44]. In addition, evidence indicates that the mean number of ZO strands in absorptive cell junctions decreases along the villus to crypt mucosal axis and increases in the duodenal to ileal direction [43].

Functionally, ZO structural characteristics are usually considered in terms of their effect on paracellular electrolyte fluxes and associated transepithelial resistance properties of the epithelium [21,55,64]. The ZO also plays an important role in the segregation of apical and basolateral plasma membrane components, thereby contributing to the establishment and maintenance of apical/basolateral epithelial polarity [60]. Recent studies indicate that the ZO is a dynamic structure that may by altered by physiological conditions, such as transient hyperosmolality and during glucose absorption. These studies suggest a possible role in antigen penetration across the intestinal epithelium as discussed later [3,39,41].

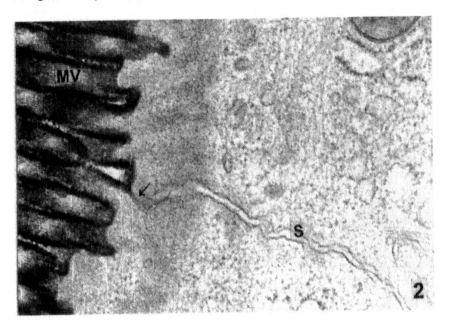

FIGURE 2 Electron micrograph of the apical portion of two absorptive epithelial cells, illustrating the macromolecular barrier function of the tight junction. The material is from an experiment in which the intestinal lumen of an adult rat was perfused with a 40,000 molecular weight (mw) glycoprotein tracer, horseradish peroxidase (HRP). In the micrograph the HRP is seen to be adherent to the microvillus (MV) surface, but it does not enter or diffuse into the tight junctional zone (arrow). HRP is also seen to be excluded from deeper portions of the intercellular space (S), between the epithelial cells. ×57,000.

Structural Mechanisms: Adult Mucosal Lysosomal Barrier

In addition to the ZO, lysosomes in the epithelial cell cytoplasm readily degrade a large majority of the macromolecules entering the cells by endocytosis from either the apical or the basolateral surface. Classically, the uptake of nonspecific potential luminal antigens into absorptive epithelial cells involves endocytosis into small vesicles at the base of microvilli. These endocytotic vesicles fuse with and deposit their contents into one of several intracellular compartments: these include endosomes, multivesicular bodies (MVBs) and lysosomes [2,29,58,70,72]. Endosomes are membrane bound cytoplasmic vacuoles with an acidic pH that receive endocytosed ligands, receptors, and other macromolecules. MVBs are also acidic vacuoles that receive endocytosed materials; they also contain internal

vesicles derived from the MVB membrane and they are destined to be converted
to active lysosomes after fusion with small acid hydrolase containing vesicles
originating in the Golgi apparatus. Lysosomes are also an acidic pH vacuolar
compartment. Morphologically they are pleomorphic and can degrade virtually
all classes of macromolecules with hydrolases that have maximal activity at an
acidic pH [29]. The products of lysosomal protein degradation include amino
acids and di- and tripeptides [29]. Some partially degraded peptides may escape
complete lysosomal degradation and cross the epithelium. As noted, experimental
evidence suggests that such partially degraded peptides have decreased immunogenicity and are less likely to elicit an immune response [23,45,52]. Antigens or
partially degraded peptides that manage to traverse the mucosa may then encounter lamina propria macrophages or Kupffer cells in the liver; all of these have
the capacity to endocytose and degrade potentially antigenic molecules.

NORMAL ANTIGEN ABSORPTION ACROSS THE GUT BARRIER

In Neonatal Mammals

In adult absorptive cells apical endocytosis operates at very low levels. In neonatal mammals the ZO structural barrier is intact; however, the mucosal lysosomal
barrier may not be fully mature and there can be receptor-mediated and nonspecific uptake of macromolecules (Fig. 3) [1,2,58,59,70,74]. The extent and importance of this neonatal macromolecular absorption are usually related to the
maturity of the intestine at birth [51]. In altricial mammals, born with an immature small intestine, such as the mouse or rat, there are very high levels of endocytosis and a receptor-mediated transcytosis of antibody (IgG) from maternal milk
across the jejunal epithelium that provides the neonate with passive immunity
(Fig. 3) [2,6,51,59]. IgG binds to an IgG Fc receptor at the base of microvilli.
Vesicles and tubules with IgG enter apical endosomal compartments. There, IgG
is segregated from nonspecific molecules that may also have been taken up in the
endocytotic vesicle. Bound to the Fc receptor, the IgG is then released in vesicles
at the basolateral surface by exocytosis [2,6]. Although nonspecific macromolecules are frequently degraded by the lysosomal barrier in neonatal absorptive
cells, there can be a low but detectable level of absorption of this component
across the epithelium [2,70,74]. In addition to immunoglobulins and nonspecific
macromolecules, trophic peptides from maternal milk, such as epidermal growth
factor and nerve growth factor, also appear to be absorbed across the maturing
neonatal intestine by a receptor-mediated process [7,36,62,63,80]. These trophic
agents may act directly on the mucosal epithelium or they may be transported to
distant sites, as is likely to be true for nerve growth factor.

At weaning, IgG immunoglobulin absorption virtually ceases and Fc receptor synthesis declines during a process called "closure." Nonspecific antigen ab-

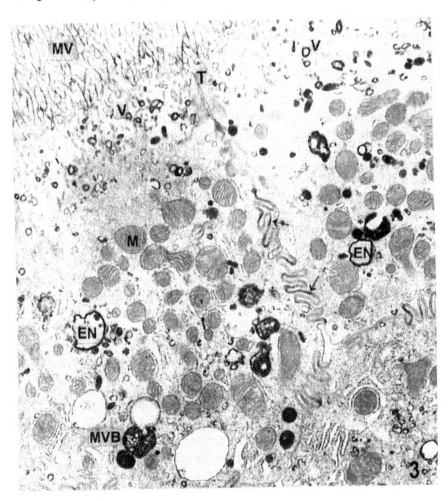

FIGURE 3 Electron micrograph of the apical portion of several intestinal epithelial cells from an immature 17 day old rat pup, illustrating the extensive uptake of macromolecules at this neonatal stage of development, prior to weaning. As in Figure 2, horseradish peroxidase (HRP), a 40,000 mw glycoprotein, was perfused through the intestinal lumen. In the neonatal animal there is extensive endocytosis of HRP into vesicles (V), endosomes (EN), and multivesicular bodies (MVBs). Some HRP is also seen in the intercellular space between the cells (arrow). Since HRP is not evident in the tight junctional zone, it is likely that the tracer reached the intercellular space by transcytosis; apical endocytosis, then exocytosis at the lateral cell surface. Note the relative lack of HRP on the microvilli as compared to that seen in adults. ×14,250.

sorption also markedly decreases. Maturation of the gut barrier, during closure, is associated with a marked decrease in apical endocytosis and disappearance of the large apical cytoplasmic endosomal compartment [2,59,70,74]. Lysosomal hydrolytic enzyme activity increases during the neonatal period; however, levels of the enzymes do not necessarily parallel closure and rises in their level may occur earlier. Changes in nonspecific uptake may reflect alterations in the microvillus membrane with development, as seen in the disappearance of the Fc receptor in the case of IgG uptake. Studies with horseradish peroxidase, a net cationic glycoprotein, show an increasing affinity of the macromolecule for binding at the microvillus brush border as closure proceeds. In earlier stages when uptake into vesicles is very extensive, binding on the microvilli is very poor. In this case the binding affinity to microvilli appears inversely related to the amount of the molecule taken up by the cells. This is likely to reflect known developmental alterations in the microvillus membrane during this period.

Some data suggest that the timing of closure may be hormone-dependent and influenced by neonatal nutritional status. In experimental rats, early closure can be induced by corticosteroids, administered by the oral route and at a concentration like that reported in rat maternal milk [68,74]. The timing of closure is also dependent on nutritional factors. It is delayed in undernourished animals raised in large litters and undersized for age (unpublished observations). Closure is also delayed by premature weaning from maternal milk to formula feedings in rat and rabbit animal models [51,70,74,75]. The relationships among nutrition, hormones, and the timing of closure in experimental animals need to be further clarified.

In more precoccial species, born with a mature intestine, passive immunity is in large part conveyed transplacentally. Placetal trophoblasts also utilize an Fc receptor for the transcytosis of maternal IgG [62]. In these mammals, neonatal macromolecular absorption is less marked and closure occurs much earlier [51]. However, even in comparatively precoccial human infants, antigens such as lactalbumin are transferred from maternal milk to the neonate [4,22]. The amount of antigen transmitted is increased in underweight premature infants, gradually declining in amount over the first 2 years of life [4,10]. In addition to maternal milk antigens, other dietary molecules, such as egg and cow's milk proteins, are transmitted to the human neonate [18,24,33]. The evidence indicates that some of the antigens absorbed by neonates are those initially consumed by the mother. These observations are relevant to food allergies reported in breast fed infants and to other intestinal pathological states, such as colic, reported in breast fed babies of mothers consuming cow's milk [22,33]. In this context, it is of interest that some experimental studies show increased dietary antigen absorption in lactating dams [26].

The consequences of nonspecific neonatal antigen absorption in the neonatal period are dependent in part on the development stage [66,67,85]. Antigens entering by the oral route, at a sufficiently mature stage of neonatal development, as well as in some adults, play a key role in the acquisition of systemic immune tolerance to those antigens [34,67,83–85]. Classic experimental studies have documented that prior oral feeding of an antigen can prevent a subsequent systemic anaphylactic response to the same antigen [37,83]. Systemic immune tolerance, induced via the oral route, can be developed against directly consumed dietary antigens and antigens transmitted to neonates in maternal milk [84,85]. On the other hand, some evidence from rodent studies suggests that neonatal immaturity may predispose to priming and an enhanced systemic immune response, rather than tolerance [67].

Absorption in Adults

Even under normal physiological conditions, in the absence of gastrointestinal disease, the intestinal barrier to foreign antigens in adult mammals is incomplete. Relatively low levels of intact or partially fragmented macromolecules cross the mucosa from the gut lumen. The antigens either enter the circulation, are engulfed, and are degraded by local macrophages or enter local antigen presenting cells [34,61]. This low level of absorption can occur at a number of sites, including the absorptive epithelium and across microfold ("M") epithelial cells overlying Peyer's patch lymphoid follicles [20,47,48,49,61,68].

In the absorptive epithelium, cytochemical studies with horseradish peroxidase suggest that the continual shedding of dying epithelial cells from the tip of villi provides a minor open pathway for gut antigen penetration. This may occur by diffusion across dying cells whose plasma membranes have lost their selective permeability characteristics or by the paracellular route between the cells [19,71,72]. Low levels of antigen may cross absorptive cells of the intestinal mucosa by transcytosis from the apical to the basolateral surfaces [71,73]. Cup cells, specialized mucosal epithelial cells, also endocytose appreciable amounts of macromolecules. However, evidence appears to indicate that antigens are retained and degraded within the cup cell cytoplasm [38].

As noted, some evidence has been reported for paracellular diffusion of antigens, or fragmented peptides, across a transiently dilated ZO during intestinal absorption of glucose or other organic nonelectrolyte nutrients [3,42]. Paracellular diffusion of macromolecules across junctions of crypt ileal epithelium has been reported during cholinergic stimulation [54]. The probability that a transiently open paracellular route allows some antigen absorption is consistent with the reported dynamic property of the ZO, and with the high degree of variability in strand number reported for the small intesine [30,39,40]. However, the physiological role of the paracellular route for organic nonelectrolyte absorption, coupled with antigen uptake, remains to be confirmed and is still a subject of investigation [5].

Possibly the most significant pathway for intestinal antigen absorption, sampling, and processing by lymphoid tissue concerns the endocytosis into and across thin ileal epithelial M or microfold cells overlying Peyer's patches in the ileum [47–49,66,86]. This epithelium forms a thin sheet, with scant microvilli, and has a basal invagination that lymphoid cells enter. The M cell surface binds antigens, and certain microbes, such as reovirus and strains of *Escherichia coli* [86]. Antigens are able to traverse the very thin epithelial cell cytoplasm efficiently, eluding lysosomal degradation, and are then released basally by exocytosis to be processed by underlying lymphoid tissue. The follicle beneath the epithelium contains T lymphocytes, S-IgA-producing B lymphocytes, dendritic cells, and macrophages [31,34,47,66]. Local macrophages may participate by either degrading antigens or processing and presenting antigens for an immune response. After antigen sampling and presentation, stimulated B lymphocytes can migrate and synthesize S-IgA at local and distant intestinal sites, as well as other epithelial mucosal surfaces, including the breast [34,65,66]. As detailed, this is the underlying process by with the neonate receives S-IgA against maternal dietary antigens.

PATHOLOGICAL ANTIGEN ABSORPTION

Under pathophysiological gastrointestinal conditions, like those encountered during infectious gastroenteritis, malabsorption, and bacterial overgrowth syndromes, the permeability of the intestine to macromolecluar antigens appears to be enhanced [8,9,45,56,76]. Pathophysiological consequences of this increase in antigen absorption may include food protein sensitivity, with consequent local effector cell (mast cells and eosinophils) mediated local damage to the intestinal mucosa. This can lead to further nonspecific luminal antigen uptake from the gut [9,22,27,28,45,53,61,65]. Some of the pathophysiological conditions that may promote enhanced absorption of antigenic molecules across the intestinal mucosa are outlined in Table 1. These can be divided into conditions in which luminal antigen concentrations are elevated and those in which the mucosal barrier is damaged. Ensuant abnormality, such as sensitization and atopic illness, resulting from increased antigen uptake also depend in part upon host genetic factors.

Luminal Antigen Elevation

Pathological compromise of any of the physiological gut barrier components, including inhibition of luminal digestion by pancreatic proteases, achlorohydria, or S-IgA deficiency, will lead to an elevation of intact antigen levels in the gut lumen. Clinical studies in patients with S-IgA deficiency and achlorhydria, as well as experimental studies on digestive enzyme deficiencies, have provided evidence for enhanced antigen absorption under these conditions, with deleterious consquences for the host. In children this often involves sensitization to cow's milk proteins, but it can include other dietary antigens as well [17,27,79,82]. Antigen levels may also be elevated as a result of motility and peristaltic defects that prolong gut transit time and thereby elevate the duration of exposure of the antigen to the gut surface.

TABLE 1 Penetration of the Gut Barrier to Macromolecules

A. **Conditions elevating luminal antigen concentration**
  1. Pancreatic and digestive enzyme insufficiency
  2. Achlorhydria
  3. Secretory immunoglobulin A deficiency
  4. Peristalsis or motility defects
B. **Conditions damaging intestinal mucosal integrity**
  1. Bacterial proliferation and metabolic products (deconjugated bile salts, fatty acids, alcohols)
  2. Acute viral, invasive bacterial, or protozoal gastroenteritis
  3. Dietary antigen-induced local anaphylaxis
  4. Malabsorption and persistent luminal hyperosmolality
  5. Dietary antigen sensitivity and local anaphylaxis
  6. Malnutrition

Mucosal Damage

An additional consequence of decreased peristalsis and motiliity may be to permit the proliferation of bacterial microbes into the more proximal portions of the small intestinal lumen. Proliferation of normal bacterial flora in the upper small intestine can lead to release in the gut lumen of a variety of metabolic by-products; these include deconjugated bile salts, fatty acids, and alcohol. Some of these are surface active agents with hydrophobic properties, which can damage the intestinal mucosa [68,88]. For example, several experimental studies have reported that luminal dihydroxy deconjugated bile salts in the upper small intestine promote enhanced macromolecular absorption from the intestinal lumen [19,69,72].

Other pathological gastrointestinal conditions, including microbial overgrowth, infection of mature absorptive cells with viral agents such as rotavirus, as well as gastroenteritis due to adherent, invasive, or toxigenic bacterial agents, can damage the gut barrier and allow enhanced antigen absorption [8,23,24,32,35,76]. After bouts of gastroenteritis increased levels and kinds of dietary antigens, including egg proteins and albumin, are seen in the serum of infants [24]. Although some evidence suggests that many of the macromolecules absorbed under pathological conditions are partially degraded and have lost antigenic properties, significant deleterious immunological consequences can occur under these conditions [23,32,45].

Pathological states that lead to nutrient malabsorption may also result in damage to the integrity of the gut barrier. Persistent luminal hypertonicity, like that seen in malabsorption syndromes, may result in structural ZO alterations that permit focal diffusion of intact antigens across the mucosa [15,46]. Experimental studies have also shown that the integrity of the gut barrier may also be experimentally altered by prolonged protein energy malnutrition or moderate protein energy malnutrition in a combined setting with bacterial overgrowth [69,87] as well as in small for gestational age human infants [4,10].

Clinical Consequences

The experimental observations that undernutrition compromises the gut barrier and enhances antigen absorption may be very relevant to problems of chronic diarrhea in underdeveloped third world countries. It is now well known that the diarrhea–malnutrition syndrome is a vicious cycle in children, particularly in many underdeveloped parts of the world where hygienc and economic conditions are substandard for much of the population. As noted, when the absorption of antigen results in local immunologic hypersensitivity in the gut, as seen in cow's milk protein–sensitive enteropathy, consequent pathophysiological alterations may promote absorption of additional antigens [9,18,24,45,56,66,82]. These rapid hypersensitivity reactions are usually mediated by IgE antibody. IgE binding to local mast cells can result in mediator and protease release, which further damages the mucosa and leads to additional antigen absorption [11,28,50,53,61]. In a potentially sensitizable host this kind of phenomenon could result in additional food protein sensitivities. Such a process is likely to complicate the treatment of gastroenteritis, which often consists of dietary exclusion or formula substitution [9,56]. Clinically, in the pediatric age group this may be manifest in the subsets of patients who fail to thrive on more than one infant formula. In the underdeveloped world, this sequence of events may lead to the protraction of diarrheal illness to a chronic phase and increase the rate of mortality.

In some populations dietary antigen absorption can result in atopic illness [12,13,22]. This is likely to be in part dependent on host genetic predispositional factors. Several studies suggest that diet can affect whether or not a potentially sensitized individual manifests disease due to antigen absorption. Research on experimental animals provided evidence that nonspecific antigen absorption is increased and closure delayed in animals fed artificial formula diets [32,51,70,74,75]. Well controlled clinical studies indicate that the frequency of symptoms and emergence of atopic clinical disease in children at high risk for antigen-mediated atopic disease can be prevented by one of two dietary treatments [12,13]. One approach is the elimination of potentially sensitizing antigens from the diet of a breast feeding mother; this is based on the premise that the mother's milk will contain antigens from her diet that will be transmitted to the child, and the observation that breast feeding without dietary restriction is of limited value. A second approach is formula feeding, with a processed protein hydrolysate formula, that is low in immunogenicity. These studies highlight the fact that breast feeding of infants at risk for atopic illness, though generally beneficial, requires maternal dietary control. This is likely to be due in part to the enhanced protein uptake by mothers during lactation [26].

SUMMARY

There is elevated uptake of antigens from the small intestine early in life in many mammals. This varies dramatically between species and is inversely dependent in quantity and duration on the maturity of the intestine at birth; antigen absorption is higher in altricial species born with an immature intestine than in precoccial mammals. Neonatal antigen absorption serves positive functions, including (a) the acquisition of protective passive immunity by the gut at a time when the neonatal capacity to mount an appropriate response may be immature; (b) the acquisition of systemic immune tolerance to the absorbed antigens, (c) the acquisition of trophic substances, such as EGF and nerve growth factor (NGF), from maternal milk. Negative consequences may include priming of the immune system and atopic illness; this is likely to be dependent in part upon host genetic and developmental factors. The mature gut barrier consisits of physiological (peristalsis, motility, mucus, gastric acidity, proteases), immunological (S-IgA), and structural components. Structural features of the barrier include the zonula occludens or tight junction, formed by strands of intramembranous particles that prevent paracellular antigen diffusion between the gut lumen and the internal mileu. The cellular barrier to antigen absorption also includes the epithelial cell lysosmal system, which degrades antigens absorbed by endocytosis. The normal development of the gut barrier is in part dependent upon adequate nutrition and may be hormonally regulated. Alterations in components of the barrier include secretory immune deficiency or other conditions that increase the luminal antigen concentration or prolong contact with the mucosal surface, such as defects in digestion or peristalsis. Damage to the epithelial barrier also leads to enhanced antigen absorption; the intestinal mucosa can be damaged during infectious gastroenteritis, in malabsorption, and as a consequence of damaging bacterial metabolic products. Further alterations can also occur econdary to initial sensitization, as a consequence of local effector cell substances; this can lead to multiple food sensitivities that complicate treatment and may result in chronic diarrhea.

REFERENCES

1. Abrahamson DR, Powers A, Rodewald R. Intestinal absorption of immune complexes by neonatal rats: a route of antigen transfer from mother to young. Science 1979; 206:567–569.
2. Abrahamson DR, Rodewald R. Intestinal absorption for the sorting of endocytotic vesicle contents during the receptor mediated transport of IgG across the newborn rat intestine. J Cell Biol 1981; 91:270–280.

3. Atisook K, Madara JL. An oligopeptide permates intestinal tight juctions at glucose-elicited dilations: implications for oligopeptide absorption. Gastroenterolgy 1991; 100:719–724.

4. Axelsson I, Jakobsson I, Linderg T, Polberger S, Benediktsson B, Raiha N. Macromolecular absorption in preterm and term infants. Acta Paediatr Scand 1989; 78:532–537.

5. Ballard ST, Hunter JH, Taylor AE. Regulation of tight junction permeability during nutrient absorption across the intestinal epithelium. Annu Rev Nutr 1995; 15:35–55.

6. Berryman M, Rodewald R. Beta 2-microglobulin co-distributes with the heavy chain of the intestinal IgG-Fc receptor throughout the transepithelial transport pathway of the neonatal rat. J Cell Sci 1995; 108:2347–2360.

7. Berseth CL, Michner SR, Norkyke CK, Vay liang WG. Postpartum changes in pattern of gastrointestinal regulatory peptides in human milk. Am J Clin Nutr 1990; 51:985–990.

8. Bloch KJ, Bloch DB, Stearns M, Walker WA. Intestinal uptake of macromolecules. VI. Uptake of protein antigen in vivo in normal rats and in rats infected with *Nippostrongylus brasiliensis* or subjected to mild systemic anaphylaxis. Gastroenterology 1979; 77:1039–1044.

9. Bloch KJ, Walker WA. Effect of locally induced intestinal anaphylaxis on the uptake of a bystander antigen. J Allergy Clin Immunol 1981; 67:312–316.

10. Boehm G, Jakobsson I, Mansson M, Raiha NCR. Macromolecular absorption in small-for-gestational-age infants. Acta Paediatr 1992; 81:864–867.

11. Catto-Smith AG, Ribber JL. Mucosal mast cells and developmental changes in gastric absorption. Am J Physiol 1995; 268:G121–G127.

12. Chandra RK, Gukrkirpal S, Shridhara B. Effect of feeding whey hydrolysate, soy and conventional cow milk formulas on incidence of atopic disease in high risk infants. Ann Allergy 1989; 63:102–106.

13. Chandra RK, Shakuntla P, Azza H. Influence of maternal diet during lactation and use of formula feeds on development of atopic eczema in high risk infants. Br Med J 1989; 299:228–230.

14. Citi S. The molecular organizaiton of tight junctions. J Cell Biol 1993; 121:485–489.

15. Cooper M, Teichberg S, Lifshitz F. Alterations in rat jejunal permeability to a macromolecular tracer during a hyperosmotic load. Lab Invest 1978; 38:447–454.

16. Cruz JR, Garcia B, Urritia J, Carlsson B, Hanson L. Food antibodies in milk from Guatemalen women. J Pediatr 1981; 99:600–602.

17. Cunningham-Rundles C, Brandeis WE, Good RA. Bovine antigens and the formation of circulating inmune compleses in selective immunoglobulin A deficiency. J Clin Invest 1979; 64:272–279.

18. Eastham EJ, Lichauco T, Grady MI, Walker WA. Antigenicity of infant formulas: role of immature intestine on protein permeability. J Pediatr 1978; 93:561–564.

19. Fagundes-Neto U, Teichberg S, Bayne MA, Morton B, Lifshitz F. Bile salt enhanced rat jejunal absorption of a macromolecular tracer. Lab Invest 1981; 44:18–6.

20. Frieri M. IgE/IgA-bearing cells in gut lymphoid tissue with special emphasis on food allergy. In Chariaramonte LT, Schneider AT, Lifshitz F, eds. Food Allergy: A Practical Approach to Diagnosis and Management. New York: Marcel Dekker 1988, pp 45–70.

21. Frizzel RA, Schultz SG. Ionic conductances of extracellular shunt pathway in rabbit ileum. J Gen Physiol 1972; 59:318–346.
22. Gerrard JW. Allergy in breast fed babies to ingredients in breast milk. Ann Allergy 1979; 42:69–72.
23. Gotteland M, Isolauri E, Heyman M, Tome D, Desjeux J-F. Antigen absorption in bacterial diarrhea: in vivo intestinal transport of B-lactoglobulin in rabbits infected with the enteroadherent *Eschericia coli* strain RDEC-1. Pediatr Res 1989; 26:237–240.
24. Gruskay FL, Cooke RE. The gastrointestinal absorption of unaltered protein in normal infants and in infants recovering from diarrhea. Pediatrics 1955; 16:763–768.
25. Hanson LA, Ashraf R, Cruz JR, Hahn-Zoric M, Jalil F, Nave M, Reimer M, Zaman S, Carlsson B. Immunity related to exposition and bacterial colonization of the infant. Acta Pediatr Scandi Suppl 1990; 365:38–45.
26. Harmatz PR, Bloch KJ, Brown M, Walker WA, Kleinman RE. Intestinal adaptation during lactation in the mouse. I. Enhanced intestinaal uptake of dietary protein antigen. Immunology 1989; 67:92–95.
27. Harrison M, Kilby A, Walker-Smith JA, France NE, Wood CBS. Cow's milk protein intolerance: a possible association with gastroenteritis, lactose intolerance, and IgA deficiency. Br Med J 1976; 1:1501–1504.
28. Hatz RA, Bloch KJ, Harmatz PR, Gonnella PA, Ariniello PD, Walker WA, Kleinman RE. Divalent apten-induced intestinal anaphylaxis in the mouse enhances macromolecular uptake from the stomach. Gastroenterology 1990; 98:894–900.
29. Holtzman E. Lysosomes: A Survey. Vienna: Springer Verlag, 1976.
30. Hyun CS, Chen CWP, Shinowara NL, Palaia T, Martello LS, Mueenuddin M, Donovan V, Teichberg S. Morphological factors influencing conductance in a rabbit model of ileitis. Gastroenterology 1995; 109:13–23.
31. Insoft RM, Sanderson IR, Walker WA. Development of immune fuction in the intestine and its role in neonatal diseases. Pediatr Clin North Am 1996; 43:551–571.
32. Isolauri E, Kaile M, Arvola T, Majamaa H, Rantala I, VirtanenE, Arvilommi H. Diet during roavirus enteritis affects jejunal permeability to macromolecules in suckling rats. Pediatr Res 1993; 33:548–553.
33. Jakobsson I, Lindberg T. Cow's milk proteins cause infantile colic in breast fed infants: a double-blind crossover study. Pediatrics 1983; 71:268–271.
34. Kagnoff MF. Immunology of the digestive system. In: Johnson LR, ed. Physiology of the Gastrointestinal Tract. 2nd ed. New York: Raven Press, 1987, pp 1699–1728.
35. Keljo DJ, Butler DG, Hamilton JR. Altered jejunal permeability to macromolecules during viral enteritis in the piglet. Gastroenterology 1985; 88:998–1004.
36. Koldovsky O, Thornburg W. Hormones in milk. Pediatr Gastroenterol 1987; 6:172–196.
37. Lafont S, Andre C, Andre F, Gillon J, Fargier M-C. Abrogation by subsequent feeding of antibody response including IgE, in parenterally immunized mice. J Exp Med 1982; 155:1573–1578.
38. Madara JL. Cup cells: structure and distribution of a unique class of epithelial cells in guinea pig, rabbit, and monkey small intestine. Gastroenterology 1982; 83:981–994.

39. Madara JL. Increases in guinea pig small intestianl transepithelial resistance in-duced by osmotic loads are accompanied by rapid alterations in absorptive-cell tight junction structure. J Cell Biol 1983; 97:125–136.

40. Madara JL. Contributions of the paracellular pathway to secretion, absorption and barrier function in the epithelium of the small intestine. In Lebenthal E, Duffey M, eds. Textbook of Secretory Diarrhea 1990. New York: Raven Press, 1990, pp 125–138.

41. Madara JL, Carlson S. Supraphysiologic L-tryptophan elicits cytoskeletal and macromolecular permeability alterations in hamster small intestinal epithelium in vitro. J Clin Invest 1991; 87:454–462.

42. Madara JL, Pappenheimer J. The structural basis for physiologic regulation of para-cellular pathways in intestinal epithelia. J Membrane Biology 1987; 100:149–164.

43. Madara JL, Trier JS, Neutra MR. Structural changes in the plasma membrane acco-manying differentiation of epithelial cells in human and monkey small intestine. Gastroenterology 1980; 78:963–975.

44. Madara JL, Trier JS. Structure and permeability of goblet cell tight junctions in rat small intestine. J Membr Biol 1982; 66:145–157.

45. Majamaa H, Isolauri E. Evaluation of the gut mucosal barrier: evidence for in-creased antigen transfer in children with atopic eczema. J Allergy Clin Immunol 1996; 97:985–990.

46. Marcial KA, Madara JL. Analysis of absorptive cell occluding junction structure–function relationships in a state of enhanced junctional permeability. Lab Invest 1987; 56:424–433.

47. Neutra MR, Frey A, Kraehenbuhl J-P. Epithelial M cells: gateways for mucosal in-fection and immunization. Cell 1996; 86:345–348.

48. Owen RL, Jones AL. Epithelial cell specialization withing human Peyer's patches of mouse ileum. Gastroenterology 1977; 72:440–451.

49. Owen RL. Sequential uptake of horseradish peroxidase by lymphoid follicle epithe-lium of Peyer's patches in the normal unobstructed mouse intestine: an ultrastruc-tural study. Lab Invest 1977; 72:440–448.

50. Patrick MK, Dunn IJ, Buret A, Miller HRP, Huntley JF, Gibson S, Gall DG. Mast cell protease release and mucosal ultrastructure during intestinal anaphylaxis in the rat. Gastroenterology 1988; 94:1–9.

51. Patt JA. Factors affecting the duration of intestinal permeability to macromolecules in newborn animals. Biol Rev 1977; 52:411–429.

52. Peng HJ, Chang ZN, Han SH, Won WH, Huang BT. Chemical denaturation of oval-bumin abrogates the induction of oral tolerance of specific IgG antibody and DTH responses in mice. Scand J Immunol 1995; 42:297–304.

53. Perdue MH, Chung M, Gall DG. Effect of intestinal anaphylaxis on gut function in the rat. Gastroenterology 1984; 86:391–397.

54. Phillips TE, Phillips TL, Neutra MR. Macromolecules can pass through occluding junctions of rat ileal epithelium during cholinergic stimulation. Cell Tissue Res 1987; 247:547–554.

55. Powell D. Barrier function of epithelia. Am J Physiol 1981; 241:G275–G278.

56. Powell GK. Milk and soy induced enterocolitis of infancy. J Pediatr 1978; 93:553–560.

57. Robinson G, Volovitz B, Passwell JH. Identification of a secretroy IgA receptor on breast milk macrophages: evidence for specific activation via these receptors. Pediatr Res 1991; 29:429–434.
58. Rodewald R. Selective antibody transport in the proximal small intestine of the neonatal rat. J Cell Biol 1970; 45:635–640.
59. Rodewald R. Distribution of immunoglobulin G receptors in the small intestine of the young rat. J Cell Biol 1980; 85:18–32.
60. Rodriguez-Boulan E, Powell SK. Polarity of epithelial and neuronal cells. Annu Rev Cell Biol 1992; 8:395–427.
61. Sanderson IR and Walker WA. Uptake and transport of macromolecules by the intestine: possible role in clinical disorders (an update). Gastroenterology 1993; 104:622–639.
62. Sedmak DD, Davis DH, Singh U, van der Winkel JG. Expression of IgG Fc receptors in placenta and on endothelial cells in humans. Am J Pathol 1991; 138:175–181.
63. Siminoski K, Gonnlla P, Bernanke J, Owen L, Neutra M, Murphy RA. Uptake and transepithelial transport of nerve growth factor in suckling rat ileum. J Cell Biol 1986; 103:1979–1990.
64. Spring K. Mechanism of fluid transport by epithelia. In: Handbook of Physiology. Vol. 6. Washington DC: American Physiologicical Society, 1991, pp 195–207.
65. Strober W, Brown WR. The mucosal immune system. Samter M, Talmage DW, Frank MM, Austen KF, Claman HN, eds. In: Immunological Diseases. 4th ed. Boston: Little Brown, 1988, pp 79–140.
66. Stroebel S. Immunologically mediated damage to the intestial mucosa. Acta Paediatr Scand Suppl 1990; 365:46–57.
67. Stroebel S, Ferguson A. Immune responses to fed protein antigens in mice. III. Systemic tolerance or priming is related to age at which antigen is first encountered. Pediatr Res 1984; 18:588–594.
68. Teichberg S. Intestinal absorption of potentially antigenic macromolecules. In: Food Allergy; a practical approach to diagnosis and management. Chiaramonte LT, A Schneider A, Lifshitz F, eds. New York: Marcel Dekker, 1988, pp 71–86.
69. Teichberg S, Fagundes-Neto U, Baybe MA, Lifshitz F. Jejunal macromolecular absorption and bile salt deconjugation in protein-energy malnourished rats. Am J Clin Nutr 1981; 34:1281–1291.
70. Teichberg S, Isolauri E, Wapnir RA, Roberts B, Lifshitz F. Development of the neonatal rat small intestinal barrier to nonspecific macromolecular absorption: effect of early weaning to artificial diets. Pediatr Res 1990; 28:31–37.
71. Teichberg S, Lifshitz F, Bayne MA, Fagundes-Neto U, Wapnir RA, McGarvey E. Disaccharide feedings enhance rat jejunal macromolecular absorption. Pediatr Res 1983; 17:381–389.
72. Teichberg S, McGarvey E, Bayne MA, Lifshitz F. Altered jejeunal macromolecular barrier induced by alpha dihydroxy deconjugated bile salts. Am J Physiol 1983; 245:G122–G132.
73. Teichberg S, Wapnir RA, Zdanowicz M, Roberts B, da Costa Ribeiro H, Jr., Lifshitz F. Morphologic and functional alterations in absorptive epithelial cells during L-tryptophan induced inhibition of net sodium and fluid absorption in the rat ileum. Lab Invest 1989; 60:88–101.

74. Teichberg S, Wapnir RA, Moyse J, Lifshitz F. Development of the neonatal rat small intestinal barrier to nonspecific macromolecular absorption. II. Role of dietary corticosterone. Pediatr Res 1992. 32:50–57.

75. Udall JN, Colony PA, Fritze L, Pand K, Trier J, Walker WA. Development of gastrointestinal mucosal barrier. II. The effect of natural versus artificial feeding on intestinal permeability to macromolecules. Pedatr Res 1981; 15:245–249.

76. Uhnoo IS, Freihorst J, Riepenhoff-Talty M, Fisher JE, Ogra PL. Effect of rotavirus infection and malnutrition on uptake of a dietary antigen in the intestine. Pediatr Res 1990; 27:153–160.

77. Walker WA, Wu M, Isselbacker KJ, Bloch KJ. Intestinal uptake of macromolecules. I. The effect of pancreatic duct ligation on the breakdown of antigen and antigen–antibody complexes on the intestinal surface. Gastroenterology 1981; 69:1223–1229.

78. Walker WA, Wu M, Bloch KJ. Stimulation by immune complexes of mucus release from goblet cells of the rat small intestine. Science 1977; 197:370–372.

79. Walker-Smith JA, Digeon B, Phillips AD. Evaluation of a casein and whey hydrolysate for treatment of cow's milk sensitive enteropathy. Eur J Pediatr 1989; 149:68–71.

80. Weaver LT, Gonnella PA, Israel EJ, Walker WA. Uptake and transport of epidermal growth factor by the small intestinal epithelium of the fetal rat. Gastroenterology 1990; 98:828–837.

81. Weaver LT, Koritz TN, Coombs RRA. Tolerance to orally induced anaphylactic sensitization to cow's milk proteins and patency of the intestinal mucosa in the neonatal guinea pig. Int Arch Allergy Appl Immunol 1987; 83:220–222.

82. Weaver LT, Walker WA. Uptake of macromolecules in the neonate. In: Human Gastrointestinal Development. Lebenthal E, ed. New York: Raven Press. 1989, pp 731–748.

83. Wells HG, Osborne TB. The biological reactions of vegetable proteins. J Infect Dis 1911; 8:66–123.

84. Wold AE, Dahlgren UIH, Ahsstedt S, Hanson LA. Lack of IgA antibody response in secretions of rat dams during long term ovalbumin feedings. Int Arch Allergy Appl Immunol 1987; 84:332–338.

85. Wold AE, Dahlgren UIH, Ahlstedt S, Hanson LA. Rats are sensitive to induction of tolerance by feeding only at young age. Monogr Allergy 1988; 24:251–252.

86. Wolff JL, Bye WA. The membranous epithelial (M) cell and the mucosal immune system. Annu Rev Med 1984; 35:95–112.

87. Worthington BS, Boatman ES, Kenney GE. Intestinal absorption of intact proteins in normal and protein deficient rats. Am J Clin Nutr 1974; 27:276–286.

88. Worthington BS, Meserole L, Syrotuck JA. Effect of dailiy ethanol ingestion on intestinal permeability to macromolecules. Dig Dis 1978; 239:23–32.

4

Food Allergens

GERALD REESE AND SAMUEL B. LEHRER
Tulane University Medical Center, New Orleans, Louisiana

INTRODUCTION

The mortality and morbidity resulting from hypersensitivity reactions to foods [1] demonstrate that food allergy can be a very serious problem. Avoidance, usually recommended as "traditional treatment" for food allergies, may not always be possible since some food products contain components that are seemingly unrelated to their original source. For example, fish protein–based surimi used as imitation sausage in pizza toppings [2] contains allergenic proteins that can trigger allergic reactions in fish-allergic subjects. Furthermore, there is concern about the safety and potential allergenicity of newly developed transgenic crops since these genetically altered plants and their products may contain unknown allergens [3,4]. Despite heightened interest in food allergy, the immunologic analysis of food allergens lags behind that of insect venom allergens and aeroallergens. Thus, it is important to identify and characterize food allergens in order to elucidate the structural features that separate food allergens from non-allergens.

DIFFICULTIES IN CHARACTERIZATION OF FOOD ALLERGEN–SPECIFIC IMMUNE RESPONSES

Food allergy can be defined as an immunological and pathological reaction to foods. In general, allergens induce the production of allergen-specific antibodies of the immunoglobulin E (IgE) isotype. These antibodies bind to the high-affinity Fc_ε receptor on mast cells and basophils via their Fc segment, thus sensitizing the cells. When allergens bridge cell-bound IgE antibodies, mast cells and basophils degranulate and release preformed mediators including histamine and bradykinin and newly formed mediators such as prostaglandins, leukotrienes, and platelet activating factor (PAF). These events result in urticaria, rhinitis, asthma, or anaphylactic shock within an hour of food exposure.

Unfortunately, most food extracts used for skin testing, in vitro detection of specific IgE, and food challenge are not well characterized or standardized in regard to their allergen content and biologic activity. This can even limit the accuracy of the gold standard for the diagnosis of food allergy, the double-blind placebo-controlled food challenge [5,6]. Furthermore, the clinical relevance of allergen cross-reactivity is an intensely debated issue since cross-reactivities of foods and proteins from closely related and unrelated sources have been described [7–9]. The question, Does in vitro detection of specific IgE or demonstration of a positive skin test result constitute clinical relevant multisensitization?, must be answered on a case to case basis [10–12].

Food allergens are often exposed to conditions that usually alter the conformation or destroy the structure of proteins. The impact of heat and digestion, for example, on the antigenicity or allergenicity is not understood. Further, the question of whether the denatured/digested protein or the native protein is responsible for induction of food allergies is unanswered. Last, the immune response of the gut-associated lymphoid tissue (GALT) to allergens has not been well studied.

MOLECULAR, STRUCTURAL, AND IMMUNOLOGICAL PROPERTIES OF SELECTED COMMON FOOD ALLERGENS

Allergen Nomenclature

In light of increased characterization of allergens using recombinant deoxyribonucleic acid (DNA) techniques, the nomenclature system for allergens has been revised recently [13,14]. Allergens are designated according to the accepted taxonomic name of their source: the first three letters of the genus, a space, the first letter of the species, a space, and the arabic number. Names are no longer italicized. Numbers are assigned to allergens in the order that they were identified; the same number is generally used to designate homologous allergens from related species. For example, the first allergen described in brown shrimp, *Penaeus aztecus,* was designated Pen a 1, and the homologous allergens in Indian shrimp, *P. indicus,* and greasyback shrimp (*Metapenaeus ensis*) are named Pen i 1 and Met e 1, respectively. However, these nomenclature rules are not strictly applied to all major allergens. For example, the well-characterized milk allergen β-lactalbumin is still referred to by its biochemical name.

Allergens that have similar sequences are grouped according to the degree of similarity. Allergens that have similar molecular size, identical biologic function, and at least 67% amino acid sequence identity are called isoallergens. Examples are the major allergens Pen a 1, Pen i 1, and Met i 1 from brown shrimp (*Penaeus aztecus*), Indian shrimp (*P. indicus*), and greasyback shrimp (*Metapenaeus ensis*). They are all tropomyosins all have molecular weight approximately 36 kD, and sequence identities range from 89.9% between Pen i 1 and Met i 1 to 99.6% between Pen a 1 and Met e 1.

Another classification system that is frequently used is the division of allergens into major and minor allergens. In this system, allergens are classified according to their IgE reactivity as major or minor. These categories refer to the frequency with which a particular protein is detected by specific IgE. According to this definition, major allergens are defined as allergens to which more than 50% of the allergic subjects react.

General Properties of Food Allergens

Foods contain a large number of different proteins. Only a few, however, elicit allergic reactions. Although most features and structural properties that are responsible for the allergenicity of a protein are generally still poorly defined; some very broad characteristics of food allergens have been identified. These include abundance of a given protein in a particular food; physicochemical properties, such as molecular weight (10–70 kD) [8], acidic isoelectric point, and glycosylation; and resistance to heat and digestion. These characteristics have been associated with the allergenicity of proteins; however, many of these properties characterize a vast number of nonallergenic proteins as well and thus are not unique to food allergens.

Abundance

Food allergens frequently account for a major fraction of the total protein content within a given food. For example, in plant seeds, such as peanuts and soybeans [15,16], important allergens appear to be major storage proteins. Similarly, the major shrimp allergen Pen a 1 accounts for about 25%–30% of the total shrimp tail muscle protein [17,18]. An exception to this rule is the major allergen of codfish *Gadus callarias,* Gad c 1; this protein, identified as parvalbumin, is not a dominant protein in cod muscle [19].

Molecular Size

There are three reasons why molecular size is important for protein allergenicity. First, the molecule must be large enough to elicit an immune response. Second, it must be of sufficient size for at least two IgE binding sites to bridge mast cell–bound IgE; third, the protein must be small enough to cross the gut mucosal membrane barrier. Most known food allergens have molecular weights between 10 and 70 kD, thus fulfilling these requirements. The molecular weight of 10 kD probably represents a lower limit of immunogenicity [8]; the upper limit of 70 kD probably reflects restricted mucosal absorption of large molecules [8]. However, there are exceptions to these size restrictions. For example, In their native form, the peanut allergens Ara h 1 and Ara h 2 are large polymers with molecular weight between 200 and 300 kD [20,21]. It is not known whether the polymer itself or the subunits cleave during digestion act as allergens. In contrast, mellitin, a 21 amino acid residue peptide from bee venom, induces histamine release from basophils and mast cells [22]. Even though this 3 kD peptide is not a food allergen, it demonstrates that a protein smaller than 10 kD can act as an allergen: it induces an immune response, binds specific IgE, and causes mast cell and basophil degranulation.

Acidic Isoelectric Point and Glycosylation

Most allergens are glycoproteins with an acidic isoelectric point (pI). However, these characteristics are not unique to allergens and many nonallergenic proteins also exhibit them.

Heat Resistance

Heat resistance is probably the most common feature of potent food allergens. The fact that heat denaturation may cause loss of the native protein's conformation, yet patients' IgE antibodies still react with these denatured food proteins, indicates that the native conformation may not always be crucial for IgE binding. Thus, food allergens may contain a large number of nonconformational, sequential epitopes. In some cases, heat treatment may even increase the allergenicity of food protein as described for soybean, rice, and celery.

Resistance to Digestion

The ability of food allergen to cross the mucosal membrane of the intestinal tract is most likely an important feature. As mentioned earlier, size is one parameter in this context; another may be a resistance to digestion. The results of a study that used a gastric model of mammalian digestion to study the digestibility of food allergens point in this direction [23]. In the study, the digestibility of allergens from egg, milk, peanut, soybean, and mustard was evaluated. Food allergens tested resisted digestion for up to 1 hr, whereas nonallergens were digested within 1 min. However, there is still insufficient information to conclude that the resistance to digestion is the most important property that characterizes a food allergen.

Examples of Common Food Allergens

This section describes common allergenic foods and their identified allergens. Major allergens that have been sequenced are summarized in Table 1.

Cow's Milk Allergens

Cow's milk is one of the most common food allergens. It is estimated that between 0.3% and 7.5% of infants and young children suffer from cow's milk allergy [24,25]. Cow's milk is a very complex mixture of proteins; two major groups of cow's milk proteins, caseins and β-lactoglobulin, have been identified as major allergens [25–27]. Caseins are phosphoproteins that precipitate from raw skim milk upon acidification to pH 4.6 at 20°C. They constitute 80% of the total milk protein. Whey proteins are those proteins remaining in the fluid ("serum") after casein precipitation [28].

The biochemical properties of milk proteins have been extensively studied [28,29]. Many cow's milk proteins have been sequenced [28,29], and computer-based molecular modeling of the three-dimensional structure of several milk proteins has also been reported [30–32]. Surprisingly, even though cow's milk is a major food allergen and the structures of cow's milk allergens are well studied, the major IgE binding sites and T cell epitopes of milk allergens have not been determined in humans.

Several milk proteins are allergenic. Caseins and β-lactoglobulin appear to be the major allergens in cow's milk [33–35]. The caseins are a family of chemically related proteins. The frequency of reactivity to different casein variants has not been systematically studied. α-S1 Casein has at least five genetic variants, with varying degrees of postranslational phosphorylation, and four α-S2 caseins variants have been identified. β-Caseins are a group of proteins that have one major component with seven genetic variants and eight minor components that are proteolytic fragments of the major component. The molecular weight of the major component is 24 kD. β-Lactoglobulin is a whey protein that composes approximately 20% of total milk proteins. It has a molecular weight of 18 kD, and at least six genetic variants have been identified. The primary structure has been determined [36,37] and has a 91% sequence homology with egg β-lactoglobulin [38].

The whey proteins α-lactalbumin and bovine serum albumin (BSA) have

TABLE 1 Identified Major Allergens

Allergen	Source	Molecular weight	Sequence	Comments	References
Api g 1	*Apium graveolens* (celery) bulb and leaf	16.3 kDa	P	Major allergen; belongs to the B et v 1 family of a pathogenesis-related proteins	149
Ara h 1	*Arachis hypogaea* (peanut)	16.5 kDa	P	Similarity to 7S seed storage proteins (phaseolin, vicilin, convicilin, conglycinin, etc.)	93
Ara h 2	*Arachis hypogaea* (peanut)	17.0 kDa	P	Conglutin; seed storage protein	21
Ber e 1	*Bertholletia excelsa* (Brazil nut)	12.0 kDa	C	High-methionine 2S protein, homologous to high-methionine protein from castor bean and rapeseed	120
Bra j 1	*Brassica juncea* (leaf mustard, indian mustard) seed	14.6 kDa	C	Mature protein consisting of a small and large chain connected by two disulfide bonds; similarity to the 2S albumins from different plants	159
Hor v 1	*Hordeum vulgare* (barley)	14.5 kDa	C	Member of the multigene family of inhibitors of cereal α-amylase/trypsin	161
Mal d 1	*Malus domestica* (apple) Granny Smith, Golden Delicious	17.5 kDa	C	Belongs to the Bet v 1 family of pathogenesis-related proteins	142
Ory s 1	*Oryza sativa* (rice) seed	14.8 kDa	C	Similarity to members of the cereal trypsin/α-amylase inhibitor family	110, 111

Allergen	Species	MW		Description	References
Sin a 1	*Sinapis alba* (yellow mustard) seed	14.2 kDa	C	Protein consisting of two chains linked by disulfide bonds; similarity to 2S albumins from different plants	160
Gad c 1	*Gadus callarias* (baltic cod)	12.1 kDa	C	Major allergen, parvalbumin beta, allergen M	19, 66, 68
Gal d 1	*Gallus domesticus* (chicken)	22.6 kDa	C	Ovomucoid	150, 151
Gal d 2	*Gallus domesticus* (chicken)	42.8 kDa	C	Ovalbumin	152–154
Gal d 3	*Gallus domesticus* (chicken)	77.8 kDa	C	Ovotransferrin, conalbumin	155, 156
Gal d 4	*Gallus domesticus* (chicken)	16.2 kDa	C	Lysozyme C	157, 158
Met e 1	*Metapenaeus ensis* (greasyback shrimp)	34.0 kDa	C	Major allergen, tropomyosin	84
Pen a 1	*Penaeus aztecus* (brown shrimp)	36.0 kDa	P	Major allergen, tropomyosin	83, 134
Pen i 1	*Penaeus indicus* (Indian shrimp)	34.0 kDa	P	Major allergen, tropomyosin	14

P, partially sequenced; C, completely sequenced.

been identified as minor cow's milk allergens [39]. α-Lactalbumin has a molecular weight of 14 kD, and its amino acid sequence has been determined [36,37,40]. BSA has a molecular weight of 67 kD and composes 1% of total milk protein.

Egg Allergens

Food allergy to proteins from egg of the domestic chicken (*Gallus domesticus*) is one of the most frequently implicated causes of immediate food allergic reactions in children in the United States and Europe [41]. Frequently, egg sensitivity disappears by the fourth or fifth year of life; however, one-third of individuals have clinical sensitivity that lasts over 6 years [41]. The egg white (albumin) appears to be more allergenic than yolk. Egg white proteins have been extensively studied, and most have been purified and their amino acid sequences determined [42].

Major Egg Allergens

Ovomucoid has been identified as the major egg white allergen Gal d 1. It is a glycoprotein with a molecular weight of 28 kD and an isoelectric point of 4.1. Its amino acid sequence has been determined [43]. It contains a polypeptide chain of 186 amino acids. The tertiary structure consists of three tandem domains, each homologous to the pancreatic secretory trypsin inhibitor.

Ovalbumin has been identified as the major egg white allergen Gal d 2 [44,45]. It is a monomeric phosphoglycoprotein with a molecular weight between 43 and 45 kD and an isoelectric point of 4.5 [46]. Its amino acid sequence has been determined. Gal d 2 contains 385 amino acid residues [47,48].

Ovotransferrin or conalbumin has been identified as the major allergen from egg white Gal d 3 with a molecular weight of 77 kD and an isoelectric point of 6.0. Its amino acid sequence (686 residues) has been determined by both amino acid sequencing and cDNA cloning [49,50].

Lysozyme from egg has been identified as the allergen Gal d 4. It has a molecular weight of 14.3 kD and an isoelectric point of 10.7. The amino acid sequence has been determined; Gal d 4 contains 129 amino acid residues in a single polypeptide chain cross-linked by four disulfide bonds [51]. The importance of Gal d 4 as an allergen is still not well established. In one study, lysozyme was found to be a major allergen by skin testing, whereas in another study no sera from egg-allergic patients had positive IgE reactivity to Gal d 4 as determined by cross-radioimmunoelectrophoresis (CRIE). In contrast, a third study showed that about half of the egg-sensitive patients reacted to lysozyme by radioallergosorbent test (RAST).

Minor Egg Allergens

In addition, a variety of other egg proteins have been described as minor allergens. These include ovomucin, a complex glycoprotein with two subunits of 180 kD and 400 kD [52]. Ovoinhibitor is a 44 kD protein whose cDNA sequence and amino acid sequence have been determined [53]. Ovaflavoprotein (riboflavin-binding protein) has been found in both egg white and egg yolk. In addition to egg white proteins, yolk proteins may also be allergenic [54–57]. Apovitellenin I derives from the low-density lipoprotein fraction of the yolk [58,59]; it is a 9 kD protein, and apovitellenin VI is a 170 kD protein composing 2% of egg yolk proteins [52]. They have been found to be major allergens for some egg-sensitive individuals [52]. Other members of this family, apovitellenins III, V, and VI, were identified as minor allergens [52]. Phosvitin, an iron-binding protein that constitutes approximately 10% of total egg yolk protein, was considered nonallergenic [8] until Walsh and coworkers implicated it as an allergen [52,60,61].

Epitopes of Egg Allergens

The T cell epitopes of ovalbumin have not been wall studied in humans. However, a peptide comprising the amino acid residues 323 to 339 binds human IgE and stimulates rabbit T cells and was used to induce immediate hypersensitivity responses in BALB/c mice [62,63]. B cell epitopes of ovalbumin have been studied in more detail. In an analysis of the reactivity to peptides obtained by cyanogen bromide cleavage, ovalbumin demonstrated IgE binding to peptide sequences 41 to 172 and 301 to 385 [64]. Ovotransferrin (Gal d 3) has been studied and seven continuous epitopes identified [65]. It appears that IgE binds to the glycosylated domains but not the nonglycosylated domains. However, it is still a question whether the carbohydrate moiety acts as an IgE binding epitope.

Fish Allergens

The consumption of fish [66] is a frequent cause of IgE-mediated reactions. Fish is one among the most commonly implicated allergenic foods and has been incriminated in fatal anaphylactic reactions [1]. Species-specific analysis of IgE reactivities has not been performed, and most studies refer only to cod or generally to fish.

The Major Allergen Gad c 1 from Baltic Cod (Gadus callarias)

One of the first and most comprehensive analyses of a food allergen was the purification and characterization of the major codfish allergen, Gad c 1. Gad c 1, originally designated allergen M, from Baltic cod, *Gadus callarias,* has been documented to be the major codfish allergen. It belongs to a group of muscle proteins called parvalbumins [19] and constitutes approximately 0.05% to 0.1% of the white cod muscle tissue. Gad c 1 has a molecular weight of 12.3 kD and an isoelectric point of 4.75. Its amino acid sequence has been established; it contains 113 amino acid residues [19,67–69]. Gad c 1 contains at least five IgE binding sides [70]. Studies using synthetic peptides established that region 49 to 64 encircled two repetitive sequences. These two tetrapeptides appear to be mutually important for IgE binding as region 49–64 showed relatively high RAST inhibition compared with that of Gad c 1 and could produce Prausnitz-Küstner reaction.

Minor Fish Allergens

Minor cod fish allergens distinct from Gad c 1 [71] were identified by CRIE but were not further characterized. Twenty-five percent of fish-allergic subjects detected an allergen designated as Ag-17-cod [71] and approximately 10% of cod-allergic individuals reacted to a cod blood serum protein [72]. Protamine sulfate, a low-molecular-weight sperm protein of fish species belonging to the families Salmonidae and Clueidea, has been implicated as an fish allergen. On the basis of the results of several studies [73–76], it can be concluded that protamine sulfate is rarely allergenic for fish-allergic subjects.

Crustacea Allergens

The class Crustacea belongs to the phylum Arthropoda and includes shrimp, prawns, crabs, lobster, and crawfish. Crustacea are common causes of hypersensitivity. Like that of fish, a higher incidence of crustacea allergy would be expected in geographic areas where more shellfish is consumed on a regular basis.

Early Studies: Antigen 1, Antigen 2, SA-I, SA-II

Hoffman and coworkers [77] were the first to characterize shrimp allergens (SAs). Antigen 1 is a heat-labile allergen composed of two noncovalently bound subunits with a molecular weight of 21 kD. Antigen 2, the heat-stable shrimp allergen, has a molecular weight of 38.3 kD and an isoelectric point of 5.4 to 5.8; it is composed of 431 amino acid residues and has 4% carbohydrate. Another group described SA-I and SA-II as two heat-stable shrimp allergens [78]. SA-I has a molecular weight of 8.2 kD; further information about this allergen is not available. The second antigen, SA-II, is composed of 301 amino acid residues and has a molecular weight of 38 kD; it appears to be similar to antigen 2 isolated by Hoffman and colleagues [77] but has not been reported to possess any carbohydrate moieties.

In contrast to the previously described protein allergens, a ribonucleic acid (tRNA) moiety has been implicated as a shrimp allergen [79] although its clinical relevance is yet to be demonstrated. The tRNA preparation contained residual protein that could be reduced but not eliminated through proteinase treatment. This study is the only example implicating a nucleic acid as an allergen, and these findings must be further substantiated.

Shrimp Tropomyosin (Pen a 1, Pen i 1, Met e 1)

A 36 kD allergen, designated Pen a 1, was isolated from boiled brown shrimp, *Penaeus aztecus,* which is similar in size and amino acid composition to SA-II and antigen 2. Sequencing of a 21 amino acid Lys-C peptide of Pen a 1 demonstrated significant homology (60%–85%) with tropomyosin from various species consistent with the conclusion that Pen a 1 is tropomyosin [80]. The greatest homology occurred in region 129–149, 70%–87% with fruitfly (*Drosophila melanogaster*) tropomyosin and 60%–62% with tropomyosin from various mammalian species. The high homology with the tropomyosin from the fruitfly can be regarded as being indicative of the phylogenic relationship between the two arthropods shrimp and fruitfly. Pen a 1 constitutes 20% of the soluble protein and crude cooked shrimp extract inhibited IgE reactivity of pooled shrimp-sensitive subject serum to whole shrimp meat extract by 75% [81]. Eighty-two percent of allergic subjects reacted to this allergen [80]. Pen a 1 was cloned and sequenced recently; its cDNA sequence showed 26 base pair substitutions when compared with the sequence of Met e 1; these base pair substitutions resulted in only one amino acid substitution in position 69 (Fig. 1).

Pen i 1, isolated from Indian shrimp *Penaeus indicus* [82], was identified as tropomyosin as well. Two peptides, 17 and 9 amino acid residues each, obtained by trypsin digestion of purified Pen i were identified as important IgE-binding epitopes, since they inhibited more than 50% of specific IgE reactivity to Pen i 1. Four IgE-binding Pen a 1 epitopes were identified recently [83]. One of two IgE-reactive peptides, previously identified in Indian shrimp, *P. indicus,* as peptide 153–161 [82], partially overlaps with IgE-reactive peptide from *P. aztecus* 157–166 [83], indicating that this part of shrimp tropomyosins is a major IgE binding site (Fig. 1).

Met e 1 is the third shrimp tropomyosin identified as a major allergen. Recombinant Met e 1 was identified in a cDNA library of greasyback shrimp, *Metapenaeus ensis* [84]. The allergen has 281 amino acid residues and is similar in amino acid composition to Pen a 1 and Pen i 1. It has a molecular weight of 34 kD. Immunoblot analysis with human sera showed that five of eight individuals reacted with recombinant Met e 1. These studies confirmed previous observations that identified the 36 kD allergen as shrimp tropomyosin.

Legumes

The seeds of plants from the botanical family Papilionaceae are called legumes. This group contains important foods such as peas, beans, soybeans, and peanuts.

Peanut Allergens

Peanut ranks first as the cause of severe and lethal reactions to foods. Even small amounts may be sufficient to trigger an allergic reaction; thus the consumption of peanut protein containing foods, such as chocolate or candy bars, can be life threatening in some individuals. Both raw and roasted peanuts contain allergens [85], even though heat-resistant allergens are considered to be clinically the most relevant allergens, since products made from roasted peanuts are probably the

```
                  10        20        30        40        50        60        70        80        90       100
Drom Tm  MDAIKKKMQAVKLEKDNAIDKADTCENQAKDANSRADKLNEEVRDLEKKFVQVEIDLVTAKEQLEKANTELEEKKLLTATESEVATLNRKVQQTEDLE
Pen i 1                                      AEKSEEAVHELQRMIQTUBEDELDVTQESLLKANIQLVEKDKALSNAEGEVAALNRRIQLLEEDLE
Pen a 1                         DRADTLEQQNKEANNRAEKSEEEVHNLQKRMQQLENDLDQVQESLLKANIQLVEKDKALSNAEGEVAALNRRIQLLEEDLE
Met e 1               MKLEKDNAMDRADTLEQQNKEANNRAEKSEEEVHNLQKRMQQLENDLDQVQESLLKANNQLVEKDKALSNAEGEVAALNRRIQLLEEDLE
                                                                 Pen i 1
                                                              50 ───── 66

                  110       120       130       140       150       160       170       180       190       300
Drom Tm  KSBERSTTAQQKLLEATQSADENNRMCKVLENRSQQDEERMDQLTNQLKEARMLAEDADTKSDEVSRKLAFVEDELEVAEDRVRSGESKIMELEEELKVV
Pen i 1  R    LAEASQAADESER                          FLAEEADRKYDEVAR            ERAEQGESKIVELEEELRVV
Pen a 1  RSEERLNTATTKLAEASQAADESERMRKVLENRSLSDEERMDALENQLKEARFLAEEADRKYDEVARKLAMVEADLERAEEERAETGESKIVELEEELRVV
Met e 1  RSEERLNTATTKLAEASQAADESERMRKVLENRSLSDEERMDALENQLKEARFLAEEADRKYDEVARKLAMVEADLERAEEERAETGESKIVELEEELRVV
                         Pen a 1        Pen i 1         Pen a 1
                     136 ─── 148    153 ─── 157     169 ─── 179
                                        161  167

                  210       220       230       240       250       260       270       280  284
DromTm   GNSLKSLEVSBEKANQRVBEFKREMKTLSIKLKBAEQRAEHAEKQVKRLQKEVDDLEDRLFNBKEKYKAICDDLDQTPAELTGY
Peni1    GNNLK   NKRBEEYKNQIK    AEFAER         DELVNEKBKYKQ
Pena1    GNNLKSLEVSBEKANQREBAYKEQIKTLTNKLKAAEARAEFAERSVQKLQKEVDRLEDELVNEKEKYKSITDELDQTFSELSGY
Mete1    GNNLKSLEVSBEKANQREBAYKEQIKTLTNKLKAAEARAEFAERSVQKLQKEVDRLEDELVNEKEKYKSITDELDQTFSELSGY
                                                          Pen a 1
                                                      262 ───── 282
```

FIGURE 1 Sequence comparison of shrimp allergens Pen i 1, Pen a 1, and Met e 1. Pen i 1 and Pen a 1 epitopes are marked.

greater source of sensitization. Peanut allergens are subject to intense analysis because of their high allergenic potential and the economic importance of peanuts as a protein source for the food-processing industry. Peanuts contain a large number of allergens [85–87]; up to 37 [86] allergenic components have been identified. Four peanut allergens have been described as major allergens, peanut 1, concanavalin A–reactive protein, Ara h 1, and Ara h 2. Ongoing studies focus on Ara h 1 and Ara h 2.

Early Studies: Several peanut allergens have been described. The peanut 1 fraction, isolated from raw peanuts [88], has an isoelectric point (pI) of 5.25–5.75; two major bands, with molecular weights of 20 and 30 kD, and several minor bands, with higher and lower molecular weights, were identified. The concanavalin A–reactive glycoprotein was identified as a major peanut allergen; it is a heat-stable 65 kD glycoprotein with an isoelectric point of 4.6 [89] and contains 2.4% carbohydrate. Removal of the carbohydrate moieties reduced but did not eliminate the allergenic activity [90]. In another study, three major allergens, with molecular weights of 15, 20, and 66 kD, were identified by immunoblot analysis; the identity of the 66 kD and the concanavalin A–reactive glycoprotein, however, was not evaluated. Another well-characterized peanut protein is the peanut agglutinin (PNA). IgE reactivity to PNA was first considered nonspecific [85]. A more recent study, however, showed IgE binding to PNA by immunoblotting and classified PNA as a minor peanut allergen [91].

Ara h 1: Burks and coworkers [92] identified a 63.5 kD molecular weight glycoprotein as the major allergen Ara h 1. It has an isoelectric point of 4.55; its primary structure has been recently identified [93]. It is the peanut storage protein, vitellin, a major protein from the globulin fraction [94]. The epitopes of Ara h 1 were investigated with Ara h 1–specific IgE and seven monoclonal antibodies raised against Ara h 1. The monoclonal antibodies identified four different antigenic sites on Ara h 1, and the human IgE identified three similar epitopes [95,96]. The identity of Ara h 1 and the concanavalin A–reactive glycoprotein was suspected, though Ara h 1 did not bind to concanavalin A.

Ara h 2: A second major peanut allergen was identified, purified, and characterized by Burks and coworkers [21]. It is smaller than Ara h 1 with a molecular weight of 17 kD and an isoelectric point of 5.2 [97]. The epitopes of Ara h 2 were investigated similarly to those of Ara h 1 [98]. Monoclonal antibodies were raised against purified Ara h 2. The Ara h 2–specific monoclonal antibodies identified two different antigenic sites on Ara h 2. In similar studies with pooled human IgE serum from peanut-allergic subjects two closely related IgE-binding epitopes were identified.

Soybean Allergens

Similarly to peanuts, soybeans contain multiple allergens. A study of three atopic dermatitis subjects and one asthmatic soy-allergic subject suggested the 2S-globulin fraction as a major source of allergens [99]. Another study showed significant levels of IgE binding to the 7S globulin fraction [100].

Gly m 1:   IgE-reactive bands with molecular weights between 14 and 70 kD were identified in the 7S fraction with major binding to a 30 kD band [100] designated as Gly m 1. The native protein has a molecular weight of more than 300 kD, indicating a polymeric structure. The 15 amino acid N-terminal sequence of Gly m 1 has been determined and is identical with the 34 kD oil body–associated protein from soybean. This soybean protein also reacts with human IgE and Gly m 1–specific monoclonal antibodies. Sixty-five percent of soybean-reactive subjects had specific Gly m 1–specific IgE antibodies; however, none of these individuals experienced severe or anaphylactic reactions to soybeans.

Other Soybean Allergens: The Kunitz soybean trypsin inhibitor was identified as a soybean allergen by skin test, RAST, and RAST inhibition in a soybean-allergic subject [101]; the IgE reactivity to soybean was inhibited completely by the Kunitz soybean trypsin inhibitor. However, the RAST reactivity of two other sera from soy-allergic individuals indicates that the Kunitz soybean trypsin inhibitor is a relatively minor allergen.

A 68 kD allergen was identified as a minor soy allergen [102]. It reacted with sera from approximately 25% of soy-allergic subjects and was identified as the α subunit of β-conglycinin. IgE only bound to the α subunit, not to the α_1 and β subunits, even though these structures are highly homologous.

A 20 kD IgE-binding protein from soybean was described [103] and designated as S-II. Two serum samples from subjects allergic to soy showed IgE binding to this 20 kD band. Roasting seemed to enhance IgE binding to the 20 kD allergen. One serum from a soy-allergic subject showed IgE binding only to a 14 kD band; sera from subjects allergic to both soybeans and peanuts showed IgE binding to several bands in the range of 50–70 kD, apparently β-conglycinin subunits. No differences in IgE binding of raw soybeans of different varieties were observed. These IgE binding proteins were not further characterized.

Other Legume Allergens

Peas: Peas (*Pisum sativum*) belong taxonomically in the same family as peanuts and soybeans. All pea allergens described so far are albumins, which constitute 14%–42% of the total protein [104] and retained their allergenic activity when heated or boiled. The other major constituents of peas, the globulins legumin (11S) and vitellin (7S), did not produce positive skin test reactions [105]. A green pea allergen with a 1.8 kD approximate molecular weight by sodium dodecyl sulfate polyacrylamide gel electrophoresis (SDS-PAGE) and a carbohydrate content of 30% was purified from pea dialysate [106], but was not further characterized.

Lupin: Lupin is primarily used as feed or as a natural fertilizer. Hefle and coworkers [107] reported the adverse reactions of a peanut-allergic child to a lupin-fortified pasta product. The IgE-binding proteins of the lupin have an approximate molecular weight of 21 kD and 35–55 kD and are heat-stable.

Cereal Grains

Cereal grains such as wheat, maize (corn), rice, barley, oats, rye, sorghum, and millet account for approximately 72% of protein consumed in the world. Their proteins can be fractionated into water-soluble albumins, the saline-soluble globulins, the 70% aqueous ethanol-soluble prolamins, and the acid- or alkali-soluble glutelins.

Wheat Allergens

Adverse reaction to wheat is considered an important food allergy. Celiac disease (gluten-sensitive enteropathy) is regarded as an immune response to wheat gluten. Wheat proteins include water-soluble albumins, saline-soluble globulins, and glutens. Gluten represents approximately 85% of the total wheat protein. It is a mixture of gliadin (28%–42%), the major prolamin protein of wheat, and glutenins (42%–62.5%), the major glutelin proteins in wheat. Gliadin is most likely responsible for gluten-sensitive enteropathy. Gliadins have molecular weights ranging from 10 to 70 kD and have common amino acid sequences.

Rice

The major rice allergens are encoded by a multigene family [108] resulting in molecular weights ranging from 14 to 60 kD [109]. Rice allergens are resistant to heat and proteolysis. The cDNA sequence coding for the major rice allergen Ory s 1 has been determined [110,111]. The mature protein has a molecular weight of approximately 14 kD, and its amino acid sequence has homology of 20% and 40% with the barley trypsin inhibitor and the wheat α-amylase inhibitor, respectively. Since a single protein seems to account for most of the allergenic activity of rice, attempts have been made to select hypoallergenic strains [112]. Protease treatment was used to reduce the allergenicity of the rice [113]. However, this process requires large amounts of enzyme. Another attempt to reduce the allergenicity of rice is repression of allergenic protein synthesis [114]. Matsuda and colleagues have cloned and sequenced a 16 kD rice seed protein kD that was identified as the major rice allergen. On the basis of its nucleotide sequence, an antisense RNA strategy was applied to repress expression of this allergen in maturing rice seeds. Seeds from transgenic plants with the antisense gene have substantially reduced amounts of the allergen [109,110,113,114].

Corn

In a recent study, the IgE-binding proteins in corn were investigated [115,116]. As do most cereals, corn contains mostly alcohol-soluble proteins. These proteins have not been considered in terms of their allergenicity. In order to assess this, aqueous and alcohol extracts of corn seeds were prepared according to established biochemical procedures and analyzed by immunoblotting. Forty-seven sera of corn-reactive individuals were tested. Individuals were considered corn-reactive if they met two of three criteria: a history of food allergy consistent with corn allergy, positive skin test result to corn, or positive IgE response to corn. Two-thirds of these subjects had significant IgE antibodies to proteins present in aqueous extracts, and, more interestingly, approximately 60% of the corn-reactive subjects also showed significant reactivity to proteins in the alcohol extracts. The reactivity to alcohol-soluble proteins did not necessarily correlate with that to proteins present in the aqueous extract. Twenty and eight IgE-reactive bands were identified in the aqueous and the alcohol exract, respectively. Two proteins of the aqueous corn fraction with molecular weights of 28 kD and 10 kD reacted with more than 50% of the subjects' sera, whereas one 28 kD band of the alcohol fraction can be considered a major allergen. These results demonstrate the need for using proper extraction methods for the preparation of food allergen extracts that are based on properties of the proteins present rather than just employing historically standard extraction procedures and reactivities to corn proteins in allergic subjects. However, to analyze the clinical relevance of these IgE reactivities double-blind placebo-controlled food challenges have to be performed.

Nuts

Almonds

In almonds, two major allergens were identified by immunoblotting. The first is a 70 kD heat-labile protein, the second is a 45–50 kD heat-stable protein [112]. A large number of minor allergens with molecular weight ranging from 38 to 70 kD were detected.

Brazil Nuts

Brazil nuts can cause systemic anaphylaxis in some individuals. Several allergenic fractions were identified by immunoblotting using sera from Brazil nut–allergic subjects [118]. The major allergen from Brazil nut, Ber e 1, is a high-methionine 2S protein [119] with a molecular weight of 12 kD. Ber e 1 is a dimer that consists of a 9 kD and a 3 kD subunit. The cDNA sequence of Ber e 1 was determined [120] and its amino acid sequence deduced. Ber e 1 is homologous to the N-terminal end of the high-methionine protein from castor bean and from rapeseed.

Chestnut

Chestnut has been shown to produce allergic reactions in patients with latex allergy [121]. Allergens identified by immunoblotting techniques had molecular weights of 14 kD and 25–30 kD. Using a latex solid phase, IgE binding was inhibited by approximately 28% with the chestnut extract in a RAST inhibition assay.

Pistachio

Pistachio is a member of the cashew and mango family (Anacardiacea). A prominent IgE-binding protein of 34 kD has been identified [122]. Other allergens range in molecular weight from 41 to 60 kD. Some cross-reactivity has been demonstrated with peanut, walnut, and sunflower.

FOOD CROSS-REACTIVITIES

Cross-reactivities are found among foods of related phylogenetic origin and foods seemingly unrelated to nonfood allergens. Legumes, cereal grains, fishes, fruits, and tree nuts are examples of phylogenetically related cross-reacting allergens existing in certain food families. Nonfood allergens that cross-react with foods are pollens, latex, and dust mites.

The origin of food allergen cross-reactivity is still unknown; it could be due to either single or multiple sensitization to similar proteins in cross-reacting foods. The clinical relevance of food allergen cross-reactivity depends on the food in question. For example, the cross-reactivities among crustacea are thought to be clinically relevant—shrimp-allergic subjects can react with lobster and crab—whereas cross-reactivities among legumes seem to be of less clinical importance: peanut-allergic subjects usually do not react with beans or peas [123].

Legumes and Cereal Grains

Peanut is a member of the Leguminosae family and one of the most potent food allergens. Positive skin reactions and positive RAST results to other Leguminosae such as soybean, peas, and beans are frequently observed [123–127]. However, multiple positive skin test results to different Leguminosae were not correlated with positive oral provocation [123], and the IgE reactivities to different leguminosae, analyzed by Western blotting, were not correlated with clinically relevant symptoms [125].

The clinical relevance of cross-reactivities among grains seems to be limited as well. In a recent study testing different grains [128] 84% of the children reacted with wheat only; approximately 20 of these children reacted to more than one grain.

Fishes

The majority of fishes consumed belong to one of five taxonomic orders [129]: Perciformes (e.g., mackerel, tuna), Gadiformes (e.g., cod), Pleuronectiformes (e.g., flounder), Cypriniformes (e.g., carp, catfish) and Clupeiformes (e.g., trout, salmon, herring). The reactivity to different fishes by RAST and skin test suggests cross-reactivity; however, the majority of fish-allergic subjects could eat other fish species or did not react during food challenge [130,131], indicating that the in vitro cross-reactivity may be of limited clinical relevance.

Crustacea

The substantial cross-reactivity among Crustacea appears to be clinically important [132,133]; shrimp-allergic subjects can react to other crustaceans without additional sensitization. The cause of this cross-reactivity is probably the major allergen tropomyosin, a highly conserved muscle protein. Tropomyosin has been identified in three shrimp species: brown shrimp (*Penaeus aztecus*) [134,80], Indian shrimp (*P. indicus*), and greasyback shrimp (*Metapenaeus ensis*) [85]. Pen a 1–like proteins were detected in crab, crawfish, and lobster using sera of shrimp-allergic subjects and Pen a 1–specific monoclonal antibodies [134,80]. The amino acid sequence similarity among these different shrimp tropomyosins is very high; for example, the amino acid sequences of Met e 1 and Pen a 1 only differ in one position (Fig. 1) [83,84].

Cross-Reactivity between Foods and Pollens

Birch, mugwort, and ragweed pollen have been associated with various food allergies. For example, ragweed pollen cross-reacts with melons and bananas [135,136]; grass and mugwort pollens, with celery and a variety of vegetables [137,139,140]; and birch pollen, with a number of fruits [137,138]. As the interest in cross-reactivity between foods and nonfood allergens has increased, more and more information about the structural basis of cross-reactivity has become available and these cross-reactivities are now the best studied examples of the cross-reactions between food and nonfood allergens.

The association of allergic reactions to pollen allergens and apple, hazelnut, potatoes, celery, and carrots has been attributed to cross-reactivities to pathogenesis-related plant proteins and profilin. The structural relationship of birch pathogenesis-related plant protein (Bet v 1) and profilin (Bet v 2) and the reactivity to fruits has been studied in more detail [141–145]. The structural and immunologic homology of the major apple allergen Mal d 1 and Bet v 1 has been demonstrated [141–144]. Sequence comparison of Mal d 1 with Bet v 1 revealed 64.5% identity on the amino acid level and 55.6% identity on the nucleic acid level. The immunologic properties of recombinant Mal d 1 were tested, and cross-reactivity with Bet v 1 was shown by inhibition assays [142]. The association between celery, apple, peanut, and kiwi fruit and mugwort pollen was ascribed to the homologous mugwort allergen Art v 1 [146] and pollen profilins [147,148]. The major allergenic protein of celery, Api g 1, was recently cloned and sequenced [149]. The 153 amino acid residue long recombinant Api g 1 has a molecular mass of 16.2 kD, 40% identity, and 60% similarity to Bet v 1, emphasizing the molecular origin of cross-reactivity between foods and pollens.

NEW CHALLENGES IN FOOD ALLERGEN RESEARCH: TRANSGENIC CROPS

New crop varieties of fruits, vegetables, and grains are currently being developed using recombinant DNA technologies [3,4]. Specific genetic modifications based on these techniques have been made, including transfer of proteins into plants from other species, which cannot be ordinarily achieved by traditional breeding techniques. Since the genes governing these new traits code for proteins that are ordinarily not present in a particular food crop, there is concern about the effect of the transferred proteins on the consumer, particularly, in regard to potential allergenicity of these proteins.

The evaluation of transgenic crops expressing proteins of a known allergen source is relatively easy. The transgenic product can be evaluated with subjects' sera or allergen-specific monoclonal antibodies. For example, the major methionine-rich allergen from Brazil nut was transferred to soybeans to increase their nutritional value [120]. The transgenic soybean expresses the allergen with its allergenicity intact as shown by immunoblot and RAST inhibition studies.

To assess proteins of unknown allergenic potency is much more challenging. The question, What structural features are responsible for the allergenicity of a protein?, is still unanswered. As discussed earlier, no specific properties that uniquely characterize food allergens have been identified. More information about the primary and tertiary structures of food allergens and allergenic epitopes is needed to understand the relationship between protein structure and allergenicity, to provide insights into the basic mechanisms of food allergy, and to use this knowledge to address the immunologic safety of transgenic crops.

REFERENCES

1. Yunginger JW, Sweeney KG, Sturner WQ, Giannandrea LA, Teigland, JD, Bray M, Benson PA, York JA, Biedrzycki L, Squillace DL, Helm RM. Fatal food induced anaphylaxis. JAMA 1988; 260:1450–1452.
2. Musmand JJ, Helbling A, El-Dahr, JM, Haydel, RD, Lehrer. Surimi: a hidden, potentially serious cause of fish allergy. Ann Allergy 1993; 70:53.

3. Kessler OA, Taylor MR, Maryanski JH, Flamm EL, Kahl LS. The safety of foods developed by biotechnology. Science 1992; 256:1747–1832.
4. Harlander SK. Biotechnology: a means for improving our food supply. Food Technol 1991; 45:841, 86, 91–92, 95.
5. Atkins RM, Steinberg SS, Metcalfe DD. Evaluation of immediate adverse reactions to foods in adults. I. Correlation of demographic, laboratory, and prick skin test data with response to controlled oral food challenge. J Allergy Clin Immunol 1985; 75:348.
6. Sampson HA, Metcalfe DD. Immediate reactions to foods. In:DD Metcalfe DD, Sampson HA, Simon RA, eds. Food Allergy: Adverse Reactions to Foods and Food Additives. Oxford: Blackwell Scientific Publications, 1991, pp 99–112.
7. Yunginger JW. Food antigens. In: Metcalfe DD, Sampson HA, Simon RA, eds. Food Allergy: Adversrse Reactions to Foods and Food Additives. Boston: Blackwell Scientific Publications, 1991 pp 36–51.
8. Taylor SL, Lemanski RF, Bush RK, Busse WW. Food allergens: structure and immunologic properties. Ann Allergy 1987; 59:93–99.
9. Barnett D, Bonhan B, Howden WEH. Allergenic cross-reactions among legume foods-in vitro study. J Allergy Clin Immunol 1987; 79:443–438.
10. Waring NP, deShazo RD, Daul CB, McCants M, Lehrer SB. Hypersensitivity reactions to ingested crustacea: clinical evaluation and diagnostic studies in shrimp sensitive individuals. J Allergy Clin Immunol 1985; 76:440–445.
11. Daul CB, Morgan JE, Waring NP, McCants ML, Hughes J, Lehrer SB. Immunological evaluation of shrimp-allergic individuals. J Allergy Clin Immunol 1987; 80:716–722.
12. Bernhisel-Broadbent J, Scanlon SM, Sampson HA. Fish hypersensitivity. I. In vitro and oral challenge results in fish-allergic patients. J Allergy Clin Immunol 1989; 83:435–440.
13. Marsh DG, Goodfriend I, King TP, Løwenstein H, Platts-Mills TAE. Allergen nomenclature. J Allergy Clin Immunol 1987; 80:639–645.
14. King, TP, Hoffman D, Lowenstein H, Marsh DG, Platts-Mills TAE, Thomas W. Allergen nomenclature. Allergy Clin Immunol News 1994; 6:38–44.
15. Burks AW, Cockrell G, Stanley JS, Helm RM, Bannon GA. Isolation, identification, and characterization of clones encoding antigens responsible for peanut hypersensitivity. Int Arch Allergy Immunol 1995; 107:248–250.
16. Burks AW, Cockrell G, Stanley JS, Helm RM, Bannon GA. Recombinant peanut allergen Ara h I expression and IgE binding in patients with peanut hypersensitivity. J Clin Invest 1995; 96:1715–1721.
17. Daul CB, Slattery M, Morgan JE Lehrer SB. Identification of a common major crustacea allergen (abstr). J Allergy Clin Immunol 1992; 89:194.
18. Daul CB, Slattery M, Morgan JE Lehrer SB. Isolation and characterization of an important 36 kD shrimp allergen (abstract). J Allergy Clin Immunol 1991; 87:192.
19. Elsayed S, Bennich H: The primary structure of allergen M from cod. Scand J Immunol 1975; 4:203–208.
20. Burks AW, Williams LW, Helm RM, Connaughton C, Cockrell G O'Brien T. Iden-

tification of a major peanut allergen, *Ara h* I, in patients with topic dermatitis and positive peanut challenges. J Allergy Clin Immunol 1991; 88:172–179.

21. Burks AW, Williams LW, Connaughton C, Cockrell G, O'Brien TJ Helm RM. Identification and characterization of a second major peanut allergen, *Ara h* II with use of the sera of patients with atopic dermatitis and positive peanut challenge. J Allergy Clin Immunol 1992; 900:962–969.

22. King TP, Coscia MR, Kochoumian. Structure-immunogenicity relationship of a peptide allergen, mellitin. In: Kraft, Sehon, eds. Molecular Biology and Immunology of Allergens. Boca Raton: FL: CRC Press, 1993, pp 11–20.

23. Fuchs RL, Astwood JD. Allergenicity assessment of foods derived from genetically modified foods. Food Technol 1996; 50:83–88.

24. Wershil BK, Walker WA. Milk allergens and other food allergies in children. Immunol Allergy Clin North Am 1988; 8:485–504.

25. Amonette MS, Rosenfeld SI, Schwartz RH. Serum IgE antibodies to cow's milk proteins in children with differing degrees of IgE-mediated cow's milk allergy; analysis by immunoblotting. Pediatr Asthma Allergy Immunol 1992; 7:99–109

26. Savilathi E, Kuitonen M. Allergenicity of cow's milk proteins. J Pediatr 1992; 121:S12–S20.

27. Savilathi E. Cow's milk allergy. Allergy 1981; 36:73–88.

28. Whitney RM. Proteins of milk. In: Wong NP, Jernes R, Keeney M, Marth EH, eds. Fundamentals of Diary Chemistry, 3rd ed. New York: Van Nostrand Reinhold, 1988, pp 81–169.

29. Swaisgood HE. 1985. Characterization of edible fluids of animal origin: milk. In: Fennema OR, ed. Food chemistry, 2nd ed. New York: Marcel Dekker, 1985, pp 791–827.

30. Kumosinski TF, Brown EM, Farrell HM. Three-dimensional molecular modelling of bovine caseins: kappa-caseins. J Dairy Sci 1991; 74:2879–2887.

31. Kumosinski TF, Brown EM, Farrell HM. Three-dimensional molecular modelling of bovine caseins: an energy-minimizing β-casein structure. J Dairy Sci 1993; 76:931–945.

32. Kumosinski RF, Brown EM, Farell HM. Three-dimensional molecular modelling of bovine caseins: α_{s1}-casein. J Dairy Sci 1991; 74:2889–2895.

33. Savilathi E. Cow's milk allergy. Allergy 1991; 36:73–88.

34. Savilathi E, Kuitunen M. Allergenicity of cow milk proteins. J Pediatr 1992; 121:S12–S20.

35. Amonette MS, Rosenfeld SI Schwartz RH. Serum IgE antibodies to cow's milk proteins in children with differing degrees of IgE-mediated cow's milk allergy: analysis by immunoblotting. Pediatr Asthma Allergy Immunol 1993; 7:99–109.

36. Whitney RM. Proteins of milk. In: Wong NP, Jernes R, Keeney M, Marth EH, eds. Fundamentals of Dairy Chemistry. New York: Van Nostrand Reinhold, 1988.

37. Swaisgood HE. Characterization of edible fluids of animal origins: milk, In: Fennema OR, ed. Food Chemistry. New York: Marcel Dekker, 1985.

38. Alexander LJ, Hayes G, Pearse MJ, Beattie CW, Stewart AF, Willis IM, Mackinlay AG. Complete sequence of the bovine beta-lactoglobulin cDNA. Nucleic Acids Res 1989; 17:6739–6745.

39. Goldman AS, Sellars WA, Halpern SR, Anderson DW, Furlow TE, Johnson CH. Milk allergy. II. Skin testing of allergic and normal children with purified milk proteins. Pediatrics 1963; 32:572–579.

40. Hurley WL, Schuler LA. Molecular cloning and nucleotide sequence of bovine α-lactalbumin. Gene 1987; 61:119–122.

41. Crespo JF, Pascual C, Ferrer A, Burks AW, Diaz Pena JM, Esteban MM. Egg white-specific IgE level as a tolerance marker in the IgE level as a tolerance marker in the follow-up of egg allergy. Allergy Proc 1994; 15:73–76.

42. Yunginger JW. Classical food allergens. Allergy Proc 1990; 11:7–9.

43. Kato I, Schrode J, Kohr WJ, Laskowski M. Chicken ovomucoid: determination of its amino acid sequence, determination of the trypsin reactive site, and preparation of all three of its domains. Biochemistry 1987; 26:193–201.

44. Langeland T. A clinical and immunological study of allergy to hen's egg white. III. Allergens in hens' egg white studied by cross radio immunoelectrophoresis, Allergy 1983; 37:500–521.

45. Langeland T. A clinical and immunological study of allergy to hen's egg white. IV. Specific IgE antibodies to individual allergens in hen's egg white related to clinical and immunological parameters in egg-allergic patients. Allergy 1983; 38:493–500.

46. Nisbet AD, Saundry RH, Moir AJ, Fothergill LA, Fothergill JE. The complete amino-acid sequence of hen ovalbumin. Eur J Biochem 1981; 115(2):335–345.

47. Nisbet AD, Saundry RH, Moir AJG, Fothergill LA, Fothergill JE. The complete amino acid sequence of hen ovalbumin. Eur J Biochem 1981; 115:335–345.

48. McReynolds L, O'Malley BW, Nisbet AD, Fothergill JE, Givol D, Fields S, Roberson M, Bownlee GG. Sequence of chicken ovalbumin mRNA. Nature 1978; 273:723–728.

49. Williams J, Elleman TC, Kingston IB, Wilkens AG, Kuhn KA. The primary structure of hen ovotransferrin. Eur J Biochem 1982: 122:297–303

50. Jeltsch JM, Chambon P: The complete sequence of the chicken ovotransferrin mRNA. Eur J Biochem 1982; 122:291–295.

51. Canfield RE: The amino acid sequence of egg white lysozyme. J Biol Chem 1963; 238:2698–2707.

52. Walsh BJ, Barnett D, Burley RW, Elliott C, Hill DJ, Howden MEH. New allergens from hen's egg white and egg yolk: *in vitro* studies of ovomucin, apovitellin I and VI, and phosvitin. Int Arch Allergy Appl Immunol 1988; 87:81–86.

53. Scott MJ, Huckaby CS, Kato I, Kohr WJ, Laskowski M, Tsai MJ, O'Malley BW. Ovoinhibitor introns specify functional domains as in the related and linked ovomucoid gene. J Biol Chem 1987; 262:5899–5907.

54. Szepfalusi Z, Ebner C, Pandjaitan R, Orlicek F, Scheiner O, Boltz-Nitulescu G, Kraft D, Ebner H. Egg yolk alpha-livetin (chicken serum albumin) is a cross-reactive allergen in the bird-egg syndrome. J Allergy Clin Immunol 1994; 93:932–942.

55. de Blay F, Hoyet C, Candolfi E, Thierry R, Pauli G. Identification of alpha livetin as a cross reacting allergen in a bird-egg syndrome. Allergy Proc 1994; 15:77–78.

56. Hoffman DR, Guenther DM. Occupational allergy to avian proteins presenting as allergy to ingestion of egg yolk. J Allergy Clin Immunol 1988; 81:484–488.

57. Anet J, Back JF, Baker RS, Barnett D, Burley RW, Howden ME. Allergens in the white and yolk of hen's egg. A study of IgE binding by egg proteins. Int Arch Allergy Appl Immunol 1985; 77:364–371.

58. Burley RW. Studies on the apoproteins of the major lipoprotein of the yolk of hen's eggs. I. Isolation and properties of the low-molecular-weight apoproteins. Aust J Biol Sci 1975; 28:121–132.

59. Burley RW, Evans AJ, Pearson JA. Molecular aspects of the synthesis and deposition of hens' egg yolk with special reference to low density lipoprotein. Poult Sci 1993; 72:850–855.

60. Walsh BJ, Elliott C, Baker RS, Barnett D, Burley RW, Hill DJ, Howden MEH. Allergenic cross-reactivity of egg-white and egg-yolk proteins. Int Arch Allergy Appl Immunol 1987; 84:228–232.

61. Walsh BJ, Barnett D, Barley RW, Elliott C, Hill DJ, Howden MEH. New allergens from hen's egg white and egg yolk. Int Arch Allergy Appl Immunol 1988; 37:81–86.

62. Johnsen G, Elsayed S. Antigenic and allergenic determinants of ovalbumin. III. MHC la-binding peptide (OA-323-339) interacts with human and rabbit specific antibodies. Mol Immunol 1990; 27:821–827.

63. Renz Bradley K, Larsen GL, McCall C, Gelfand EW. Comparison of the allergenicity of ovalbumin and ovalbumin peptide 323–339: differential expression of V β-expressing T-cell populations. J Immunol 1993; 151:7206–7213.

64. Kahlert H, Petersen A, Becker WM, Schlaak M. Epitope analysis of the allergen ovalbumin (Gal d III) with monoclonal antibodies and patients' IgE. Mol Immunol 1992; 29:1191–1201.

65. Church WR, Brown SA, Mason AB. Monoclonal antibodies to the amino- and carboxyl-terminal domains of ovotransferrin. Hybridoma 1988; 7:471–484.

66. Elsayed S, Aas K, Slette K, Johansson SGO. Tryptic cleavage of a homogenous cod fish allergen and isolation of two active polypeptide fragments. Immunochemistry 1972; 9:647–661.

67. Elsayed S, von Bahr-Lindstrom H, Bennich H. The primary structure of fragment TM2 of allergen M from cod. Scand J Immunol 1974; 3:683–686.

68. Elsayed S, Aas K. Characterization of a major allergen (cod): chemical composition and immunological properties. Int Arch Allergy Appl Immunol 1970; 38:536–448.

69. Elsayed, SM, Apold S, Aas K, Bennich H. The allergenic structure of allergen M from cod: tryptic peptides of fragment TM1. Int Arch Allergy Appl Immunol 1976; 52:59–63.

70. Elsayed S, Apold J. Immunological analysis of cod fish allergen M: locations of the immunoglobulin binding sites as demonstrated by native and synthetic peptides. Allergy 1983; 449–459.

71. Aukrust L, Apold J, Elsayed S, Aas K. Crossed immunoelectro-phoretic and crossed radioimmunoelectrophoretic studies employing a model allergen from codfish. Int Arch Allergy Appl Immunol 1978; 57:253–262.

72. Aas K, Elsayed S. Physicochemical properties and specific activity of a purified allergen (codfish). Dev Biol Stand 1975; 29:90–98.

73. Knape JTA, Schuller JL, De Haan P, de Jong AP, Bovill JG. An anaphylactic reaction to protamine in a patient allergic to fish. Anaethesiology 1981; 55:324–325.
74. Greenberger PA, Patterson R, Tobin MC, Liota JL, Roberts M. Am J Med Sci 1989; 298:104–108.
75. Caplan SN Beckman EM. Protamine sulfate and fish allergy. N Engl J Med 1976; 295:172.
76. Levy JH, Schwieger IM, Zaidan JR, Faraj BA, Weintraub WS. Evaluation of patients at risk for protamine reactions. J Thorac Cardiovasc Surg 1989; 98:200–204.
77. Hoffman DR, Day ED Miller JS. The major heat stable allergen of shrimp. Ann Allergy 1981; 47:17–22.
78. Nagpal S, Rajappa L, Metcalfe DD Rao PV. Isolation and characterization of heat-stable allergens from shrimp (*Penaeus indicus*). J Allergy Clin Immunol 1989; 83:26–36.
79. Nagpal S, Mecalfe DD, Rao PV. Identification of a shrimp-derived allergen as tRNA .J Immunol 1987; 138:4169–4174.
80. Daul CB, Slattery M, Reese G, Lehrer SB. Identification of the major brown shrimp (*Penaeus aztecus*) allergen as the muscle protein tropomyosin. Int Arch Allergy Immunol 1994; 105:49–55.
81. Morgan JE, Daul CB, Lehrer SB. Characterization of important shrimp allergens by immunoblot analysis. J Allergy Clin Immunol 1990; 85:170 (abstract).
82. Shatin KN, Martin BM, Nagpal S, Metcalfe DD, Sabba-Rao PV. Identification of tropomyosin as the major shrimp allergen and characterization of its IgE binding epitopes. J Immunol 1993; 151:5354–5363.
83. Reese G, Jeoung B-J, Daul CB, Lehrer SB. Characterization of recombinant shrimp allergen Pen a 1 (tropomyosin). Int Arch Allergy Clin Immunol (in press).
84. Leung PSC, Chu KH, Chow WK, Aftab A, Bandea CI, Kwan HS, Nagy SM, Gershwin ME. Cloning, expression, and primary structure of *Metapenaeus ensis* tropomyosin, the major heat-stable shrimp allergen. J Allergy Clin Immunol 1994; 92:837–845.
85. Barnett D, Baldo BA, Howden MEH. Multiplicity of allergens in peanuts. J Allergy Clin Immunol 1983; 72:61–68.
86. Bush RK, Voss M, Taylor SL, Nordlee J, Busse W Yunginger JW. Detection of peanut allergens by crossed radioimmuno-electrophoresis (CRIE) (abstr). J Allergy Clin Immunol 1983; 71:95.
87. Meier-Davis S, Taylor SL, Nordlee J Bush RK. Identification of peanut allergens by immunoblotting (abstr). J Allergy Clin Immunol 1987; 79:218.
88. Sachs MI, Jones RT Yunginger JW. Isolation and partial characterization of a major peanut allergen. J Allergy Clin Immunol 1981; 67:27–34.
89. Gleeson PA, Jermyn MA. Leguminous seed glycoproteins that interact with concanavalin A. Aust J Plant Physiol 1977; 4:25–37.
90. Barnett D. Howden WEH. Partial characterization of an allergenic glycoprotein from peanut (*Arachis hypogaea* L.). Biochem Biophys Acta 1986; 882:97–105.
91. Burks AW, Cockrell G, Connaughton C, Guin J, Allen W, Helm RM. Identification

of peanut agglutinin and soybean trypsin inhibitor as minor legume allergens. Int Arch Allergy Immunol 1994; 105:143–149.

92. Burks AW, Williams LW, Helm RM, Connaughton C, Cockrell G, O'Brien T. Identification of a major peanut allergen, *Ara h* I, in patients with topic dermatitis and positive peanut challenges. J Allergy Clin Immunol 1991; 88:172–179.

93. Burks AW, Cockrell G, Stanley JS, Helm RM, Bannon GA. Recombinant peanut allergen Ara h I expression and IgE binding in patients with peanut hypersensitivity. J Clin Invest 1995; 96:1715–1721.

94. Burks AW, Helm RM, Cockrell G, Stanley J, Bannon GA. The identification of a family of vicilin-like gene encoding allergens responsible for peanut hypersensitivity (abstr). J Allergy Clin Immunol 1995; 96:332.

95. Burks AW, Cockrell G, Connaughton C, Helm RM. Epitope specificity and immunoaffinity purification of the major peanut allergen, Ara h I. J Allergy Clin Immunol 1994; 93:743–750.

96. Stanley JS, Burks AW, Helm RM, Cockrell G, Bannon GA. Ara h I, a major allergen involved in peanut hypersensitivity, has multiple IgE binding sites (abstr). J Allergy Clin Immunol 1995; 95:333.

97. Burks AW, Williams LW, Connaughton C, Cockrell G, O'Brien TJ, Helm RM. Identification and characterization of a second major peanut allergen, Ara h II, with use of the sera of patients with atopic dermatitis and positive peanut challenge. J Allergy Clin Immunol 1992; 90:962–969.

98. Burks AW, Cockrell G, Connaughton C, Karpas A, Helm RM. Epitope specificity of the major peanut allergen, Ara h II. J Allergy Clin Immunol 1995; 95:607–611.

99. Shibasaki M, Suzuki S, Tajima S, Nemoto H, Kuroume T. Allergenicity of major component proteins of soybeans. Int Arch Allergy Appl Immunol 1980; 61:441–448.

100. Ogawa T, Bando N, Tsuji H, Okajima H, Nishikawa K, Sasoka K. Investigation of the IgE-binding proteins in soybeans by immunoblotting with the sera of soybean-sensitive patients with atopic dermatitis. J Nutr Sci Vitaminol 1991; 37:555–565.

101. Moroz LA, Yang WH. Kunitz soybean trypsin inhibitor, a specific allergen in food anaphylaxis. N Engl J Med 1980; 302:1126–1128.

102. Ogawa T, Bando N, Tsuji H, Nishikawa K, Kitamura K. α-Subunit of β-conglycinin, an allergenic protein recognized by IgE of soybean-sensitive patients with atopic dermatitis. Biosci Biotech Biochem 1995; 59:831–833.

103. Herian AM, Taylor SL, Bush RK. Identification of soybean allergens by immunoblotting with sera from soy-allergic adults. Int Arch Allergy Appl Immunol 1990; 92:193–198.

104. Grant DR, Sumner AK, Johnson J. An investigation of pea seed albumins. J Can Inst Food Technol 1976; 9:84–91.

105. Malley A, Baecher L, Mackler B Perlman F. The isolation of allergens from the green pea. J Allergy Clin Immunol 1975; 56:282–290.

106. Malley A, Baecher L, Mackler B Perlman F. Further characterization of a low molecular weight allergen fragment isolate from green pea. Clin Exp Immunol 1976; 25:159–164.

107. Hefle SL, Bush RK. Adverse reaction to lupin. J Allergy Clin Immunol 1994; 94:167–172.

108. Adachi T, Izumi H, Yamada T, Tanaka K, Takeuchi S, Nakamura R, Matsuda T. Gene structure and expression of rice seed allergenic proteins belonging to the α-amylase/trypsin inhibitor family. Plant Mol Biol 1993; 21:239–248.

109. Matsuda T, Alvarez AM, Tada Y, Adachi T, Nakamura R. Gene engineering for hypo-allergenic rice: repression of allergenic protein synthesis in seeds of trans-genic rice plant by antisense RNA. Proceedings of the International Workshop on Life Science in Production and Food-Consumption of Agricultural Products, Tsukuba, Japan, 1993 Session 4.

110. Izumi H, Adachi T, Fujii N, Matsuda T, Nakamura R, Tanaka K, Urisu A, Kuro-sawa Y. Nucleotide sequence of a cDNA clone encoding a major allergenic protein in rice seeds: homology of the deduced amino acid sequence with member of α-amylase/trypsin inhibitor family. FEBS 1992; 302:213–216.

111. Adachi T, Izumi H, Yamada T, Tanaka K, Takeuchi S, Nakamura R, Matsuda T. Gene structure and expression of rice seed allergenic proteins belonging to the α-amylase/trypsin inhibitor family. Plant Mol Biol 1993; 21:239–248.

112. Nakamura R, Matsuda T. Rice allergenic protein and molecular-genetic approach for hypoallergenic rice. Biosci Biotechnol Biochem 1996; 60:1215–1221.

113. Watanabe M. Hypoallergenic rice as a physiologically functional food. Trends Food Sci Tech 1993; 4:125–128.

114. Matsuda T, Nakamura R. Molecular structure and immunological properties of food allergens. Trends Food Sci Technol 1993; 4:289–293.

115. Lehrer SB, Reese G, Ortega H, El-Dahr JM, Goldberg B, Malo J-L. IgE antibody reactivity to aqueous-soluble, alcohol-soluble and transgenic corn proteins. J Allergy Clin Immunol 1997; 99:S147 (abstract).

116. Lehrer SB, Reese G. Recombinant proteins in newly developed foods: identification of allergenic activity. Int Arch Allergy Immunol 1997; 113:122–124.

117. Bargman TJ, Rupnow JH, Taylor SL. IgE-binding proteins in almonds (*Prunus amygdalus*): identification by immunoblotting with sera from almond-allergic adults. J Food Sci 1992; 57:717–720.

118. Arshad SH, Malmberg E, Krapt K, Hide DW. Clinical and immunological charac-teristics of Brazil nut allergy. Clin Exp Allergy 1991; 21:373–376.

119. Nordlee JA Taylor SL, Townsend JA. Thomas LA: High methinone Brazil nut pro-tein binds human IgE (abstr). J allergy Clin Immunol 1994; 93:209.

120. Altenbach SB, Pearson KW, Leung FW, Sun SSM. Cloning and sequence analysis of a cDNA encoding a Brazil nut protein exceptionally rich in methione. Plant Mol Biol 1987; 8:239–259.

121. Anibarro B, Garcia-Ara C, Ojeda JA. Bird-egg syndrome in children. J Allergy Clin Immunol 1993; 92:628–630.

122. Parra FM, Cuevas M, Lezaun A, Alonso MD, Beristain AM, Losada E. Pistachio nut hypersensitivity: identification of pistachio nut allergens. Clin Exp Allergy 1993; 23:996–1001.

123. Bernhisel-Broadbent J, Sampson HA. Cross-allergenicity in the legume botanical family in children with food hypersensitivity. J Allergy Clin Immunol 1989; 83:435–440.

124. Bernhisel-Broadbent J. Allergenic cross-reactivity of foods and characterization of food allergens and extracts. Ann Allergy Asthma Immunol 1995; 95:295–303.

125. Bernhisel-Broadbent J, Taylor S, Sampson HA. Cross-allergenicity in the legume botanical family in children with food hypersensitivity. II. Laboratory correlates. J Allergy Clin Immunol 1989; 84:701–709.

126. Bock SA, Atkins. Patterns of food hypersensitivity during sixteen years of double-blind, placebo-controlled food challenges. J Pediatr 1990; 117:561–567.

127. Barnett D, Bonhan B, Howden WEH. Allergenic cross-reactions among legume foods—in vitro study. J. Allergy Clin Immunol 1987; 79:443–438.

128. Jones MM, Magnolfi C, Cooke, Sampson HA. Immunologic cross-reactivity among cereal grains and grasses in children with food hypersensitivity. J Allergy Clin Immunol 1995; 96:341–351.

129. Moody MW, Roberts KJ, Huner JV. Phylogeny of commercially important seafood and description of the seafood industry. Clin Rev Allergy 1993; 11:159–181.

130. Aas K. Studies of hypersensitivity to fish: a clinical study. Int Arch Allergy Clin Immunol 1966; 29:346–363.

131. Bernhisel-Broadbent J, Scanlon SM, Sampson HA. Fish hypersensitivity. I. In vitro and oral challenge results in fish-allergic patients. J Allergy Clin Immunol 1992; 89:730–737.

132. Waring NP, deShazo RD, Daul CB, McCants M, Lehrer SB. Hypersensitivity reactions to ingested crustacean: clinical evaluation and diagnostic studies in shrimp sensitive individuals. J Allergy Clin Immunol 1985; 76:440–445.

133. Daul CB, Morgan JE, Waring NP, McCants ML, Hughes J, Lehrer SB. Immunological evaluation of shrimp-allergic individuals. J Allergy Clin Immunol 1987; 80:716–722.

134. Daul CB, Slattery M, Morgan JE, Lehrer SB. Common crustacea allergens: identification of B cell epitopes with the shrimp specific monoclonal antibodies. In: Kraft D, Sehon A, eds. Molecular Biology and Immunology of Allergens. pp 291–294.

135. Anderson LB, Dreyfuss EM, Logan J, Johnston DE. Melon and banana sensitivity coincident with ragweed pollinosis. J Allergy Clin Immunol 1970; 45:310–319.

136. Enberg RN, Leickley FE, McCoullough J, Bailey J, Ownby DR. Watermelon and ragweed share allergens. J Allergy Clin Immunol 1987; 79:867–875.

137. Calkhoven PG, Aalbers M, Koshte VL, Schilte PP, Yntema JL, Griffioen RW, Van Nierop JC, Oranje AP, Aalberse RC. Relationship between IgG1 and IgE4 antibodies to foods and the development of IgE antibodies to inhalant allergens. II. Increased levels of IgG antibodies to foods in children who subsequently develop IgE antibodies to inhalant allergens. Clin Exp Allergy 1991; 21:99–107.

138. Halmepuro, L, Vuontela K, Kalimo K, Björlstén. Cross-reactivity of IgE antibodies with allergens in birch pollen, fruits and vegetables. Int Arch Allergy Appl Immunol 1984; 74:235–240.

139. Calkhoven PG, Aalbers M, Koshte VL, Pos O, Oei HD, Aalberse RC. Cross-reactivity among birch pollen, vegetables and fruits as detected by IgE antibodies is due to at least three distinct cross-reactive structures. Allergy 1987; 42:382–390.

140. Wütrich B, Dietschi R. The celery-carrot-mugwort-condiment syndrome: skin test and RAST results. Schweiz Med Wochenschr 1985; 115:258–264.

141. Vieths S, Janek K, Aulepp H, Petersen A. Isolation and characterization of the 18-kDa major apple allergen and comparison with the major birch pollen allergen (Bet v I). Allergy 1995; 50:421–430

142. Vanek-Krebitz M, Hoffmann-Sommergruber K, Laimer da Camara Machado M, Susani M, Ebner C, Kraft D, Scheiner O, Breiteneder H. Cloning and sequencing of Mal d 1, the major allergen from apple (*Malus domestica*), and its immunological relationship to Bet v 1, the major birch pollen allergen. Biochem Biophys Res Commun 1995; 14; 214:538–551.

143. Fahlbusch B, Rudeschko O, Müller WD, Schlenvoigt G, Vettermann S, Jäger L. Purification and characterization of the major allergen from apple and its allergenic cross-reactivity with Bet v 1. Int Arch Allergy Immunol 1995; 108:119–126.

144. Vieths S, Schoning B, Petersen A. Characterization of the 18-kDa apple allergen by two-dimensional immunoblotting and microsequencing. Int Arch Allergy Immunol 1994; 104:399–404.

145. Ebner C, Hirschwehr R, Bauer L, Breiteneder H, Valenta R, Ebner H, Kraft D, Scheiner O. Identification of allergens in fruits and vegetables: IgE cross-reactivities with the important birch pollen allergens Bet v 1 and Bet v 2 (birch profilin). J Allergy Clin Immunol 1995; 95:962–969.

146. Valenta R, Kraft D. Type I allergic reactions to plant-derived food: a consequence of primary sensitization to pollen allergens. J Allergy Clin Immunol 1995; 95:893–895.

147. Vallier P, DeChamp C, Valenta R, Vial O, Deviller P. Purification and characterization of an allergen from celery immunochemically related to an allergen present in several other plant species: identification as a profilin. Clin Exp Allergy 1992; 22:774–782

148. Valenta R, Duchene M, Ebner C, Valent P, Sillaber C, Deviller P, Ferreira F, Tejkl M, Edelmann H, Kraft D, Scheiner O. Profilins constitute a novel family of functional plant pan-allergens. J Exp Med 1992; 175:377–385.

149. Breiteneder H, Hoffmann-Sommergruber K, O'Riordain G, Susani M, Ahorn H, Ebner C, Kraft D, Scheiner O. Molecular characterization of Api g 1, the major allergen of celery (*Apium graveolens*), and its immunological and structural relationships to a group of 17 kDa tree pollen allergens. Eur J Biochem 1995;233:484–489

150. Catterall JF, Stein JP, Kristo P, Means AR, O'Malley BW. The primary sequence of ovomucoid messenger RNA as determined from cloned complementry DNA. J Cell Biol 1980; 87:480–487.

151. Kato I, Schrode J, Kohr WJ, Laskowski M JR. Chicken ovomucoid: determination of its amino acid sequene, determination of the trypsin reactive site, and preparation of all three of its domains. Biochemistry 1987; 26:193–201.

152. Woo SLC, Beattie WG, Catterall JF, Dugaiczyk A, Staden R, Brownlee GG, O'-Malley BW. Complete nucleotide sequence of the chicken chromosomal ovalbumin and its biological significance. Biochemistry 1981; 20:6437–6446.

153. McReynolds L, O'Malley BW, Nisbet AD, Fothergill JE, Givol D, Fields S,

    Robertson M, Brownlee GG. Sequence of chicken ovalbumin mRNA. Nature
    1978; 273:723–728.

154. Catterall JF, O'Malley BW, Robertson MA, Staden R, Tanaka Y, Brownlee GG.
     Nucleotide sequence homology at 12 intro-exon junctions in the chick ovalbumin
     gene. Nature 1978; 275:510–513.

155. Jeltsch J-M, Chambon P. The complete nucleotide sequence of the chicken ovo-
     transferrin mRNA. Eur J Biochem 1982; 122:291–295.

156. Jeltsch J-M, Hen R, Maroteaux L, Garnier J-M, Chambon P. Sequence of the
     chicken ovotransferrin gene. Nucleic Acids Res 1987; 15:7643–7645.

157. Jung A, Sippel AE, Grez M, Schutz G. Exons encode functional and structural
     units of chicken lysozyme. Proc Natl Acad Sci USA 1980; 77:5759–5763.

158. Palmiter RD, Gagnon J, Ericsson LH, Walsh KA. Precursor of egg white
     lysozyme. J Biol Chem 1977; 252:6386–6393.

159. Monslave RE, Gonzalez de la Pena MA, Menendez-Arias L, Lopez-Otin C, Vil-
     lalba M, Rodriguez R. Characterization of a new mustard allergen, Bra j IE: detec-
     tion of an allergenic epitope. Biochem J 1993; 294:625–632.

160. Menendez-Arias L, Moneo I, Dominguez J, Rodriquez R. Primary structure of the
     major allergen of yellow mustard (*Sinapis alba*) seed, Sin a 1. Eur J Biochem
     1988; 177:159–166.

161. Mena M, Sanchez-Monge R, Gomez L, Salcedo, Carbonero P. A major barley al-
     lergen associated with baker's asthma disease is a glycosylated monomeric in-
     hibitor of insect α-amylase: cDNA cloning and chromosomal location of the gene.
     Plant Mol Biol 1992; 20:451–458.

5

Cow's Milk Allergy

Arne Høst
Odense University Hospital, Odense, Denmark

Sami L. Bahna
University of South Florida, All Children's Hospital, St. Petersburg, Florida

INTRODUCTION

Historical Background

Reproducible adverse reactions to cow's milk (CM) were first described by Hippocrates (prior to 370 B.C.), who reported that CM could cause urticaria and gastric upset [1]. About 500 years later, Galen described a case of cow's milk allergy (CMA) [2]. In the first decades of this century, reports on adverse reactions to CM protein were published in the German literature [3]. In these reports adverse reactions to CM protein were described as "idiosyncrasy." Wernstedt, in Sweden, was probably the first to refer to such reactions as allergy, indicating a state of changed reactivity [4]. In 1916, the American pediatrician Talbot described the relation between "idiosyncrasy" and anaphylaxis to CM [5]. In 1938, an allergic reaction to inhalation of CM in a Danish dairy worker was described [6]. Until the second half of this century, CMA seemed to be infrequent. Since the

1950s, an increasing frequency has been reported, possibly caused by a decrease in breast feeding and an increase in CM-based infant formula feeding [7,8]. In the recent decades, CMA has become the most common food allergy in early childhood, and about 5%–15% of infants are suspected of having CMA during the first year of life [3]. Many reviews [3,7–14] have elucidated varying aspects of CMA, but still much controversy exists regarding its prevalence, spectrum of manifestations, and diagnostic methods [3].

Definition and Diagnosis

The term "allergy" is commonly used for immunologically mediated reactions, whereas non–immunologically mediated reactions are often referred to as "intolerance," a rather general term that can actually encompass any type of adverse reaction. Like food allergy in general, CMA can be divided into immunoglobulin E– (IgE)-mediated or type I, and non-IgE-mediated reactions, mainly type III (immune complexes) and type IV (cell-mediated), and very rarely type II (cytotoxic) [14,15]. It is noteworthy that many studies on "milk allergy" have not investigated the immunologic basis of the clinical manifestations. Since none of the manifestations of CMA is pathognomonic and laboratory or skin tests are not confirmatory, the diagnosis must be based on strict, well-defined food elimination and challenge procedures, preferably in a double-blind, placebo-controlled manner in patients beyond infancy [16,17]. In young infants, open challenges can be reliable when performed under medical observation [18,19]. Gastrointestinal symptoms related to milk can be due to either milk protein hypersensitivity or cow's milk intolerance (CMI) secondary to lactase enzyme deficiency. It is important to differentiate between these two conditions [20].

In order to prevent overdiagnosis the following diagnostic criteria should be fulfilled:

1. Definite disappearance of symptoms after strict dietary elimination of CM, preferably on two occasions
2. Recurrence of symptoms after challenge
3. Exclusion of lactose intolerance or intercurrent infection, especially when the symptoms are limited to the gastrointestinal tract

In young infants, these diagnostic criteria will usually be sufficient, provided that challenge procedures are performed under medical observation [3]. In solely breast fed infants, elimination and challenge procedures should be performed via regulation of the mother's intake of cow's milk. In any case a well define standardized challenge schedule should be followed [3]. In older children and in adults blind challenges [17,19,21] will often be necessary in order to exclude psychological or casual reactions. However, it should be stressed that double-blind, placebo-controlled food challenge (DBPCFC) is not practical in patients with delayed reactions, because prolonged double-blind, controlled administration of CM or placebo in high doses (equivalent to normal daily intake of the food) for possibly several days will be difficult to accomplish. Therefore, if the result of DBPCFC is negative, an open controlled challenge including normal intake of the food protein in question should be carried out while watching for the occurrence of delayed reactions.

PREVALENCE

Estimates of the prevalence of CMA varied widely from 1.8% to 7.5% depending on the study design, population studied, manifestations included, and diagnostic criteria [22–28]. In prospective longitudinal studies of unselected newborns, infants with symptoms suggestive of adverse reactions to CM have varied from 5% to 15% [3]. However, in infants suspected of having CMA, the diagnosis was only proved in about one-third using controlled elimination-challenge tests; i.e., the actual prevalence is between 1.9% and 7.5% (Table 1). Two prospective longitudinal studies have documented an association between early introduction of CM or CM-based formula and development of CMA/CMI [22,27]. In exclusively breast fed infants the incidence of CMA/CMI during the first year of life was found to be about 0.5% [24,27].

ETIOLOGY

Development of CMA depends on both genetic predisposition and environmental exposure.

TABLE 1   Prevalence of Cow's Milk Allergy/Intolerance During the First Year of Life According to Seven Prospective Studies

Authors, Year	Prevalence
Halpern et al., 1973	20/1084 (1.8%)
Gerrard et al., 1973	59/787 (7.5%)
Jakobsson and Lindberg, 1979	20/1079 (1.9%)
Hide and Guyer, 1983	15/609 (2.5%)
Bock, 1987	25/480 (5.2%)[a]
Høst et al., 1988	39/1749 (2.2%)
Schrander et al., 1993	26/1158 (2.3%)

[a] When double-blind, placebo-controlled food challenge (DBPCFC) was used, 11/480 (2.2%).

Atopy

In prospective studies on CMA, an increased frequency of atopy among first-degree relatives has been noted, with estimates between 40% and 80% [3]. A pronounced atopic predisposition has been documented in one study, in which atopy in both parents was noted in 23% versus 3% in the general population [18]. Genetic factors are of great importance for the development of IgE-mediated reactions [29]. Infants with a pronounced atopic predisposition and increased risk for development of CMA may have a primary immunoregulatory defect [30], which can be identified by elevated cord blood total IgE [31,32], high levels of specific IgE, low numbers of T cells [33], disturbed T-helper/T-suppressor cell ratio [34,35], or delayed postnatal maturation of T-cell competence [36].

Allergenicity of Cow's Milk Proteins

Food allergy/intolerance is principally a problem in infancy and early childhood and the causative foods will depend on dietary habits. In developed countries, CM is usually the first foreign food given to infants. Cow's milk protein includes more than 40 fractions, any of which can act as an allergen [37]. Cow's milk contains 30–35 g/l of total protein, of which about 80% is casein (24–28 g/l) and about 20% is whey (5–7 g/l). Formation of antibodies to cow's milk proteins is a physiologic response and can be demonstrated in normal subjects, with the highest levels being during infancy [3]. It can be concluded that CM proteins are antigenic in humans. The humoral immune response to foods involves the formation of IgG, IgA, and IgM antibodies. These antibodies as well as low levels of IgE antibodies are usually harmless, whereas high levels of IgE antibodies to foods are supportive of development of allergic disease [38]. T-cell-mediated reactions in the gut have been documented in several reports, and active immune responses can be detected and measured in humans, as well as in animals. There is evidence that T-cell-mediated reactions in the small bowel mucosa can cause immune mediated damage and malabsorption. Lymphokine detecting assays and lymphoblast stimulation tests have demonstrated a pathogenic role of T-cell-mediated reactions to CM proteins [3,39,40].

The allergenicity of cow's milk proteins may be altered by technologic processing, especially by digestion. Enzymatic digestion (hydrolysis) denatures the sequential epitopes, whereas low heat treatment (low pasteurization at 75°C for 15 sec) only ensures bacteriologic quality of milk and does not cause any significant reduction of its antigenicity or allergenicity. However, strong heat treatment (121°C for 20 min) may destroy the allergenicity of the whey proteins (mainly the conformational epitopes) but only reduces that of caseins. In general, heat treatment only reduces but does not eliminate the allergenicity of milk proteins. As regards antigenicity/allergenicity, no significant difference has been found in comparative studies between unhomogenized and pasteurized/homogenized milk in children with CMA [41].

On the basis of determination of specific IgE to individual cow's milk proteins in patients with CMA, the major allergens in infancy seem to be bovine serum albumin, β-lactoglobulin, and bovine immunoglobulin, whereas in older children β-lactoglobulin, caseins, and α-lactalbumin may be more reactive. In general, most patients react to two or more proteins [3].

Exposure to CM

Exposure to CM proteins may occur *prenatally,* considering that high-molecular-weight milk proteins may cross the placenta, stimulate the fetal immune system, and elicit specific IgE response, as indicated by the demonstration of food-specific IgE antibodies in cord blood [42].

Postnatally, breast fed infants are exposed to CM and other food proteins that are ingested by the mother and are excreted by the mammary gland [43]. Bovine β-lactoglobulin can be detected in the breast milk in 95% of lactating women in quantities ranging from 0.9 to 150 μg/l [43]. With the introduction of CM-based formula into the infants' diet, the antigenic load of CM proteins becomes enormous during the first year of life, amounting to about 10–15 g/day (or 3.6–5.5 kg/yr) considering that normal CM formula contains about 15 g/l. CM proteins are absorbed from the gut and can be measured in the blood in quantities of micrograms per liter, in both children and adults [44,45]. Macromolecular absorption is increased in preterm infants and in newborns and has also been demonstrated in infants with CMA. Whether increased macromolecular absorption is a part of an allergic constitution/heredity or is due to temporal mucosal damage is not clarified and the relevance of increased absorption to development of clinical disease is unclear [3].

Sensitization to Cow's Milk

Prenatal Sensitization

Previously, only a few studies have reported specific IgE antibodies against cow's milk proteins by the allergosorbent test (RAST) in 0%–3.7% of newborns [3]. Recently, specific IgE against individual cow's milk proteins was demonstrated by means of cross-radioimmunoelectrophoresis (CRIE) analysis in 76% of a selected group of infants in whom CMA/CMI later developed. By means of another very sensitive method (Magic Lite SQ-System) specific IgE against individual CM proteins was detected in cord blood of newborns with and without atopic predisposition in 11% and 9%, respectively [46]. These data indicate that *prenatal sensitization* occurs and may play a role in the pathogenesis of food allergy. Other authors have demonstrated fetal T-cell proliferative responses to specific inhalant and ingestant allergens, providing further evidence of intrauterine sensitization [47].

Postnatal Sensitization

Exclusively breast fed infants in whom CMA develops may react to minute amounts of CM protein in *human milk*. Also, sensitization to foods during exclusive breast feeding is likely to result from ingestion of hidden CM protein and possibly from inhalation or skin contact. The extent of the role played by such routes may be appreciated if one considers that just 1 ml of CM contains 35 mg of protein, of which about 3 mg is β-lactoglobulin, which is equivalent to the amount expected from about 2 months' feeding 1 liter human milk/day. The very small amounts of cow's milk protein in breast milk may rather induce tolerance than allergic sensitization and development of allergic disease. On the other hand, a significant relationship exists between early neonatal exposure to *CM formula* feeding and subsequent development of CMA [3,22,27].

Development of Clinical Disease

There is increasing evidence that intrauterine sensitization to foods as well as to inhalants may occur. However, such weak intrauterine sensitization may be a normal phenomenon as is the well known weak postnatal IgE response in infants without allergic disease [38]. Neonatal exposure to a "high dose" of foreign protein may be necessary for development of allergic disease [3]. Clinical symptoms of CMA/CMI may appear during the period of breast feeding, but most infants have symptoms shortly after introduction of CM formula [3]. Many studies have shown that CMA develops mostly during early infancy and rarely afterward [3].

MANIFESTATIONS

A broad spectrum of symptoms in children may be caused by CMA (Table 2). In early infancy the reactions are mostly gastrointestinal (about 60%), but it may also affect other systems such as the skin (about 50%–60%) or the respiratory tract (about 20%–30%) [3]. Systemic anaphylaxis has been reported in up to 9% of milk-sensitive children [48].

In general, the symptoms may occur within a few minutes to 1 hr after milk ingestion (immediate reactions) or after a few hours (late reactions). In some cases the symptoms develop after days (delayed reactions). On the basis of clinical and immunologic types of reactions, some authors have classified patients into three groups, as immediate, intermediate, and late reactors [49–52]. Children with IgE-mediated reactions to CM mostly show immediate reactions, whereas those with non-IgE-mediated reactions are mostly late or delayed. A substantial degree of overlap between these groups exists. It is noteworthy that

TABLE 2 Manifestations of Cow's Milk Allergy

System Involved	IgE-Mediated	Non-IgE-Mediated
Gastrointestinal	Oral allergy syndrome Vomiting Colic Diarrhea	Bleeding (occult or gross) Eosinophilic gastroenteropathy Enterocolitis Protein-losing enteropathy Gastroesophageal reflux Constipation
Dermatologic	Atopic dermatitis Urticaria Angioedema	Contact rash Atopic dermatitis Vasculitis
Respiratory	Rhinoconjunctivitis Laryngeal edema Cough Asthma Otitis media[a]	Chronic pulmonary disease (Heiner syndrome) Pulmonary hemosiderosis
Systemic anaphylaxis **Rare manifestations**	Most anaphylaxis	Postprandial exercise-induced Headache/migraine Irritability Vasculitis Arthropathy Nephropathy Thrombocytopenia

[a] Probably secondary to eustachian tube dysfunction and/or allergic rhinitis.

the majority of infants with CMA has more than one symptom in one or more systems [3]. In exclusively breast fed infants the symptoms are similar to those in formula fed infants, except for atopic dermatitis, which tends to be severe in the first group [3].

TREATMENT

Avoidance

The basic treatment of CMA is complete avoidance of CM and its products. A hypoallergenic formula can be the only diet for infants up to 6 months of age (see Appendix). Afterward milk-free solid foods can be gradually introduced. Commercially available foods may contain small quantities of milk proteins not listed on the labels or listed under unfamiliar names, such as whey, casein, or caseinate [53]. An experienced dietitian is often needed to ensure a correct milk-free diet and adequate nutrition.

Previously various non-milk-based formulas were used in the treatment of

CMA/CMI. However, soy formula allergy may occur in about 17% to 47% of children [3]. Goat's or sheep's milk should not be recommended as a CM substitute because most of the protein fractions in the milk of these animals are identical [3]. Pasteurization, spray drying, evaporation, and other procedures ordinarily used in the production of commercial formulas and other milk products may only reduce the allergenicity of milk proteins.

In conclusion, only proven hypoallergenic formulas should be used in infants with CMA. The extensively hydrolyzed formulas (eHFs) have been found substantially less antigenic and less allergenic than the partially hydrolyzed formulas (pHFs). Exquisitely sensitive individuals, however, may react to small quantities of residual high-molecular-weight peptides, even in eHF, indicating that none of these "hypoallergenic" formulas is "nonallergenic" [54,55]. It has been recommended that a hypoallergenic formula should fulfill the criteria of 90% clinical tolerance (with 95% confidence limits) in infants with proven CMA [55,56]. Before recommending a particular formula to a highly milk-sensitive subject, it would be prudent to perform a skin prick test with a fresh sample of the recommended ready-to-feed formula, followed by an open supervised challenge to confirm its safety. In patients who react to eHF or do not accept the taste, an amino acid–derived elemental formula (see Appendix) should be used [57].

Desensitization

Very limited trials reported a possible successful effect of oral desensitization with cow's milk [58]. Such trials have several limitations [59], and the current information indicates that this procedure does not have sufficient reliability. There is a definite need for well designed placebo-controlled trials. Likewise, no convincing effect has been demonstrated in preliminary studies on the effect of immunotherapy by intracutaneous or subcutaneous injection [60].

Reintroduction

Because of the usually favorable prognosis of CMA, it is important to prevent an unnecessarily long-lasting milk-free diet. Therefore, controlled rechallenges are recommended at intervals of about 6–12 months in early childhood up to 3 years of age, and in older children at intervals of 1–2 years. Such challenges are preferably performed under medical supervision in case severe reactions occur. However, in many patients, accidental exposure may determine the degree of clinical tolerance.

PREVENTION

There is sufficient evidence that the mode of early infant feeding influences the development of food allergy, especially in infants with hereditary atopic predisposition (physician's diagnosed atopic disease in first-degree relatives).

A significant association between early neonatal exposure to cow's milk formula feeding and subsequent development of CMA has been documented [3]. When breast milk is insufficient or lacking, a hypoallergenic formula is needed. Several recent prospective studies showed a preventive effect of feeding high-risk infants an extensively hydrolyzed formula and avoiding cow's milk and solid foods for at least the first 4 months of life [55]. Partially hydrolyzed formulas may be effective in allergy prevention [61], but because of the high content of such formulas of intact protein and high-molecular-weight peptides, there is much concern about such practice and further evidence is needed.

Regarding maternal diet, avoidance of the most common allergenic foods did not seem to have a preventive effect during late pregnancy [62]. However, a significant effect was noted in exclusively breast fed infants whose mothers followed an elimination diet during lactation [63].

PROGNOSIS

The prognosis of CMA has recently been reviewed [3,64]. The main findings are summarized in Table 3. Overall, the prognosis is good, particularly in infancy and early childhood, with a remission rate of about 45%–55% at 1 year, 60%–75% at 2 years, and 85%–90% at 3 years [3]. With increasing age, tolerance will develop in a lower proportion of milk-intolerant children [64]. Infants with IgE-mediated CMA have a significantly lower rate of recovery than infants with non-IgE-mediated reactions [64]. Regarding the non-IgE-mediated gastrointestinal reactions (e.g., enteropathy, enterocolitis, and colitis) the prognosis is excellent with total recovery within 1–2 years on a milk-free diet.

Development of adverse reactions to other foods, mostly egg, soy, peanut, citrus, fish, and cereals, occurs very often in milk-allergic infants [3]. Development of allergy against environmental inhalant allergens has been reported to appear in about 50% by 3 years and in about 80% before puberty [3,64]. In general, the increased risk of development of other allergies seems to be confined to the

TABLE 3 Prognosis of Cow's Milk Allergy

	Recovery	Other Food Allergy	Inhalant Allergy
Prospective unselected series 0–3 yr	84%–87%	54%–60%	28%[a]
Prospective selected series 2–4 yr	33%–38%	41%–75%	40%–43%[b]

[a] Among infants with CMA (IgE-mediated reactions) in 48% inhalant allergy developed by 3 years. CMA, cow's milk allergy; IgE, immunoglobulin E.
[b] In one study in 80% inhalant allergy developed before puberty.

group of infants with evidence of early IgE-mediated reactions against CM protein. Therefore, in cases of early development of CMA, especially of the IgE-mediated type, it would be prudent to apply preventive measures against common environmental allergens and irritants, particularly pets, house dust mites, mold, and tobacco smoke.

ACKNOWLEDGMENT

The authors thank Sylvia King for her assistance in preparation of this chapter.

REFERENCES

1. Chabot R. Pediatric Allergy. New York: McGraw-Hill, 1951.
2. O'Keefe ES. The history of infants feeding. II. Seventeenth and eighteenth centuries. Arch Dis Child 1953; 28:232–240.
3. Høst A. Cow's milk protein allergy and intolerance in infancy: some clinical, epidemiological and immunological aspects. Pediatr Allergy Immunol 1994; 5(suppl):5–36.
4. Wernstedt W. Zur Frage der Kuhmilchdidiosynkrasie im Säuglingsalter. Monatsschr Kinderheilk 1910; 9:25–26.
5. Talbot FB. Idiosyncrasy to cow's milk: its relation to anaphylaxis. Boston Med Surg J 1916; 175:409–410.
6. Hansen P. Urticaria provoked by inhalation of milk protein (in Danish). Ugeskr Laeger 1938; 100–226.
7. Savilahti E. Cow's milk allergy. Allergy 1981; 36:73–88.
8. Hamburger RN. Introduction: a brief history of food allergy with definitions of terminology in food intolerance. In: Hamburger RN, ed. Food Intolerance in Infancy. New York: Raven Press, 1989, pp 1–6.
9. Bahna SL, Gandhi MD. Milk hypersensitivity. II. Practical aspects of diagnosis, treatment and prevention. Allergy 1983; 50:295–301.
10. Hill DJ. Cow's milk allergy in infants: some clinical and immunologic features. Ann Allergy 1986; 57:225–228.
11. Walker-Smith JA. Milk intolerance in children. Clin Allergy 1986; 16:83–90.
12. Bahna SL. Milk allergy in infancy. Ann Allergy 1987; 59:131–136.
13. Wilson NW, Hamburger RN. Allergy to cow's milk in the first year of life and its prevention. Ann Allergy 1988; 61:323–327.
14. Bahna SL. Pathogenesis of milk hypersensitivity. Immunol Today 1985; 6:153–153.
15. Bruinjzeel-Koomen CAFM, Ortolani C, Aas K, Bindslev-Jensen C, Björkstén B, Moneret Vautrin DA, Wütrich B. Adverse reactions to foods: positions paper. Allergy 1995; 50:623–636.
16. Bahna SL. Practical considerations in food challenge testing. Immunol Allergy Clin North Am 1991; 11:843–850.
17. Metcalfe DD, Sampson HA. Workshop on experimental methodology for clinical

studies of adverse reactions to foods and food additives. J Allergy Clin Immunol 1990; 86:421–442.

18. Høst A, Halken S. A prospective study of cow milk allergy in Danish infants during the first 3 years of life: clinical course in relation to clinical and immunological type of hypersensitivity reaction. Allergy 1990; 45:587–596.

19. Bahna SL. Food challenge procedures in research and in clinical practice. Pediatr Allergy Immunol 1995; 6(suppl 8):49–53.

20. Bahna SL. Is it milk allergy or lactose intolerance? Immunol Allergy Clin North Am 1996; 16:187–198.

21. Bock SA, Sampson HA, Atkins RM, Zeiger RS, Lehrer S, Sachs M, Bush RK, Metcalfe DD. Double-blind placebo controlled food challenge as an office procedure: a manual. J Allergy Clin Immunol 1988; 82:986–997.

22. Halpern SR, Sellars WA, Johnson RB, Anderson DW, Saperstein S, Reisch JS. Development of childhood allergy in infants fed breast, soy or cow milk. J Allergy Clin Immunol 1973; 51:139–151.

23. Gerrard JW, Mackenzie JWA, Goluboff N, Garson JZ, Maningas CS. Cow's milk allergy: prevalence and manifestations in an unselected series of newborn. Acta Paediatr Scand 1973; (suppl 234):1–21.

24. Jacobsson O, Lindberg T. A prospective study of cow's milk protein intolerance in Swedish infants. Acta Paediatr Scand 1979; 68:853–859.

25. Hide DW, Guyer BM. Cow's milk intolerance in Isle of Wight infants. Br J Clin Pract 1983; 37:285–287.

26. Bock SA. Prospective appraisal of complaints of adverse reactions to foods in children during the first 3 years of life. Pediatrics 1987; 79:683–688.

27. Høst A, Husby S, Østerballe O. A prospective study of cow's milk allergy in exclusively breast-fed infants: incidence, pathogenetic role of early inadvertent exposure to cow's milk formula, and characterization of bovine milk protein in human milk. Acta Paediatr Scand 1988; 77:663–670.

28. Schrander JJP, Bogart JHP, Forget PP, Schrander-Stumpel CTRM, Kuiten RH, Krester ADM. Cow's milk protein intolerance in infants under 1 year of age: a prospective epidemiological study. Eur J Pediatr 1993; 152:640–644.

29. Zeiger RS, Heller S, Mellon MH, Helsey JF, Hamburger RN, Sampson HA. Genetic and environmental factors affecting the development of atopy through age 4 in children of atopic parents: a prospective randomized study of food allergen avoidance. Pediatr Allergy Immunol 1992; 3:110–127.

30. Björkstén B. Does breastfeeding prevent the development of allergy? Immunol Today 1983; 215–217.

31. Businco L, Marchetti F, Pellegrini G, Perlini R. Predictive value of cord blood IgE levels in "at risk" newborn babies and influence of type of feeding. Clin Allergy 1983; 13:503–508.

32. Chandra RK, Puri S, Cheema PS. Predictive value of cord blood IgE in the development of atopic diseases and role of breastfeeding in its prevention. Clin Allergy 1985; 15:517–522.

33. Juto P, Björkstén B. Serum IgE in infants and influence of type of feeding. Clin Allergy 1980; 10:593–600.

34. Strannegård I. Strannegård IL. T lymphocyte numbers and function in humane IgE-mediated allergy. Immunol Rev 1978; 41:149–170.

35. Juto P, Möller C, Engberg S, Björkstén B. Influence of type of feeding on lymphocyte function and development of infantile allergy. Clin Allergy 1982; 12:409–416.

36. Holt PG, Clough JB, Holt BJ, Baron-Hay MJ, Rose AH, Robinson BW, Thomas WR. Genetic "risk" for atopy is associated with delayed postnatal maturation of T-cell competence. Clin Exp Allergy 1992; 22:1093–1099.

37. Gjesing B, Lowenstein H. Immunochemistry of food antigens. Ann Allergy 1984; 53:602–608.

38. Hattevig G, Kjellman B, Björkstén B. Clinical symptoms and IgE responses to common food proteins and inhalations in the first 7 years of life. Clin Allergy 1987; 17:571–578.

39. Frieri M, Martinez S, Agarwal K, Trotta P. A preliminary study of interleukin 4 detection in atopic pediatric and adult patients: effect of dietary modification. Pediatr Asthma Allergy Immunol 1993; 7:27–35.

40. Knapik M, Frieri M. Altered cytokine production in atopic dermatitis: a preliminary study. Pediatr Asthma Allergy Immunol 1993; 7:127–133.

41. Høst A. Samuelsson E-G. Allergic reactions to raw, pasteurized and homogenized/pasteurized cow milk: a comparison. Allergy 1988; 43:113–118.

42. Høst A, Husby S, Gjesing B, Larsen JN, Løwenstein H. Prospective estimation of IgG subclass and IgE antibodies to dietary proteins in infants with cow milk allergy: levels of antibodies to whole milk proteins, BLG and ovalbumin in relation to repeated milk challenge and clinical course of cow milk allergy. Allergy 1992; 47:218–229.

43. Høst A, Husby S, Hansen LK, Østerballe O. Bovine beta-lactoglobulin in human milk from atopic and non-atopic mothers: relationship to maternal intake of homogenized and unhomogenized milk. Clin Exp Allergy 1990; 20:383–387.

44. Husby S. Dietary antigens: uptake and humoral immunity in man. APMIS 1988; 96(suppl):1–40.

45. Husby S, Høst A Teisner B, Svehag S-E. Infants and children with cow milk allergy/intolerance: investigation of the uptake of cow milk protein and activation of the complement system. Allergy 1990; 45:547–551.

46. Halken S, Høst A. Prevention of allergic disease: exposure to food allergens and dietetic intervention. Pediatr Allergy Immunol 1996; 7 (9 Suppl):102–107.

47. Jones AC, Miles EA, Warner JA, Warner JO. IFN-gamma and proliferative responses from foetal leucocytes during second and third trimester of pregnancy. J Allergy Clin Immunol 1995; 95:83.

48. Goldman AS, Anderson JR DW, Sellers WA, Saperstein S, Kniker WT, Halpern SR. Milk allergy. I. Oral challenge with milk and isolated milk proteins in allergic children. Pediatrics 1963; 32:425–443.

49. Hill DJ, Ball G, Hoskings CS. Clinical manifestations of cow's milk allergy in childhood. I. Association with in vitro cellular immune responses. Clin Allergy 1988; 18:469–479.

50. Hill DJ, Firer MA, Shelton MJ, Hosking CS. Manifestations of milk allergy in infancy: clinical and immunological findings. J Pediatr 1986; 109:270–276.

51. Hill DJ, Ford RPK, Shelton MH, Hosking CS. A study of 100 infants and young children with cow's milk allergy. Clin Rev Allergy 1984; 2:125–142.
52. Hill DJ, Duke AM, Hosking CS, Hudson IL. Clinical manifestations of cow's milk allergy in childhood. II. The diagnostic value of skin tests and RAST. Clin Allergy 1988; 18:81–90.
53. Gern JE, Yang E, Evrard HM, Sampson HA. Allergic reactions to milk-contaminated nondairy products. N Engl J Med 1991; 324:976–979.
54. Saylor JD, Bahna SL. Anaphylaxis to casein hydrolysate formula. J Pediatr 1991; 118:71–74.
55. Businco L, Dreborg S, Einarsson R, Giampietro PG, Høst A, Keller KM, Strobel S, Wahn U, Biorksten B, Kjellman MN. Hydrolysed cow's milk formulae: allergenicity and use in treatment and prevention: an ESPACI position paper. Pediatr Allergy Immunol 1993; 4:101–111.
56. Kleinman RE, Bahna S, Powell GF, Sampson HA. Use of infant formulas in infants with cow milk allergy: a review and recommendations. Pediatr Allergy Immunol 1991; 2:146–155.
57. Sampson HA, James JM, Bernhisel-Broadbent J. Safety of an amino-acid derived infants formula in children allergic to cow milk. Pediatrics 1992; 90:463–465.
58. Wüthrich B. Oral desensitization with cow's milk in cow's milk allergy: Pro! In: Wüthrich B, Ortolani C, eds. Highlights in Food Allergy, Monogr Allergy, Vol. 32. Basel: Karger, 1996, pp 236–240.
59. Bahna SL. Oral desensitization with cow's milk in IgE-mediated cow's milk allergy: Contra! In: Wüthrich B, Ortolani C, eds. Highlights in Food Allergy, Monogr Allergy, Vol. 32. Basel: Karger, 1996, pp 233–235.
60. American Academy of Allergy & Immunology. Position statements: unproven procedures for diagnosis and treatment of allergic and immunologic diseases. J Allergy Clin Immunol 1986; 78:275–277.
61. Chandra RK, Singh G, Shridhara B. Effect of feeding whey hydrolysate, soy and conventional cow milk formulas on incidence of atopic disease in high risk infants. Ann Allergy 1989; 63:102–105.
62. Falth-Magnusson F, Kjellman N-IM. Allergy prevention by maternal elimination diet during late pregnancy-A five year follow-up of a randomized study. J Allergy Clin Immunol 1992; 89:709–713.
63. Hattevig G, Kjellman B, Sigurs N, Grodinsky E, Hed J, Bjorksten B. The effect of maternal avoidance of eggs, cow's milk, and fish during lactation on the development of IgE, IgG, and IgA antibodies in infants. J Allergy Clin Immunol 1990; 85:108–115.
64. Høst A, Jacobsen HP, Halken S, Holmenlund D. The natural history of cow's milk protein allergy/intolerance. Eur J Clin Nutr 1995; 49 (suppl 1): 13–18.

6

Adverse Reactions to Food Additives

IRA FINEGOLD
St. Luke's-Roosevelt Medical Center, New York, New York

Food additives, for the most part, are necessary improvements to the foods in our diet. Substances have been added to foods for thousands of years. Salting foods was an early means of preservation, as were pickling and exposing the food to smoke. Adding substances to foods is a necessity for the transportation and marketing of foods from remote farms and food production facilities to distant consumers. Not infrequently the food products may even originate from other continents of the globe. Thus there is a need to add substances that retard or prevent spoilage of food products. Other additives enhance appearance and consistency of foods or improve their nutritional value. As with any substance that enters the human body, there is a potential for untoward reactions. This chapter deals with the variety of additives most people knowingly or unknowingly ingest and the scope and nature of the reactions that may ensue whether they be through allergic or other mechanisms.

Knowledge that additives may cause allergic reactions is not new and was reported more than 50 years ago. Almost any of these products is capable of causing an allergic reaction. The reactions may vary in intensity and effect. Some of these reactions may not be true immunoglobulin E–(IgE)-mediated reactions but may be toxic, hypersensitive, or irritant reactions. The true incidence of allergic reactions to food additives is unknown. At one time food additive reactions were believed to be quite common; however, more recent studies suggest that they are less frequent than originally suspected. Wuthrich estimates a prevalence rate of 0.03%–0.23% [1]. When reactions of atopic children were tested to coloring agents, preservatives, citric acid, and flavoring agents in a double-blinded fashion, 6 of 335 or 2% were found to have a positive reaction [2]. Food additive intolerance in adults is estimated to be less than 0.15% [3].

Food additives are regulated by the Food and Drug Administration (FDA). Modern food law is based on the Federal Food, Drug and Cosmetic Act of 1938 and the Food Additives Amendment passed in 1958. This amendment requires the manufacturer to prove an additive's safety. Substances that were extensively used as additives prior to 1958 were classified as Generally Regarded as Safe (GRAS). In 1960 similar legislation was passed regulating color dyes, the Color Additive Amendment. Safety had to be demonstrated for all color dyes in order to stay in use. The Delaney Amendment excludes from use additives and/or dyes that have been shown to be carcinogenic in animals or humans. Many of the additives and dyes have been linked to human illness from modest skin eruptions to anaphylaxis and death.

Diagnosis is frequently by a process of evaluation, deduction, and then elimination of the offending agent. Reintroduction of the agent in a double-blinded placebo-controlled fashion with the reappearance of the symptoms would confirm the original hypothesis. Unfortunately only a few additives are able to be evaluated through diagnostic skin or in vitro tests.

Additives may be classified into the following categories according to their main use:

Product consistency enhancers
Thickening agents
Nutritional value
Palatability and wholesomeness
Leavening agents
Flavors and dyes

Examples of commonly used additives that have presented problems to susceptible individuals follow:

Product consistency enhancers
    Emulsifiers
        Gum arabic
    Stabilizers
        Ethylenediamine tetraacetic acid (EDTA)
Thickening agents and fillers
    Thickening agents

Vegetable gums, arabic (acacia), karaya, tragacanth
Fillers
Propyleneglycol
Nutrition enhancers
Vitamins
Minerals
Soy protein
Milk protein
Palatability and wholesomeness
Antioxidants
Butylated hydroxy anisol (BHA)
Butylated hydroxy toluene (BHT)
Preservatives
Benzoates
Citrates
Nitrates
Nitrites
Parabens
Sulfites
Leavening and pH control
Baking soda
Flavors and dyes
Food colors
Certified dyes
Amaranth (red #5)
Erythocine (red #3)
Indigotin (blue #2)
Ponceau (red #4)
Sunset yellow (yellow #6)
Tartrazine (yellow #5)
Flavoring agents
Carvone
Vanillin
Flavor enhancers
Monosodium glutamate (MSG)
Sweeteners
Aspartame
Saccharin
Sorbitol

This section describes in detail allergic and other untoward effects of these food additives in humans. To some extent the relative importance of each item is reflected in the length of discussion of that additive.

PRODUCT CONSISTENCY ENHANCERS

Product consistency enhancers include emulsifiers and stabilizers. Some foods spoil because of enzymatic reactions that are catalyzed by either metals or trace metallic compounds. EDTA is a potent metal chelator and acts through that mechanism to retard spoilage. There is apparently little toxicity unless it is used in large amounts and chelates ingested metals. In this manner zinc, calcium, and other metal deficiencies may occur [4].

THICKENING AGENTS AND FILLERS

Vegetable gums are used in foods to thicken such products as ice cream, cream cheese, beverages, candies, and many other products. It is important to note that since these are natural products the label may read *no artificial ingredients.* The most common vegetable gum is gum arabic. It is a product of the *Acacia senegal* tree. Gum arabic has been an article of commerce for more than 2000 years. Originally it was sent to Arabian ports from the Sudan, hence the name gum arabic [5]. The most important gums are gum arabic, tragacanth, and karaya. They are available as skin test reagents. Of lesser importance are India, locust, guar, and carrageenan gums. Allergic reactions to the gums were first described more than 50 years ago [6–7]. Reactions to gums include eczema, asthma, perennial rhinitis, and urticaria [8].

Propylene glycol is a surfactant that may also be used as a filler. It is not toxic but may lead to untoward effects in patients with renal disease [9]. Huriez et al. have reported immediate-type allergic reactions to propylene glycol–containing liquid medication [10].

NUTRITION ENHANCERS

Nutrition enhancers include vitamins, minerals, soy protein, and milk protein. Most of these substances are discussed elsewhere in this text.

PALATABILITY AND WHOLESOMENESS

Antioxidants and preservatives are used to enhance palatability and to ensure wholesomeness.

Butylated hydroxy anisol (BHA) and butylated hydroxy toluene (BHT) are antioxidants used to retard spoilage of oils and fats. They are ubiquitous, especially in breakfast cereals. Chronic urticaria in some patients has been attributed to them [11].

Benzoates are frequently used as preservatives in foods and beverages. Annual consumption is more than 10 million pounds by the food industry world-wide [12]. While testing patients with aspirin sensitivity Juhlin et al. found that all seven patients reacted to some type of benzoic acid product in a single-blinded fashion [13]. Other investigators have found varying positive reactions to benzoic acid or benzoate challenges [14–17]. Other studies suggest that these substances are not important in patients with chronic urticaria [18] or perennial asthma [19]. Benzoic acid products have been implicated in cases of allergic vasculitis but very uncommonly [20].

Another group of preservatives are the citrates. In a study of 472 Danish children citric acid was found to exacerbate atopic dermatitis and to produce gastrointestinal symptoms [21].

Nitrates were used originally to cure meats. However, it was found that their active ingredient was nitrite.

Nitrites are added to meats to retard spoilage. Most cured luncheon meats and frankfurters contain nitrites. Although there have been no documented allergic reactions to these substances, doses from 0.5 mg to 10 mg can cause headaches and facial flushing in susceptible individuals [22].

Parabens are esters of parahydroxybenzoate. They have antifungal and antibacterial properties. They do not seem important with regard to ingested food reactions, although there are a number of reports of topical sensitization [23].

Use of sulfites as antioxidants was common until 1986. After a number of reports of patients whose asthma was aggravated by sulfite ingestion, in 1986, the FDA required that when the sulfite residues exceed 10 parts per million, that information must be declared on the label. Since sulfites are used to stop fermentation, the Bureau of Alcohol, Tobacco and Firearms enforced similar requirements for wine labeling. The Environmental Protection Agency also regulates sulfite residues on grapes, which cannot be imported into the United States with detectable sulfite residues. However, sulfites are still used in the food and beverage industries. Foods with high sulfite content include dried fruit (but not brown raisins and prunes), nonfrozen lemon juice, nonfrozen lime juice, wine, molasses, sauerkraut juice, and white, pink, and sparkling grape juices. Medium-content sulfite-containing foods include dried potatoes, wine vinegar, some gravies and sauces, fruit toppings, maraschino cherries, pectin, fresh shrimp, sauerkraut, pickled peppers, cocktail onions, pickles, and relishes [24].

Sulfites have been linked to a number of allergic reactions. Patients with asthma seem to be more sensitive to sulfites when a solution is swallowed [25]. This may be due to a cholinergic mechanism since atropine can block or diminish bronchoconstriction from sulfites [26]. Although some authors have found evidence that sulfite sensitivity may be mediated by an IgE mechanism [24,27], others have not [28]. Specific antibodies to IgE have not been demonstrated [24].

Asthmatic reactions to sulfites were first suspected by Kochen [29]. Such reactions were demonstrated by Freedman with open challenges without placebo controls [30], and sulfites were shown conclusively by Stevenson and Simon and others to be substances capable of provoking asthmatic reactions [28,31]. The sulfite-sensitive asthmatic patients tend to be corticosteroid-dependent and provoked by nonatopic factors such as respiratory tract infections, irritants, and exercise. Frequently vasomotor rhinosinusitis is present but not aspirin sensitivity [24]. Sulfite challenges to 203 asthmatics found an overall prevalence of 8 reactive patients, 1 of the 120 patients who were not receiving corticosteroids and 7 in the corticosteroid-dependent group, indicating an overall prevalence rate of 3.9% for all the asthmatic patients in this study [32].

In the past sulfite challenges were done to diagnose sensitivity in asthmatics. However, since federal legislation to eliminate sulfites was passed, there are fewer instances when this is necessary. Sample challenge protocols may be found in recent reviews of this subject [24,33].

A number of other untoward reactions have been ascribed to ingestion of sulfites. These include urticaria, pruritis, and angioedema [27,34]. Most of them have been tested with open challenges or represent case reports. When patients with idiopathic anaphylaxis to restaurant meals were tested by Sonin and Patterson, none was reactive [35]. Taylor et al. conclude that for the nonatopic nonasthmatic subject the risk from sulfite ingestion is low [33].

The best treatment for reactions to sulfites is avoidance. There appears to be no evidence of concern for small amounts of sulfites (less than 10 parts per million) in products. For severe anaphylactic or asthmatic reactions epinephrine may be given even though some forms of epinephrine contain sulfite as a preservative [33].

LEAVENING AND pH CONTROL

Baking soda is the chief agent used in leavening. Yeast is not considered an additive. Most of these additives are simple chemicals, such as sodium bicarbonate and tend to be non-allergenic.

FLAVORS AND DYES

Food colors are produced by certified dyes: amaranth (red #5), erythrocine (red #3), indigotin (blue #2), ponceau (red #4), sunset yellow (yellow #6), and tartrazine (yellow #5).

Although there have been anecdotal reports for practically all certified dyes, the one that has generated the most studies and controversy has been tartrazine. Forty years ago, Lockey first described urticarial reactions from ingestion of this dye [36]. A number of other papers soon followed, but as better techniques for testing and provoking reactions to these substances developed, they appeared to be uncommon agents in provoking anaphylaxis, angioedema, urticaria, or asthmatic reactions. Stevenson et al. studied 24 patients with a history of urticaria or angioedema; in only 1 did urticaria secondary to tartrazine actually develop [37]. They concluded that tartrazine uncommonly contributed to chronic urticaria. Weber et al. looked at the incidence of bronchoconstriction due to azo and nonazo dyes in patients with perennial asthma. Forty-five patients were initially tested by an open single-blinded challenge with repeat double-blinded testing afterward. Seven of 44 patients tested with tartrazine had a significant decrease in pulmonary function on the open challenge. However, this was not confirmed on the double-blinded challenge in all 7 patients. Forty-three patients were similarly tested to a mix of azo (amaranth, ponceau, sunset yellow) and nonazo (brilliant blue, erythrosine, indigotin) dyes. Four patients reacted initially but only 1 had a positive reaction to ponceau on the double-blinded challenge. Of the 42 patients tested with the nonazo dye mix, 3 had positive results on the open challenge, but only 1 to erthrosine on the closed challenge. The authors concluded that clinically important intolerance to dyes is uncommon in patients with severe perennial asthma [19].

There have been rare reports of reactions to the other dyes, such as sunset yellow, amaranth, erythrosine, and ponceau [38].

Behavioral reactions to foods and additives remain a controversial subject. Initially, Feingold suggested that learning disorders, hyperactivity, attention deficit disorder, and other behavioral problems might be related to ingested foods, chemicals, and coloring agents [39]. A number of studies followed with primarily negative results. However, reports showed an occasional patient appeared to respond with behavioral improvement after dietary manipulation. Recently two studies have suggested, once again, that behavior may be influenced by diet. Boris and Mandel tested 26 patients; 16 patients completed their protocol. Four of these patients responded with a positive result to a double-blind placebo-controlled food challenge to colors [40]. Rowe and Rowe began with a cohort of 800 children, with 200 participating in an open trial of a synthetic coloring agent–free diet. The parents of 150 children noted improvement. From this group they studied 34 children with 20 control patients. Nineteen of 23 children whose parents claimed were reactors had positive challenge results, 3 of 11 were uncertain reactors, and 2 of 20 controls also had positive challenge results. Furthermore, a dose-dependent effect was noted as the amount of tartrazine in the blinded challenges increased from 1 to 50 mg [41].

Flavoring agents are added to food to enhance its taste. Carvone is the major ingredient of spearmint flavoring. It has been associated with asthma [42]. and the Melkersson–Rosenthal syndrome (lip/facial swelling, fissuring of the tongue, and seventh nerve palsy) [43]. A more recent study looked at six patients with this syndrome and found no reactions to double-blinded placebo-controlled oral challenges to MSG, tartrazine, sulfites, erythrosine, paraoxybenzoate, sodium benzoate, lactose, aspirin, and annate [44].

Synthetic vanillin is used to impart a vanilla flavor. It is a parahydroxybenzaldehyde structurally resembling benzoic acid. There is one report of a patient in whom asthma developed after ingestion of vanilla-flavored food [45].

The flavor enhancer monosodium glutamate is a common food additive and for most individuals carries little risk of adverse reactions. However, for some it may present a problem. MSG is categorized by the FDA as "generally regarded as safe" (GRAS). At one time MSG was thought to have a salutary effect and was even added to baby foods. This practice was discontinued in the late 1970s as the potential for MSG to induce brain damage in experimental subjects was demonstrated [46]. The addition of MSG may be noted on the label; however, the amount is seldom mentioned, and MSG may also masquerade as "hydrolyzed vegetable protein." It may also be in "secret recipes" of fast foods [24].

Adverse reactions to MSG drew national attention after the report by Kwok describing the Chinese restaurant syndrome [47]. Symptoms of headache, burning sensations on the back of the neck, chest tightness, nausea, and sweating may occur within hours after eating a meal containing large amounts of MSG. Absorption is increased when food is eaten on an empty stomach; frequently Chinese soup containing up to 5 grams of MSG per bowl is eaten as the first course. By the end of the dinner the Chinese restaurant syndrome may occur in susceptible individuals.

Asthma may be caused by MSG. There appears to be an early reaction occurring 1–2 hr after MSG is eaten with a delayed reaction occurring 10–14 hr

TABLE 1 An Example of an Additive-Free Diet

Allowed	Not permitted[a]
Cereals and breads in fresh state	Cereals with BHA, BHT
Fats: butter, olive oil	Margarine with color or preservatives
Meats: all fresh, fresh eggs	Bacon or luncheon meats
Fish, fresh in small quantities	Smoked or canned fish
Vegetables: all fresh except those listed in next column; tomatoes in moderation.	Carrots, cabbage, beans, spinach, sauerkraut
Condiments: cane sugar, salt, pepper, others as dried leaves	Vinegar (unless preservative-free), mayonnaise, prepared dressing
Sweets: homemade without additives	Ice cream, ready-made desserts
Beverages: fresh milk, tea, coffee, fruit juice, mineral water	Wines, alcohol, soda, colored beverages

[a]Avoid: colored toothpaste, colored cosmetics, artificial sweeteners. BHA, butylated hydroxy anisol; BHT, butylated hydroxy toluene.
Source: Modified from Ref. 17.

later [46,48]. Simon reports that their group has not seen a positive early or late reaction in his Scripps Clinic asthma population during double-blind placebo-controlled challenges [24]. There is one case report by Squire concerning angioedema after ingestion of soup containing MSG [49].

Aspartame, saccharin, and sorbitol are used to sweeten the flavor of foods.

Aspartame (L-aspartyl-L-phenylalanine methyl ester) is a dipeptide composed of two amino acids, phenyl alanine and aspartic acid. It is much sweeter than sugar. It cannot be given to patients with phenylketonuria. Urticaria has been reported as a result of ingestion of aspartame [50].

Saccharin (1,2-benzisothiazol-3-one 1,1-dioxide) is a member of the sulfonamide group. Considering its widespread use as a sweetening agent there have been relatively few reports of allergic reactions. Miller et al. reported one patient who reacted in a single-blinded study to 40 mg of saccharin with pruritis and wheals [51].

Sorbitol is the most common sweetener in many sugar-free candies and gums. The main reactions are abdominal pain, bloating, and diarrhea from the laxative effect of this polyalcohol taken in excess of 3 grams in children and 10 grams in adults [52].

SUMMARY

It is clear that there may be many types of reactions to food additives. Some of these are classical IgE-mediated reactions. Others may be mediated through other immune and or nonimmune mechanisms. Over the past 50 years additives have seemed to cause everything and then practically nothing depending upon the rigor of the investigation. An additive-free diet such as that in Table 1 may be a first start, but the best method of approaching suspected reactions to these substances is submitting the patient to an oral provocative test using a double-blinded placebo-controlled method. Table 2 lists challenge dose ranges.

TABLE 2 Challenge Dosing for Oral Provocation

Aspartame	150[a] mg
BHA/BHT	100[a] mg
Sodium benzoate	10–500, 100[a] mg
Methylparaben	10–100[a] mg
Monosodium glutamate	5[a]–200 mg
Sulfites	5–200[a] mg
Tartrazine	5–50[a] mg

[a]Suggested maximun doses from Ref. 24.

REFERENCES

1. Wuthrich B. Adverse reactions to food additives. *Ann Allergy 1993; 71:*379.
2. Fuglsang G, Madsen G, Halken S, Jorgensen S, Ostergaard PA, Osterballe O. Adverse reactions to food additives in children with atopic symptoms. *Allergy 1994; 49:*31.
3. Madsen C. Prevalence of food additive intolerance. *Hum Exp Toxicol 1994; 13:*393.
4. Weiner M, Bernstein IL. *Adverse Reactions to Drug Formulation Agents: A Handbook of Excipients.* New York: Marcel Dekker, 1989, pp 183–184.
5. Howes FN. *Vegetable Gums and Resins.* Waltham, MA: Chronica Botanica, 1949, p 17.
6 Brown EB, Crepea SB. Allergy (asthma) to ingested gum tragacanth. *J Allergy 1947; 18:*214.
7. Gelfand HH. The vegetable gums by ingestion in the etiology of allergic disorders. *J Allergy 1949; 20:*311.
8. Vaughan WT. *Practice of Allergy.* Saint Louis: CV Mosby, 1939, p 395.
9. Cate JC, Hedrick R. Propylene glycol intoxication and lactic acidosis. *N Engl J Med 1980; 03:*1237.
10. Huriez C, Agache P, Martin P. Allergy to propylene glycol. *Rev Fr Allergy 1966; 6:*200.
11. Juhlin L. Recurrent urticaria: clinical investigation of 330 patients. *Br J Dermatol 1981; 104:*369.
12. Jacobsen DW. Adverse reactions to benzoates and parabens. In: *Food Allergy Adverse Reactions to Foods and Food Additives.* Metcalfe DD, Sampson HA, Simon RA, eds. Boston: Blackwell Scientific, 1991, p 277.
13. Juhlin L, Michaelsson G, Zetterstrom O. Urticaria and asthma induced by food-and-drug additives in patients with aspirin hypersensitivity. *J Allergy Clin Immunol 1972; 50:*92.
14. Doeglas HMG. Reactions to aspirin and food additives in patients with chronic urticaria, including the physical urticarias. *Br J Dermatol 1975; 93:*135.
15. Ros A-M, Juhlin L, Michaelsson G. A following study of patients with recurrent urticaria and hypersensitivity to aspirin, benzoates and azo dyes. *Br J Dermatol* 1976; 95:19.
16. Ortolani C, Pastorello E, Luraghi MT, Della Torre F, Ballani M, Zanussi C. Diagnosis and intolerance to food additives. *Ann Allergy 1984; 53:*587.
17. Genton C, Frei PC, Pecoud A. Value of oral provocation tests to aspirin and food additives in the routine investigation of asthma and chronic urticaria. *J Allergy Clin Immunol 1985; 76:*40.
18. Lahti A, Hannuksela M, Is benzoic acid really harmful in cases of atopy and urticaria? *Lancet 1981; 2:*1055.
19. Weber RW, Hoffman M, Raine DA, Nelson HS. Incidence of bronchoconstriction due to aspirin, azo dyes, non-azo dyes, and preservatives in a population of perennial asthmatics. *J Allergy Clin Immunol 1979; 64:*32.
20. Michaelsson G, Petersson L, Juhlin L. Purpura caused by food and drug additives. *Arch Dermatol 1974; 109:*49.

21. Fuglsang G, Madsen G, Halken S, Jorgensen S. et al. Adverse reactions to food additives in children with atopic symptoms. *Allergy 1994; 49:*31.
22. Henderson WR, Raskin NH. "Hot-dog" headache: individual susceptibility to nitrite. *Lancet 1972; 2:*1162.
23. Weiner M, Bernstein IL. *Adverse Reactions to Drug Formulation Agents: A Handbook of Excipients.* New York: Marcel Dekker, 1989, p 298.
24. Simon RA. Adverse reactions to food and drug additives. *Immunol Allergy Clin North Am 1996; 16:*137.
25. Delohery J, Simmul R, Castle WD, Allen DH. The relationship of inhaled sulfur dioxide reactivity to ingested metabisulfite sensitivity in patients with asthma. *Am Rev Respir Dis 1984; 130:*1027.
26. Simon R, Godfarb G, Jacobsen D. Blocking studies in sulfite sensitive asthmatics (SSA). *J Allergy Clin Immunol 1984; 73:*136.
27. Prenner BM, Stevens JJ. Anaphylaxis after ingestion of sodium bisulfite. *Ann Allergy 1976; 37:*180.
28. Stevenson DD, Simon RA. Sensitivity to ingested metabisulfites in asthmatic subjects. *J Allergy Clin Immunol 1981; 68:*26.
29. Kochen J. Sulfur dioxide, a respiratory tract irritant even if ingested (letter). *Pediatrics 1973; 52:*145.
30. Freedman BJ. Asthma induced by sulphur dioxide, benzoate and tartrazine contained in orange drinks. *Clin Allergy 1977; 7:*407.
31. Baker GJ, Colette P, Allen DH, Bronchospasm induced by metabisulfite-containing foods and drugs. *Med J Aust 1981; 2:*614.
32. Bush RK, Taylor SL, Holden K. Prevalence of sensitivity to sulfiting agentsin asthmatic patients. *Am J Med 1986; 81:*816.
33. Taylor SL, Bush RK, Nordlee JA Sulfites. In: *Food Allergy Adverse Reactions to Foods and Food Additives.* Metcalfe DD, Sampson HA, Simon RA, eds. Boston: Blackwell Scientific 1991, p 239.
34. Yang WH, Purchase ECR, Rivington RN. Positive skin tests and Prausnitz-Kustner reactions in metabisulfite-sensitive subjects. *J Allergy Clin Immunol 1986; 78:*443.
35. Sonin L, Patterson R. Metabisulfite challenge in patients with idiopathic anaphylaxis. *J. Allergy Clin Immunol 1985; 75:*67.
36. Lockey SD. Allergic reactions due to FD & C yellow no. 5 tartrazine, an aniline dye used as a coloring and identifying agent in various steroids. *Ann Allergy 1959; 17:*719.
37. Stevenson DD, Simon RA, Lumry WR, Mathison DA. Adverse reactions to tartrazine. *J Allergy Clin Immunol 1986; 78:*182.
38. Weiner M, Bernstein IL. *Adverse Reactions to Drug Formulation Agents: A Handbook of Excipients.* New York: Marcel Dekker, 1989, p 274.
39. Feingold BF. *Why Is Your Child Hyperactive?* New York: Random House, 1975.
40. Boris M, Mandel FS. Foods and additives are common causes of the attention deficit hyperactive disorder in children. *Ann Allergy 1994; 72:*462.
41. Rowe KS, Rowe KJ. Synthetic food coloring and behavior: a dose response effect in a double blind placebo-controlled, repeated-measures study. *J Pediatr 1994; 125:*691.
42. Subiza J, Subiza JL, Valdivieso R, Escribano PM, Garcia R, Jerez M, Subiza E. Toothpaste flavor-induced asthma. *J Allergy Clin Immunol 1992; 90:*1004.

43. Patton DW, Ferguson MM, Forsyth A, James J. Oro-facial granulomatosis: a possible allergic basis. *Br J Oral Maxillofac Surg 1985; 23:*235.
44. Morales C, Penarrocha M, Bagan JV, Burches E, Palaez A. Immunological study of Melkersson-Rosenthal syndrome: lack of response to food additive challenge. *Clin Exp Allergy 1995; 25:*260.
45. van Assendelft AHW. Bronchospasm induced by vanillin and lactose. *Eur J Respir Dis 1984; 65:*468.
46. Allen DH. Monosodium glutamate. In: *Food Allergy Adverse Reactions to Foods and Food Additives.* Metcalfe DD, Sampson HA, Simon RA, eds. Boston: Blackwell Scientific 1991, p 261.
47. Kwok RHM. Chinese restaurant syndrome. *N Engl J Med 1968; 278:*796.
48. Allen DH, Delohery J, Baker G. Monosodium 1-glutamate-induced asthma. *J Allergy Clin Immunol 1987; 78:*530.
49. Squire EN. Angio-edema and monosodium glutamate. *Lancet 1987; 1:*988.
50. Kulczycki A, Jr. Aspartame induced urticaria: brief reports. *Ann Intern Med 1986; 104:*207.
51. Miller R, White LW, Schwartz HJ. A case of episodic urticaria due to saccharin ingestion. *J Allergy Clin Immunol 1974; 53:*240.
52. Weiner M, Bernstein IL. *Adverse Reactions to Drug Formulation Agents: A Handbook of Excipients.* New York: Marcel Dekker, 1989, pp 205–206.

7

Cross-Reactive and Hidden Allergies

MARIANNE FRIERI

Nassau County Medical Center, East Meadow, and State University of New York at Stony Brook, Stony Brook, New York

INTRODUCTION

Animal and vegetable phylogenetic tables for food cross-allergenicity appear in several reference texts. Practically, most patients experience more cross-reactivity between fish and crustaceans than within vegetable food groups. However, individuals with anaphylactic reactions should be cautioned to avoid certain foods, and the increasing reports of latex-related and hidden food reactions should alert physicians and dietitians to these emerging issues. Selective avoidance diets have been used for the treatment of food hypersensitivity. However, such diets are frequently too restrictive, and a better dietary formulation of these diets will require improved diagnosis, training of dietitians to assist patients, and additional research [1].

CROSS-REACTIVITY

The concept of cross-reactivity of food and botanical groups originated in the 1920s [2]. Cross-reactivity is a concern in the development of selective avoidance diets [1]. Authors of an early study in patients with poorly documented legume allergy reported that multiple sensitization was common in the legume family [3]. Barnett et al., using in vitro studies, reiterated this theory [4], which was disproved by studies of Bernhisel-Broadbent et al. [5,6]. Other studies reported fruit and vegetable hypersensitivity within the same botanical family, such as apple and pear, stone fruits, and nut fruits [7–11]. Oral itching was reported in 1943 in a birch pollen–allergic patient who ingested an apple [12]. In 1970, Anderson et al. noted melon and banana sensitivity coincident with ragweed pollinosis [13].

THE ORAL ALLERGY SYNDROME

The oral allergy syndrome with symptoms of oral pruritus; irritation; swelling of the lip, tongue, palate, and throat; and oral mucosal blistering was described in patients with ragweed and birch pollinosis reacting to fresh melon, bananas, fresh apples, and hazelnuts [14]. In a more recent study on the oral allergy syndrome, one of the most frequent clusters of associations in Italy was fruit hypersensitivity to the Prunoideae subfamily [15]. No association between allergy to peach, apricot, plum, or any type of pollinosis was found even though fruit and vegetable hypersensitivity is reported to be clinically associated with allergic rhinitis caused by pollens such as those of grasses, mugwort, and birch [9,10,14,15].

Using radioallergosorbent test (RAST) inhibition, DeMartino et al. demonstrated common structures in grass pollen, tomato, and peanut antigens [16]. Wuthrich et al. confirmed the presence of common allergens among celery, birch, and mugwort by RAST inhibition [17].

In an in vivo and in vitro study conducted in Italy and Sweden, allergenic cross-reactivity among peach, apricot, plum, and cherry in patients with the oral allergy syndrome was found to be due to a common 131 kDa immunoglobulin E– (IgE)-binding component not shared with grass and birch pollen [18]. Thus, the clinical observation of a cluster of hypersensitivity to the Prunoideae fruit subfamily has a solid immunochemical basis [18]. Allergenic cross-reactivity of foods and characterization of food allergens and extracts were reviewed by Bernhisel-Broadbent [19]. This article stated that patients with pollinosis and the oral allergy syndrome have IgE binding that cross-reacts with highly homologous proteins in various unrelated pollens, foods, and commercial extracts that are currently nonstandardized and not well characterized [18]. Although cross-allergenicity in food families is commonly demonstrated in vitro or by skin testing with clinical relevance using oral challenge, dietary restrictions of entire food families are rarely necessary [19]. Thus, accurate diagnosis of food hypersensitivity is essential because of the potential for serious adverse reactions, but this should not lead to the unnecessary use of overly restricted diets based entirely on results of in vitro or skin testing [19].

A study of pollen immunotherapy alleviating oral symptoms in a few patients with the oral allergy syndrome was reported [20].

EGGS

Cross-reactions are also known to occur among various eggs, milk, and crustacea. Langeland showed that the allergens in chicken egg white cross-react with proteins in the egg white of turkey, duck, goose, and seagull, as well as chicken sera and flesh [21]. The major egg white allergens have been identified as ovomucoid, ovalbumin, ovomucin, and ovotransferrin [19]. Ovomucoid or Gal d III has been shown to be more antigenic and allergenic than ovalbumin or Gal d in egg-allergic children [22]. An association was reported between allergic reactions to egg and respiratory symptoms in bird keepers exposed to their birds [23]. Of interest, the major cross-reactive allergen found in egg yolk and an extract of bird feathers was shown to consist of a 70 kDa protein, α-livetin or chicken serum albumin [24].

MILK

Cow's milk, as the most common food allergen in infants, can cause mild or systemic reactions. Juntunen and Ali-Yrkkos confirmed cow's milk allergy in 26 children by provocation, skin prick, and RAST and noted that 22 were also allergic to goat's milk [25]. In addition, most milk-allergic patients are sensitized to more than one milk protein and have been shown to react to α-lactoglobulin, β-lactoglobulin, bovine serum albumin, and bovine γ-globulin [26].

Werfel et al. demonstrated clinical reactivity to beef in cow's milk–allergic children. In this study of 335 children with atopic dermatitis, 11 were reactive to beef, and 8 were also sensitive to milk, as demonstrated in a prior double-blind placebo-controlled food challenge [27]. Three of the patients tolerated well-cooked beef and only had clinical symptoms after ingesting rare beef [27]. Soy protein is also a frequent cause of adverse food reactions in infants through soy-based infant formulas [28].

LEGUMES

In a double-blind placebo-controlled oral food challenge study in 69 children with one or more positive prick skin test results to legumes, clinical allergy was confirmed in 41, but only 5% were allergic to more than one legume [5]. In these 2 patients, after 2-year soy and peanut restriction, both lost their soy allergy but remained allergic to peanut. The authors stated that this rarity of clinically relevant cross-reactivity to legumes was in dramatic contrast to the extensive immunological cross-reactivity demonstrated in vitro with sera from the same legume-allergic patients [5]. Many patients allergic to one member of the legume family will have positive prick skin test or RAST results to other legumes but uncommonly have clinical reactivity to more than one legume member [29].

Peanut allergy is common, lifelong, hidden in many foods, and associated with severe life-threatening reactions after accidental ingestion [19]. In a study by Boch et al. of the natural history of peanut allergy in 46 patients, only 5% were allergic to another legume, and none was allergic to tree nuts [30]. An adverse reaction to lupine- (a pealike plant that is a member of the legume family) fortified pasta was reported by Hefle et al. [31]. The 5-year-old girl with peanut sensitivity experienced urticaria and angioedema after ingesting a spaghettilike pasta fortified with lupine seed flour that was extracted and used in studies in patients with peanut sensitivity [31]. Direct RAST demonstrated IgE binding in these patients.

TREE NUTS AND SHELLFISH

Proper studies of tree nut and shellfish (crustaceans such as shrimp, crab, and lobster and mollusks such as clams, oysters, and scallops) families have not yet been completed [19]. These reactions are severe and usually lifelong, but fortunately, total group elimination from the diet is generally not nutritionally hazardous [19]. Shanti et al. determined a major shrimp antigen to be a tropomyosin cross-reacting with a fruit fly extract containing an analogous tropomyosin [32].

FISH

Fish-allergic patients have been studied by many investigators; some have shown some reaction to only one fish, whereas others seem to react to multiple species such as tuna, cod, salmon, flounder, and snapper [19]. In an in vitro and oral challenge study in fish-allergic patients, prick skin test findings were positive to 10 fish species and patients were orally challenged to 4 to 6 species. Positive oral challenge responses occurred to only one specific fish in seven patients, two fish in one, and three fish in two patients, there was one nonreactive patient [33]. These authors recommend that fish-allergic patients be specifically tested by oral food challenge in a controlled environment before advice on consumption is given after a positive skin test result [19].

CEREAL GRAINS

Cereal grain allergy was studied by Jones et al. in 145 children [34]. Patients with allergy to one or more grains demonstrated extensive in vitro cross-reactivity to other grains but little to toxonomically related grasses, whereas those with grass allergy alone showed extensive in vitro cross-reactivity to both cereal grains and grasses [34]. In addition, grass-allergic patients had nonspecific binding to several wheat protein fractions. Thus in clinical practice, grass-allergic patients may have their diet inappropriately restricted as a result of positive wheat or other cereal grain RAST results that are not relevant [34].

FOOD–POLLEN ASSOCIATION

Plant profilins (14 kD) have been demonstrated to be prominent allergens in timothy grass, birch, hazel, and mugwort, carrot, and potato [35,36]. Thus, this pan-plant allergen could account for cross-reacting allergenic components from distantly related plants and food [19].

In a Finnish study of 49 patients, skin prick tests with native spices, coriander, caraway, paprika, cayenne, mustard, and white pepper were performed, along with determination of spice-specific serum IgE levels [37]. Three-fourths of the patients with positive skin test responses to native spices had positive responses to birch pollen, one-half to a vegetable; mild clinical symptoms from spices were reported by one-third [37].

Celery–carrot–mugwort–spice syndrome is well recognized in Europe. Helbling et al. studied the cross-reactivity of carrot, stalk celery, and spices, all members of the Apiaceae botanical family, and birch pollen in a patient with laryngeal edema and bronchospasm after shredding or eating several of these foods [38]. RAST inhibition demonstrated some cross-reactivity among raw carrot, stalk celery, and other members of the Apiaceae. Immunoprint inhibition revealed common allergic epitopes on a 17 kDa band shown by carrot, celery, and birch pollen, suggesting carrot hypersensitivity can be associated with birch pollen allergy [32]. Kiwi fruit has also been suggested to represent another birch pollen–associated food hypersensitivity [39].

A German and Swedish study utilizing serum electrophoretic separation and immunoblotting found the degree of cross-reactivity among kiwi, sesame seeds, poppy seeds, hazelnuts, and rye grain very high in eight patients with atopic dermatitis, some with associated asthma and allergic rhinitis [40]. These patients had clinical symptoms as well as positive skin test and RAST results [40].

A Spanish study of 262 patients sensitized to pollen, suggesting the existence of common epitopes, revealed that melon sensitivity shared allergens with plantago (a native weed) and grass pollen [41].

Cross-allergenicity among celery, cucumber, carrot, and watermelon was evaluated in six individuals with clinical allergy [42]. Immunoblots of individual sera revealed a 15 kDa protein band in all four foods, with mutual inhibition of all bands, suggesting shared antigens in the clustering of these food allergens [42].

Cross-reactivity does not indicate clinical sensitivity, and the clinical relevance needs to be carefully examined. IgE in some human sera was shown in early studies to react with an antigen in a large number of unrelated foods: potato, spinach, wheat, buckwheat, peanut, honey, and others [42]. The antigen was also found in pollen, and antibodies reacted in vitro with bee and vespid venom induced by *Hymenoptera* stings [43]. The clinical relevance of these antibodies is not clear [43].

HIDDEN FOODS

Foods may be contaminated by a wide variety of hidden substances that can lead to reactions that may be confused with food allergy, as listed in Table 1 [44]. In patients with certain systemic mast cell or autoimmune disorders, abdominal symptoms can mimic food hypersensitivity [45–48]. In both these disorders, increased gastrointestinal mast cells are noted. A recent review of "hidden" allergens in foods by Steinman addresses the reasons for hidden allergens such as contamination of a safe food by utensils or equipment, misleading labels, and ingredient switching [49]. Various useful tables indicating the presence of egg, milk, soy, wheat, and peanut protein are included in this article, along with preventative measures [49].

Hidden allergic reactions to milk-contaminated "nondairy" products were reported with Tofulite, Oscar Meyer hot dogs, bologna, rice cream, and Acme tuna [49]. In fact, canned tuna was reported in an article by Gern et al. to contain sodium caseinate, a milk protein used to promote the packing qualities of the tuna [50]. The variety of manifestations of cow's milk allergy include urticaria, angioedema, atopic dermatitis, rhinitis, wheezing, anaphylactic reactions, various gastrointestinal syndromes, and failure to thrive [51,52]. We evaluated several patients with cow's milk allergy with many of these manifestations that improved on dietary manipulation [53–56].

Other hidden food antigens due to egg proteins can lead to severe reactions. Eggs may be hidden in root beer as a foam agent or in wine and coffee [57]. Unfamiliar hidden labels for egg derivatives can be found on labels such as albumin, ovomucin, ovomucoid, livetin, ovovitellin, and vitellin [58].

Allergic reactions due to exposure to hidden antigenic substances have been reported in the past with contamination of meat and dairy products with penicillin [59–61].

Food-induced anaphylaxis could result from hidden food proteins or the increasing incidence of cross-reactivity described with latex proteins. Hidden nuts and seeds in cakes and cookies could lead to severe reactions. Peanut butter used in chili preparation has resulted in one fatal and one near-fatal reaction of anaphylaxis in unsuspecting restaurant patrons [62]. Peanuts are the most allergenic foods and the most common cause of anaphylaxis. A fatal reaction to peanut antigen in almond icing was reported [63]. Peanut butter may be used to

TABLE 1 Diffferential Diagnosis of Food Allergy

Gastrointestinal tract disorders
  Structural abnormalities
  Hiatal hernia
  Pyloric stenosis
  Tracheoesophageal fistula
Enzyme deficiencies (primary vs. secondary)
  Disaccharidase deficiency (lactase, sucrase-isomaltase and glucoso-galactose)
  Galactosemia
  Phenylketonuria
Malignancy
Others
  Pancreatic insufficiency (cystic fibrosis)
  Gallbladder disease
  Peptic ulcer disease
Contaminants and additives
  Flavorings and preservatives
  Sulfiting agents
  Monosodium glutamate
  Nitrites/nitrates
  Aspartame, benzoates, butylated hydroxytoluene, and butylated hydroxyanisole
Dyes (Tartrazine)
Toxins
  Bacterial (*Clostridium botulinum* and *Staphylococcus aureus*)
  Fungal (aflatoxins, trichothecanes, and ergot)
  Seafood associated
  Scombroid poisoning (tuna and mackerel)
  Ciguatera poisoning (*grouper and snapper, barracuda*)
  Saxitoxin (shellfish)
Infectious organisms
  Bacteria (*Salmonella, Shigella, Escherichia coli, Yersinia,* and *Campylobacter*)
  Parasites (*Giardia* and *Trichinella*)
  Virus (hepatitis, rotavirus, and enterovirus)
Accidental contaminants
  Heavy metals (mercury and copper)
  Pesticides
  Antibiotics (penicillin)
Pharmacological agents
  Caffeine (coffee, tea, soft drinks, and cocoa)
  Theobromine (chocolate, tea)
  Histamine (fish, beer, wine, chocolate, and sauerkraut)
  Tyramine (cheeses, pickled herring, avocado, orange, banana, and tomato)
  Tryptamine (tomato and blue plum)
  Serotonin (banana, tomato, plum, avocado, and pineapple juice)
  Phenylethylamine (chocolate)
  Glycosidal alkaloid solamine (potatoes)
  Alcohol
  Psychological reactions

Source: Ref. 102.

"glue down" ends of egg rolls [64]; in addition, some individuals don't realize peanut butter is used in Oriental cooking and can be hidden in emulsifiers and flavoring in Oriental sauce [49]. Similarly, sulfites in wine, other foods, antioxidants, and medications can lead to anaphylaxis-like events [65].

Masked allergens can be present in processed food. A French group reported a patient with a history of allergy to mustard who had severe anaphylaxis to mustard masked in "chicken dips" [66]. Adverse reactions to hidden food additives can occur with tartrazine, azo, nonazo dyes, and aspartame. Urticaria, asthma, and contact dermatitis have been reported [67]. Hidden substances naturally occurring in food can lead to headache. Foods containing histamine include wine, beer, sauerkraut, and chocolate (which also contains phenylethylamine). Foods containing serotonin, tryptamine, tyramine, dopamine, or norepinephrine include banana, tomato, plum, avocado, orange, pineapple, fermented cheese, wine, pickled herring, and salt dried fish. Foods containing nitrates include spinach, beets, radishes, lettuce, and packaged meats such as sausage, bacon, luncheon meats, and hot dogs [68].

Shellfish are generally not hidden in foods, but occasionally different shellfish may be included in Asian dishes in restaurants, unknown to the persons serving them. Some seafood flavors are added to food in the form of powder from the seafood shell [49]. Soy protein may also be present in tofu, vegetable starch, or broth, and recently one report identified soy protein cross-reactive with latex.

Soy beans may be ingested as whole beans, flour, or oil, and soy bean flour is often added to cereal flour, which is used extensively in the baking industry [49]. Soy products are also used as meat substitutes in vegetarian products in catering centers, including hospital and army food services [49]. Severe allergic reactions have also occurred with cottonseed hidden in cookies [69], psyllium in drugs or cereals [70], and latex cross-reactivity [71–78]. Exercise-induced anaphylaxis has occurred with celery, shellfish, and masked wheat protein [79–81]. Wheat is the most allergenic of all cereals, and wheat gluten is frequently added to baked products made from other grains, including those from soy flour. Occupational asthma confirmed by bronchoprovocation was reported by Park et al.; it was caused by two herbal materials, Sanyak or *Discorea batatas,* and Banha or *Pinellia ternata,* which belong to the Discarreaceae and Araceae families [82]. These Oriental herbal substances are used to treat gastrointestinal and cough symptoms. Bee pollen in certain herbal preparations has also been shown to cause reactions.

LATEX

Several reports have highlighted clinical and immunochemical cross-reactivity between latex and banana, chestnut, avocado, and other fruits [71–78]. A history of allergy to certain other foods in the latex-sensitive individual has been reported for kiwi, papaya, melon, apple, pear, peach, plums, tomatoes, potatoes, cherries, figs, celery, and hazelnut [83]. Health care workers are at increased risk for latex allergy [84]. Although cross-reactive immunological food reactions can occur, they may not be clinically significant [85]. It may be necessary to counsel latex-sensitive health care workers and families of spina bifida patients about hidden or cross-reactive food proteins [86]. We evaluated 38 patients with suspected latex allergy and possible food protein cross-reactivity for in vitro reactivity to kiwi, banana, peach, cherry, walnut, chestnut, and the panplant profilin [87]. Fifteen patients reacted in vitro to latex protein with 0.4 (class II) to 25 or greater (class VI) IU/ml reaction. All the latex-positive patients were also profilin-positive, in contrast to a 45% incidence in the latex-negative group. The frequency of food-positive reactions in the latex-positive group was the following: banana, 80%; walnut, 44%; cherry, 40%; chestnut, 30%; kiwi, 27%; and peach, 20%.

Latex-negative subjects reacted only to banana protein (90%) [87]. Thus, continued exposure to these cross-reactive foods might potentially lead to clinical reactions.

A study from our center reported on systemic anaphylaxis to a hidden cross-reactive food in a surgical resident with latex hypersensitivity [88]. The patient experienced the episode when ingesting snacks that had been kept near guacamole; the reaction progressed to flushing, nasal congestion, pruritus, urticaria, facial angioedema, and wheezing, despite self-administered epinephrine [88]. Cross-reacting allergens in natural rubber latex and avocado were reviewed by Ahlroth et al [89]. These authors demonstrated a large number of inhibitable proteins in immunoblot experiments and clinical observations from skin prick tests suggesting considerable immunological cross-reactivity [89]. Additional cross-reactivities are being identified between latex and other allergens. Anaphylaxis to carrageenan, commonly ingested in milk and pharmaceutical products such as barium enema solutions, has been reported as a pseudo latex allergy [90]. Thus, carrageenan's wide distribution in common foods could account for some symptoms related to milk products or baby formula [90].

All investigations have suggested that in vitro cross-reactivity is partial and RAST inhibition does not necessarily predict clinical sensitivity. It is still unclear whether patients allergic to fruit constitute an independent risk group. Hidden food allergies account for a wide range of urticarial reactions (13%–57%); however, the role of foods is more important in acute than in chronic urticaria [91–96]. In a recent study, chronic urticaria was attributed to foods in 4% and food additives in 2.6% in a group of 226 children [97]. In another CME review article from our center on chronic steroid-resistant urticaria, foods and additives were searched for in a patient with a long history of chronic idiopathic urticaria [98].

Weak in vitro specific IgE to milk protein was noted with class I reactions to short ragweed and *Dermatophagoides farinae*. Class II reactivity was noted to storage mites that can be found in grains [98]. Of interest, anaphylaxis after ingestion of *Dermatophagoides farinae*–contaminated beignets has been reported [99]. Thus, perhaps, *D. farinae* could be considered a "hidden" food allergen as well! DeMaat-Bleeker et al. reported on a patient sensitized to house dust mite reaction after consumption of vineyard snails [100]. Specific IgE to snail (*Eobania vermiculata*) was positive and >80% inhibited by house dust mite. The authors considered this another possible example of food allergy related to primary sensitization by an aeroallergen [100].

PREVENTATIVE MEASURES

Most fatal and near-fatal food reactions occur when eating away from home [30,101]. Individuals with severe food hypersensitivity should avoid processed foods [49], and counseling for cross-reactive foods should be given to high-risk individuals [86,88]. Parents and children should carefully scrutinize food labels, and very sensitive individuals should wear a Medi-Alert bracelet and carry self-injector epinephrine [49]. Registered dietitians should work closely with allergists–immunologists in educating and counseling patients for cross-reactive and hidden foods.

REFERENCES

1. Taylor SL, Bush RK, Busse WW. Avoidance diets: How selective should we be? NER Allergy Proc 1986; 7:527–532.
2. Vaughan WT, Black JH. Practice of Allergy. St. Louis: CV Mosby, 1948, pp 278–279.
3. Vaughan WT, Black JH. Practice of Allergy. St. Louis: CV Mosby 1948, pp 290–291.
4. Barnett D, Bonham B, Howden ME. Allergenic cross-reactions among legume foods: an in vitro study. J Allergy Clin Immunol 1987; 79:433–438.
5. Bernhisel-Broadbent J, Sampson HA. Cross-allergenicity in the legume botanical family in children with food hypersensitivity. J Allergy Clin Immunol 1989; 83:435–440.
6. Bernhisel-Broadbent J, Taylor S, Sampson HA. Cross-allergenicity in the legume botanical family in children with food hypersensitivity. II. Laboratory correlates. J Allergy Clin Immunol 1989; 84:701–709.
7. Eriksson NE. Clustering of food stuffs in food hypersensitivity: an inquiry study in pollen allergic patients. Allergol Immunopathol 1984; 12:28–32.
8. Ortolani C, Pastorello EA, Farioli L et al. IgE mediated allergy from vegetable allergens. Ann Allergy 1993; 71:470–476.
9. Eriksson NE. Food sensitivity reported by patients with asthma and hay fever. Allergy 1978; 33:189–196.
10. Ebner C, Birkner T, Valenta R et al. Common epitopes of birch pollen and apples: Studies by Western and Northern blot. J Allergy Clin Immunol 1991; 88:588–595.

11. Ebner C, Hirshwehr R, Bauer L, Breiteneder H, Valenta R, Ebner H et al. Identification of allergens in fruits and vegetables: IgE cross-reactivities with the important birch pollen allergens. Bet v 1 and Bet v 2 (birch profilin). J Allergy Clin Immunol 1995; 95:962–969.

12. Juhlin-Dannfeldt C. About the occurrence of different types of pollens and its implications for diagnoses and therapy. Nardick Med 1943; 20:2328.

13. Anderson BL, Dreyfuss E, Logans et al. Melon and banana sensitivity conident with ragweed pollinosis. J Allergy 1970; 45:310–319.

14. Ortolani C, Ispano M, Pastorello EA, Bigi A, Ansaloni R. The oral allergy syndrome. Ann Allergy 1988; 61:47–52.

15. Pastorello EA, Ortolani C. In Food Allergy: Adverse Reactions to Foods and Food Additives. Metcalfe DD, Sampson HA, Simon RA, eds. Cambridge, Massachusetts: Blackwell Science 1997, pp 221–233.

16. DeMartino M, Novembre E, Cozza G et al. Sensitivity to tomato and peanut allergens in children monosensitized to grass pollen. Allergy 1988; 43:206–213.

17. Wuthrich B, Stager J, Johannson GGO. Celery allergy associated with birch and mugwort pollinosis. Allergy 1990; 45:566–571.

18. Pastorello EA, Ortolani C, Farioli L, Pravettoni V et al. Allergenic cross-reactivity among peach, apricot, plum, and cherry in patients with oral allergy syndrome: an in vivo and in vitro study. J Allergy Clin Immunol 1994; 94:699–707.

19. Bernhisel-Broadbent J. Allergenic cross-reactivity of foods and characterization of food allergens and extracts. Ann Allergy Asthma Immunol 1995; 75:295–303.

20. Kelso J, Jones R, Tellez R, Yunginger J. Oral allergy syndrome successfully treated with pollen immunotherapy. Ann Allergy Asthma Immunol 1995; 74:391–396.

21. Langeland T. A clinical and immunological study of allergy to hen's egg white. VI. Occurrence of proteins cross-reacting with allergens in hen's egg white as studied in egg white from turkey, duck, goose, seagull, and in hen egg yolk and hen and chicken sera and flesh. Allergy 1983; 39:399–412.

22. Bernhisel-Broadbent J, Dintzis HM, Dintzis RZ, Sampson HA. Allergenicity and antigenicity of chicken egg ovomucoid (Gal d III) compared with ovalbumin (Gal d I) in children with egg allergy and in mice. J Allergy Clin Immunol 1994; 93:1047–1059.

23. Mandallaz M, de Weck AL, Dahinden C. Bird-egg syndrome: Cross reactivity between bird antigens and egg-yolk livetins in IgE mediated hypersensitivity. Int Arch Allergy Appl Immunol 1988; 87:143–150.

24. Szepfalusi Z, Ebner C, Pandjaitan R, Orlicek F, Scheiner O, Boltz-Nitulescu G et al. Egg yolk a-livetin (chicken serum albumin) is a cross-reactive allergen in the bird-egg syndrome. J Allergy Clin Immunol 1994; 93:932–942.

25. Juntunen K, Ali-Yrkkos. Goat's milk for children allergic to cow's milk. Kiel Milchwirt Forschungsber 1983; 35:439.

26. Bernhisel-Broadbent J, Voker RH, Sampson HA. Allergenicity of orally administered immunoglobulin preparations in food allergic children. Pediatrics 1990; 87:208–214.

27. Werfel S, Cooke S, Sampson HA. Clinical reactivity to beef in cow milk allergic children. J Allergy Clin Immunol 1996.

28. Taylor SL, Lemanski RF, Bush RK, Busse WW. Food allergens: structure and immunologic properties. Ann Allergy 1987; 59:93–99.

29. Bernhisel-Broadbent J. Allergenic cross-reactivity of foods and characterization of food allergens and extracts. Ann Allergy Asthma Immunol 1995; 75:295–303.

30. Boch SA, Atkins FM. The natural history of peanut allergy. J Allergy Clin Immunol 1989; 83:900–904.

31. Hefle SL, Lemanski RF, Bush RK. Adverse reaction to lupine-fortified pasta. J Allergy Clin Immunol 1994; 94:167–172,

32. Shanti KN, Martin BM, Nagpal S et al. Identification of tropomyosin as the major shrimp allergen and characterization of its IgE-binding epitopes. J Immunol 1993; 151:5354–5363.

33. Bernhisel-Broadbent J, Scanlon SM, Sampson HA. Fish hypersensitivity. I. In vitro and oral challenge results in fish allergic patients. J Allergy Clin Immunol 1992; 89:730–737.

34. Jones SM, Magnolfic Cooke SA, Sampson HA. Immunologic cross-reactivity among cereal grains and grasses in children with food hypersensitivity. J Allergy Clin Immunol 1995; 96:341–351.

35. Valenta R, Duchene M, Ebner C et al. Profilins constitute a novel family of functional plant panallergens. J Exp Med 1992; 175:377–385.

36. Van Ree R, Voitenko V, van Leeuwen WA, Aalberse RC. Profilin is a cross-reactive allergen in pollen and vegetable foods. Int Arch Allergy Appl Immunol 1992; 98:97–104. 1992.

37. Niinimaki A, Hannuksela M, Makinen-Kiljunen S. Skin prick test and in vitro immunoassays with native spices and spice extracts. Ann Allergy Asthma Immunol 1995; 75:280.

38. Helbling A, Lopez M, Schwartz J, Lehrer SB. Reactivity of carrot-specific IgE antibodies with celery, apiaceous spices and birch pollen. Ann Allergy 1993; 70:495–499.

39. Gall H, Kalveram KJ, Forck G, Sterry W. Kiwi fruit allergy: a new birch pollen-associated food allergy. J Allergy Clin Immunol 1994; 94:70–76.

40. Vocks E, Borga A, Szliska C, Seifert HU et al. Common allergenic structures in hazelnut, rye grain, sesame seeds, kiwi and poppy seeds. Allergy 1993; 48:168–172.

41. Garcia Ortiz JC, Cosmes Martin P, Lopez-Asun Solo A. Melon sensitivity shares allergens with Plantago and grass pollens. Allergy 1995; 50:269–273.

42. Wagner-Jordan DL, Whisman BA, Goetz DW. Cross-allergenicity among celery, cucumber, carrot, and watermelon. Ann Allergy 1993; 71:70–79.

43. Aalhuse RC, Koshte V, Clemens JGJ. Immunoglobulin E antibodies that cross-react with vegetable foods, pollen and Hymenoptera venom. J Allergy Clin Immunol 1981; 68:356–364.

44. Sampson HA. Differential diagnosis in adverse reactions to foods. J Allergy Clin Immunol 1986; 78:212.

45. Frieri M, Steinberg SC, Metcalfe DD. A controlled trial of the effects of oral disodium cromoglycate or the combination of chlorpheniramine and cimetidine in the treatment of systemic mastocytosis. Am J Med 1985; 78:9–14.

46. Frieri M, Claus M, Martinez S et al. Fever, hemorrhagic bullae and gastritis in a 20 month old male. Ann Allergy 1989; 63:179–183.
47. Frieri M, Linn N, Schweitzer M, Angadi C et al. Lymphadenopathic mastocytosis with eosinophilia and biclonal gammopathy. J Allergy Clin Immunol 1990; 86:126–132.
48. Frieri M. Systemic sclerosis: the role of the mast cell and cytokines: CME review article. Ann Allergy 1992; 69:385–397.
49. Steinman HA. Rostrum: "hidden" allergens in foods. J Allergy Clin Immunol 1996; 98:241–250.
50. Gern JE, Yang E, Evrard HM, Sampson HA. Allergic reactions to milk contaminated "non-dairy" products. N Engl J Med 1991; 324:976.
51. Goldman AS, Anderson DW Jr., Sellers NA et al. Milk allergy. I. Oral challenge with milk and isolated milk proteins in allergic children. Pediatrics 1963; 32:425.
52. Sampson HA. Food allergy. J Allergy Clin Immunol 1989; 84:1062.
53. Frieri M, Martinez S, Agarwal K et al. Cytokine detection and effect of dietary modification in food hypersensitivity. Presented at the VII International Food Allergy Symposium, July 1990.
54. Frieri M, Martinez S, Young R et al. Preliminary investigation of interleukin-4 in food hypersensitivity in atopic patients. Clin Res 1990; 38:486a.
55. Frieri, M, Martinez S, Agarwal K, Trotta P. A preliminary study of interleukin-4 detection in atopic pediatric and young adult patients Pediatr Asthma Allergy Immunol 1993; 7;27–35.
56. Martinez S, Dominquez J, Klotz, SD, Frieri M. Atopic dermatitis with extremely elevated IgE, Ann Allergy 1995; p4: p28.
57. Criep LH. Etiology of atopy. In: LH Criep, ed. Allergy and Clinical Immunology. New York: Grune & Stratton, 1976, pp 147–160.
58. Greenberg LE, Moses NS. Egg-free and corn-free diets. In: Chiarmonte LT, Schneider AT, Lifshitz F; eds. Food Allergy. New York: Marcel Dekker, 1988, pp 441–452.
59. Seigel BB. Hidden contacts with penicillin. Bull World Health Organ 1959; 21;703–713.
60. Dewdney JM, Edwards RG. Penicillin hypersensitivity: is milk a significant hazard? A review. JR Soc Med 1986; 77;866–877.
61. Friend BA, Shahani KM. Antibiotics in foods. In: Finley JW, Schwass DE, eds. Xenobiotics in foods and feeds. Washington DC: American Chemical Society, 1986, pp 47–61.
62. FDA Ad Hoc Committee on Hypersensitivity to Food Constituents. Report. Washington, DC:U.S. Food & Drug Administration, 1986.
63. Evans S, Skea D, Dolovich J. Fatal reaction to peanut antigen in almond icing. Can Med Assoc J 1988; 139:231–232.
64. Loza C, Brostoff J. Peanut allergy (review). Clin Exp Allergy 1995; 25:493–502.
65. Taylor SL, Bush RK, Nardlee JA. Chapter 17. In: Metcalfe DD, Sampson HA, Simon RA, eds. Food Allergy. Cambridge, MA: Blackwell Scientific, 1991, pp 239–260.
66. Kanny G, Fremont S, Talhouarne G et al. Anaphylaxis to mustard as a masked allergen in chicken dips. Ann Allergy Asthma Immunol 1995;75:340.

67. Stevenson DD. Tartrazine, azo and non-azodyes. In: Food Allergy. Metcalfe DD, Sampson HA, Simon RA, eds. Cambridge, MA: 1991, Blackwell Science pp 267–275.
68. Condemi J. Foods and Headache. ACAAI 45th Annual Congress Syllabus, 1988, pp 105–107.
69. Atkins FM, Wilson M, Bock SA. Cottonseed hypersensitivity: new concerns over an old problem. J Allergy Clin Immunol 1988; 82:242.
70. Posner LH, Mandarano C, Zitt MJ, Frieri M et al. Recurrent bronchospasm in a nurse. Ann Allergy 1986; 56:14.
71. M'Raihi L, Charpin D, Pons A, Bongrand P, Vervloet D. Cross-reactivity between latex and banana. J Allergy Clin Immunol 1991; 87:129–130.
72. Young MC, Osleeb C, Slater J. Latex and banana anaphylaxis (abstr). J Allergy Clin Immunol 1992; 89:226.
73. Ross BD, McCullough J, Ownby DR. Partial cross-reactivity between latex and banana allergens. J Allergy Clin Immunol 1992; 90:409–410.
74. Lavaud F, Cossart C, Reiter V, Bernard J, Deltour G, Holmquist I. Latex allergy in patient with allergy to fruit (letter). Lancet 1992; 339:492–493.
75. Ceuppens JL, Van Durme P, Dooms-Goossens A. Latex allergy in patient with allergy to fruit (letter). Lancet 1992; 339–493.
76. deCorres LF, Moneo I, Munoz D, Bernaola G, Fernandez E, Audicana M, Urrutia I. Sensitization from chestnuts and bananas in patients with urticaria and anaphylaxis from contact with latex. Ann Allergy 1993; 70:35–39.
77. Rodriquez M, Vega F, Garcia MT, Panizo C, Laffond E, Montalvo A, Cuevas M. Hypersensitivity to latex, chestnut, and banana. Ann Allergy 1993; 70:31–34.
78. Makinen-Kiljunen S, Alenius H, Ahlroth M, Turjanmaa K, Palosuo T, Reunala T. Immunoblot inhibition detects several common allergens in rubber latex and banana (abstr) J Allergy Clin Immunol 1993; 91:242.
79. Silverstein SR, Frommer DA, Dobozin B, Rosen P. Celery-dependent exercise-induced anaphylaxis. J Emerg Med 1986; 4:195–199.
80. Maulitz RM, Pratt DA, Schocket AL. Exercise-induced anaphylactic reaction to shellfish. J Allergy Clin Immunol 1979; 63(6):433–434.
81. Kushimoto H, Aoki T. Masked type I wheat allergy. Arch Dermatol 1985; 121:355–360.
82. Park HS, Kim MJ, Moon HB. Occupational asthma caused by two herb materials, *Dioscorea batatas* and *Pinellia ternata*. Clin Exp Allergy 1994; 24:575–581.
83. Blanco C, Carrillo T, Castillo R, Quiralte J et al. Latex allergy: clinical features and cross-reactivity with fruits. Ann Allergy 1994; 73(4):309–314.
84. Frieri M. Latex hypersensitivity in health care workers and high risk patients Nassau County Medical Center proceedings. 1997; 24:1–6.
85. Frieri M. Food allergy. In: Kaliner MA, ed. Current Review of Allergic Diseases, Current Medicine, 1999, pp 173–182 Blackwell Science.
86. Fitzgerald D, Chavarria V, Cosachov J, Zitt M, Frieri M. Evaluation and counseling of latex allergic subjects. J Allergy Clin Immunol 1994; 93:7a.
87. Tillah F, Therattil J, Mitrache I, Dellavechia D, Frieri M. Latex allergy and food cross-reactivity in an outpatient setting. Ann Allergy Asthma Immunol 1998; 80:A.

88. Therattil J, Frieri M. Systemic anaphylaxis to a hidden cross-reactive food in a surgical resident with latex hypersensitivity. Pediatr Asthma Allergy Immunology, 1997;11:141–146.
89. Ahlroth M, Alenius H, Turjanmaa K et al. Cross-reacting allergens in natural rubber latex and avocado. J Allergy Clin Immunol 1995; 96:167–173.
90. Tarlo SM, Dolovich J, Listgarten C. Anaphylaxis to carrageenan: a pseudo-latex allergy. J Allergy Clin Immunol 1995; 95:933–936.
91. Sehgal VN, Rege VL. An interrogative study of 158 urticaria patients. Ann Allergy 1973; 31:279–283.
92. Nizami RM, Baboo MT, Sehgal VN, Rege VL. Office management of patients 55: an interrogative study of 158 urticaria patients. Ann Allergy 1973; 31:279–283.
93. Kauppinen K, Juntunen K, Lanki H. Urticaria in children: retrospective evaluation and follow-up. Allergy 1984; 39:469–472.
94. Halpern SR. Chronic hives in children: an analysis of 75 cases. Ann Allergy 1965; 23:589–599.
95. Champion RH, Roberts SOB, Carpenter RG, Roger JH. Urticaria and angioedema: a review of 554 patients. Br J Dermatol 1969; 81:588–597.
96. Harris A, Twarog FJ, Geha RF. Chronic urticaria in childhood: natural course and etiology. Ann Allergy 1983; 51:161–165.
97. Volonakis M, Katsari Katsarou A, Stratigos J. Etiologic factors in childhood chronic urticaria. Ann Allergy 1992; 69:61.
98. Frieri M, Madden J. Chronic steroid resistant urticaria. Ann Allergy 1993; 70:1–7.
99. Erken A, Rodriques JL, McCullough J et al. Anaphylaxis following ingestion of *D. farinae* contaminated beignet. J Allergy Clin Immunol 1992; 208a.
100. DeMaat-Bleeker F, Akkerdaas JH, Van Ree R et al. Vineyard snail allergy possibly induced by sensitization to house dust mite (Dermatophagoides pteronyssinus). Allergy 1995; 50:438–440.
101. Sampson HA, Mendelson L, Rosen JP. Fatal and near-fatal-induced anaphylaxis. N Engl J Med 1992; 327:380–384.
102. Simpson HA, Buckley RH, Metcalfe DD. Food allergy. JAMA 1987; 258:2886–2890.

8

Allergylike Intoxications from Foods

STEVE L. TAYLOR AND SUSAN L. HEFLE
University of Nebraska, Lincoln, Nebraska

DISTINCTIONS BETWEEN TRUE FOOD ALLERGIES AND ALLERGYLIKE INTOXICATIONS

True food allergies involve abnormal responses of the immune system to substances, usually proteins, in foods. Immunoglobulin E– (IgE) mediated food allergies are the most familiar example. True food allergies affect only a small portion of the population. The tolerance level for the offending food in true food allergies is not precisely known, but allergic individuals are unable, in many cases, to tolerate even very small amounts of the offending food.

Allergylike intoxications mimic true food allergies in terms of symptoms and onset times. However, these illnesses do not involve responses of the immune system. Although some differences may exist in the degree of susceptibility of individuals, everyone is susceptible to allergylike intoxications. However, in contrast to true food allergies, tolerances do exist for the offending substances so that the ingestion of small amounts does not elicit any adverse reaction.

HISTAMINE INTOXICATION

Histamine poisoning is the most commonly encountered allergylike intoxication. Outbreaks of histamine intoxication, sometimes referred to as scombroid fish poisoning, occur with some frequency in the United States, Europe, Japan, and other countries. Histamine intoxication is thought to be caused by the ingestion of foods containing high levels of histamine, a substance that is not normally present in foods at such elevated levels. Several recent studies have questioned the role of food-borne histamine in scombroid fish poisoning.

Clinical Features

Symptoms

Since histamine is one of the primary mediators released from mast cells in IgE-mediated food allergies, the similarity in symptoms between histamine intoxication and IgE-mediated food allergy should not be surprising. However, like IgE-mediated food allergies, the symptoms can be variable and are not particularly definitive. A wide variety of symptoms can occur in cases of histamine intoxication, although the illness is typically rather mild [1,2]. Gastrointestinal complaints such as nausea, vomiting, diarrhea, and abdominal cramps are common. Tingling, itching, and burning sensations often occur in the mouth and can be accompanied by flushing, urticaria, and angioedema. Often, urticaria and other itchy rashes appear systemically as well. Hypotension is a common manifestation. Other common symptoms include headache and palpitations. Most patients suffer only a few of these symptoms. In the study of a large series of outbreaks in the United Kingdom, the most common symptoms were rash, diarrhea, flushing and sweating, and headache [3]. Such symptoms are not particularly definitive; as a result, misdiagnosis of histamine intoxication is common.

Although histamine intoxication is usually rather mild, serious cardiac and respiratory complications can occur on rare occasions [4,5]. These more serious, life-threatening conditions seem to occur in individuals who have preexisting cardiac and respiratory conditions. We are aware of one alleged death from histamine poisoning in an individual with preexisting cardiac problems and a colostomy. Russell and Maretic [4] described the case of a young asthmatic child who experienced respiratory collapse after consuming fish contaminated with high levels of histamine.

Onset Time and Duration

Histamine poisoning is a typical acute chemical intoxication with symptoms appearing within minutes to a few hours after ingestion of the offending food [1]. The oral symptoms, when they occur, are often noted first and frequently occur while the food is being masticated. Histamine intoxication is a self-limited illness. Even without treatment, symptoms usually subside within a few hours. However, if left untreated, symptoms can persist for as long as 24 to 48 hr [6]. The duration of the symptoms may be a function of the dose of exposure and/or the susceptibility of the affected individual. Effective treatment leads to a prompt resolution of the symptoms.

Diagnosis

The diagnosis of histamine poisoning is contingent upon the association of the ingestion of one of the more commonly implicated foods with the rapid onset of symptoms typical of histamine intoxication [1,2]. Recognition of the symptoms of histamine poisoning will often arouse suspicion regarding this possible diagnosis. However, as noted earlier, the symptoms of histamine intoxication are not definitive, although the development of allergylike symptoms such as urticaria or other rashes would eliminate many other possible diagnoses. The physician must be thorough in inquiring about the symptoms experienced by the patient. Symptoms such as an oral burning sensation (sometimes characterized as a peppery taste), tingling, flushing, and even mild headache may be ignored by the patient but can be quite helpful in making the correct diagnosis [2]. Even when the patient only experiences gastrointestinal complaints, the short onset time of histamine intoxication would allow differentiation between this illness and many of the food-borne bacterial and viral infections with longer incubation periods. If histamine poisoning is even remotely suspected, the physician should inquire about foods eaten at the most recent meal. The identification of one of the foods commonly implicated in histamine intoxication, such as certain fish or cheeses, would strengthen the likelihood of histamine intoxication as the diagnosis. A beneficial response of the patient to antihistamines would further strengthen the diagnosis [6–8].

A diagnosis of histamine intoxication can be confirmed only by analysis of the suspect food with the detection of unusually high levels of histamine [1,2]. Samples of the incriminated food should be sought immediately whenever histamine intoxication is suspected. Since histamine poisoning often occurs in food service facilities, the assistance of local health departments should be sought for obtaining the appropriate samples where necessary. In cases involving food service facilities, the local health authorities should be contacted because of the potential for a more widespread outbreak of histamine poisoning. The accepted procedure for the analysis of histamine in the incriminated food involves extraction, cleanup, and fluorometric analysis [9]. Although this analytical procedure is not difficult, many laboratories have little, if any, experience in the analysis of foods for histamine. In cases where food samples are not available, the confirmation of the diagnosis of histamine is probably impossible. Vomitus and/or stomach contents could be analyzed for histamine, but baseline data on histamine levels in these materials are not readily available [2]. Blood analysis for histamine could be attempted, but the rapid metabolism of histamine would be expected to complicate this approach unless samples could be obtained soon after ingestion of the incriminated food. Urine analysis for histamine and its metabolites would be another potential approach [1,10], but it has not been attempted to our knowledge.

Histamine poisoning is often misdiagnosed as an allergic reaction to food because of the similarities in symptoms and the beneficial effects of antihistamines on both conditions. However, histamine intoxications can be easily distinguished from IgE-mediated food allergies [1,6]. In cases of histamine intoxication, the patient typically has no prior history of allergic reactions to the implicated food and may not even have any sort of allergic history. By contrast, the patient usually is well aware of existing IgE-mediated food allergies. In addition, skin prick tests with commercial extracts of the food will have negative results if no IgE-mediated allergy exists in the patient. But if an extract is made of the actual incriminated food, the skin prick test finding can be positive as a result of the presence of histamine in the extract. Also, the patient should be asked whether others consuming the same meal experienced similar symptoms. With histamine intoxication, the attack rates in group outbreaks are often 50%–100%. With IgE-mediated food allergies, in contrast, it would be rare to encounter two individuals sharing the same meal who would experience the same food allergy. If the reaction occurred in a restaurant, the local health authorities may be helpful in locating other patrons who purchased the same meal, especially if they were also subsequently treated for symptoms of histamine intoxication. Finally, histamine intoxication can be distinguished from IgE-mediated food allergy by analysis of the incriminated food and detection of abnormally high levels of histamine.

Treatment

The administration of antihistamines is the most effective treatment in patients suffering from histamine intoxication. The H_1 antagonists such as diphenhydramine and chlorpheniramine are the usual choices for treatment [7]. However, H_2 antagonists such as cimetidine are also effective [8]. Even without treatment, the symptoms of histamine intoxication will usually subside within a few hours. However, treatment with antihistamines will shorten the duration of the illness and lessen the discomfort experienced by the patient.

Foods Associated with Histamine Intoxication

Fish

Fish are the foods most commonly implicated in outbreaks of histamine intoxication [1,11]. This food-borne disease is sometimes referred to as scombroid fish poisoning because of the frequent assocation with fish from the families

Scomberesocidae and Scombridae. Tuna, skipjack, mackerel, bonito, and albacore are common types of scombroid fish, although albacore have not been implicated in cases of histamine intoxication to our knowledge. Tuna, skipjack, and mackerel are very frequently involved in cases of histamine intoxication. However, certain types of nonscombroid fish are also commonly involved. Examples include mahi-mahi, bluefish, jack mackerel, sardines, yellowtail, anchovies, and herring. In the United States, mahi-mahi has become one of the most frequent offending foods in cases of histamine intoxication. Sardines, anchovies, and herring have been occasionally implicated in Europe, but, thus far, histamine poisoning episodes in the United States have not involved these species. These species of fish do not elicit histamine poisoning unless they contain elevated levels of histamine. The Food and Drug Administration considers 50 mg of histamine per 100 g of fish to be hazardous for tuna on the basis of the investigation of numerous outbreaks [12]. Occasionally, other fish species are identified in isolated cases of histamine intoxication. However, unless the fish has been identified by experts, the accuracy of these identifications could be questioned. Evidence for the involvement of fish other than those mentioned is questionable. The total lack of involvement of freshwater fish in histamine intoxication is noteworthy.

Cheeses

Outbreaks of histamine poisoning from cheese are much less frequent than outbreaks involving fish [2]. Swiss cheese has been implicated in several outbreaks of histamine intoxication in the United States [2,13,14]. All of these episodes involved the ingestion of Swiss cheese containing in excess of 100 mg of histamine per 100 g of cheese [2]. Few retail Swiss cheese samples contain such elevated levels [15]. Cheddar and Gouda cheeses have been implicated in single incidents of histamine poisoning [6,17], but histamine content of these cheeses is typically quite low.

Other Foods

Other foods, beyond fish and cheese, are rarely, if ever, implicated in cases of histamine intoxication. Chicken, sauerkraut, shellfish, and ham have individually been implicated in one incident [1,18]. However, firm evidence linking the ingestion of these foods to histamine intoxication was missing in all of these episodes. Confirmed episodes including the detection of high levels of histamine in the implicated products will be necessary to establish a definite role for these foods in histamine intoxication.

Histamine may be a cause of wine intolerance [19]. In a challenge study with 125 ml of red wine containing 50 µg of histamine, 22 of 28 patients experienced a significant rise in plasma histamine level within 30 min along with some symptoms consistent with histamine intoxication [19].

Certain other foods, especially fermented foods, are known to contain high levels of histamine [1,13]. Beer; fermented sausages, e.g., salami and pepperoni; sauerkraut, and other fermented vegetables; various fermented soy products; and fermented fish products do contain elevated levels of histamine [1,13]. However, the levels are often lower than the levels found in cheese and spoiled fish products. None of these products, with the exception of the single case involving sauerkraut, has ever been associated with histamine poisoning.

Formation of Histamine in Foods

Histamine formation in foods is associated with the growth of bacteria possessing the enzyme histidine decarboxylase (Fig. 1). These bacteria are able to convert the amino acid histidine into histamine. Only a few species of bacteria are capable of the prolific levels of histamine formation necessary to develop hazardous food products. In fish, *Morganella morganii* and *Klebsiella pneumoniae* are two species with such capabilities [1,20,21]. If fish are contaminated with such histamine-producing bacteria (and most are not), the bacteria can convert large amounts of histidine to histamine in a relatively short period when the fish are held at elevated temperatures. Such fish will not necessarily appear to be spoiled even though they contain hazardous levels of histamine. Tuna and related species may be especially susceptible to histamine formation because they have high levels of free histidine in their tissues [22].

In cheese, certain species of lactobacilli are probably responsible for histamine formation. Histamine formation is a rather unusual trait among lactobacilli [2]; however, some strains of *Lactobacillus buchneri, L. delbreuckii, L. brevis, L. fermentum, L. lactis,* and *L. helviticus* have been identified as prolific histamine-producing bacteria capable of growth in cheeses [15,23,24]. Several factors may contribute to histamine formation in cheese, including higher ripening temperatures, excessive proteolysis, high pH, and low salt concentration [15,25]. The process used to make Swiss cheese is especially conducive to histamine formation, and the levels of histamine in Swiss cheese appear to be dependent primarily on the number of histamine-producing bacteria in the raw milk supply [25].

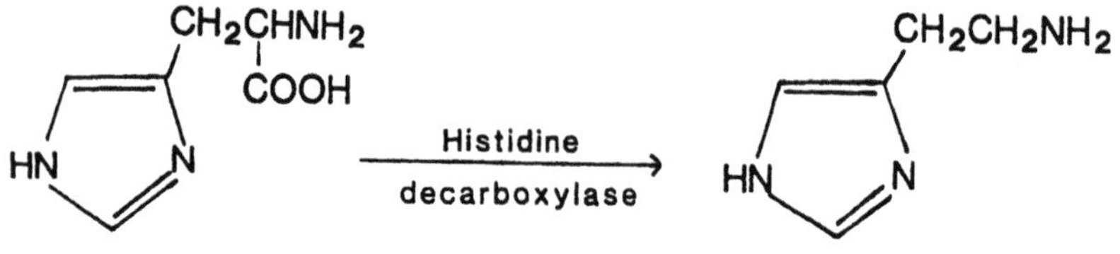

FIGURE 1 The histidine decarboxylase reaction.

Toxicological Properties of Histamine

Fortunately, histamine is much less potent when taken orally than it is when released or administered intravenously [1]. Humans can tolerate milligram levels of histamine orally without untoward effects, whereas microgram amounts administered intravenously will elicit symptoms [26]. Challenges with humans have indicated no adverse effects at doses up to 180 mg of pure histamine [26], only mild symptoms at doses of 100 to 180 mg with good quality tuna [27], mild symptoms at doses of 300 mg with good quality mackerel [28], and mild, subjective symptoms at doses of 90 mg with herring that had been incubated with a histamine-producing bacterium [29]. The lack of toxicity of orally administered histamine is not particularly surprising since humans have several enzymes in the intestinal mucosa, diamine oxidase and histamine-N-methyltransferase, that are capable of detoxifying histamine [1]. The toxicity of histamine may be increased by ingesting histamine in red wine: Wantke et al. [19] observed symptoms after challenge with 50 µg of histamine in 125 ml of wine, although the reasons for this increased toxicity are not known.

In fact, the role of food-borne histamine in scombroid fish poisoning has been questioned by some investigators [30,31]. Volunteers consumed mackerel samples that had been implicated in outbreaks of scombroid fish poisoning, and no correlation was observed between the dose of histamine and the likelihood of an adverse reaction [30,31]. The lowest dose of histamine eliciting a positive reaction was 0.3 mg/kg body weight; the highest dose that did not produce a reaction in a previously susceptible person was 2.8 mg/kg [30]. However, chlorpheniramine abolished the adverse effects observed in some individuals with specific samples of spoiled mackerel [31]. Thus, Ijomah et al. [31] postulated that spoiled fish contain an as-yet-unidentified substance that induces the degranulation of mast cells such that scombroid fish poisoning is caused by the release of endogenous histamine rather than the ingestion of exogenous histamine. Thus, the mechanism may be an anaphylactoid reaction. In contrast, Morrow et al. [32] asserted that exogenous histamine was the likely causative agent in scombroid fish poisoning. These investigators found high levels of histamine and one of its metabolites, N-methylhistamine, in the urine of three individuals experiencing scombroid fish poisoning from marlin [32]. They were unable to find elevated urinary levels of the prostaglandin D_2 metabolite, 9α, 11β-dihydroxy-15-oxo-2,3,18,19-tetranorprost-5-ene-1, 20-dioic acid, suggesting that mast cell degranulation had not occurred [32]. The use of tryptase as a measure of mast cell degranulation would have been preferable, but to our knowledge that has never been done.

Although the role of food-borne histamine in this syndrome has not been completely resolved, there is little dispute that histamine plays a critical role in this illness. For the physician, whether scombroid fish poisoning is caused by endogenous histamine or exogenous histamine, treatment with antihistamines remains appropriate.

Some individual variability is likely in susceptibility to histamine poisoning [2]. Clifford et al. [30] noted considerable differences in individual susceptibility to ingestion of mackerel fillets that had been implicated in a scombroid fish poisoning outbreak. Certainly, it is well known that some individuals may be compromised in their ability to detoxify and excrete histamine [2]. Several drugs including isoniazid can inhibit the detoxification of histamine and are likely to increase sensitivity to histamine. Isoniazid has been implicated as a contributing factor in several outbreaks of histamine poisoning [33,34]. Alternatively, individuals taking antihistamines for various reasons may be protected to some extent from the effects of histamine [2].

Preventive Measures

Although the role of exogenous histamine remains controversial, a key to the prevention of histamine intoxication is prevention of spoilage and histamine formation. Although efforts have focused on prevention of histamine formation, the mast cell–degranulating factor, if present, must also be formed during spoilage because freshly caught and/or properly refrigerated/frozen fish do not cause illness. Holding fish at temperatures below 5°C prevents histamine formation [1].

Another important approach is the elimination of the source of histamine. Good hygienic practices may be important in the control of histamine formation [1]. Since most of the histamine-producing bacteria in fish are enteric bacteria, human handling of the fish after catch may be the source of contamination. Good hygienic practices should be maintained during distribution, storage, handling, processing, and preparation to prevent contamination of the fish. With cheese, the control of histamine formation seems tied to the reduction in the number of histamine-producing bacteria in the raw milk [25]. Thus, the risk should be quite small in any cheese made from pasteurized milk.

MONOAMINE INTOXICATION

A wide variety of monoamines occur in foods, but only a few have been implicated in food-borne disease. The structures of several of these important monoamines are shown in Figure 2.

Clinical Features

The majority of monoamine intoxications have been associated with tyramine, a decarboxylation product of tyrosine [35]. Other monoamines of some importance in monoamine intoxications include 2-phenylethylamine, tryptamine, serotonin, and dopamine.

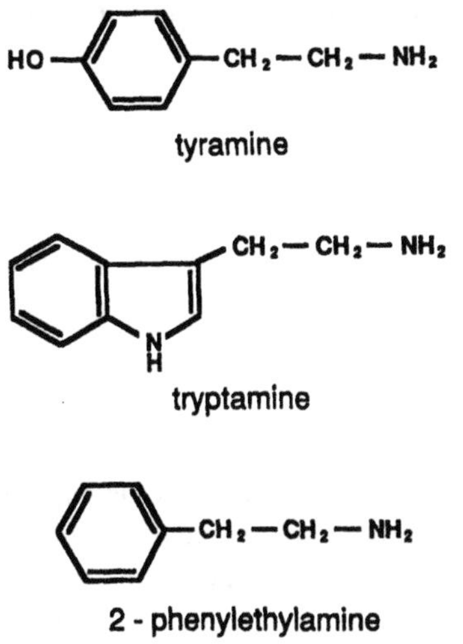

HO—⟨benzene ring⟩—CH_2—CH_2—NH_2

tyramine

⟨indole ring⟩ CH_2—CH_2—NH_2

tryptamine

⟨benzene ring⟩—CH_2—CH_2—NH_2

2 - phenylethylamine

FIGURE 2 Structures of several important food-borne monoamines.

The symptoms of monoamine intoxication include severe headache, hypertension, palpitations, flushing, profuse perspiration, stiff neck, nausea, vomiting, and prostration [35]. The type and severity of symptoms vary from case to case and are dependent upon individual susceptibility and the dose of exposure. Severe headache and hypertension are the most definitive symptoms, and their development after the ingestion of certain foods, especially among certain susceptible individuals, should lead to a tentative diagnosis of monoamine intoxication. These monoamines are often known as pressor amines because of their ability to elicit increases in blood pressure.

The symptoms of monoamine intoxication typically appear within minutes to a few hours after ingestion of the incriminated food [35]. Symptoms can last from 10 min to about 6 hr. Although symptoms can be treated, prevention is the primary strategy.

Foods Associated with Monoamine Intoxication

The food most commonly involved in episodes of monoamine intoxication is cheese, particularly aged cheddar cheese [35]. Numerous episodes of hypertension and headache associated with the ingestion of cheeses were recorded in the early 1960s [36]. Cheeses, especially cheddar cheese, can contain considerable quantities of tyramine, although lesser amounts of tryptamine and 2-phenylethylamine are also present. The level of the various monoamines in cheeses is quite variable, but cheddar cheese can contain up to 1800 ppm of tyramine [35]. Tyramine and the other monoamines are formed in cheese by bacteria (discussed later) during the fermentation process.

Tyramine intoxication has also resulted from ingestion of pickled herring, yeast extract (a British product often known as Vegemite), and chicken livers [35,36]. Other monoamines have been implicated in a few isolated incidents of monoamine intoxication including 2-phenylethylamine in chocolate and dopamine in broad beans [35]. Other foods may also serve as good sources of these and other monoamines, but actual intoxication has not been recorded.

Formation of Monoamines in Foods

Monoamines are formed in foods from the decarboxylation of amino acids; the general reaction is depicted in Figure 3. These decarboxylation reactions are catalyzed by a variety of different amino acid decarboxylase enzymes found in certain bacteria [35]. Small quantities of a wide variety of monoamines occur naturally in plants, probably as a result of their formation by amino acid decarboxylases found in plants [37]. However, the levels of monoamines found in plants are usually far below any level that is hazardous to consumers.

Tyramine is formed in foods by the action of bacterial tyrosine decarboxylase [35]. Tyrosine decarboxylase is found in several types of bacteria, including most clostridia, a few lactobacilli, the group D streptococci, *Leuconostoc cremoris,* some strains of *Escherichia coli,* and some strains of various *Proteus* species [35]. The group D streptococci are the most common source of tyramine in cheeses.

Phenylalanine decarboxylase, which catalyzes the formation of 2-phenylethylamine, occurs rarely in bacteria [35]. Hence, it is found infrequently and at relatively low levels in most foods. Phenylalanine decarboxylase is only known to occur in some strains of *Enterococcus faecalis* and a few unusual *Pseudomonas* species [35].

The distribution of tryptophan decarboxylase, the enzyme responsible for tryptamine formation, in bacteria has not been studied. Since small quantities of tryptamine are found in most food products, this enzyme is not likely to be widely distributed.

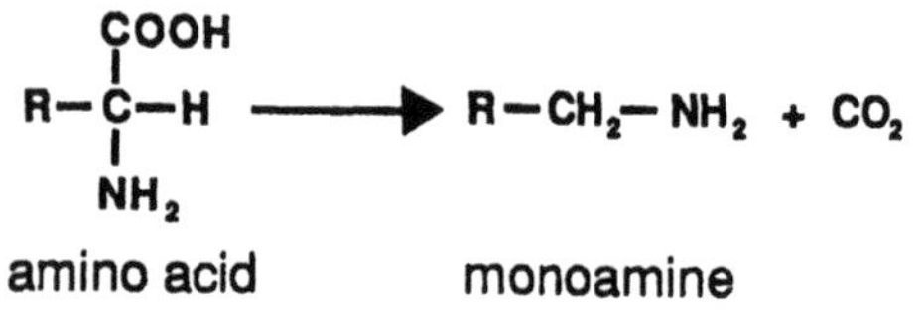

$$R-\underset{\underset{NH_2}{|}}{\overset{\overset{COOH}{|}}{C}}-H \longrightarrow R-CH_2-NH_2 + CO_2$$

amino acid   monoamine

FIGURE 3   The general reaction for the formation of monoamines.

Toxicological Properties of Ingested Monoamines

Monoamine intoxications occur infrequently. Rather large quantities of monoamines can be safely ingested by most individuals; for example, up to 80 mg of tyramine can be taken orally with no elevation of blood pressure in normal individuals [35,36]. The lack of oral toxicity of the monoamines is due to the fact that they are detoxified in the intestinal tract [35]. Monoamine oxidase is the primary enzyme involved in this detoxification process. Certain individuals who are taking certain types of therapeutic drugs have impaired ability to detoxify the monoamines. Among the drugs that are known inhibitors of monoamine oxidase are tranylcypromine, pargyline, and iproniazid [35,36]. When tranylcypromine and pargyline were introduced in the late 1950s for the treatment of depression, hypertensive crises began to be noticed in patients who had consumed cheeses while taking the drugs [35,36]. This led to the discovery of this classic food–drug interaction. In the early 1960s, several severe reactions and deaths occurred before this association was made [36]. Drugs known to be inhibitors of monoamine oxidase now contain label warnings to avoid eating foods that serve as significant sources of monoamines. The *Physician's Desk Reference* lists a variety of foods that should be avoided by individuals taking monoamine oxidase–inhibiting drugs including cheese, pickled herring, yeast extract, chicken liver, broad beans, chocolate, sour cream, wine, beer, sherry, canned figs, raisins, bananas, avocados, soy sauce, and meats treated with tenderizer. Although all of these foods would contain monoamines, it is not clear whether all of them would contain sufficient quantities of monoamines to elicit adverse reactions in patients on monoamine oxidase–inhibiting drugs

Preventive Measures

Individuals taking monoamine oxidase–inhibiting drugs are probably the only consumers at risk of monoamine intoxication. These individuals should be informed of the hazards associated with the ingestion of foods that contain high levels of monoamines such as tyramine. Cheeses are a particular concern. If an avoidance diet is carefully practiced, problems should be circumvented.

REFERENCES

1. Taylor SL. Histamine food poisoning: toxicology and clinical aspects. CRC Crit Rev Toxicol 1986; 17:91–128.
2. Taylor SL, Stratton JE, Nordlee JA. Histamine poisoning (scombroid fish poisoning): an allergy-like intoxication. Clin Toxicol 1989; 27:225–240.
3. Bartholomew BA, Berry PR, Rodhouse JC, Gilbert RJ. Scombrotoxic fish poisoning in Britain: features of over 250 suspected incidents from 1976 to 1986. Epidemiol Infect 1987; 99:775–782.

4. Russell FE, Maretic Z. Scombroid poisoning: mini-review with case histories. Toxicon 1986; 24: 967–973.
5. Borysiewicz L, Krikler D. Scombrotoxic atrial flutter. Br Med J 1981; 282:1434.
6. Lerke PA, Werner SB, Taylor SL, Guthertz LS. Scombroid poisoning: report of an outbreak. West J Med 1978; 129:381–386.
7. Dickinson G. Scombroid fish poisoning syndrome. Ann Emerg Med 1982; 11:487–489.
8. Blakesley ML. Scombroid poisoning: prompt resolution of symptoms with cimetidine. Ann Emerg Med 1983; 12:104–106.
9. Histamine in seafood: fluorometric method. In: Helrich K, ed. Official Methods of Analysis of the Association of Analytical Chemists, 15th ed. Arlington, VA: Association of Official Analytical Chemists, 1990, pp 876–877.
10. Hui JY, Taylor SL. Inhibition of in vivo histamine metabolism in rats by foodborne and pharmacologic inhibitors of diamine oxidase, histamine N-methyltransferase, and monoamine oxidase. Toxicol Appl Pharmacol 1985; 81:241–249.
11. Taylor SL, Bush RK. Allergy by ingestion of seafoods. In: Tu AT, ed. Handbook of Natural Toxins, Vol. 3, Marine Toxins and Venoms. New York: Marcel Dekker, 1988, pp 149–183.
12. Food and Drug Administration. Decomposition and histamine: raw, frozen tuna and mahi-mahi; canned tuna; and related species. Compliance Policy Guide 7108.24 1995.
13. Stratton JE, Hutkins RW, Taylor SL. Biogenic amines in cheese and other fermented foods: a review. J Food Prot 1991; 54:460–470.
14. Taylor SL, Keefe TJ, Windham ES, Howell JF. Outbreak of histamine poisoning associated with consumption of Swiss cheese. J Food Prot 1982; 45:455–457.
15. Stratton JE, Hutkins RW, Sumner SS, Taylor SL. Histamine and histamine-producing bacteria in retail Swiss and low-salt cheeses. J Food Prot 1992; 55:435–439.
16. Kahana LM, Todd E. Histamine poisoning in a patient on isoniazid. Can Dis Wkly Rpt 1981; 7:79–80.
17. Doeglas HMG, Huisman J, Nater JP. Histamine intoxication after cheese. Lancet 1967; 2:1361–1362.
18. Mayer K, Pause G. Biogene amines in sauerkraut. Leben Wiss Technol 1972; 5:108–109.
19. Wantke F, Gotz M, Jarisch R. The red wine provocation test: intolerance to histamine as a model for food intolerance. N Engl Reg Allergy Proc 1994; 15:27–32.
20. Eitenmiller RR, Wallis JW, Orr JH, Phillips RD. Production of histidine decarboxylase and histamine by *Proteus morganii*. J Food Prot 1981; 44:815–820.
21. Taylor SL, Guthertz LS, Leatherwood M, Lieber ER. Histamine production by *Klebsiella pneumoniae* and an incident of scombroid fish poisoning. Appl Environ Microbiol 1979; 37:274–278.
22. Lukton A, Olcott HS. Content of free imidazole compounds in the muscle tissue of aquatic animals. Food Res 1958; 23:611–618.
23. Sumner SS, Speckhard MW, Somers EB, Taylor SL. Isolation of histamine-producing *Lactobacillus buchneri* from Swiss cheese implicated in a food poisoning outbreak. Appl Environ Microbiol 1985; 50:1094–1096.

24. Halasz A, Barath A, Simon-Sarkadi L, Holzapfel W. Biogenic amines and their production by microorganisms in food. Trends Food Sci Technol 1994; 5:42–49.
25. Sumner SS, Roche F, Taylor SL. Factors controlling histamine formation in Swiss cheese inoculated with *Lactobacillus buchneri*. J Dairy Sci 1990; 73:3050–3058.
26. Weiss S, Robb GP, Ellis LB. The systemic effects of histamine in man. Arch Intern Med 1932; 49:360–362.
27. Motil KJ, Scrimshaw NS. The role of exogenous histamine in scombroid poisoning. Toxicol Lett 1979; 3:219–223.
28. Clifford MN, Walker R, Wright J, Hardy R, Murray CK. Studies with volunteers on the role of histamine in suspected scombrotoxicosis. J Sci Food Agric 1989; 47:365–375.
29. van Gelderen CEM, Savelkoul TJF, van Ginkel LA, van Dokkum W. The effects of histamine administered in fish samples to healthy volunteers. Clin Toxicol 1992; 30:585–596.
30. Clifford MN, Walker R, Ijomah P, Wright J, Murray CK, Hardy R. Is there a role for amines other than histamines in the aetiology of scombrotoxicosis? Food Addit Contam 1991; 8:641–652.
31. Ijomah P, Clifford MN, Walker R, Wright J, Hardy R, Murray CK. The importance of endogenous histamine relative to dietary histamine in the aetiology of scombrotoxicosis. Food Add Contam 1991; 8:531–542.
32. Morrow JD, Margolies GR, Rowland J, Roberts LJ II. Evidence that histamine is the causative toxin of scombroid-fish poisoning. N Engl J Med 1991; 324:716–720.
33. Uragoda CG, Kottegoda SR. Adverse reactions to isoniazid on ingestion of fish with a high histamine content. Tubercle 1977; 58:83–89.
34. Senanayake N, Vyravanathan S. Histamine reactions to ingestion of tuna fish (*Thunnus argentivittatus*) in patients on anti-tuberculosis therapy. Toxicon 1981; 19:184–185.
35. Taylor SL. Other microbial intoxications. In: Cliver DO, ed. Foodborne Diseases. San Diego: Academic Press, 1990, pp 159–170.
36. Marley E, Blackwell B. Interactions of monoamine oxidase inhibitors, amines, and foodstuffs. Adv Pharmacol Chemother 1970; 8:185–249.
37. Maga JA. Amines in foods. CRC Crit Rev Food Sci Nutr 1978; 10:373–403.

9

Food Allergy Perception and Reality

Lawrence T. Chiaramonte, Clifford W. Bassett, and Daryl R. Altman
Little Neck, New York

There is a marked difference between the general public's perception that food allergy is common and the food reactions that physicians can really confirm with double-blind placebo-controlled food challenge (DBPCFC) tests. About 7% of individuals believe they have food allergy, but less than 2% of adults have a DBPCFC confirmed food reaction. Some of this confusion can be explained by the lumping of food allergy or hypersensitivity (immunological reaction) and food intolerance in the lay press. The term *adverse food reaction* can be applied to both.

The food allergy perception/reality disparity is not a peculiarly American phenomenon. When a random sample of 1483 Dutch adults was polled, 12.4% claimed to have food allergy [1]. Food allergy was confirmed by DBPCFC in only 12 of 73 individuals who completed the protocol. This indicated a probable 2.4% prevalence of true food allergy in the Dutch adult population, assuming that allergy was equal in participants, nonparticipants, and dropouts. In response, the Dutch government created a national information bureau to focus on public education about food allergy and intolerance.

A food allergy questionnaire was sent to 15,000 British households, half chosen from the electoral registers, half from the Wycombe Health Authority [2]. This represented an estimated 20,000 individuals. The overall response rate was 47%. Of the initial responding individuals, 19.9% reported food allergy. Of 93 individuals undergoing DBPCFCs, 18 (19.4%) had a positive result for the suspected foods. A second, more brief survey elicited additional responses from those households that did not initially respond to the original food allergy survey. The response rate to the second survey was 17.4 %, with 6.4 % reporting food allergy, none of whom were challenged. Assuming that this second group would also have a 19.4% positive challenge rate, and making corrections for those who did not respond to any survey, the investigators estimated a 1.4%–1.7% prevalence of food allergy in the British population [2]. In both European studies, women had a higher prevalence of self-reported food allergy and, in the British study, confirmed food allergy as well.

We will discuss the current orthodox guidelines for the diagnosis of food allergy and our view of their limitations. Fatal food reactions do occur. Attention will be paid to the circumstances surrounding them with an emphasis on prevention. The concept of pseudo food allergy as an eating disorder will be reviewed. Our clinical experience in running a food allergy center, as well as what we feel are significant papers from the literature have been used in the formation of the concepts presented in this chapter. We have seen some patients with severe allergic reactions, in whom extensive history taking and testing did not reveal any causative agent: food, drugs, nor stinging insects. We have found Dr. Patterson's approach to idiopathic anaphylaxis quiet useful [3]. A few cases have resolved with the removal of angiotensin converting enzyme (ACE) inhibitors [4].

A short, simple question about food allergy (Fig. 1) was incorporated into a broader self-reported, mailed consumer questionnaire administered by the NPD Group of Marketing and Research Companies, Port Washington, New York, in May 1989, June 1992, and June 1993.

The technique used was a quota sample, a type of nonprobability sample. Quota samples are used to poll a survey population that is representative, with respect to certain defined characteristics, of the population at large. This study population was constructed to represent the demographics of the United States. Unlike random probability samples, quota samples are not subject to standard statistical tests. Despite this, they provide a valid technique, widely employed by the market research industry.

For each of these quota samples, a different representative group of 5000 American households was surveyed. The demographic factors (quotas) controlled for were household size, household income, age of householder, household socioeconomic status, education of householder, and population density within each geographic region, as determined by the U.S. Census [5]. These characteristics were chosen because they are considered to be the best predictors

ABOUT FOOD ALLERGIES

1. Does anyone in your household have a food allergy

    Yes ☐ 8-1   No ☐ 2 → (Go to the next section)

    If "Yes", let me know their age and sex, as well as their allergy:

Age	Sex 1 2 M☐ F☐	Describe allergy(s) such as milk, shellfish, peanuts, etc.
____	1 2 M☐ F☐	_____ 9-13
____	1 2 M☐ F☐	_____ 14-18
____	1 2 M☐ F☐	_____ 19-23

FIGURE 1 Food allergy question incorporated into a broad consumer questionnaire.

of consumer behavior [6]. Known group response rates were considered in the panel design so that the demographic characteristics of respondents would reflect the demographics of the U.S. population at large.

Of the 5000 households polled in 1989, 1992, and 1993, the response rates were, respectively, 79%, 75%, and 74%, largely, we believe, because of the simplicity of the questions and the public's interest in this subject. Overall 16.2%, 16.6%, and 13.9%, respectively, of responding households reported at least 1 individual in the home with a food allergy, with an average of 1.17 persons in each household believing he or she had a food reaction.

When viewed by region of the United States (Fig. 2), geographic differences were apparent in the percentages of households reporting individuals with food allergy (Fig. 3). The highest percentage of households reporting a positive perception were from the Pacific region. The lowest percentage reporting food reactions was the South East Central region of the United States.

Twice as many females as males reported food allergy in all years studied. Figure 4 shows the age and sex distribution of individuals reported as having food allergy in 1993. The distribution among males was skewed toward younger individuals; this age predilection was not apparent among females. These patterns were consistent over the 4-year period.

The most frequently reported foods causing allergic reactions were milk (29.3 %) fish/seafood (21%), vegetables (19.7), fruits (19.7%), and chocolate

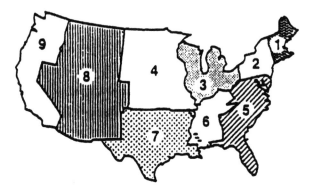

FIGURE 2 Geographic regions of the United States.

(11.1). Table 1 shows the foods implicated as being responsible for the reported food allergies [7]. Peanut allergy is the most common food allergy in adults. In the view of physicians, using DBPCFC was reported as a problem in only 5.5% of individuals in this survey of the public's perception.

This survey along with other studies shows that the public's perception of food allergy is greater than that which can be proved by DBPCFC. Some of this can be explained by the limitations of the orthodox approach to food allergy and some by the existence of pseudo food allergy, which will be discussed later in this chapter.

The orthodox diagnosis approach to food reactions begins with a complete history. Suspected food allergy can be further explored with diet diaries, elimination diets, or even elemental diets. Open changes and provocative diets can be attempted when safety issues have been addressed.

A positive skin test result by prick method to a food demonstrates only the potential for a clinically relevant immunoglobulin E– (IgE)-mediated reaction. It does not prove that the food is the cause of an allergic reaction. This can be only confirmed by a double-blind placebo-controlled DBPCFC.

The present orthodox approach recommends a challenge test to skin test positive foods and no challenge test to skin test negative foods. As with many "general rules," the physician must consider modifying factors. How safe is a challenge test in this patient with this food? Is the suspect food eaten frequently? If not, is the challenge worth the time and effort? We also have a concern for situations in which the prick skin test finding is negative and the history is clearly positive for a food reaction. This happens in our opinion quiet frequently in milk and wheat allergy. Individual antigen testing is more productive than testing with the whole food. These foods are complex mixtures of many antigens. Allergy extracts of foods are not subject to the same requirements of standardization as in-

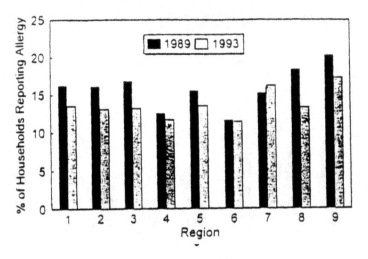

FIGURE 3 Percentage of households in each geographic region reporting at least one allergic individual.

halant antigens. We have used fresh vegetables and fruit juices as additional testing materials with some success.

Before a DBPCFC can be attempted, there must be agreement on a simple food that is suspected to be responsible for the symptoms the patient is having. The primary or target symptom must be identified. The interval between the ingestion of the food and the appearance of the symptom must be noted. Finally, the quantity of food causing the reaction described must be estimated. The influence of variables such as season and exercise is not clear.

Roughly half of the quantity of food suspected of causing the reaction is given to the patient in disguised form. The patient is observed for a time greater than twice the interval occurring in the history. If the single identified target symptom does not occur, this process is repeated with incrementally greater amounts of food until the quantity exceeds twice the amount causing the reaction in the history. When the changes of a correct guess have been statistically eliminated by repetition, a positive double-blind challenge finding confirms a positive food reaction, although not necessarily an immunological one. A negative challenge result fails to confirm food allergy; that is not quite the same as proving that food allergy does not exist. Negatives are always difficult to prove. The orthodox approach to this dilemma is to follow a negative DBPCFC result with an open challenge. The food is given in open fashion to gauge the patient's reaction. There are some difficulties with this approach. It assumes that food reactions are consistent and independent of many extraneous factors. We know that patients lose some food allergies with time. Exercise

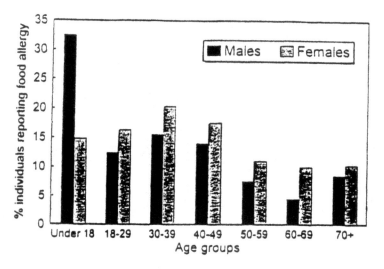

FIGURE 4 Age distribution of individuals identified as food allergic in 1993.

has been shown to increase food allergy. Other factors are suspected of having a similar role. Of course the patient who is emotionally committed to believing he or she has food allergy can discover modifying factors that are required to produce a positive result after a negative challenge, finding. One solution to this latter problem is to have a written agreement describing the clinical situation surrounding the food reaction. Then attempt to duplicate this in the challenge. As the time between the ingestion of the food and symptom increases, the DBPCFC becomes more difficult to accomplish. If a satisfactory marker of an allergic reaction in the blood or urine could be found, it would be a useful confirmation to the DBPCFC.

When vague reactions to food additives in one person are difficult to prove by DBPCFC, a cross over study can be useful: dividing those people with symptoms into two groups and following both groups, one on placebo, one on the additive, for at least three symptom cycles. The groups are given an adequate washout period, then switched. This will not be useful in proving anything in the individual patient—but can explore the role of the additive in causing complaints.

In 1988 a multicenter experience with DBPCFC was reported on the patients who had a positive history and skin test finding to a food [8]. Only 20%–40% had a positive result on double-blind challenge. In 1990 Allen Bock, M.D., a pioneer in the development of the DBPCFC, reported on 16 years of experience with 1014 challenges in 480 children. Most of the children with a positive DBPCFC result were skin test–positive to that food. Only about 25% of

TABLE 1 Foods Indicated as Responsible for Allergy in Reported Allergic Individuals

Food	Percentage Of Individuals Identifying Food	
	1989	1993
Milk	29.3	30.7
Fruit	19.7	21.8
Vegetables	19.9	19.2
Seafood/shellfish	16.9	16.5
Dairy (except "milk")	10.2	9.7
Chocolate	11.1	8.3
Eggs	6.8	7.2
Peanuts	5.5	7.2
Meat/poultry	6.7	4.7
Nuts	3.3	4.5
Fish	4.1	3.2
Wheat	3.7	3.0
Monosodium glutamate (MSG)	1.7	2.7
Yeast	1.1	1.2
Spices/seasonings	2.0	1.2
Food dyes/colorings	1.6	1.2
Caffeine	1.1	1.2
Sugar	1.7	1.0
All others	3.4	1.8

the patients with a history and skin test were confirmed on DBPCFC. Peanut was the greatest proven offender in the children over 3 years of age. Eggs, nuts, and milk followed in order of decreasing frequency. In the children under 3 years of age, cow's milk was the food most frequently positive on DBPCFC. Eggs, peanut, and soy followed in order of decreasing frequency. Corn, often reported as an offender by patients, was almost always negative on DBPCFC. Dr. Bock found that seldom were patients proved to be positive to many foods [9]. Even patients with proven food allergy to one food may incorrectly that they are allergic to many foods. DBPCFC. with these foods usually has a negative outcome. This is clinically useful information. It can help to focus dietary restriction on only relevant foods.

It has been our experience with patients with food allergy complaints that most complaining of food reactions do not have a provable food reaction. This is a great dilemma for the honest clinician. If the patient and family are not adequately supported while their belief system is challenged, they will vote with their feet. They will walk to the nearest uninformed practitioner or seek out "alternative medicine." These alternative practitioners diagnose food reactions that really do not exist and allow the patient to eat what he or she by using ineffective treatments for allergies that do not exist. We have found that close corroboration with a dietician and a family therapist while a food investigation is proceeding is useful.

We have reported DBPCFCs on individuals who claimed to suffer from monosodium glutamate– (MSG)-induced reactions [10]. Subjects were recruited by extensive advertising in local and regional newspapers, fliers in Chinese restaurants, letters to area allergists, and announcements at local allergy society meetings, over $2^1/_2$ year period. The estimated reach of these attempts was 1.5 million households. A stipend was offered. Forty-seven people who claimed to have MSG reactions were given DBPCFC with MSG at 1.5: 3, 6 grams in a liquid vehicle. The doses were administered in the doctor's office after an overnight fast in random fashion. This challenge was repeated by using self-administered capsules at home. Of the 26 people completing the study, 11 subjects reported symptoms after both MSG and placebo and 2 after placebo only. Six had no symptoms after any dose. Seven subjects reported symptoms after MSG but in two cases symptoms occurred at 3 grams but not at 6 grams. Of the 16 who went on to take MSG at home 10 subjects reported symptoms after both MSG and placebo and 3 after MSG only. Three subjects had no symptoms. The symptoms were of rapid onset and short duration. Although no statistical conclusions can be reached, the DBPCFC was valuable in demonstrating that more people report MSG reactions than can be proved. These studies are still in progress.

Parker et al. investigated 45 patients with food complaints by history, skin tests, and DBPCFC. Patients were divided into two groups, those with provable food allergy and those with pseudo food allergy, and the characteristics of both groups were compared [11].

The patients with probable food allergy identified a mean of 5.2 foods as a cause of difficulty, compared to the probably negative group, who had a mean of 25.5 foods. The difference between the two groups was statistically significant. The group with pseudo food allergy complained of more problematic foods. Identifying the cause due to milk, white sugar, wheat, eggs, cured meat, and yeast. The patients with probable food allergy reported peanut, shrimp, fish, and mixed nuts as sources of difficulty; that report is supported by the data of Bock et al. [8].

The group with probable food allergy had significantly more positive food skin test results as would be predicted. They also had an early age of onset of food-related symptoms.

The pattern of symptoms in the two groups overlapped to some degree. Swelling and respiratory problems were statistically reported more often in the probable food allergic group, whereas the pseudo food allergic group had statistically more vague nonspecific complaints. They were also more influenced by nontraditional medicine and had family members who seemed to have more commonly long-standing food-related complaints.

With these findings in Parker's paper being significant in only 45 patients, we felt that the building of a computer data base with greater numbers of patients would more accurately define these differences. The value of any data base is only as good as the data entered, and we have progressed to the point of agreeing on how and which data to input. We hope that if this concept is successful, patients can be sorted out with greater refinement.

Patients proved to be allergic to a food are not always allergic to that food for the rest of their lifetime. Infants seem to have immature gastrointestinal (GI) tracks that allow for frequent food reactions. The prevalence of milk allergy seems to decrease with age. Some food allergic reactions are remarkably persistent, such as shellfish and nut allergy. The role of dietary avoidance and the ingestion of related foods must be studied in the development of tolerance. A data base that is developed must follow a person's food reactions over time.

People rarely die of food allergy. The lay press dramatizes these relatively rare events, and this emphasis falsely influences the public perception of food allergy [12]. Hugh Sampson studied 13 patients with severe food reactions, 6 who died and 7 who had near-fatal reactions. Most of these patients could be identified as high-risk children. They were atopic and asthmatic and had prior food reactions. The affecting food most of the time had been already identified as causing difficulty but was ingested accidentally. Peanut, as in other studies, was a major offender. The anaphylactic reactions observed in this study lasted 4 to 6 hr. Some reactions had a biphasic component. The major difference between the patients who died and the ones that survived was the interval between the onset of respiratory symptoms and the injection of adrenalin. Those who survived received adrenalin early in the reaction.

In conclusion, food reactions can be frighteningly real or ridiculously imagined in the minds of patients, with many variations between these two extremes. The orthodox clinician must attempt to categorize the reported reaction and patient, but treat each patient with respect and without prejudice. We do not always recognize those with vague late-phase reaction to many foods. Some may have a form of eating disorder, signifying emotional problems. This may be a pattern as food can be the social glue of a family. Gentle handling by allergist is required to encourage these patients to accept a family systems approach and abandon their beliefs. The alternative is nonorthodox medicine, which treats nonexistent food allergy with ineffective therapies. Avoidance is the only accepted treatment for the prevention of food allergy.

Most fatal food reactions usually occur in prediagnosed individuals who have had previous reactions with the offending food [12–15]. The clinician must be certain that the patient is aware of situations in which the offending food can be accidentally ingested. At our center a college student with peanut allergy died when she ate chili containing peanut butter: Adrenaline, Adrenaline, Adrenaline! We cannot emphasize this enough for the treatment of the acute reactions. Patients must be taught how to self-inject adrenaline in case of hidden accidental ingestion of a food to which they are extremely allergic. They must be reminded to keep a current EpiPen with them at all times.

REFERENCES

1. Jansen JJ, Kardinaal AF, Huijbers G, Vlieg-Boerstra BJ, Martens BP, Ockhuizen T. Prevalence of food allergy and intolerance in the adult Dutch population. J Allergy Clin Immunol 1994; 93:446–456.
2. Young E, Stoneham MD, Petruckevitch A et al. A population study of food intolerance. Lancet 1994; 343:1127–131.
3. Wiggins CA, Dykewicz MS, Patterson R. Idiopathic anaphylaxis: classification, evaluation, and treatment of 123 patients. J Allergy Clin Immunol 1988; 82 (5 Pt 1):849–855.
4. Patterson R, Stoloff RS, Greenberger PA, Grammar LC, Harris KE. Algorithms for the diagnosis and management of idiopathic anaphylaxis. Ann Allergy 1993; 71(1):40–44.
5. US Bureau of the Census. Statistical Abstract of the United States, 11th ed. Washington, DC, 1991.
6. Berkman HW, Gilson C. Consumer Behavior: Concepts and Strategies. 3rd ed. Boston: Kent, 1986, pp 41–93.
7. Altman DR, Cerement LT. Public perception of food allergy. J Allergy Clin Immunol 1996; 97:
8. Bock SA, Sampson HA, Atkins FM, Zeiger RS, Lehrer S, Sachs M, Bush RK, Metcalfe DD. Double-blind, placebo-controlled food challenge (DBPCFC) as an office procedure: a manual. J Allergy Clin Immunol 1988; 82:986–997.
9. Bock SA, Atkins FM. Patterns of food hypersensitivity during sixteen years of double-blind placebo-controlled food challenges. J Pediatr 1990; 117(4):561–567.
10. Altman DR, Fitzgerald T, Chiaramonte LT. Double-blind placebo-controlled challenge (DBPCC) of persons reporting adverse reactions to monosodium glutamate (MSG). Am Acad Allergy Immunol 1994;
11. Parker SL, Leznoff A, Sussman GL, Tarlo SM, Krondl M. Characteristics of patients with food-related complaints. J Allergy Clin Immunol 1990; 86:503–511.
12. Sampson HA, Mendelson L, Rosen JP. Fatal and near-fatal anaphylactic reactions to food in children and adolesecents. N Engl J Med 1992; 327(6):380–384.
13. Yunginger JW, Sweeney KG, Sturner WQ, Giannandrea LA, Teigland JD, Bray M, Benson PA, York JA, Biedrzycki L, Squillace DL et al. Fatal food-induced anaphylaxis. JAMA 1988; 260(10):1450–1452.
14. Patterson R, Clayton DE, Booth BH, Greenberger PA, Grammar LC, Harris KE. Fatal and near fatal idiopathic anaphylaxis. Allergy Proc 1995; 16(3):103–108.
15. Sampson HA, Metcalfe DD. Immediate reactions to foods. In: Metcalfe DD, Sampson HA, Simon RA, eds. Food Allergy Adverse Reactions to Foods and Food Additives. Boston: Blackwell Scientific, 1991, p 100.

10

Delayed and Non-IgE-Mediated Reactions

WILLIAM T. KNIKER

University of Texas Health Science Center at San Antonio,
San Antonio, Texas

INTRODUCTION

The subject of adverse reactions to foods is one of the most controversial areas of medicine. There is considerable disagreement on incidence and prevalence, possible clinical manifestations, and utility of various diagnostic approaches. In two recent European studies of adults, 12.4%–20% felt they had food allergy or food intolerance; double-blind placebo-controlled food challenge (DBPCFC) in selected subjects suggested a true prevalence of at least 1.4% to 2.4% in the populations [1,2]. In school age children in Denmark 10% of the atopics had positive open challenge results to a mixture of food additives as compared to none of the nonatopic controls. The prevalence of intolerance to additives in the children was estimated to be 1%–2% [3]. In all three studies there was a wide range of clinical reactions in terms of time elapsed after ingestion, organ systems involved, and nature of foodstuff triggers.

It is clinically useful to divide adverse reactions to foods temporally, into those occurring within 2 hr after ingestion (immediate) and those occurring more than 2 hr later (delayed) (Table 1). Immediate reactions generally are classically allergic, triggered by specific immunoglobulin E (IgE) complexing with relatively small doses of antigen [4,5]. Such reactions have been widely studied, are well understood, and are covered extensively in other sections of this book. Delayed reactions, particularly those not known to be associated with IgE triggering, are not well studied. There is much ignorance about pathogenic mechanisms, nature of triggering, possible clinical manifestations, and diagnostic approaches.

Before examining what is known about delayed and non-IgE-mediated reactions to foodstuffs, it is useful to remember that adverse reactions to food may occur at two levels. The first is the gastrointestinal tract itself; in some cases, the entire reaction is limited to that organ system. The second level, accounting for the bulk of clinically relevant reactions, is outside the gut. Intact food or partially digested food molecules or additives are absorbed, circulate in the blood, and gain access to virtually any part of the body where the opportunity for sensitization and triggering of disease exists.

TABLE 1 Times after Ingestion for Adverse Reactions to Foodstuffs

	Immediate (< 2 hr)	Delayed (> 2 hr)
Triggering mechanisms	IgE in atopic individuals; also idiosyncratic	Type I IgE and other immunological hypersensitivities; nonimmunological
Clinical manifestations	Classical allergic disorders: anaphylaxis, vomiting, cramps, diarrhea, urticaria/angioedema, pruritis, oral allergy syndrome, rhinitis, asthma, CNS aberrations	Classical allergic disorders plus variable involvement of single or multiple organ systems: colic, constipation, atopic dermatitis, otitis media, arthralgias, vasculitis, headaches, CNS aberrations
Diagnostic points	History usually identifies agent; specific IgE test (skin, in vitro) results usually positive; positive oral food challenge response definitive; small dose may be adequate	History of limited help; specific IgE test results usually negative; other in vitro test results unreliable positive oral food challenge response definitive; large dose often required

CLASSIFICATION OF ADVERSE REACTIONS TO FOODS OR ADDITIVES

Possible Triggering Mechanisms

Adverse reactions can be divided conveniently into two groups on the basis of triggering mechanisms after ingestion of foodstuffs (Fig. 1). The first is the true food hypersensitivity group, in which immunological triggering is assumed but rarely proved [5,6]. A further division into IgE-mediated or "allergic" (Gell and Coombs' type I) versus type II, III, or IV hypersensitivity mechanisms can be made. It is clear from many published reports later cited that delayed reactions to foods can be associated with any of these immunological pathways, including the late phase of classical IgE-mediated responses in atopic individuals.

In these immunologically triggered reactions foodstuffs themselves serve as antigens in one form or other [6]. The food may be a complete antigen or may be haptenic when combined with a carrier protein (Table 2A). The antigenicity may be present in many forms of the food or be limited to the raw, processed, cooked, or partially digested phase. Food antigen may be cross-reactive with antigens in other members of the same group (not common) or with unrelated substances. The oral allergy syndrome, urticaria and angioedema, has frequently been seen in pollen-sensitive individuals eating certain foods: birch with fruits, nuts, carrots, potatoes, and other foods [7]; mugwort with celery, spices, carrots; ragweed with melons and bananas; and grass pollen with tomato and peanut allergens [7,8]. In a sense, inhaled pollen may cause delayed adverse reactions, e.g., asthma, much as a food does in sensitized subjects! Whereas smaller partially solubilized pollen grains can cause immediate respiratory allergic responses, the bulk of larger pollen grains is ultimately

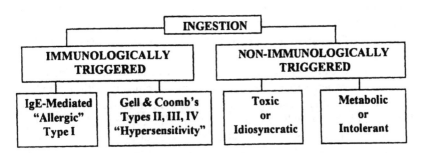

FIGURE 1 Possible triggering mechanisms for adverse reactions to ingested foods and additives.

TABLE 2   How Foodstuffs May Cause Disease

1. As antigens in immunologically mediated hypersensitivity reactions:
    -Complete or haptenic
    -Form: raw, processed, cooked, partially digested
    -Cross-reactive: other foodstuffs, pollens, other agents
    -Concomitant triggers: foodstuffs, inhalants (persorption), chemicals, stress, exercise, infections, etc.
    -Variable hypersensitivity mechanisms: I, II, III, IV
    -Variable immunomodulation, between immunological tolerance and immune responsiveness
2. As immune modulators, e.g., lectins. (Freed[a])
3. Through pharmacological effects, as by caffeine, vasoactive amines including histamine, tyramine, and exorphins. (Finn[a])
4. Through toxic effects, including additives, pesticides (Seba et al.[a])
5. By "idiosyncratic" direct activation of mediators of inflammation
6. In metabolic aberrations, including enzyme abnormalities (Brostoff[a]):
    (a) deficiencies, e.g. lactase; (b) abnormal detoxification, cytochrome P-450 system, (c) slowed activity, e.g., Phenol sulfotransferase, and headaches
7. Through nonspecific irritation or inflammation.

[a]Authors of relevant chapters in Ref. 259.
Source: Ref. 259.

swallowed and partially digested. Solubilized pollen antigen is absorbed from the gut and delivered by blood (persorption) to virtually any sensitized tissue in the body [9,10].

It appears that food antigens can trigger disease not every time eaten, but only when ingested in association with concomitant trigger factors [5,6,11]. These include the eating of certain other foodstuffs, exposure to chemicals, stress, vigorous exercise, and the presence of infection. In most people immunological tolerance to most foods develops during early infancy. It is not clear why some have a lifelong extreme sensitivity to certain foods, generally IgE-mediated with anaphylaxis potential, and why others lose their tolerance to single or many foods at some point later in life.

The second category of triggering mechanism is nonimmunological, as the foodstuff does not serve as antigen binding specifically with antibody or lymphocyte (Fig. 1 and Table 2B). Many foods contain lectins, resistant to digestion, which have multiple effects on growth cell receptors and immunological and hormonal functions in the gut and throughout the body [12]. Lectins immunoregulate several classes of lymphocytes, stimulate antibody production (especially IgE and IgG), and enhance cytotoxicity [13]. Possible adverse effects of lectins include agglutination of any type of blood cell, activation and mediator release from mast cells and basophiles, malabsorption in the gut, and potentiation of chronic inflammatory disorders. Some foodstuffs induce phamacological effects that are dose-related [14]. Caffeine is associated with chronic anxiety, insomnia, palpitations, headache, and gastrointestinal stimulation. Vasoactive amines act on blood vessels, histamine (in strawberries) causing flushing and urticaria and tyramine (in some cheese and chocolate) causing migraine headaches or hypertension. Although opioid-like exorphins derived from gluten have been found in brain tissue, their effects are unknown [15]. Hundreds of potentially toxic chemicals have been measured in drinking water, food, breast milk, blood, and urine. Unfortunately, except for a few substances like lead, it has been difficult to ascertain the pathological effects of such ingested agents, if any [16]. Among the thousands of food additives widely used, some are known to cause adverse reactions [17,18]. It is clear that many of these "idiosyncratic" reactions involve activation of mast cells and release of typical "allergic" mediators of inflammation [19]. Monosodium glutamate (MSG) is noteworthy because it is intrinsic in many foods as well as a component of food seasonings. The familiar delayed symptoms of "Chinese restaurant syndrome" are caused by possible neurotoxic and neuroexcitatory mechanisms [20]. Des, preservatives, salicylates, yeast products, and sugars have been popularly associated with a variety of adverse reactions, but the true incidence is unknown. It is estimated, on the basis of double-blind challenges, that 2% of atopic children react adversely to additives, as compared to less than 1% of nonatopic adults of children [21]. Bisulfates are added as preservatives to a wide variety of foods and beverages. Acute or delayed urticaria, angioedema, and asthma reactions are not uncommon; a delayed eczematoid reaction in food handlers also may be seen [22,23].

Metabolic aberrations, including enzyme abnormalities, can lead to problems in association with foods [11]. First, deficiency of digestive enzymes such as lactase leads to a variety of gastrointestinal symptoms in affected children and adults. Second, genetic abnormalities in the debrisoquine locus of the cytochrome P-450 system can be associated with reduced oxidative detoxification of drugs and foods. Third, phenolsulfotransferase deficiency may lead to impaired metabolism of phenolic compounds in foods, resulting in a variety of reactions, e.g., headache.

The difficulties in understanding the mechanisms of food sensitivity is illustrated by celiac disease (CD). It is a malabsorption disorder manifested by diarrhea, streatorrhea, malnutrition, abdominal distension, hypoproteinemia, and anemia [24]. The jejunal mucosa typically shows flat mosaic appearance, villous atrophy, and intraepithelial lymphocytes. CD is caused by ingestion of gluten, the major protein in wheat and other grains. Some data suggest that CD is a food "allergy" (hypersensitivity): there is lymphocytic inflammation in the gut, antibody sensitization to gliadin and various tissue autoantigens, and immunoflourescent demonstration of presumed gliadin–antibody complexes in the intestinal wall [25]. Others feel that the evidence for an "allergic" cause of CD is extremely weak, and that the pathogenic mechanism for the gluten-induced enteropathy is unknown [24].

Times After Ingestion for Adverse Reactions

A useful clinical differentiation between patients having adverse reactions is based on the time elapsed since ingestion of the offending food [5] (Table 1).

Immediate Reactions

Symptoms occur less than 2 hr after eating or drinking a relatively small portion of foodstuff. The patient usually recognizes the causal relationship and attempts to prevent future reactions by avoiding the offending food. Most of the individuals are atopic and there is high correlation among oral challenge, immediate skin test, and in vitro radioallergosorbent test (RAST) results. Typical disorders include the following:

- Classic allergic diseases such as allergic rhinitis, asthma, urticaria, angioedema
- Allergic reactions of the gastrointestinal system such as the oral allergy syndrome [26], vomiting, cramps, diarrhea, allergic gastroenteritis
- Anaphylaxis, sometimes concomitant with exercise or idiopathic [24]
- Heiner–Kniker–Sears syndrome
- Atopic dermatitis (eczema)
- Grain dust allergy [27]
- Snow crab–processing worker's disease [28]

Epidemiologically, most "true," e.g., IgE-mediated, food allergies occur in infants and small children. Eight foods account for 93% of the reactions proved by DBPCFC: egg, peanut, cow milk, soy, tree nuts, crustacean shellfish, true fish, and wheat [26]. However, in 112 adults in whom food allergy developed after 10 years of age, fruits and vegetables were the main allergens responsible, and milk and eggs were the least common [29]. They all had immediate clinical food reactions and positive skin test and DBPCFC results to one or more foods. The most common symptoms were urticaria, often accompanied by rhinitis. Some individuals are so exquisitely sensitized that they have immediate symptoms, such as asthma or anaphylaxis, after breathing vapors from food (meat, crustaceans, lentils, etc.) cooking on a stove [30,31]. Anaphylaxis associated with food in either adults or children is uncommon, mostly related to ingestion of peanut, true nut, seafood, egg, or milk [32,33].

Delayed Reactions

Delayed adverse reactions to foods are exceedingly diverse and may involve virtually any organ system [4,5,34]. Many reactions are classically allergic, reflecting the late phase of IgE-mediated triggering, often in the absence of a discernible immediate-phase clinical response. Others involve a single organ system (e.g., the gastrointestinal tract in celiac disease) or multiple organ systems (e.g., the respiratory, skin, gastrointestinal, muscloskeletal, and central nervous systems) in a puzzling array of symptoms.

Symptoms occur at least 2 hr after ingesting the offending agent, or even days later. Large doses or even repeated feedings of the food may be necessary. Accordingly, the diagnosis can be very difficult since the patient is unaware of a relationship between eating of certain foods and subsequent disease. The prevalence of delayed food sensitivities is unknown but has been estimated to be at least that of immediate reactions, if not higher.

Diagnosis is also hampered by the absence of reliable laboratory tests. Skin tests or in vitro tests measuring IgE specific for a given food usually have negative findings. In vitro tests of other antibody (IgG, IgG_4, IgA) and lymphocyte sensitization to foods are unreliable because they do not distinguish between normal individuals and food reactors. Indeed, for both immediate and delayed reactions to food, the only reliable and definitive diagnostic test is a positive clinical response to oral food challenge.

GENERAL ASPECTS OF DELAYED REACTIONS

Pathogenic Mechanisms

For most food sensitivity reactions, the nature of the triggering and the immunological and inflammatory mechanisms are not known or understood. Although antibody or lymphocyte sensitization to specific food antigen may be demonstrated, it is difficult to prove that the binding of immune reactant with antigen actually evokes clinical disease. Indeed, in atopics with bona fide IgE-mediated food sensitivities, the majority of skin test–positive foods do *not* cause disease on ingestion [4,5,11,34]! Inability to show immunological sensitization to a putative food antigen may mean that (a) the test is insensitive and yields falsely negative results; (b) the appropriate test to demonstrate sensitization has not been selected; or (c) no immune sensitization exists and any adverse reaction is triggered by a nonimmune mechanism.

TABLE 3 Some Foods and Additives Reported to Cause
Nonimmunological Adverse Reactions[a]

	Agent	Reaction	Mechanism
Toxic or idiosyncratic	Monosodium glutamate	Chinese restaurant syndrome	Unknown
	Bisulfites	Asthma, urticaria	Converts to SO_2
	Dyes, preservatives, and salicylates	Asthma, urticaria, CNS aberrations	Variable
	Nutmeg	Hallucinations	LSD-like psychotrope
	Histamine	Flushing, urticaria	Dose related
	Sucrose	Hypertension	Unknown
	Yeast products, sugars, alcohol	Variable	Unknown
Metabolic or intolerance	Sugars (mono- or disaccharide)	Gastrointestinal and variable	Deficiency of digestive enzyme
	Glutens and gliadins	Celiac disease and dermatitis herpetiformis	Some aspects of inflammatory reaction to glutens and gliadins
	Tyramine, tryptophane	Migraine headaches, hypertension	Lowered plasma (e.g., MAO) oxidase levels

[a]CNS, central nervous system; LSD, lysergic acid diethylamide; MAO, monoamine oxidase.

Immunological Phenomena in the Gut: Sensitization versus Tolerance

Considering the large amounts of foreign potentially antigenic substances eaten everyday, it is a wonder that all of us don't suffer continuously from food sensitivities. Indeed, in the first 6 months of life, a number of factors predispose the infant to sensitization and disease: (a) relatively indiscriminate absorption of macromolecules including foodstuffs from the gut; (b) immature surface immunity with low IgA "gatekeeper" function; and (c) maturing but low levels of digestive enzymes [5,35,36]. At this age, and in anyone older with intestinal inflammation, the enhanced absorption of antigenic food molecules does lead to high levels of specific antibodies of various classes and lymphocyte sensitization systemically. Fortunately, these responses usually are inconsequential or protective, and only in a minority of cases are they pathogenic [6]. From later infancy

onward, the immunoregulative responses to ingested foodstuffs favor immunological tolerance [36,37]. However, allergic reactions, infections, inflammation,
immune dysregulation, or toxic agents in the gut disturb the delicate balance
with the possible sequelae of intestinal dysfunctions, malabsorption, loss of immunological tolerance, and adverse reactions in any tissue where reactive food
molecules are delivered.

Hypersensitivity Mechanisms

Type I: IgE-Mediated

In delayed reactions associated with IgE food antigen triggering, it is likely that
immediate-phase reactions take place subclinically in the gut and other target tissues [34]. Even in nonallergic individuals, triggering of mast cells in the gut occurs with subsequent immediate release of mediators of inflammation and
increased albumin and hyaluronan into the gut lumen [38]. Mucosal specific IgE
seems to be less pathogenic if "balanced" by protective levels of specific secre-
tary IgA [36,39,40].

Late-phase or delayed IgE-associated mechanisms have been suggested
in a host of gastrointestinal disorders (allergic enteropathies, malabsorption
syndromes), respiratory disorders (asthma, rhinitis, Heiner's syndrome),
atopic dermatitis, and migraine [5,6,34]. The likelihood of occurrence of a
late-phase-type reaction is supported by the finding of elevated plasma histamine levels, but not tryptase levels, at the time of onset of delayed symptoms
after oral challenge in food-allergic children [41]. This suggests basophil, but
not mast cell, activation. In the same study, children with immediate reactions
to food showed elevated plasma levels of histamine and tryptase within 2 hr
of oral challenge, suggestive of mast cell activation in the immediate phase.
In a study at the Nassau County Medical Center, interleukin 4 and plasma histamine levels changed after food challenge suggesting other markers for objective data [42].

Type II: Antibody-Mediated Cell Injury

As previously stated, most individuals have measurable serum levels of antibodies of various classes to different foods, simply reflecting a normal inconsequential response to absorbed food antigens [6,36]. Higher titers of such antibodies
and circulatory antigen-specific B cells tend to be found in patients with actual
food sensitivities [43]. target tissues outside the gut. A notable example is the
Heiner syndrome, manifested by failure to thrive, pulmonary infiltrates with
eosinophilia, bleeding in the gut and lung, and anemia [48]. Arthus-type complexes may be present in some patients with food-induced dermatitis herpetiformis accompanying celiac disease, recurrent otitis media with effusion, and
arthritis/arthralgia [5,6].

Type IV: T Cell–Mediated Delayed-Type Hypersensitivity

T lymphocytes are a normal part of the gut-associated lymphoid tissue (GALT) system, residing in high numbers especially at the intraepithelial level [36]. It is widely recognized that T cell sensitization to food antigens and haptenic materials is universal, beginning in early infancy [6]. As expected, the in vitro demonstration of lymphocyte blastogenesis in the presence of specific foods is usually not helpful in distinguishing normal individuals from those with presumed food-induced disease. Two groups suggest that T cell function in relation to food is largely inhibitory in the gut, leading to a state of relative tolerance to foods [49,50]. When infections, toxic agents, inflammation, or allergic reactions occur, a breakdown of tolerance can cause activation of T cells with release of interleukins and cytokines leading to mucosal inflammation and malabsorption [34].

In the gut the delayed hypensensitivity Type IV mechanism has been postulated to operate in celiac disease, protein-losing enteropathies, eosinophilic gastroenteritis, and inflammatory bowel disorders, e.g., ulcerative colitis [6,34,36]. Proving such a role has become difficult in view of the complexities of the CD4+ T cell system. In food-related atopic dermatitis (AD), inflammatory skin lesions are infiltrated both with TH-1 cells (which produce interleukin 2 [IL-2] and interferon gamma [γ-IFN]) and TH-2 cells (which produce IL-3, 4, 5, 6, 10, and granulocyte macrophage colony-stimulating factor [GM-CSF] [51]. In many studies, the TH-2 cells associated with type I hypersensitivity predominate, in part as a result of the putative suppressive effect of IL-10 on the TH-1 cells, which would ordinarily induce "delayed hypersensitivity" reactions. In a recent study of cow's milk allergy (CMA), lymphocyte suppressor activity and γ-IFN levels were low before reacting to antigen challenge; months later, after recovery/remission, suppressor and γ-IFN were both high, in the range of normal individuals [52]. However, other studies of food-related atopic dermatitis (AD) show the opposite, namely, TH-1 cell enhanced activity following specific food lymphocyte stimulation (elevated IL-2 and IFN-γ, reduced IL-4 level) as compared to healthy controls or those with exclusive immediate allergic reactions [53–55]. In a study of children with "food allergic" delayed reactions, *both* IL-4 and IFN-γ serum levels were elevated, along with that of specific IgE, as compared to those of non-food-allergic controls [56]. The lymphocytes from patients with food-associated AD also produce high levels of monocyte chemotactic factor [57] and CD4+CD45RO+ T cells with a concomitant decrease in L-selection expression as compared to those of controls [58].

Varieties of Clinical Manifestations

Subjective responses that follow food ingestion are symptoms recognized only by the patient and have no measurable functional or inflammatory changes. They might be psychosomatic and could be discounted unless accompanied by convincing historical, physical, or laboratory data. D.W., a 38-year-old male, is illustrative (Table 4). He had subjective chronic and recurrent ringing in his ears, abdominal pain, and headache as well as observable flushing, urticaria, behavioral changes, and a vertical forehead skin crease. After dietitian supervised elimination diet and open foodstuff challenges, it was clear that he had immediate or delayed symptoms after virtually all additives and many processed foods. He was nonatopic and RAST-negative to eight foods, some of which he couldn't tolerate. He remained free of all symptoms if he stuck to home cooking and avoided all known foodstuff offenders.

Functional changes in tissues or organs are stronger evidence of food-related disease, particularly when they follow provocative food challenge [5]. Examples of smooth muscle dysfunction include those affecting the bladder detrusor muscle (enuresis), bronchioles (asthma), and intestine (hyperperistalsis). Increased vascular permeability is seen in milk-induced nephrotic syndrome, and in anaphylactic shock. Malabsorption is common in the gut [36]. Central nervous system dysfunction appears to be uncommon, ranging from irritability, sleep disturbance, lethargy, and behavioral changes to hyperactivity, seizures, depression, and psychotic manifestations [59,60]. Certainly many examples of dysfunction associated with eating food cannot be documented until a quantifiable abnormal function can be measured (e.g., reduced spirometric values) after a careful open food challenge or blinded challenge.

TABLE 4   D.W., 38 Year Old Male #0606 5536[a]

SX:	1½ years constant ringing in ears and episodic urticaria, flushing, abdominal pain, headache; behavioral/mood change, forehead skin crease
HX:	Immediate or delayed SX after MSG, citrus, caffeine, fast foods, processed foods, nitrites. "Food" intolerance in mother, siblings, children
FINDINGS:	Total IgE 130. RAST result negative to banana,[b] beef,[b] lemon,[b] milk, potato, soy, wheat, egg.
SUBSEQUENT COURSE:	Dietitian supervised elimination and challenge: sensitive to many additives in fast food and processed foods; few SX on home cooking and food avoidance; SX with foods outside home largely prevented by Gastrocrom but not by pancreatic enzymes.

[a]MSG, monosodium glutamate; IgE, immunoglobulin E; RAST, radioallergosorbent test.
[b]Not tolerated.

Morphological and Inflammatory Changes

Morphological and inflammatory alterations in tissues, as seen in biopsy samples, that are present during periods of food ingestion and that disappear during elimination of food and clinical remission can be strong evidences of food-induced disease. In Heiner's syndrome immune complexes containing milk antigen are localized in lung vascular structures, leading to pneumonitis, hemorrhage, and hemosiderosis [61,62]. Arteritis, thrombophelitis, and vasculitis at times have been reported to be food related [63,64]. Thrombocytopenia and other blood dyscrasias, sometimes with lupuslike symptoms, have uncommonly been connected to food allergy [5,34,65,66]. Other examples of food-associated pathological changes are discussed in organ system sections that follow.

DISORDERS OF INFANTS AND TODDLERS

General Aspects, Emphasizing Cow's Milk Allergy (CMA)

Probably 3%–5% of infants suffer from food allergy; cow's milk is the leading offender, far and away [5,67,68]. There are two reaction patterns: one in which the baby is exquisitely sensitive, having an immediate classic allergic reactions (usually IgE-mediated) after ingesting small amounts of milk; and another in which delayed reactions of a wider spectrum follow ingestion of relatively larger amounts of food [69–71]. In the first 6 months of life, a number of factors predispose the infant to sensitization and disease. These include a relatively indiscriminate absorption of macromolecules from the gut, low levels of digestible enzymes, and immature gut surface immunity with lessened "gatekeeper" IgA functions and undeveloped immunological tolerance to various foodstuffs [5,72,73].

Largely because CMA is relatively common, most clinical and basic studies of infant food sensitivity involve cow's milk. Many babies appear to be sensitized in utero, with milk-specific IgE level measurable in cord blood [66]. Some emphasize the multiplicity of over 20 constituent proteins theoretically capable of inducing IgE [67]. The clinical manifestations of CMA are highly variable. Although many cases are type I, easily identified by immediate reactions on challenge, many are not so easily diagnosed, requiring extended challenges with greater amounts of milk and likely involving type II, III, or IV hypersensitivity and nonimmunological mechanisms [67,68,71].

The studies of D. J. Hill and colleagues in Melbourne, Australia, since the mid-1980s have been particularly edifying [74–78]. They have identified three distinct reaction patterns in over a hundred cases that illustrate the diversity of CMA (see Table 5). The first group, approximately one-fourth of the total, is typically atopic reacting to a relatively small milk challenge usually in under an hour. Many have vomiting/diarrhea, and some show urticaria/angioedema and/or

TABLE 5 Reaction Patterns in Infants and Toddlers with Cow's Milk Allergy[a]

	Immediate (27%)	Intermediate (53%)	Late (20%)
Time of onset	< 2 hr	2–24 hr	1–5 Days
Milk dose required	Smallest	Larger	Largest, often repeated
Manifestations			
Gastrointestinal	Vomiting, diarrhea, colic	Vomiting, often severe; diarrhea, often severe; colic; failure to thrive	Diarrhea, often severe; failure to thrive; colic; intolerance of other foods
Skin	Urticaria, angioedema	—	Atopic eczema
Respiratory	Rhinitis, occasional; asthma, occasional	—	Rhinitis common; asthma common
Immunological parameters[a]			
IgE sensitization to milk Ags	Usually present (atopic)	Only in a minority	Only in those with eczema
Other immunoglobulins	—	Some IgA deficiency	↑ IgM in some
T-cell reactivity to milk Ags in vitro	—	—	↑ Lymphocyte response in vitro, e.g., ↑LIF

[a]IgE, immunoglobulin.
Source: According to Dr. J. Hill and colleagues, Melbourne, Australia.

rhinitis/asthma. IgE sensitization to bovine proteins is usual. The intermediate group (half of the total) reacts to a larger milk dose after 2 to 24 hr. Gastrointestinal reactions are prominent, frequently with failure to thrive. IgE sensitization to milk is present in less than a third; some have IgA deficiency. The third category comprises the 20% that react after 24 hr up to 5 days, generally after repeated milk feedings. Severe gastrointestinal symptoms and failure to thrive are common, as is the tendency for intolerance of other foods. Atopic eczema is common; only these individuals have elevated total serum IgE and milk-specific IgE levels. Rhinitis and asthma are common, and often severe. A minority of these children have elevated serum IgM level. Most show increased in vitro lymphocyte responsiveness to bovine antigens, e.g., elevated LIF release [77].

A 1996 report by Baehler et al. reaches a similar conclusion [71]. Sixty-nine children with history suggestive of CMA whose condition was resolved on a milk-free diet were studied. IgE sensitization to milk was measured by skin test and in vitro assay, and a two-stage DBPCFC with milk was carried out over several days.

About a one-fourth reacted in under 2 hr with typical allergic symptoms; average age was 36 months. Over two-thirds of these were IgE-sensitized, with 83% specificity. The other group, three-quarters of the total, had delayed reactions, 2 hr to 6 days after first challenge. Average age was 17 months. Symptoms were mostly gastrointestinal; the positive DBPCFC result usually required repeated challenges. None of this group had milk-positive IgE sensitization; specificity was 97%. They concluded that IgE-antibody determination cannot predict the outcome of DBPCFC in delayed reactors, and that a thorough clinical history was the most helpful tool.

Food Sensitivity in Infants

Symptoms most commonly appear in the first 2 months of life and are often overlooked [5,34,79,80]. Although CMA accounts for most reactions, soy, egg, and wheat also are important. The *gastrointestinal system* is most frequently involved; chronic diarrhea (sometimes bloody) is the most common manifestation [36,80]. Buccal/oral involvement (angioedema, stomatitis), vomiting, colic, distension, malabsorption, occult bleeding, constipation, eosinophilic gastritis–enteritis–colitis, and failure to thrive also may be seen. A possible association between hypertrophic pyloric stenosis, atopy, and CMA has been suggested [81]. Recently, gastroesophageal reflux secondary to intolerance to milk and other foods has been recognized [82]

Next, in order of frequency, is the *respiratory system.* Upper respiratory disorders include chronic rhinitis with associated chronic or recurrent sinusitis and otitis media, often with effusion. "Frequent colds" and chronic nasal congestion/obstruction are common. Lower respiratory manifestations include asthmalike symptoms (frequent cough, chest congestion, wheezing) and inflammatory/infectious responses ("bronchitis," "pneumonitis") that probably are asthma equivalents in many cases. A special form of recurrent pneumonitis is the Heiner syndrome, already described, associated with type I, III, and possibly IV responses to bovine antigens. Findings include failure to thrive, gastrointestinal reactions, fever, dyspnea, malabsorption, and anemia secondary to gastrointestinal bleeding; iron malabsorption; and bleeding at affected lung sites (hemosiderosis) [5,34,80].

In babies with sensitivity to milk and other foods, the *skin* is next most often involved. Atopic dermatitis (eczema) is a particular problem, discussed later; urticaria and angioedema are less common. The *central nervous system* follows in frequency, with a spectrum including irritability, fussiness, behavioral changes, and sleep disturbances, especially insomnia [80,85]. Systemic *anaphylaxis* to foods is relatively uncommon.

Diagnosis of food sensitivity in infants is relatively easy, once the physician considers the possibility [68]. Any array of symptoms suggestive of "allergy" (especially gastrointestinal, respiratory, or cutaneous) *automatically* should provoke work-up for food triggers, since inhalant allergens play a lesser in the first year of life. The diagnostic steps are the following:

- Interdict all or most solid foods.
- Maintain nutrition exclusively or mostly with a cow's milk substitute.
  - If breast milk, mother may need to interdict highly allergenic foods in her diet.
  - If a proprietary "hypoallergenic" formula, casein hydrolysates are more reliable than the relatively allergenic soy-based formulas.
- Remission of most/all symptoms occurs within 2 weeks if food-sensitive.
- Reintroduce interdicted foods, including milk formula, one at a time, to provoke symptoms (positive challenge result) and identify whichever foods are to be eliminated in subsequent diet.
- To be certain, all steps can be repeated.

The role of testing for IgE sensitization to specific foods is problematic in infants with suspected adverse reactions to foods. As previously discussed, skin sensitivity is relatively low, not becoming fully developed for allergen testing until several years later. Further, skin tests or in vitro tests usually yield negative results for most tested foods, particularly those causing delayed reactions. In infants with known food "allergies," skin testing or RAST testing to a food never before ingested (e.g., egg) can help predict in which infants symptoms, even delayed, will develop, on subsequent initial oral challenge [84]. In 16 infants with documented CMA (two or more positive challenge results), IgE plasma cells were found in 9 small bowel mucosal biopsy samples and in only 1 of 15 nonsensitive controls ($P < 0.01$) [85]. RAST for cow's milk had a positive result in only 6 of the 16 allergic infants, and in 2 of the 15 controls; 5 of the 9 babies with CMA and mucosal IgE plasma cells had negative RAST findings for cow's milk.

Management of infants with sensitivity to milk or other foods ordinarily is relatively simple. Once the baby is on breast milk or hypoallergenic formula and a diet eliminating all major food offenders, the clinical course is calm except for occasional symptoms that follow dietary indiscretions. However, a number of special situations deserve comment.

Maternal Factors: Intrauterine Sensitization and Breast Milk Feeding

It is widely appreciated that immunogenic fractions of foods ingested by pregnant females circulate in their blood and gain access to the placental circulation. Genetically susceptible fetuses become sensitized in utero, so that neonatally [5,80,86] or some days or weeks thereafter, adverse reactions occur upon ingestion of cow's milk or other foodstuffs. In 210 studied "allergy-risk" infants, maternal avoidance of cow's milk and egg during pregnancy had no effect on food antibodies in cord serum, but the mother's intake of these foods during lactation had an effect [87]. Elimination of cow's milk in the maternal diet during lactation lowered specific antibody levels in their babies and delayed atopic symptoms, as compared to infants of control mothers drinking cow's milk. In another study, some babies were fed cow's milk formula, others were exclusively breast fed; a third group received both [88]. By 4 months of age, the formula-fed babies had elevated IgE and IgG antibodies to milk proteins and had more CMA-related disease than did the breast milk group. Of note, CMA symptoms were not significantly related to the presence of specific antibody!

It has been documented that human breast milk contains significant (not necessarily trace) amounts of maternal ingested foods such as bovine milk proteins and egg allergens [89]. Generally the low levels of food macromolecule are inconsequential or may favor immune tolerance; breast milk generally is associated with prevention of allergic disease, as compared to cow's milk formula [90,91]. However, occasional babies are so exquisitely sensitized and/or susceptible that the minute amounts of food(s) in breast milk induce disease. When 18 of 19 mothers of breast-fed infants with colic went on a cow's milk–free diet, the colic disappeared promptly in 13. In all but 1, reintroduction of milk in the mother's diet resulted in recurrence of colic [92]. Other workers studying 20 similar patients reached different conclusions: avoidance of cow's milk by lactating mothers did not reduce colic, but increasing the number of other foods in their diet increased attacks of colic in the infants [93]. In a study of 57 babies exclusively fed breast milk allergic disease developed in 11 [94]. The breast milk from mothers of these allergic infants contained lower total IgA ($p < 0.01$) and IgA specific for cow's milk proteins ($p < .001$) than milk from mothers of healthy babies. Inadequate levels of possibly protective specific IgA were more closely associated with allergic disease than was parental atopic history! β-Lactoglobulin was detectable in almost half of the maternal milk donors, for up to 3 days after dietary milk exclusion. An Italian study by Cavagni et al. convincingly demonstrated that in babies with atopic dermatitis who were exclusively breast fed, maternally ingested bovine lactoglobulin is regularly transported from breast milk into the sera of the babies [95]. Maternal milk elimination diet improved eczema in 11 of 13 infants and maternal milk challenge worsened the disease in 9 of 9.

The Utility of Hypoallergenic Formulas

In most infants with cow's milk allergy, a so-called hypoallergenic formula will be substituted rather than breast milk. Soy formulas were introduced in the 1950s as a practical and relatively inexpensive substitute for cow's milk. Unfortunately their allergenicity rivals that of cow's milk formulas, and many babies allergic to bovine milk proteins are allergic to soy proteins as well

[96,97]. The preferred milk substitutes are casein hydrolysates in which the proteins have been extensively hydrolyzed to relatively small poorly immunogenic molecules [98], available whey protein products are only partially hydrolyzed [96,98]. When casein hydrolysates are adequately hydrolyzed they are quite safe, are well tolerated by almost all milk-allergic infants, and are immunologically nonreactive in sensitized animals or sensitive in vitro test [99,100].

Multiple Food Protein Intolerance and the Need for Elemental Formulas

Unfortunately, 1%–2% of infants with CMA cannot tolerate casein hydrolysates such as Nutramigen or Pregestemil. Frequently they have multiple food sensitivities, as well. In such cases, amino acid formula Neocate, SHS North America, has proved to be well tolerated, palatable, and associated with excellent growth [98,101,102]. More recently, an extremely serious condition called multiple food protein intolerance (MFPI) has been recognized, characterized by irritability, vomiting, diarrhea, colitis, severe generalized eczema, and growth failure [98,103]. Babies are intolerant of most or all protein-containing foods; IgE sensitization is present for some but not most, and reactions may be immediate or, more commonly, delayed. One such patient in my practice (see Table 6) was intolerant of several hypoallergenic formulas, all foods, and several medications. MFPI seems to be the cause of reflux esophagitis in many infants unresponsive to hypoallergenic formulas, H_2 antagonists and prokinetic agents [104]. In all the situations associated with multiple or universal food intolerances, Neocate proved to be efficacious and tolerated, virtually without exception.

TABLE 6 K. H., 8 Month Old Male #0607 4549[a]

SX:	Severe atopic dermatitis and mild rhinitis, rash unresponsive to medical management and diet manipulation
HX:	Virtually all foods and all hypoallergenic formulas cause immediate or delayed flaring of eczema, flushing, fussiness, sleeplessness.
Findings:	IgE 216; RAST response positive to two foods and negative to five foods and four inhalants, gut endoscopy finding normal with normal biopsy samples of stomach, small intestine, colon
Course to 24 months:	Nutramigen, Pregestamil, Neocate one-Plus, Hydroxyzine, Prelone, Gastrocrom, Tylenol. not tolerated. Only Elemental Formula Neocate (SHS) tolerated, associated with remission of disease and make up growth; small amounts of many foods now safely supplement Neocate after 16 months of age

[a]IgE, immunoglobulin E; RAST, radioallergosorbent test.

Protective Effect of Hypoallergenic Formulas or Breast Milk in Newborns at Risk for Allergic Disease

Babies born in families in which one or both parents are allergic have a greatly increased risk for development of allergic disease in the first year or so of life. When such newborns are placed on a prophylactic regimen of breast milk or hypoallergenic formula, early exclusion of commonly allergenic foods, and control of perennial indoor inhalant allergens (e.g., dust mite, cat), most studies show significant protection against allergic disease lasting at least 2 and up to 5 years [105–107]. For example, Zeiger et al. showed that babies on (Nutramigen) casein hydrolysate and restricted diet had a 16% incidence of allergic disease as compared to 27% in babies fed cow's milk formula and nonrestricted diet [108]. Interestingly, the incidence of positive skin prick test (SPT) results to milk antigen was 12% in controls and only 1% in the prophylactic group ($p = 0.0001$), suggesting that allergic reactions in the latter group often were not IgE-related in the usual sense and likely delayed. Chandra et al. also studied a newborn population at high risk for allergy [109]. They found later atopic manifestations to be lowest in babies fed a whey–protein hydrolysate, Goodstart (7%), or breast milk (20%). Those fed milk formula, Similac, or soy formula, Isomil, had equally higher rates of allergic disease (36%–37%). In symptomatic babies, the SPT response to milk antigens was positive in 58% of breast fed (!), 66% of Similac, and 80% of the Goodstart group, again suggesting that some reactions were likely delayed and unrelated to IgE.

FOOD SENSITIVITY IN TODDLERS AND PRESCHOOL CHILDREN

Common manifestations of food sensitivity and associated immunological phenomena in this age group have already been described in the preceding section, General Aspects Emphasizing Milk Allergy (Table 5). When 97 of the original 100 in the Australian group were followed for up to 99 months, one-fourth (28%) tolerated cow's milk at 2 years, half (56%) by 4 years, and three-fourths (78%) by age 6 [110]. Only one-fourth (25%) were allergic to milk alone; 58% were sensitive to egg, 47% to soy milk, and 34% to peanut. At final follow-up, in 40% asthma had developed and allergic rhinitis in 45%. Similarly, Businco's group in Italy found that two-thirds (25 of 37) of children with cow's milk–induced chronic diarrhea followed 4 to 10 years tolerated milk by 6 years; the median age of recovery was age 2 [111]. In the majority inhalant allergies developed as well. In Host's review of the natural course of CMA, recovery occurred earlier than in other studies: 45%–56% by 1 year; 60%–77% by age 2; and 71%–87% by only age 3 [68]. Only one-fourth (28%) had experienced inhalant allergies by age 3, and 80% before puberty, particularly those showing an early, brisk IgE response to milk proteins.

Two conditions that have been frequently associated with food sensitivity deserve special mention. One is *chronic or recurrent otitis media with effusion (OME),* often in combination with sinusitis and rhinitis. Refractory/recurrent OME has been associated with allergy, either to inhalants or less commonly to foods, at an incidence of 23%–80% [112], 4%–90% [113] or 33% [114]. Startling work by Nsouli et al. at first reported in 1994 suggests that refractory OME in children (median age 4.6 years) is causally related to food allergy 78% of the time [115,116]! Of 104 individuals, 81 (78%) had IgE sensitization to foods and an allergic history. Of these 81, 70 (86%) had significant amelioration of their OME clinically and by tympanometry when placed on a food elimination diet for 16 weeks. Of these 70, 66 (94%) experienced recurrence of OME when IgE-positive foods were replaced in their diet (open challenge). In one control group of similar allergic children with OME sensitized to foods, but not placed on a diet, only 25% improved ($p < 0.01$); in a second control group with OME, nonallergic, only 11% improved over 16 weeks.

In all the food-allergic children [115,116], the order of frequency for the main offending foods was the following: milk (38%), wheat, egg white, peanut, soy, corn, and orange (10%). Eighty-one percent of cases were sensitized to one to four foods, 14% to only one, and 5% to five or more. The study has been criticized because of loose diagnostic criteria for food allergy and the use of open food challenge other than DBPCFC [117]; it is likely that food sensitivity in most patients with OME is uncommon, but that it is far more prevalent in the subpopulation with refractory/chronic OME.

Atopic dermatitis (eczema) (AD) is the second disorder in preschool children that is often associated with food sensitivities. AD is most common in the first years of life (85% of cases by age 5) with the prevalence and severity falling off markedly thereafter [112]. The incidence in the pediatric population is estimated to be 12% [118]. Most of these affected are highly atopic, sensitized to many inhalant and food antigens, and manifesting allergic rhinitis in 20% and asthma in 45% of cases [112,118–120]. The incidence of food sensitivity in AD has been reported to be 33%–60% of cases on the basic of studies of relatively severe AD employing DBPCFC techniques [5,121,122]. IgE mechanisms for immediate and some delayed reactions are supported by the frequent correlation of specific IgE sensitization to foods causing immediate flaring of eczema [119–123], release of histamine and prostaglandin D_2 (PGD_2) into skin blister chambers after SPT-positive food epicutaneous challenges [124], and high rates of spontaneous histamine release from peripheral blood basophils as compared to that of normal controls or AD patients on elimination diets [125]. In addition, delayed-type T cell mechanisms seem to be operative in AD, related at times to delayed reactions to foods, the cellular infiltrate in skin and gut mucosal lesions, regulation of IgE synthesis, and activation of mast cells [5,119,125]. Agata et al. found that the increased deoxyribonucleic acid (DNA) synthesis in blood mononuclear cells stimulated by food in vitro and the high serum specific IgE levels dropped markedly when AD food, sensitive patients were placed on an elimination diet [126]. Leung suggested that eczema skin lesions include an expansion of TH-2 cells after stimulation by specific antigens, with the potential for IL-4 and IL-5 production and increase of IgE and accumulation of eosinophils [127]. The allergic gastrointestinal mucosal inflammation associated with AD seems to relate to the not-infrequent gastrointestnal symptoms in AD patients [5,121,128,129] and the indiscriminate absorption into the blood of relatively large molecules (e.g., food) from the intestine [130].

Results of many studies, often employing DBPCFC, suggest that the majority of food reactions in AD are delayed [5,74–78,112,131], although immediate reactions are common. Some studies find that the ratio of delayed to immediate reactions is half and half [5,132]. Sampson's group, on the other hand, reports that the large majority of reactions are immediate, possibly reflecting unusually high levels of atopy in their population [118,120,122,123]. Egg, soy, milk, peanut, and wheat tend to be the most prominent offenders [5,121,123,112]; the number is limited to one or two in most patients of Sampson's group [123] and commonly four or more in other studies [5,74–78,112,131,132,109,128,129].

A work-up for food sensitivity should be considered in any AD patient not responding well to comprehensive medical management [121]. The diagnosis of food sensitivity is dependent on elimination of suspect foods and subsequent challenge with each individually [5,112,131]. In clinical practice open challenge often will suffice, but for research purposes or most dependable results, DBPCFC is recommended [119,122,123,133,134]. The history is unreliable except for identifying potential food offenders [5,131]. SPT/in vitro testing suffers from variable sensitivity and low specificity and is mainly useful to identify foods that yield "positive" results to be included in elimination and challenge [112,131,132,135]. A Finnish DBPCFC report suggests that a patch test for delayed food reactions may additionally be helpful. Immediate reactions to food SPT were positive 67% of the time, and the patch test result was always negative; in delayed reactions the patch test finding was positive 89% of the time and the SPT result often positive [132].

The relevance of food sensitivity in AD is best demonstrated by the fact that high numbers of food-sensitive AD patients improve significantly on long-term elimination diets and suffer exacerbation on rechallenge with known food offenders [5,94,112,112,123]. It should be remembered that food additives and simple nutrients, e.g., citric or malic acid, can also trigger eczema [136,137] and that those with reactions to breast milk and many or most foods (and even some medications) may require an elemental diet [5,95,98,103,138]. Sampson et al. followed 25 of their food-sensitive severe AD patients on long-term elimination diets [139]. After 1 year, 25% lost all signs of clinical food reactivity by DBPCFC. After 2 years, 91% continued to have persistently positive re-

sponses to one or two offending foods, and after the third challenge, 100%. Total or specific IgE levels did not correlate with loss or retention of food sensitivity over time.

DISORDERS IN OLDER CHILDREN AND ADULTS

Because the *gastrointestinal tract* is the first site where ingestants interact with
body constituents it is no surprise that vomiting, diarrhea, distension, hyperperi-
staris, and constipation are common manifestations of foodstuff sensitivity. The
diagnosis of a food-induced gastroenteropathy should be entertained in anyone
with chronic diarrhea, malabsorption, hypoproteinemia, anemia, or failure to
thrive that is otherwise unexplained [34]. It could be predicted that adverse reactions to foods could involve every level of the gastrointestinal tract, and that is
the case. Some reactions are IgE-mediated and usually immediate; these include
the oral allergy syndrome, gastrointestinal (GI) anaphylaxis, and a subset of allergic eosinophilic gastroenteritis (AEG). The others, named later, are often non-
IgE-mediated and frequently delayed [140,141].

Moving downward from the mouth, oral lesions include the oral allergy
syndrome after ingestion of fresh fruits and vegetables (at times associated with
concomitant inhalant allergy and allergic disease elsewhere in the body
[142,143], apthous ulcers, pruritis, and chronic mucosal fissuring [140,144].
AEG manifests postprandial nausea and vomiting, abdominal pain,
diarrhea/streatorrhea, and failure to thrive or weight loss. Eosinophilic inflammation involves the mucosal, muscular, and/or serocal layers of the stomach or
small intestine [4,140,147]. The small intestine is the site of milk- or soy-induced enteropathy; mucosal injury [145], manifesting as anemia secondary to
blood loss, GI protein loss, edema, and hypoproterinemia; and chronic diarrhea
with malabsorption [4,34,140]. Gluten-induced enteropathy is similar. The diagnosis is made by the finding of typical villous atrophy and chronic inflammation
on intestinal biopsy with histological and clinical resolution after a gluten-free
diet [4,34,140,141]. Dermatitis herpetiformis, with characteristic deposited granular IgA deposits, is often associated [4,146]. Food-induced colitis syndromes,
commonly showing diarrhea, cramping, and bleeding, also are described, especially in children [4,140,141].

Food sensitivity has been postulated as a cause in two other disorders; the
evidence for both is tenuous. Irritable bowel syndrome is characterized by dyspepsia, abdominal distension and pain, constipation, and/or diarrhea and a high incidence of psychiatric disorders [147]. It appears to be a condition in which the gut is
hyperreactive to a variety of nonspecific mechanical and chemical stimuli perhaps
secondary to increased numbers and activation states of mast cells and other effector cells and augmentation of some neuralgic reflex mechanisms [148–150]. Inflammatory bowel disease such as ulcerative colitis or Crohn's disease similarly

has not been demonstrated to be disorders of food sensitivity causally, but the poorly understood inflammatory conditions with immunological involvement that often improve significantly on exclusion or elemental diets [151–153]. In bona fide GI adverse reactions to foods, aggressive factors such as IgA deficiency, alterations in the mucosal barrier (e.g., inflammation), decreased mucosal viability, constipation, and decreased pancreatic enzymes may tip the balance away from the "tolerance" promoted by immune defenses via GALT, and nonimmune defenses such as normal enteric flora, enteric secretions and mucus, acid secretions, and digestive enzymes [154,155]. Conversely, the Gell and Coombs' triggering mechanisms, mast cell activation, histamine/mediator release, cytokine and interleukin release, and chronic inflammation can bring about immediate and delayed gastrointestinal responses, malabsorption, transient loss of tolerance to certain foods (e.g., carbohydrates), and nonspecific gut irritability [34,140,155–157].

Adverse reactions to foods involving the *respiratory system* have attracted much attention. Oehling's group in Spain found that 18.5% of food-allergic patients had symptoms limited exclusively to the respiratory tract; most were atopic and appeared to be sensitive to one food [158]. Boccafogli et al. studied 219 Italian adults with rhinitis, asthma, or both [159]. Of the 169 monosensitized to grass pollen, 48% had respiratory symptoms after food ingestion (and sometimes OAS, urticaria, or GI symptoms), whereas of the 50 monosensitized to house dust mites, only 6% reacted to food according to detailed history, $p <$ 0.0000001! Of the 38% having a positive food challenge result in the grass group, a third of the reactions were immediate and IgE related and two-thirds were delayed and not IgE-related, very comparable to the results of Hill's CMA infants and toddlers in Australia [72–76]. In pollen-sensitive European patients with respiratory allergy, as many as 47% are sensitized to food allergens; in about a fourth of these rhinitis and OAS develop, and about one-fifth manifest asthma and development of urticaria [7,160].

Heiner suggested that rhinitis is the most common respiratory symptom of food sensitivity and that it is frequently associated with asthma, secretory otitis media, and tonsillar/adenoidal hypertrophy [161]. In studies of several hundred unselected rhinitis-affected adults in Milan, foodstuffs evoked rhinitis symptoms in about 25% [159]. In a DBPCFC study of 320 highly atopic children nasal symptoms developed after 166 (70%) of 236 positive food challenge results [162]. In Holland, Pelikan studied 142 perennial allergic rhinitis patients with SPT to foods, rhinomanometry, and food histories [163]. Of 47 with positive food "allergy" histories, 41 (90%) had positive nasal responses to 65 of 72 food challenges. The overall incidence of food sensitivity causing rhinitis was 29%. Of 95 rhinitics with questionable food allergy by history, 54 had positive food challenge responses, most of which were late, delayed, dual immediate/late, or delayed as opposed to immediate.

The reported incidence of food-induced *asthma* is quite variable because of selection of patients (atopic versus unselected) and differing diagnostic criteria. Using DBPCFC, food sensitivity was found to cause asthma in 2% [161] and 5.7% [162] of atopic European cases. Oehling and Gagnani found the incidence to be 8.5% of asthmatic children, generally in response to a single food [166]. In Denmark, Hoj et al. placed 37 comparable chronic severe asthmatics on a double-blind diet for 2 weeks [167]. Nine of 21 (43%) on an elemental Vivenex-like product improved greatly, whereas only 1 of 16 on a blended ordinary diet did so ($p < .05$). Two-thirds of the 9 elemental diet reponders were considered "intrinsic" asthmatics; the author concluded that all severe asthmatic patients deserve a diagnostic evaluation for food/additive sensitivity. At the National Jewish Center in Denver, 279 had a history of food-induced asthma; there were positive food challenge findings in 168 (60%) of these, including 67 (24%) who had positive DBPCFC results associated with wheezing [168]. In a 1987 Holland study of 107 perennial asthmatic subjects, 15 of 21 (71%) with food allergy history showed a positive asthmatic response to food challenge [169]. Indeed, 45 of 86 (56%) without food allergy history also showed positive bronchial responses on food challenge. About a fourth of the asthmatic responses were immediate; the rest were late, delayed, or dual. There was poor correlation with SPT or in vitro food sensitization. In a contemporary study of adults with DBPCFC proven food-induced asthma, 5 reactions were immediate, 18 late or delayed, and 4 dual [170]. Recently, James et al. demonstrated 22 positive DBPCFC reactions among 26 asthmatics with food allergy [171]. Twelve reactions were typically asthmatic and 10 were nonpulmonary, involving the larynx, GI tract, or skin. Finally, it should be mentioned that individuals with atopic dermatitis have a high rate of asthmatic responses to DBPCFC, 26% inBusinco's group [172] and 27% in a Johns Hopkins study [167].

Pulmonary hemosiderosis with infiltrates and eosinophilia occurs uncommonly in older children, generally as a result of cow's milk sensitization [173] but to other foods as well, such as buckwheat [174].

Urticaria occurs at least once in 20% of the population; a minority of individuals have chronic urticaria lasting over 6 weeks [175]. Lesions of chronic urticaria exhibit vascular dilatation with infiltrates suggestive of the typical late-phase "allergic" reaction [175,176]; T cell activation with cytokine release occurs [177]. Allergic contact dermatitis, acute or delayed, associated with food sensitivity and recognized by patch testing has also been described [175,178]. It has long been recognized that chronic urticaria (and angioedema) is at times causally associated with many foods and additives [5,175,179–181]. The incidence of foodstuff-induced urticaria is reported to be 11%–55% of cases, measured by improvement on strict elimination diet and provocation of symptoms by DBPCFC. Most patients are not atopic, and SPT- or RAST-type tests [182] to foods are not helpful in most cases. It would appear that additives such as dyes, flavorings, salicylates, and preservatives are more frequent offenders than foods per se [5,175,179,181]. The patient L.M. (Table 7) is illustrative: urticaria, present for 6 years and associated with atopy and possible silicone–rubber–kiwi, banana, and avocado cross-reactivity, disappeared on a strict elimination diet. Except to caffeine, urticarial reactions to foods or additive challenges were delayed 6–8 hr.

Recurrent or chronic *arthralgia,* usually without serological evidence of rheumatoid arthritis or of permanent joint changes, is a not uncommon manifestation of delayed food reactions at times in association with other "allergic" symptoms [5,183,184]. Paganelli et al. studied 24 subjects with chronic urticaria/angioedema, 13 of whom had frequent arthralgia, and were treated with an aligoantigenic diet [185]. Twenty-four (two-thirds) went into remission, including the majority of those with arthralgia. They had increased absorption of bovine lactoglobulin (BLG) after milk ingestion, suggesting that circulating BLG–antibody complexes were playing a role. None had milk-specific IgE detected! Carini et al. studied 10 "allergic" patients who suffered from arthralgia; dietary exclusion of foods relieved the symptoms and food challenge reproduced them [186]. Levels of IgG anti-IgE autoantibodies and immune complexes were high in serum and synovial fluid as compared to those of controls and patients with other arthritis disorders. In a similar group of patients, Brostoff et al. found that the appearance of immune complexes and joint symptoms could be prevented by pretreatment with oral cromolyn before food, e.g., milk, challenge [183]. Table 8 illustrates the role of food sensitivity in a 15 year old girl with $1^1/_2$ years of recurrent arthralgia and associated myalgia, headaches, and abdominal pain. All symptoms appeared within a month of starting a vegetarian diet, very high in milk and wheat products. Her disease remitted on diet eliminating milk,

TABLE 7   L.M., 47 Year Old Female #0625-8663[a]

SX:	6 Years of chronic urticaria, daily, worse with heat and baths
HX:	Allergic rhinitis in early adult years; hives in past from contact with rubber products; silicone breast implants 22 years ago; ruptured 6 years ago and removed a year later; high doses of antihistamines give negligible relief
Findings:	Bananas, avocados, tomatoes, kiwi, Big Red, coffee, tea, soy cause hives; as does running; RAST response positive for wheat, oat, corn, peanut, soy, tomato, avocado, negative for 15 other foods
Course:	Dietitian supervised elimination and open challenges: caffeine, all legumes, and some additives are offenders. Except for caffeine, urticaria delayed 6–8 hr after offending food or additive ingestion; doing well on strict elimination diet; oral cromolyn before meals reduces breakthrough hives

[a]RAST, radiallergosorbent test.

TABLE 8   M.Z., 15 Year Old Female[a]

SX:	1$\frac{1}{2}$ Years of chronic, recurrent arthralgia involving multiple joints; no crippling; myalgia, headaches, and abdominal pain also present
HX:	Multiple allergies and food sensitivities as infant; asthma since age 10; started vegetarian diet (high dairy and wheat products) 1-month before onset of SX; now seronegative, sed rate in 80s and DX of atypical rheumatoid arthritis
Findings:	Dietitian supervised elimination diet and open challenges showed milk, wheat, several other foods to trigger GI SX (4 hr) and arthralgia, headaches, CNS dysfunction (next day)
Course:	Remission of disease with minimal to no SX on strict elimination diet

[a]GI, gatrointestinal; CNS, central nervous System.

wheat, and other trigger foods; most symptoms including arthralgia appeared on the day after food challenge!

A possible role of food sensitivity in *rheumatoid arthritis* has been controversial, with scattered case reports suggesting a causative role. In one blind, placebo-controlled British study of 45 patients with rheumatoid arthritis, 33 (73%) considered their arthritis after 6 weeks of dietary exclusion to be significantly better [187]. Panush et al. have developed rabbit models of food- (e.g., milk) induced "rheumatoid arthritis," with circulating and localized milk–antibody complexes associated with typical synovial pathological conditions that offer promise for better understanding of the problem [188]. In a study by Fueri et al., increased interleuken 4 production was observed in response to mast cell mediators and human type I collagen in patients with rheumatoid arthritis [189].

The possible role of food sensitivity in *central nervous system* (CNS) disorders has enjoyed a great deal of attention and controversy in recent decades. Earlier largely unsubstantiated notions concerning food "allergy" and CNS dysfunction (e.g., tension fatigue syndrome of Speer and Crook [190] increasingly have been supplanted by a more scientific approach involving carefully designed and implemented studies [191]. Ten years ago Heiner stated that individuals "with food-induced chronic diseases are likely to be fretful, depressed, restless, sleepless, or to have other manifestations of CNS dysfunction" [192]. Evidence for this assertion continues to accumulate. In Belgium, of 17 preschool children with severe unexplained insomnia, restlessness, and agitation 15 resolved completely on a milk-free diet and all but 1 manifested exacerbations on DBPCFC with milk [193].

According to Egger, *migraine* is best regarded as a neurovascular syndrome with a generalized vasomotor instability and vulnerability to multiple factors [191]. The earlier hypothesis of tyramine/vasoactive amine triggering in association with monamine oxidase deficiency seems less tenable than that of food sensitivity in which allergens or vasoactive substances absorbed from the gut trigger headaches centrally. In a 1983 study, Egger et al. found that 93% of 88 children with severe and frequent migraine benefited from an oligoantigenic diet [194]. In a DBPCFC cross-over trial, 90% of these responders relapsed with one or more foods, far more than to placebos ($p < .001$). Headaches generally were delayed, usually 2–3 days. In an earlier study, Monro et al. found that two-thirds of severe migraneurs improved on elimination diets (RAST findings often positive to offending foods) and usually relapsed on challenge [195]. Oral cromolyn before challenge often protected subjects from expected challenge headaches. In a study of 12 children with abdominal migraine, a broad elimination diet effected improvement in 10 [196]. Only 4 were atopic and RASTs to various foods were not helpful in any of the cases.

CNS dysfunctions, including cognitive and behavioral defects, hyperactivity, ADHD, and other problems, have long been associated with foods [5,190–192]. In the 1970s Feingold claimed that 40%–70% of hyperkinetic children benefited from diets free of additives, natural salicylates, and some foods, e.g., sugar and chocolate [5,191]; his findings were anecdotal and lacking in objective evidence. Dozens of studies [5,191,197,198] and an NIH consensus conference [199] suggest that Feingold's claims were exaggerated and that reactions to foods or additives account for a relatively small percentage of ADHD and hyperactivity cases. However, these studies are difficult to compare and many are flawed scientifically, particularly when only one or two arbitrary test substances (e.g., a dye or a preservative) were used for elimination and challenge. In 1989, Wilson and Scott studied 19 children with "alleged" food allergy involving the CNS and other organ systems [200]. Using double-blind cross-over diets testing four different additives, they found three children (16%) had serious reactions: urticaria from tartrazine and sunset yellow colors; abnormal behavior induced by sodium metabisulfite and sodium benzoate (preservatives) and abdominal pain from both sets of additives.

Three relatively recent well-constructed studies make a convincing case for a relatively common role of foodstuffs in the causation of ADHD, hyperactivity, and other severe CNS dysfunctions. The first report is by Kaplan et al., Calgary, Canada, in 1989 [201]. Twenty-four hyperactive preschool boys underwent placebo-controlled, blinded cross-over diets. The experimental diet eliminated all additives, caffeine, suspected food offenders, and sugar. On the test diet over half had marked improvement in hyperactivity, sleep disturbance, etc., although the placebo diet showed negligible effects. In the second study, by Boris and Mandel, in 1994, 26 children with ADHD were treated with a multiple item elimination diet [198]. Nineteen responded favorably (73%), $p < 0.001$. On open challenge all 19 reacted to many foods and additives. DBPCFC was completed in 16 children; there was significant improvement on placebo days, as compared to challenge days ($p = .003$). Atopics with multiple allergies responded better than nonatopics. The third study carried out in England in 1989 by Egger et al. [202] is particularly telling. Forty-five children with severe, recalcitrant epilepsy and abnormal electroencephalogram EEG findings also associated with headaches or hyperkinetic behavior or both and 18 children solely with epilepsy were studied. On oligoantigenic diet (OAD) 40 of the first group improved and the seizures disappeared or lessened markedly in 36 (80%); the other symptoms also largely disappeared. By open challenge in most and by DBPCFC, 15 of 16 had symptoms, including epilepsy, provoked by multiple foods and additives. Of the solely epileptic children, *none* improved on OAD!

Two cases dramatically illustrate the role that foodstuffs can play in complex and serious CNS disorders. M.M., a 10 year old, had ADHD with great variation in degree of hyperactivity on different days plus other variable CNS dysfunctions and local inflammatory reactions (Table 9). He was very atopic, having generalized symptoms on Multitest skin testing with inhalant and food allergens. He craved sugar so much that he scooped up and ate handfuls from bowls whenever possible; he did the same with potato chips. On challenge after elimination, these and other foods were found to cause CNS dysfunctions, asthma, facial inflammation, or throat clogging. He remained well on an elimination diet. The second case (see Table 10) is a 6 year old boy who had hard bizarre overwhelming CNS dysfunction (PDD-NOS, hyperactivity, and autistic features) since age 9 months. Excruciating headaches occurred daily. He had chronic rhinitis and recurrent otitis media. Certain foods, laden with dyes, dramatically worsened his behavior for hours. RAST test results

TABLE 9   M.M., 10 Year Old Male[a]

SX:	• ADHD—erratic hyperactivity, sleeplessness, dyslexia, reduced attention and concentration, belligerence; Ritalin no help; • Episodic sweats, edema, and erythema (painful) of face and ears, injected eyes, throat clogging

Work-up:	Milk allergy in infancy; now allergic rhinitis, asthma, mild eczema; food allergies in family; skin tests (many results positive) to inhalants and foods caused generalized SX; craving of sugar and potato chips; dietitian elimination and challenge:
	   Sugar (worst): facial, ocular, ear inflammation
	   Wheat (worst): hyperactivity
	   Tomato: belligerent behavior
	   Milk: throat clogging
	   Red food dye: asthma

Management:	Totally asymptomatic on diet rotating safe food, symptoms return on dietary indiscretion

[a]ADHD, attention deficit hyperactivity disorder.

TABLE 10 A.B.P., 6 Year Old Male #0625-8655[a]

SX:	Bizarre CNS dysfunction (PDD-NOS; hyperactivity and autistic features) since 9 months; daily excruciating headaches
HX:	Chronic rhinitis and recurrent otitis media from 2 mos Much worse on some days; some foods (e.g., Fruit Loops, Kool Aid, Skittles) dramatically worsen behavior for several hours; little help from dexedrine and Prozac
Findings:	RAST test results negative for 11 common food allergens; dietitian's elimination of additives and common foods led to 3 days of sleep "drunken" behavior followed by persisting unusually calm behavior and absence of headaches; rhinitis much improved; daily reintroduction of several test foods led to recognition of multiple offenders
Course:	On long-term elimination diet avoiding additives and known food offenders, CNS function virtually normal except for delayed development and some autistic features; no headaches, no need for psychotropic drugs, no evidence of rhinitis or otitis

[a]CNS, central nervous system; PDD-NOS, RAST, radioallergosorbent test.

were negative for many common foods. When placed on a diet eliminating many foods and all additives, he slept continuously, with drunken behavior on arousal for 3 days. Thereafter he displayed unusually calm behavior and stopped having headaches; rhinitis and otitis media disappeared. With long-term elimination diet, he seems normal except for delayed development and some autistic features.

From many published reports [112,191,198,200–202] and such illustrative cases, three clues have been identified that strongly suggest the possibility of CNS dysfunction (e.g., ADHD and hyperactivity) triggered by foods or additives:

1. The subject has a variety of associated "allergic" symptoms or conditions, e.g., rhinitis, eczema.
2. The CNS dysfunction is erratic on a day-to-day basis (one day a saint, another day a monster).
3. Certain foods or additives have been observed to provoke marked CNS dysfunction (e.g., hyperactivity, belligerence) for periods lasting several hours after ingestion.

In 1977, Sandberg et al. reported six older children with *nephrotic syndrome* and CMA [203]. Elimination of milk from the diet was associated with remission and reintroduction with exacerbation. Ten years later, Laurent et al. followed 13 patients with idiopathic nephrotic syndrome who had not responded to corticosteroids after many trials. Eight were "allergic"; IgE sensitivity to foods was present in 11 [204]. After OAD, proteinuria significantly decreased in all 13 and disappeared completely in 5.

DIAGNOSIS OF FOOD/ADDITIVE SENSITIVITY

Although this chapter is concerned with delayed/non-IgE adverse reactions to foodstuffs, any discussion of diagnosis or management must be broad enough to include immediate/IgE reactions since any patient may show both. It should also be acknowledged that the *only* definitive positive test result is an adverse reaction to reliable oral food/additive challenge. No single in vitro or in vivo test or procedure measuring sensitization to foodstuffs has sufficient sensitivity and specificity to be trustworthy in all clinical situations [205–211]. The diagnostic approach conveniently can be divided into four steps.

Step One: Appreciate the Diversity of Reactions to Foods or Additives

Because immediate reactions to foods, generally associated with positive SPT or in vitro test results showing specific IgE sensitization, are so easy to recognize, clinicians may be tempted to put all their diagnostic eggs in that basket. It must always be remembered that other immunological and nonimmunological triggering mechanisms exist (see Figure 1) and that *most* reactions are delayed and not immediate (see Table 1) [5,34,112,210,211]. Delayed reactions have a broader array of manifestations and usually follow relatively large ingestion of foodstuff to produce reactions hours or days later, not necessarily after each ingestion of offending agents.

Step Two: Acquire a High Index of Suspicion

A physician will never diagnose a condition unless he or she considers it as a reasonable possibility. Unfortunately, adverse reactions to foods often are not given serious consideration when they should be. There are two ways to raise the level of consciousness for possible food sensitivity. One is to remember that common "allergic" and other chronic/recurrent disorders can be triggered by foodstuffs not infrequently or commonly (see Table 11). A second aid is a set of clues that may suggest food sensitivity (see Table 12).

TABLE 11 Educated Guesses of the Prevalence/Incidence of Food-Related Disorders Reported in the Literature[a]

• Chronic rhinitis	25%–29%
• Atopic eczema	33%–60%
• Bronchial asthma	2%–43%
• Idiopathic urticaria	11%–55%
• Migraine headaches	20%–67%
• ADHD, other CNS aberrations	2%–73%
• Recurrent/persistent otitis media with effusion	25%–78%

[a]ADHD, attention deficit hypersensitivity disorder; CNS, central nervous system.

TABLE 12   Clues That May Suggest Food Sensitivity

• Allergic organ system disease not responding well to usual therapy; symptoms episodic, variable, erratic
• Associated "allergic" disease in other organs
• Symptoms (some or all) may be related to food(s) at times; immediate or delayed reactions after ingestion
• Dramatic improvement or worsening upon significant changes in diet; extreme cravings and dislikes of certain foods
• History of "allergic" symptoms associated with food sensitivity in early years; similar history in relatives
• Occasional association of environmental trigger factors (e.g., seasonal pollens) or exercise

---

Step Three: Identify Possible Food Offenders That Might Cause Disease

Identifying possible offenders is accomplished by detailed historical search for possible reactions to foods and specific dislikes; use of diaries, and questionnaires, and skin testing or in vitro testing for sensitization to suspect foods (see Table 13). In these and subsequent efforts, a working relationship with a dietitian is virtually indispensable. Because dietitians are not trained in adverse reactions to foods, they must have received expertise in workshops, courses, or preceptorship in a medical practice knowledgeable about adverse reactions to foods. Such a trained dietitian interacts with patients in providing and interpreting diaries and questionnaires and will largely supervise elimination diets and provocative challenge procedures and develop therapeutic long-term elimination diets.

Specific IgE-Related Tests

Physicians have long realized that tests measuring specific IgE sensitization to food can be useful to identify foods that possibly could trigger adverse reactions on challenge [208]. There is a high correlation of positive SPT or RAST test responses to milk in children with CMA who show immediate reactions (urticaria/eczema/respiratory/anaphylactic) to relatively small doses of milk [210]. Such tests can have negative results in IgE-mediated immediate reactions to food when the antigen is insoluble [217] or in an inappropriate form [209,212]. Conversely, immediate skin tests (or in vitro tests) to foods often have "falsely positive" results in subjects not reacting clinically to the food; Bock would prefer that

TABLE 13 Approaches to Identification of Possible Food Offenders That Might Cause Disease

A. **Detailed medical history**
- Are there allergic disorders unresponsive to usual therapy?
- Ask whether ingestion of any foodstuff, at any time, has ever caused immediate or delayed symptoms; repeat question several times later since patients' memories may need "jogging"
- Undue fatigue or relief of symptoms after fast or skipped meals
- Unexplained recurrent symptoms such as recurrent otitis, headaches, CNS cognitive, behavioral, or motor aberrations; abdominal pain; constipation; diarrhea; arthralgias; enuresis
- Unusual craving or extreme dislike for certain foods

B. **Dietary information from forms filled out by patient (preferably with help of dietitian)**
- *Diet Diaries:* for 2 weeks, all foods, medications, ingested agents listed and related to clinical events, if any; although suggestive association of a food with symptoms often cannot be made, diary useful for designing later elimination diets
- *Food frequency questionnaire:* very useful to rule out foods unlikely to cause disease and to identify those to be excluded on elimination diets

C. **Tests to show sensitization to specific food allergens[a]**
- Skin tests or in vitro tests that measure IgE sensitization to foods useful to support causative role of IgE; result usually positive in IgE-mediated immediate food reactions (high sensitivity) but often also positive to safe foods (low specificity); never skin test with a food known to cause anaphylaxis; substitute in vitro test, result usually negative in patients with delayed reactions to foods, and in idiosyncratic reactions to food additives

  Note: For oral allergy syndrome reactions to fruits, vegetables, or nuts, fresh food antigen may be required for positive test results
- Other in vitro tests, e.g., specific IgG, food antigen–antibody complexes, and those measuring functional changes in leukocytes and lymphocytes are either unreliable or not proved clinically practical
- In vivo sublingual or intracutaneous provocation by food extracts not considered diagnostically useful
- In vitro demonstration of IgA antigliadin and antiendomysial antibodies supports the diagnosis of celiac disease, definitive diagnosis depends upon villous atrophy and inflammation on intestinal biopsy specimen during gluten ingestion that resolves after gluten elimination

[a]IgE, immunoglobulin E.

the term *asymptomatic sensitization* be substituted [213]. Because the majority of food-sensitive children and adults have delayed and non-IgE-associated reactions, IgE-dependent tests usually yield negative results to test foods [210,212].

The in vitro histamine release assay involving blood basophils incubated with food allergens has been introduced. It has been found to be comparable in utility to SPT and RAST in most situations [214–216], although it seems more clinically useful in other studies [217]. Ohtsuka et al. measured plasma histamine and tryptase levels in food-allergic children before and after open food challenge [218]. With immediate reactions they found elevated histamine levels at 2 and 4 hr and elevated tryptase level at 4 hr suggesting mast cell activation (IgE-triggered). After delayed reactions to food challenge there were histamine level elevations but never tryptase level elevations up to 24 hr, suggesting basophil activation.

Specific IgG and IgG-Related Immune Complexes

Although some workers claim that specific IgG or IgG_4 levels to food antigens serve as valuable makers of sensitization to select foods for elimination diets [219], the majority find no practical diagnostic utility in such measurements [220,221]. Although antibody–food antigen complexes can be measured in the serum of presumably food-sensitive subjects in commercial labs [222,223], the utility of such testing has not yet been determined.

Cell-Mediated Immunity and Combined Immunological Testing

For some years, Breneman and colleague have advanced the cause of patch testing with individual foods suspended in dimethylsulfoxide (DMSO), employing immediate and delayed readings [224]. Irritant DMSO effects are controlled for by use of appropriate controls [225]; the utility of such testing awaits clinical validation. Tainio et al. studied 19 children with challenge-positive CMA; 12 (63%) with immediate reactions had elevated IgE-milk antigen test results, low IgA levels, and low lymphocyte stimulation indices to BLG and mitogen. The seven (37%) with delayed reactions had negative IgE-related test results and elevated lymphocyte stimulation to the two agents with increased CD 4/8 ratio [205]. Similar results were obtained by Rasenen et al. studying 22 children with CMA [206]. In those with immediate reactions results of IgE-related tests (SPT, RAST, histamine release) were comparably positive (55%–59%) whereas in those with delayed reactions the patch test (33%) and lymphocyte stimulation by milk antigen (77%) results were much more likely to be positive. In these last two studies [205,206], combining an IgE-related test with lymphocyte stimulation gave superior sensitivity (88%, 95%) and specificity (67%, 58%) over any test alone. In a study by Frieri et al. using lymphocyte stimulation by milk and egg antigen, specific interleukin 4 levels were shown to decline after dietary modification [226].

Impractical, Unproven, and Controversial Tests

It would seem that tests of gut function could have real value in the diagnosis of food sensitivity. However, when Ford et al. compared histological study of small bowel mucosa, mucosal disaccharidase levels, 1 hr blood Xylose test, and the lactose breath hydrogen test in 36 toddlers with suspected CMA, they found no advantage of any test over clinical observation [227]. On the other hand, two other studies of food-allergic children demonstrated that urinary levels of a high-molecular-weight sugar (lactulose or cellobiose) increased markedly after positive challenge with offending food and levels of a low-molecular-weight sugar, mannitol, decreased, signifying a pathogenic increase in gut permeability [228,229]. Although such tests could prove to be clinically useful they are not routinely available.

In the past decade the ALCAT test, which electronically measures changes in leukocyte cell volumes after in vitro incubation with food or other antigens, has been proposed as an in vitro procedure for detecting food sensitivities [230]. Using dietary elimination based on test-positive foods, marked clinical improvement occurred in certain clinical disorders [231]. Bindsler-Jensen and Paulsen point out that the procedure (which can also measure changes in platelet volumes) needs validation in carefully constructed studies before it can be considered for routine use [232]. Other procedures such as leukocytoxic testing, sublingual or subcutaneous provocation, and neutralization testing, and the neutrophil chemotactic assays have never been documented to have diagnostic utility and cannot be recommended [207,212,216,233,234].

Step Four: Employ Appropriate Dietary Manipulations to Make (or Rule Out) the Definitive Diagnosis of Food Sensitivity

Because no diagnostic procedure described in the previous section is universally reliable and all can only suggest the pathogenic potential of a foodstuff, the provocation of symptoms by a food or additive challenge is the only definitive diagnostic test [5,34,112,123,207,212,216,233]. Selection of possible foods for provocative challenge is mostly based on history of suggestive reactions but also includes positive results of food sensitization tests and knowledge of common offending foods (Table 13) [235]. Challenges are never carried out with foods likely to cause anaphylaxis or a very severe reaction [236]. Selected foods are eliminated from the diet for 10–14 days to lose adaptation and maximize reactivity; any subsequent reaction to challenge likely will take place within 4 hr [4,236] (see Table 14). For some patients, a single food may be eliminated, for others two or three foods, in some cases most foods and additives (oligoantigenic diet), and in rare cases, all foodstuffs are eliminated, the nutrition provided by an elemental diet. At the end of the elimination phase the patient should have partial or complete

relief of previous symptoms if eliminated foods were playing a significant pathogenic role. Eliminated suspect foods are reintroduced one at a time, first in a relatively tiny amount (for safety), then doubling of dose every 15–30 minutes until
a meal-size portion or full test dose has been ingested [4,5,236].

The easiest type of provocative challenge is "open" (see Table 15). It is
readily carried out in clinical practice, at patients' homes under the supervision of a dietitian; one or two foods can be tested daily. Open challenges are
appropriate for small children and responsible older children and adults
[5,236,237], and they are useful after negative DBPCFC test results, using
large doses to determine that a subject truly is nonreactive to a given food.
Open challenge should follow every negative DBPCFC result because an appreciable number will be positive, reflecting the relative insensitivity of
DBPCFC [4,207,238,239].

In the diagnosis of food sensitivity the DBPCFC, originally developed by
May and Bock, has become the "gold standard" (see Table 15) [4,216,235–239].
A detailed "manual" for DBPCFC as an office procedure was published by the
American Academy of Allergy, Asthma and Immunology in 1988 [240]. Such
testing is essential for diagnosis in difficult patients and for scholarly research
on food sensitivities. The procedure is extremely difficult to apply routinely in
clinical practice because of difficulties in obtaining necessary capsules, purified lyophilized foods, and placebo substances and in justifying the expense

TABLE 14 Appropriate Dietary Manipulations to Make (or Rule Out) the
Definitive Diagnosis of Food Sensitivity

---

1. **Eliminate single food, multiple foods, or all foods for 1–2 weeks to induce partial
   or complete remission.**[a]
   • Number and types of eliminated foods are based on history, diaries and
     questionnaires, and test results.
   • Withdrawal symptoms are common during the first days.
   • If most or all foods are eliminated, an elemental diet (e.g., Neocate one-Plus, E028,
     Peptamin can be used for nutrition
   • Rotating each presumed safe food every 4 days may permit easier recognition of
     new food offenders should symptoms follow their ingestion.

   Example of common foodstuffs
   • Cow and goat milk   • Fish and shellfish
   • Eggs   • All citrus fruits
   • Wheat   • Cocoa, chocolate, and colas
   • All legumes (beans, peas, peanut,   • Coffee and tea
     soy)   • All additives, preservatives, food
   • Nuts (true)   colorings

TABLE 14 Continued

2. **Reintroduce each eliminated food systematically to determine whether it is safe (tolerated) or unsafe (provokes typical symptoms).**

   Do not carry out challenge with any food known to cause an anaphylactic reaction.

A. **Open challenge**
   - In clinical practice, most challenges can be "open," carried out in the patient's home (if anticipated reactions are not severe) or at times in the physician's office. *Advantages:* convenient to patient/family; relatively easy; cost-effective; usually reliable. *Disadvantages:* relatively subjective and sometimes unreliable; difficult to carry out if many unsafe foods; not amenable to scientific data accumulation.
   - Challenge begins with tiny dose (e.g., 1/20 of meal-sized portion [MSP]) followed by doubling increments ever 15 minutes until a full MSP is ingested within 2 hr. If symptoms appear, halt the challenge. If no reaction, a challenge to a second food can be carried out 4 hr later on the same day.
   - When a challenge evokes significant symptoms, Alka Seltzer Gold may moderate the reaction. A purge with magnesium citrate can shorten severe reactions by expulsion of responsible foodstuff.

B. **Single- or double-blind placebo-controlled food challenge (DBPCFC)**
   - In some situations, such as when psychological factors may cloud the reliability of open challenge results, or when open challenges are too difficult at home, or when numerous positive reactions occur, it may be desirable to employ single or double-blind placebo-controlled food challenges (DBPCFC) During and after blinded food challenge, it is desirable to document and quantify the time course and nature of any reaction by quantifiable measurements of altered organ function and symptom scores.
   - Double-blind challenges in particular are difficult to carry out in clinical practice: lack of standardized test substances; lack of simple protocols; logistical complexities in blinded challenge techniques; extensive time/cost requirements for personnel, space, and supplies. Accordingly, many allergists would prefer to refer the more difficult patients to a center that regularly carries out DBPCFC procedures.
   - If the allergist elects to carry out such procedures in the office, some relatively simple steps can be followed. Meal-sized portions of food in the form usually ingested (e.g., raw, partially processed cooked) can be liquefied in a slurry, generally with some "placebo" safe agent or food that hides the taste and texture. While drinking aliquots of the food challenge mixture, clamping of the nose to prevent smelling and tasting and blindfolding reinforce the "blinding" of the challenge. After a water chaser, the blindfold and nose clamp can be removed until the next challenge dose.

ᵃPatients need to be provided with a list of presumed safe foods in all food groups and a list of synonyms for eliminated foods that appear on food labels. A nutritionist/ dietitian is virtually required in these procedures.

(personnel, equipment, supplies) of such studies [4,238,236,237,241]. In an extensive report of 16 years experience with DBPCFC, Bock and Atkins tested 480 children having a history of possible food allergy [239]. DBPCFC result was positive to food in 185 (39%) and 24% of all food challenges had positive outcomes. Although most food reactors had positive skin test reactions to the same food, the majority of positive skin test results were challenge-negative. Reactions to placebo were rare, as were reactions to multiple foods. A Japanese group tested 27 atopic dermatitis children allergic to egg with DBPCFC using egg [242]. Eleven had immediate reactions, with elevated RAST level ($p < .01$), and 16 showed delayed reactions, negative to SPT but positive to lymphocyte stimulation by egg antigen ($p < .01$).

THE MANAGEMENT OF PATIENTS WITH FOOD SENSITIVITY

Long-Term Elimination Diet

Once it is documented that food(s) or additive(s) cause a pathological clinical response, the only treatment to be considered is elimination of all major offending foodstuffs for an indefinite period (see Table 15). If one or two foods are eliminated, there is relatively little impingement on life-style. If many foods and additives are eliminated, great stresses are placed on the patient and family. A dietitian is virtually indispensable to help with food selection, reading of labels, recipes, maintenance of nutrition, etc [4,243]. With multiple sensitivities, rotating "safe" foods no more often than every 4 days may minimize reactions and reduce the likelihood of sensitization to new foods [5].

There are potential problems for any long-term elimination diet regimen. "Hidden" unsafe foods or additives in processed foods or in fast food/restaurant servings sporadically can trigger disease. Stringent dietary restrictions often foster rebellion and noncompliance. If many foods are eliminated or adverse reactions occur frequently, it may become impossible to maintain nutrition without using hypoallergenic or elemental supplements such as Neocate or Neocate-one Plus in small children or E028 in adults, all provided by SHS, North America.

Adjunctive Pharmaceutical Therapy

Pharmaceutical agents may be useful in the management of food-sensitive patients when symptoms break through at an unacceptable rate or when dietary restrictions are so profound that compliance or adequate nutrition is difficult to achieve (see Table 15). Obviously, appropriate preventive/antiinflammatory and symptom-relieving therapy is indicated for affected organ systems and short bursts of oral corticosteroid for relief of severe episodes. Preloaded epinephrine and antihistamine tablets should always be available for those

TABLE 15 Management of Patients with Food Sensitivity

Devise a dietary regimen eliminating offending foodstuffs:
- *The only primary first-line treatment is adjustment of the diet to eliminate all or at least the major foodstuff offenders, so that the patient can be essentially or predominantly free of symptoms* in ensuing months. Under these conditions, tolerance to many previously unsafe foods develops months or years later (except for those that cause anaphylaxis); challenge with these every year or so.
- Compliance with a long-term elimination diet can be difficult. The dietitian can greatly assist by providing information:
  - Where to shop
  - What foodstuffs to buy
  - How to recognize "hidden" foodstuffs in processed foods
  - Development of new recipes
  - Search for wider variety of "safe" new foods
  - Maintenance of adequate nutrition
  - Optimization of patient compliance
  - Later liberalization of the diet
- If a food has caused anaphylaxis, it must be absolutely avoided. Carrying a preloaded injectable epinephrine device and antihistamine tablets is essential.

Adjunctive pharmaceutical therapy may be indicated when symptoms break through the long-term elimination diet at an unacceptable rate. Possible medications include the following:
- Appropriate preventive/antiinflammatory and symptom-relieving treatment of affected organ systems.
- Short bursts of oral prednisone or prednisolone for severe acute episodes.
- Epinephrine from preloaded device for anaphylactic reaction to food.
- Aspirin or NSAIDs,[a] particularly for gastrointestinal reactions
- Consider 1–2 month trial of oral cromolyn (Gastrocrom) 100 or 200 mg cap dissolved in warm water, taken 15 minutes before meals and major snacks. If efficacious, continue indefinitely.
- Consider pancreatic protease/lipase oral supplement (e.g., Cotazym-S), 1–2 capsules 15 minutes before meals and major snacks. Trial of 2–4 weeks may be necessary. If efficacious, continue indefinitely.

[a]NSAID, nonsteroidal antiinflammatory drug.

who have had food-induced anaphylaxis [4]. Prostaglandin synthetase inhibitors such as aspirin and the nonsteroidal antiinflammatory drugs (NSAIDs) are useful in some patients with food sensitivities, particularly those who are nonatopic or have gastrointestinal symptoms [244]. Ciprandi et al. compared four regimens over 4–6 weeks in 80 adults with food-induced chronic urticaria/angioedema; 37 were IgE-associated and 43 were not atopic [245]. Antihistamine (H_1 antagonists) were of little help whereas combination with H_2 antagonists was effective. Oral cromolyn was helpful, particularly in the atopics; ketotifen was helpful in both groups. Ketotifen, an oral antihistamine with cromolynlike properties, has been widely used in Europe. It has been shown to prevent or inhibit IgE-mediated clinical reactions, in vitro lymphoblastogenic response to egg antigen in egg-sensitive patients, and immediate or delayed food-induced asthma [170,246].

Two medications administered orally P.O. before meals that have the potential to prevent or reduce adverse reactions and to permit liberalization of the diet deserve consideration (see Table 15). One is oral cromolyn, Gastrocrom, available in the United States as an "orphan drug." Taken prior to oral challenge with unsafe food it reduces food absorption from the gut, ameliorates the gut inflammatory response, prevents appearance of circulating food-associated immune complexes, and abolishes the anticipated adverse reaction (e.g., asthma, eczema, anaphylaxis, migraine) [5,228,247–251]. As an adjunct to elimination diet, oral cromolyn has been helpful in the chronic management of food-induced disorders, particularly IgE-mediated, such as asthma [164], atopic dermatitis [249], irritable bowel syndrome [252], eosinophilic gastroenteritis [253], and many other "allergic" reactions [254]. Between 1980 and 1990 in San Antonio, our group followed 38 patients with severe food sensitization not adequately controlled by strict elimination diet and adjunctive medications; most were atopic [255]. On open challenge, the majority were reactive to multiple foods, displaying slightly more delayed reactions than immediate. Chronic oral cromolyn therapy before meals (average of seven 100 mg capsules daily) effected good to excellent improvement in 61% with attendant liberalization of their diet. Sixteen of 17 repeatedly exacerbated on withdrawing cromolyn and regained remission on restarting the drug. Those with multiple organ system involvement did best, particularly those with atopic dermatitis or gastrointestinal symptoms. Intermediate improvement was noted for asthma, rhinitis, or CNS systems and the least improvement from cromolyn was seen with urticaria and headaches.

In the mid-1930s, Oelgoetz carried out several studies showing that the oral ingestion of pancreatic enzymes (proteases, lipase) was effective in treatment of food allergies, food intolerance, and indigestion [256,257]. Theoretically, these supplemental enzymes augment the digestion of foods, both in the gut and in the circulation after absorption, to minimize antigen availability in the gut and other tissues. In the ensuing years many clinicians anecdotally have shown that slow-release pancreatic enzymes are helpful in some cases of food sensitivity [5]. McCann and Bahna reported in 1991 that one to two capsules before each meal were quite effective in patients with multiple food sensitivities involving multiple organ systems [258]. The beneficial and virtually essential use of oral pancreatic enzymes was seen in a 6 year old female with extremely severe "allergies" (non-IgE-mediated) involving many organ systems who is intolerant of many foods and medications, including cromolyn (see Table 16).

TABLE 16 M.F., 6 Year old Female #0300 4429[a]

SX:	Chronic rhinosinusitis, asthma, abdominal pain and diarrhea, headaches, CNS dysfunction
Past HX:	In infancy intolerant of cow's milk, soy, Nutramigen; most foods; persistent otitis media with effusion until 2 years of age
Findings:	Nonatopic; negative tests reactions for inhalants and foods; dietitian elimination and challenge: intolerant of milk, soy, legumes, grains, many fruits; intolerant of Intal, Gastrocrom, quercitin, Tilade, Serevent, theophylline, Volmax
Course over 4 years:	SX generally under fair to good control: on strict elimination diet with pancreatic enzymes before meals; requires many medications, severe exacerbations after viral infections, environmental "chemical" exposure, and dietary indiscretions

[a]CNS, central nervous system.

CONCLUDING COMMENTS

Immediate reactions to foodstuffs usually are IgE-mediated and are relatively easy to diagnose, study, and treat. On the other hand, delayed reactions by their very nature are more difficult to suspect, diagnose, and document. Pathogenic mechanisms may be immunological (even IgE-mediated) or nonimmunological, and possible clinical manifestations run the gamut of virtually every organ system. A great stumbling block to the acceptance of delayed reactions to foodstuffs is our ignorance of triggering and pathogenic mechanisms generally and sparse data about true incidence (and, therefore, importance) of such reactions in various "allergic" and nonallergic disorders. When such data accumulate, it is likely that adverse reactions to ingestants will rival or surpass in importance adverse reactions to inhalants in allergy and clinical immunology.

REFERENCES

1. Young E, Stoneham MD, Petruckevitch A, Barton J, Rona R. A population study of food intolerance. Lancet 1994; 343(8906): 1127–1130.
2. Jansen JJ, Kardinaal AF, Huijbers G, Vlieg-Boerstra BJ, Martens BP, Ockhuizen T. Prevalence of food allergy and intolerance in the adult Dutch population. J Allergy Clin Immunol 1994; 93(2):446–456.
3. Fuglsang G, Madsen C, Saval P, Osterballe O. Prevalence of intolerance to food additives among Danish school children. Pediatr Allergy Immunol 1993; 4(3):123–129.
4. Rumsaeng V, Metcalfe DD. Food allergy. Semin Gastrointest Dis 1996; 7(3):134–143.

5. Kniker WT, Rodriguez LM. Non-IgE-mediated and delayed adverse reactions to food or additives. In: Breneman JC, ed. Handbook of Food Allergies. New York: Marcel Dekker, 1987, pp 125–161.
6. Kniker WT. Immunologically mediated reactions to food: state of the art. Ann Allergy 1987; 59:60.
7. Dreborg S. Food allergy in pollen-sensitive patients. Ann Allergy 1988; 61(6 Or 2):41–46.
8. De Martino M, Novembre E, Cozza G, De Marco A, Bonazza P, Vierucci A. Sensitivity to tomato and peanut allergens in children monosensitized to grass pollen. Allergy 1988; 43:206–213.
9. Wilson AF, Novey HS, Berke, RA, Surprenant EL. Deposition of inhaled pollen and pollen extract in human airways. N Engl J Med 1973; 1056–1058.
10. Baraniuk JN, Esch, RE, Buckley CE, III. J Allergy Clin Immunol 1988; 81(6):1126–1134.
11. Brostoff J. Mechanisms: an introduction. In: Brostoff J, Challacombe SJ, eds. Food Allergy and Intolerance. Eastbourne, England: Bailliere Tindall, 1987, pp 433–455.
12. Pusztai A. Dietary lectins are metabolic signals for the gut and modulate immune and hormone functions. Eur J Clin Nutr 1993; 47(10):691–699.
13. Freed DLF. Dietary lectins and disease. In: Brostoff J, Challacombe SJ, eds. Food Allergy and Intolerance. Eastbourne, England: Bailliere Tindall, 1987, pp 375–400.
14. Finn R. Pharmacological actions of foods. In: Brostoff J, Challacombe SJ, eds. Food Allergy and Intolerance. Eastbourne, England: Bailliere Tindall, 1987, 425–430.
15. Zioudrou C, Streaty RA, Klee WA. Opioid peptides derived from food proteins: the exorphins. J Biol Chem 1979; 254:2446–2449.
16. Seba DB, Milam MF, Laseter FL. Uptake, measurement and elimination of synthetic chemicals by man. In: Brostoff J, Challacombe SJ, eds. Food Allergy and Intolerance. Eastbourne, England: Bailliere Tindall, 1987, pp 401–415.
17. Wuthrich B. Adverse reactions to food additives. Ann Allergy 1993; 71:379–384.
18. Weber RW. Food additives and allergy. Ann Allergy 1993;70:183–192.
19. Ortolani C, Pastorello E, Luraghi MT, Della Torre F, Bellani M, Zanussi C. [226]. Friere M, Martinez S, Agarwal K, Trotta P. a preliminary study of interleukin 4. detection in atopic pediatric and adult patients: effect of dietary modification Pediatr. Asthma Allergy Immunal 7:27-35,1993 Diagnosis of intolerance to food additives. Ann Allergy 1984; 53(6 Pt 2):587–591.
20. Allen DH, Baker GJ. Asthma and MSG (letter). Med J Aust 1981; 2(11):576.
21. Fuglsang G, Madsen G, Halken S, Jorgensen S, Ostergaard PA, Osterballe O. Adverse reactions to food additives in children with atopic symptoms. Allergy 1994; 49(1):31–37.
22. Botey J, Cozzo M, Eseverri JL, Mar'in A. Sulfites and skin pathology in children. Allergol Immunopathol (Madr) 1987; 15(6):365–367.
23. Fisher, AA. Reactions to sulfites in foods: delayed eczematous and immediate urticarial, anaphylactoid, and asthmatic reactions, Part III. CUTIS 1989; 44: 187–190.

24.   Bahna SL. Celiac disease: a food allergy? Contra! Monogr Allergy 1996; 32:211–215.
25.   Hed J. Coeliac disease: a food allergy? Monogr Allergy 1996; 32:204–210.
26.   Anderson JA. Milestones marking the knowledge of adverse reactions to food in the decade of the 1980s. Ann Allergy 1994; 72:143–154.
27.   Belchi-Hernandez J, Mora-Gonzalez A, Inlesta-Perez J. Baker's asthma caused by *Saccharomyces cerevisiae* in dry powder form. J Allergy Clin Immunol 1996; 97(1 Pt 1):131–134.
28.   Cartier A, Malo J-L, Ghezzo H, McCants M, Lehrer SB. IgE sensitization in snow crab-processing workers. J Allergy Clin Immunol 1986; 78(2):344–348.
29.   Kivity S, Dunner K, Marian Y. The pattern of food hypersensitivity in patients with onset after 10 years of age. Clin Exp Allergy 1994; 24(1):19–22.
30.   Polasani R, Melgar L, Reisman RE, Ballow M. Hot dog vapor-induced status asthmaticus. Ann Allergy Asthma Immunol 1997; 78(1):35–36.
31.   Kalogeromitros D, Armenaka M, Galatas I, Capellou O, Katsorou A. Anaphylaxis induced by lentils. Ann Allergy Asthma Immunol 1996; 77(6):480–482.
32.   Yunginger JW, Sweeney KG, Sturner WQ, Giannandrea LA, Teigland JD, Bray M, Benson PA, York JA, Biedrzycki L, Squillace DL, Helm RM. Fatal food-induced anaphylaxis. JAMA 1988; 260(10):1450–1452.
33.   Sampson HA, Mendelson L, Rosen JP. Fatal and near-fatal anaphylactic reactions to food in children and adolescents. N Engl J Med 1992; 237:380–384.
34.   Heiner DC, Wilson JF. Delayed immunologic food reactions. New Engl Reg Allergy Proc 1986; 7(6):520–526.
35.   Eastman FJ, Lichauco T, Grade MI, Walker WA. Antigenicity of infant formulas: role of immature intestine on protein permeability. J Pediatr 1978; 93(4):561–564.
36.   Cunningham-Rundles C. Dietary antigens and immunologic disease in humans. Rheum Dis Clin North Am 1991; 17(2):287–307.
37.   Strobel S. Mechanisms of gastrointestinal immunoregulation and food induced injury to the gut. Euro J Clin Nutr 1991; 45(1):1–9.
38.   Knutson TW, Bengtsson U, Dannaeus A, Ahlstedt S, Stalenheim G, Hallgren R, Knutson L. Clinical aspects of allergic disease: intestinal reactivity in allergic and nonallergic patients: an approach to determine the complexity of the mucosal reaction. J Allergy Clin Immunol 1993; 91(2):553–559.
39.   Pastorello EA, Pravettoni V, Bigi A, Qualizza R, Vassellatti D, Schilke ML, Stocchi L, Tedeschi A, Ansaloni R, Zanussi C. IgE-mediated food allergy. Ann Allergy 1987; 59(5 Pt 2):82–89.
40.   Frieri M IgE/IgA bearing cells in gut lymphoid tissue with special emphasis on food allergy. In: Chiaramonte, Schneider A, Lifshitz F, eds. Food Allergy, a Practical Approach to Diagnosis and Management. New York: Marcel Dekker, 1988.
41.   Ohtsuka T, Matsumaru S, Uchida K, Onobori M, Matsumoto T, Kuwahata K, Arita M. Time course of plasma histamine and tryptase following food challenges in children with suspected food allergy. Ann Allergy 1993; 71:139–145
42.   Chavarua V, Young R, Zitt M, Karnik A, Kuepad C, Fitzgerald D, Frieri M. Interleukin 4 and plasma histamine in challenged food hypersensitivity patients. Ann Allergy 1994; 72:57a.

43. Ohshiba A, Yata J. Increase of ovalbumin (OVA)-specific B cells in the peripheral blood of egg-allergic patients. J Allergy Clin Immunol 1991; 87(3):729–736.
44. Caffrey EA, Sladen GE, Isaaca PET et al. Thrombocytopenia caused by cow's milk. Lancet 1981:316.
45. Scott H, Brandtzaeg P, Thorsby E et al. Mucosal and systemic immune response patterns in celiac disease. Ann Allergy 1983; 51:233–239.
46. Hofman T. IgE and IgG antibodies in children with food allergy. Rocz Akad Med Bialymst 1995; 40(3):468–473.
47. Carini C, Brostoff J, Wraith DG. IgE complexes in food allergy. Ann Allergy 1987; 59(2):110–117.
48. Lee SK, Kniker WT, Cook CD et al. Cow's milk-induced pulmonary disease in children. Adv Pediatr 1978; 25:39–57.
49. Kay RA, Ferguson A. Intestinal T cells, mucosal cell-mediated immunity and their relevance to food allergic disease. Clin Rev Allergy 1984; 2(1):55–68.
50. Ferguson A, Mowat AM, Strobel S et al. T-cell mediated immunity in food allergy. Ann Allergy 1983; 51(2 Part 2):246–248.
51. Sampson HA. Food antigen-induced lymphocyte proliferation in children with atopic dermatitis and food hypersensitivity. J Allergy Clin Immunol 1993; 91(2):549–550.
52. Suomalainen H, Isolauri E. New concepts of allergy to cow's milk. Ann Med 1994;26(4):289–296.
53. Kondo N, Fukutomi O, Agata H, Motoyoshi F, Shinoda S, Kobayashi Y, Kuwabara N, Kameyama T, Orii T. Immunodeficiency and other clinical immunology: the role of T lymphocytes in patients with food-sensitive atopic dermatitis. J Allergy Clin Immunol 1993; 91(2):658–668.
54. Szczepa'nski M, Kaczmarski M. The level of interleukine-2 (IL-2) in blood serum in children with food sensitive atopic dermatitis. Rocz Akad Med Bialymst 1995; 40(3):692–695.
55. Werfel T, Ahlers G, Schmidt P, Boeker M, Kapp A, Neumann C. Milk-responsive atopic dermatitis is associated with a casein-specific lymphocyte response in adolescent and adults patients. J Allergy Clin Immunol 1997; 99(1 Pt 1):124–133.
56. Hofman T. IL-4 and IFN-gamma level in blood serum of children with food allergy. Rocz Akad Med Bialymst 1995; 40(3):462–467.
57. Fukutomi O, Kondo N, Agata H, Shinoda S, Kuwabara N, Shinbara M, Inoue R, Orii T. Identification of monocyte chemotactic factors in supernatants of ovalbumin-stimulated lymphocytes from patients with atopic dermatitis who are sensitive to hen's egg. Clin Exp Allergy 1994; 24(4):359–366.
58. Beyer K, Niggemann B, Nasert S, Renz H, Wahn U. Severe allergic reactions to foods are predicted by increases of CD4+CD45RO+ T cells and loss of L-selectin expression. J Allergy Clin Immunol 1997; 99(4):522–529.
59. Weiss B. Food additives and environmental chemicals as sources of childhood behavior disorders. J Am Acad Child Psychiatry 1982; 21(2):144–152.
60. Hall K. Allergy of the nervous system: a review. Ann Allergy 1976; 36:49–64.
61. Heiner DC, Sears JW, Kniker WT. Multiple precipitins to cow's milk in chronic respiratory disease. Am J Dis Child 1962; 103:40–60.

62. Lee SK, Kniker WT, Cook CD, Heiner DC. Cow's milk-induced pulmonary disease in children. Adv Pediatr 1978; 25:39–57.

63. Rea WJ. Diagnosing food and chemical susceptibility. Cont Ed 1979; 57:47–59.

64. Rea WJ, Peters DW, Smiley RE, Edgar R, et al. Recurrent environmentally triggered thrombophlebitis: a five-year follow-up. Ann Allergy 1981; 47:338–344.

65. Caffrey EA, Sladen GE, Isaaca PET, Clark KGA. Thrombocytopena caused by cow's milk. Lancet 1981:316.

66. Anderson JA, Weiss L, Rebuck JW, Cabal LA, Sweet LC. Hyperactivity to cow's milk in an infant with LE and tart cell phenomenon. J Pediatr 1974; 84(1):59–67.

67. Dean T. Cow's milk allergy: therapeutic options and immunological aspects. Eur J Clin Nutr 1995; 49(suppl 1):S19–S25.

68. Host A, Jacobsen HP, Halken S, Holmenlund D. The natural history of cow's milk protein allergy/intolerance (review). Eur J Clin Nutr 1995; 49(suppl 1):S13–S8.

69. Gerrard JW, Shenassa M. Food allergy: two common types as seen in breast and formula fed babies. Ann Allergy 1983; (50):375–379.

70. Ford RP, Hill DJ, Hosking CS. Cows' milk hypersensitivity: immediate and delayed onset clinical patterns. Arch Dis Child 1983; 58(11):856–862.

71. Baehler P, Chad Z, Gurbindo C, Bonin AP, Bouthillier L, Seidman EG. Distinct patterns of cow's milk allergy in infancy defined by prolonged, two-stage double-blind, placebo-controlled food challenges. Clin Exp Allergy 1996; 26(3):254–261.

72. Husby S. Mucosal immunity. In: Metcalfe DD, Sampson HA, Simon RA, eds. Food Allergy: Adverse Reactions to Foods and Food Additives, 2nd ed. Cambridge: Blackwell Sciences, 1996 pp 3–26.

73. Strobel S. Oral tolerance: immune response to food antigens. In: Metcalfe DD, Sampson HA, Simon RA, eds. Food Allergy: Adverse Reactions to Foods and Food Additives, 2nd ed. Cambridge: Blackwell Sciences, 1996, pp 107–136.

74. Hill DJ, Firer MA, Shelton MJ, Hosking CS. Manifestations of milk allergy in infancy: clinical and immunologic findings. J Pediatr 1986; 109(2):270–276.

75. Hill DJ. Clinical recognition of the child with food allergy. Ann Allergy 1987; 59(5 Pt 2):141–145.

76. Hill DJ, Hosking CS. The cow milk allergy complex: overlapping disease profiles in infancy. Eur J Clin Nutr 1995; 49(suppl 1):S1–S12.

77. Hill DJ, Ball G, Hosking CS. Clinical manifestations of cows' milk allergy in childhood. I. Associations with in-vitro cellular immune responses. Clin Allergy 1988; 18(5):469–479.

78. Firer MA, Hoskings CS, Hill DJ. Humoral immune response to cow's milk in children with cow's milk allergy: relationship to the time of clinical repsonse to cow's milk challenge. Int Arch Allergy Appl Immunol 1987; 84(2):173–177.

79. Goldman, AS, Anderson DW, Jr., Sellers WA, Saperstein S et al. Milk allergy. I. Oral challenge with milk and isolated milk proteins in allergic children. Pediatrics 1963; 32(3):425–443.

80. Businco L, Benincori N, Cantani A. The spectrum of food allergy in infancy and childhood. Ann Allergy 1986; 57:213–218.

81. Ventura A, Ciana G, Vinci A, Davanzo R, Giannotta A, Perini R. Hypertrophic

stenosis of the pylorus: correlations with allergy to milk proteins and atopy. Pediatr Med Chir 1987; 9(6):679–683.

82. Lacono G, Carroccio A, Cavataio F, Montalto G, Kazmierska I, Lorello D, Soresi M, Notarbartolo A. Gastroesophageal reflux and cow's milk allergy in infants: a prospective study. J Allergy Clin Immunol 1996; 9:822–82.

83. Kahn A, Rebuffat E, Blum D, Casimir G, Duchateau J, Mozin MJ, Jost R. Difficulty in initiating and maintaining sleep associated with cow's milk allergy in infants. Sleep 1987; 10(2):116–121.

84. Caffarelli C, Cavagni G, Giordano S, Stapane I, Rossi C. Relationship between oral challenges with previously uningested egg and egg-specific IgE antibodies and skin prick tests in infants with food allergy. J Allergy Clin Immunol 1995; 95(6): 1215–1220.

85. Schrander JP, Dellevoet JPF, Arends JW, Forget P, Kuijten R. Small intestinal mucosa IgE plasma cells and specific anti-cow milk IgE in children with cow milk protein intolerance. Ann Allergy 1993; 70:406–409.

86. Sherman MP, Cox KL. Neonatal eosinophilic colitis. J Pediatr 1982; 100(4):587–589.

87. Falth-Magnusson K, Kjellman NI, Magnusson KE. Antibodies IgG, IgA, and IgM to food antigens during the first 18 months of life in relation to feeding and development of atopic disease. J Allergy Clin Immunol 1988; 81(4):743–749.

88. Harris MC, Kolski GB, Cambell DE, Deuber C, Marcus M, Douglas SD. Ontogeny of the antibody response to cow milk proteins. Ann Allergy 1989; 63:439–443.

89. Jakobsson I. Food antigens in human milk. Eur J Clin Nutr 1991; 45(suppl 1): 29–33.

90. Hide DW, Guyer BM. Clinical manifestations of allergy related to breast- and cow's milk-feeding. Pediatrics 1985; 76(6):973–974.

91. Gerrard JW. Allergies in breastfed babies to foods ingested by the mother. Clin Rev Allergy 1984; 2(2):143–149.

92. Jakobsson I, Lindberg T. Cow's milk as a cause of infantile colic in breast-fed infants. Lancet 1978; 437–9.

93. Evans RW, Allardyce RA, Fergusson DM, Taylor B. Maternal diet and infantile colic in breast-fed infants. Lancet, 1981:1340–1343.

94. Machtinger S, Moss R. Cow's milk allergy in breast-fed infants: the role of allergen and maternal secretory IgA antibody. J Allergy Clin Immunol 1986; 77(2):341–347.

95. Cavagni G, Paganelli R, Caffarelli C, D'Offizi GP, Bertolini P, Aiuti F, Giovannelli G. Passage of food antigens into circulation of breast-fed infants with atopic dermatitis. Ann Allergy 1988; 61(5):361–365.

96. Milla PJ. The clinical use of protein hydrolysates and soya formulae. Eur J Clin Nutr 1991; 45(suppl 1):23–28.

97. Burks AW, Casteel HB, Fiedorek SC, Williams LW, Pumphrey CL. Prospective oral food challenge study of two soybean protein isolates in patients with possible milk or soy protein enterocolitis. Pediatr Allergy Immunol 1994; 5(1):40–45.

98. Isolauri E, Sutas Y, Makinen-Kiljunen S, Oja S, Isosomppi R, Turjanmaa K. Effi-

cacy and safety of hydrolyzed cow milk and amino acid-derived formulas in infants with cow milk allergy. J Pediatr 1995; 127(4):550–557.

99. Cordle CT, Duska-McEwen G, Janas LM, Malone WT, Hirsch MA. Evaluation of the immunogenicity of protein hydrolysate formulas using laboratory animal hyperimmunization. Pediatr Allergy Immunol 1994; 5(1):14–19.

100. Restani P, Plebani A, Velon'a T, Cavagni G, Ugazio AG. Use of immunoblotting and monoclonal antibodies to evaluate the residual antigenic activity of milk protein hydrolysed formulas. Clin Exp Allergy 1996; 26(10):1182–1187.

101. Sampson JA, James JM, Bernhisel-Broadbent J. Safety of an amino acid-derived infant formula in children allergic to cow milk (abstr). Pediatrics 1992; 90(3):463–465.

102. De Boissieu D, Matarrazzo P, Dupont C. Use of a preparation with an amino acid base for children who are allergic to protein hydrolysates. Communication lors du congres annuel due Group Francophone d'Hepato Gastro Enterologie et de Nutrition Pediatrique (G.F.H.G.E.N.P.), Nancy 1996, 27–29 Mars.

103. Hill DJ, Cameron DJS, Francis DEM, Gonzalez-Andaya AM, Hosking CS. Challenge confirmation of late-onset reactions to extensively hydrolyzed formulas in infants with multiple food protein intolerance. J Allergy Clin Immunol 1995; 96(3):386–394.

104. Hill DJ, Catto-Smith ACS, Cameron DJS, Chow CW, Francis DM, Hosking CS. Is multiple food protein intolerance (MFPI) the cause of "reflux esophagitis" in distressed infants. Congress of American Academy of Allergy, Asthma and Immunology, 1996.

105. Vandenplas Y. Pathogenesis of food allergy in infants. Curr Opin Pediatr 1993; 5(5):567–572.

106. Businco L, Bruno G, Giampietro PG, Ferrara M. Is prevention of allergy worthwhile? J Invest Allergol Clin Immunol 1993; 3(5):231–236.

107. Hide DW, Matthews S, Matthews L, Stevens M, Ridout S, Twiselton R, Gant C, Arshad SH. Effect of allergen avoidance in infancy on allergic manifestations at age two years. J Allergy Clin Immunol 1994; 93(5):842–846.

108. Zeiger RS et al. Effect of maternal and infant avoidance of allergenic foods on development of food allergy was examined in a prenatally randomized, controlled trial of infants of atopic parents. J Allergy Clin Immunol 1989; 84:72–89.

109. Chandra RK, Singh G, Shridhara B. Effect of feeding whey hydrolysate, soy and conventional cow milk formulas on incidence of atopic disease in high risk infants. Ann Allergy 1989; 63(2): 102–106.

110. Bishop JM, Hill DJ, Hosking CS. Natural history of cow milk allergy: clinical outcome. J Pediatr 1990; 116(6):862–867.

111. Businco L, Benincori N, Cantani A, Tacconi L, Picarazzi A. Chronic diarrhea due to cow's milk allergy: a 4- to 10-year follow-up study. Ann Allergy 1985; 55:844–847.

112. Brostoff J, Hawk LJ. Food allergy in children. Eur J Clin Nutr 1991; 45(suppl 1):11–15.

113. Corey JP, Adham RE, Abbass AH, Seligman I. The role of IgE-mediated hypersensitivity in otitis media with effusion. Am J Otolaryngol 1994; 15(2):138–144.

114. Bernstein JM. The role of IgE-mediated hypersensitivity in the development of
      otitis media with effusion. Otolaryngol Clin North Am 1992; 25:197–211.
115. Nsouli TM, Nsouli SM, Linde RE, O'Mara F, Scanlon RT, Bellanti JA. Role of
      food allergy in serous otitis media. Ann Allergy 1994; 73:215–219.
116. Bellanti JA, Nsouli SM, Nsouli TM. Serous otitis media and food allergy. Monogr
      Allergy 1996; 32:188–194.
117. Host A. Otitis serosa: a food allergy? Monogr Allergy 1996; 32:195–197.
118. Jones SM, Sampson HA. The role of allergens in atopic dermatitis. Clin Rev Al-
      lergy 1993; 11(4):471–490.
119. Adinoff AD, Clark RAF. The allergic nature of atopic dermatitis. Immunol Allergy
      Pract 1989; XI(5):191–200.
120. Sampson HA. Late-phase response to food in atopic dermatitis. Hosp Pract 1987;
      22(12):111–118, 121, 122, 127–128.
121. Burks AW, Mallory SB, Williams LW, Shirrell MA. Atopic dermatitis: clinical rel-
      evance of food hypersensitivity reactions. J Pediatr 1988; 113(3):447–451.
122. James JM, Bernhisel-Broadbent J, Sampson HA. Respiratory reactions provoked
      by double-blind food challenges in children. Am J Respir Crit Care Med 1994;
      149(1):59–64.
123. Sampson HA. Immediate hypersensitivity reactions to foods: blinded food chal-
      lenges in children with atopic dermatitis. Ann Allergy 1986; 57(3):209–212.
124. Charlesworth EN, Kagey-Sobotka A, Norman PS, Lichtenstein LM, Sampson HA.
      Cutaneous late-phase response in food-allergic children and adolescents with
      atopic dermatitis. Clin Exp Allergy 1993; 23(5):391–397.
125. Sampson HA, Broadbent KR, Bernhisel-Broadbent J. Spontaneous release of hist-
      amine from basophiles and histamine-releasing factor in patients with atopic der-
      matitis and food hypersensitivity. N Engl J Med 1989; 321(4):228–232.
126. Agata H, Kondo N, Fukutomi O, Shinoda S, Orii T. Effect of elimination diets on
      food-specific IgE antibodies and lymphocyte proliferative responses to food anti-
      gens in atopic dermatitis patients exhibiting sensitivity to food allergens. J Allergy
      Clin Immunol 1993; 91(2):668–678.
127. Leung DY. Role of IgG in atopic dermatitis. Curr Opin Immunol 1993;
      5(6):956–962.
128. McCalla R, Savilahti E, Perkkio M, Kuitunen P, Backman A. Morphology of
      the jejunum in children with eczema due to food allergy. Allergy 1980;
      35:563–571.
129. Perkkio M. Immunohistochemical study of intestinal biopsies from children with
      atopic eczema due to food allergy. Allergy 1980; 35:573–580.
130. Jackson PG, Baker RWR, Lessof MH, Ferrett J, MacDonald DM. Intestinal per-
      meability in patients with eczema and food allergy. Lancet 1981; 1285–1286.
131. Meglio P, Farinella F, Trogolo E, Giampietro PG, Cantani A, Businco L. Immedi-
      ate reactions following challenge-tests in children with atopic dermatitis. Allerg
      Immunol 1988; 20(2):57–62.
132. Isolauri E, Turjanmaa K. Combined skin prick and patch testing enhances identifi-
      cation of food allergy in infants with atopic dermatitis. J Allergy Clin Immunol
      1996; 97(1 pt 1):9–15.

133. Taylor SL. Elimination diets in the diagnosis of atopic dermatitis. Allergy 1989; 44(suppl 9):97–100.
134. David TJ. Hazards of challenge tests in atopic dermatitis. Allergy 1989; 44 (suppl 9):101–107.
135. Hannuksela M. Diagnosis of dermatologic food allergy. Ann Allergy 1987; 59(5 pt 2):153–156.
136. Van Bever HP, Docx M, Stevens WJ. Food and food additives in severe atopic dermatitis. Allergy 1989; 44(8):588–594.
137. Walsh WE. Atopic dermatitis associated with citric and malic acid intolerance. Minn Med 1979; 62(9):637–639.
138. Hill DJ, Lynch BC. Elemental diet in the management of severe eczema in childhood. Clin Allergy 1982; 12:313–315.
139. Sampson HA, Scanlon SM. Natural history of food hypersensitivity in children with atopic dermatitis. Journal Pediatr 1989; 115 (1):23–27.
140. Proujansky R, Winter HS, Walker WA. Gastrointestinal syndromes associated with food sensitivity. Adv Pediatr 1988; 35:219–237.
141. Sampson HA. Diseases of the gastrointestinal tract of children caused by immune reactions to foods. Monogr Allergy 1996; 32:36–48.
142. Ortolani C, Ispano M, Pastorfello EA, Ansaloni R, Magri GC. Comparison of results of skin prick tests (with fresh foods and commercial food extracts) and RAST in 100 patients with oral allergy syndrome. J Allergy Clin Immunol 1989; 83(3):683–690.
143. Amlot PL, Kemeny DM, Zachary C, Parkes P, Lessof MH. Oral allergy syndrome (OAS): symptoms of IgE-mediated hypersensitivity to foods. Clin Allergy 1987; 17(1):33–42.
144. Wilson CWM. Food sensitivities, taste changes, aphthous ulcers and atopic symptoms in allergic disease. Ann Allergy 1980; 44:302–307.
145. Perkkio M, Savilahti E, Kuitunen P. Morphometric and immunohistochemical study of jejunal biopsies from children with intestinal soy allergy. Eur J Pediatr 1981; 137(1):63–69.
146. Zone JJ, LaSalle BA, Provost TT. Induction of IgA circulating immune complexes after wheat feeding in dermatitis herpetiformis patients. J Invest Dermatol 1982; 78(5):375–380.
147. Gallo C, Vighi G, Pellegrini MP, Ortolani C. Irritable bowel: a food allergy? Monogr Allergy 1996; 32:198–203.
148. Read NW. Irritable bowel syndrome (IBS): definition and pathophysiology. Scand J Gastroenterol 1987; (suppl 130).
149. Zwetchkenbaum J, Burakoff R. The irritable bowel syndrome and food hypersensitivity. Ann Allergy 1988; 61(1):47–49.
150. Swi,atkowski M, Klopocka M, Suppan K. Hypersensitivity reactions in patients with irritable colon syndrome. Wiad Lek 1993; 46(13–14):482–488.
151. Nolte H, Spjeldnaes N, Kruse A, Windelborg B. Histamine release from gut mast cells from patients with inflammatory bowel diseases. Gut 1990; 31(7):791–794.
152. Thomas AG, Taylor F, Miller V. Dietary intake and nutritional treatment in childhood Crohn's disease. J Pediatr Gastroenterol Nutr 1993; 17:75–81.

153. Riordan AM, Hunter JO, Cowan RE, Crampton JR, Davidson AR, Dickinson RJ, Dronfield MW, Fellows IW, Hishon S, Kerrigan GNW, Kennedy HJ, Mc-Gouran RCM, Neale G, Saunders JHB. Treatment of active Crohn's disease by exclusion diet: East Anglian multicentre controlled trial. Lancet 1993; 342:1131–1134.

154. Ciprandi G, Canonica GW. Incidence of digestive diseases in patients with adverse reactions to foods. Ann Allergy 1988; 61:334–336.

155. Strobel S. Mechanisms of mucusal immunology and gastrointestinal damage. Pediatr Allergy Immunol 1993; 4(suppl 3):25–32.

156. Miner PB, Jr. The role of the mast cell in clinical gastrointestinal disease with special reference to systemic mastocytosis. J Invest Dermatol 1991; 90:1–5.

157. Baenkler HW, Lux G. Antigen-induced histamine-release from duodenal biopsy in gastrointestinal food allergy. Ann Allergy 1989; 62(5):449–452.

158. Oehling A, Garcia B, Santos F, Cordoba H, Dieguez I, Fernandex M, Sanz ML. Food allergy as a cause of rhinitis and/or asthma. J Invest Allergol Clin Immunol 1992; 2(2):78–83.

159. Boccafogli A, Vincenti L, Camerani A et al. Adverse food reactions in patients with grass pollen allergic respiratory disease. Ann Allergy 1994; 73:297–304.

160. Bircher AJ, Van Melle G, Haller E, Curty B, Frei PC. IgE to food allergens are highly prevalent in patients allergic to pollens, with and without symptoms of food allergy. Clin Exp Allergy 1994; 24(4):367–374.

161. Heiner DC. Respiratory diseases and food allergy. Ann Allergy 1984; 53:657–664.

162. James JM, Bernhisel-Broadbent J, Sampson HA. Respiratory reactions provoked by double-blind food challenges in children. Am J Respir Crit Care Med 1994; 149:59–64.

163. Pelikan Z. Nasal response to food ingestion challenge. Arch Otolaryngol Head Neck Surg 1988; 114(5):525–530.

164. Onorato J, Merland N, Terral C, Michel FB, Bousquet J. Placebo-controlled double-blind food challenge in asthma. J Allergy Clin Immunol 1986; 78(6): 1139–1146.

165. Novembre E, de Martino M, Vierruci A. Foods and respiratory allergy. J Allergy Clin Immunol 1988; 81(5 pt 2): 1059–1065.

166. Oehling A, Cagnani CEB. Food allergy and child asthma. Allergol Immunopathol 1980; 8:7–14.

167. Høj L, Østerballe O, Bundgaard A, Weeke B, Weiss M. A double-blind controlled trial of elemental diet in severe, perennial asthma. Allergy 1981; 36:257–262. Medical Department TA, Rigshospitalet, Copenhagen, Denmark

168. Bock SA. Respiratory reactions induced by food challenges in children with pulmonary disease. Pediatr Allergy Immunol 1992; 3:188–194.

169. Pelikan Z, Pelikan-Filipek M. Bronchial response to the food ingestion challenge. Ann Allergy 1987; 58:164–172.

170. Furian J, Suskovic S, Rus A. The effect of food on the bronchial response in adult asthmatic patients, and the protective role of ketotifen. Allergol Immunopathol 1987; 15(2):73–81.

171. James JM, Eigenmann PA, Eggleston PA, Sampson HA. Airway reactivity

changes in asthmatic patients undergoing blinded food challenges. Am J Respir Crit Care Med 1996; 153:597–603.

172. Businco L, Falconieri P, Giampietro P et al. Food allergy and asthma. Pediatr Pulmonol Suppl 1995; 11:59–60.
173. Lee SK, Kniker WT, Cook CD, Heiner DC. Cow's milk-induced pulmonary disease in children. Adv Pediatr 1978; 25:39–57.
174. Agata H, Kondo N, Fukutomi O, Takemura M, Tashita H, Kobayashi Y, Shinoda S, Nishida T, Shinbara M, Orii T. Pulmonary hemosiderosis with hypersensitivity to buckwheat. Ann Allergy Asthma Immunol 1997; 78:233–237.
175. Lemanske RF, Jr., Sampson HA. Adverse reactions to foods and their relationship to skin diseases in children. Adv Pediatr 1988; 35:189–218.
176. Massey WA. Pathogenesis and pharmacologic modulation of the cutaneous late-phase reaction. Ann Allergy 1993; 71(6):578–584.
177. Warrington RJ, Sauder PJ, McPhillips S. Cell-mediated immune responses to artificial food additives in chronic urticaria. Clin Allergy 1986; 16(6):527–533.
178. Futrell JM, Rietschel RL. Spice allergy evaluated by results of patch tests. Cutis 1993; 52(5):288–290.
179. Antico A, Di Berardino L. The role of additives in chronic pseudo-allergic dermatopathies from food intolerance. Allerg Immunol (Paris) 1995; 27(5): 157–160.
180. Supramaniam G, Warner JO. Artificial food additive intolerance in patients with angio-edema and urticaria. Lancet 1986; 2(8512):907–909.
181. Gibson A, Clancy R. Management of chronic idiopathic urticaria by the identification and exclusion of dietary factors. Clin Allergy 1980; 10:699–704.
182. Kaeser P, Revelly ML, Frei PC. Prevalence of IgE antibodies specific for food allergens in patients with chronic urticaria of unexplained etiology. Allergy 1994; 49(8):626–629.
183. Brostoff, J, Carini C, Wraith, DG. The presence of immune complexes containing IgE following food challenge and the effect of sodium cromoglycate. Proceedings of the Second Fisons Food Allergy Workshop, Fisons Corp., Jan. 1983, pp 30–34.
184. Denman AM, Mitchell B, Ansell BM. Joint complaints and food allergic disorders. Ann Allergy 1983; 51:26–263.
185. Paganelli R, Fagiolo U, Cancian M, Scala E. Intestinal permeability in patients with chronic urticaria-angioedema with and without arthralgia. Ann Allergy 1991; 66:181–184.
186. Carini C, Fratazzi C, Aiuti F. Immune complexes in food-induced arthralgia. Ann Allergy 1987; 59(6):422–428.
187. Darlington LG, Ramsey NW, Mansfield JR. Placebo-controlled, blind study of dietary manipulation therapy in rheumatoid arthritis. Lancet 1986; 236–238.
188. Panush RS, Webster EM, Endo LP, Greer JM, Woodard JC. Food induced ("allergic") arthritis: inflammatory synovitis in rabbits. J Rheumatol 1990; 17(3):285–290.
189. Frieri M, Agarwal K, Datar A, Trotta P. Increased interleukin 4 production in response to mast cell mediators and human type I collagen in patients with rheumatoid arthritis. Ann Allergy 1994; 72:360–367.
190. Crook WG. Food allergy: the great masquerader. Pediatr Clin North Am 1975; 22(1):227–238.

191. Egger J. Psychoneurological aspects of food allergy. Eur J Clin Nutr 1991; 45(suppl 1):35–45.
192. Heiner DC, Kim K. Allergy to foods. Am J Asthma Allergy Pediatr 1987; 1(1):32–38.
193. Kahn A, Mozin MJ, Rebuffat E, Sottiaux M, Muller MF. Milk intolerance in children with persistent sleeplessness: a prospective double-blind crossover evaluation. Pediatrics 1989; 84(4):595–602.
194. Egger J, Carter CM, Wilson J et al. Is migraine food allergy? A double-blind controlled trial of oligoantigenic diet treatment. Lancet 1983; 2:865–869.
195. Monro J, Brostoff J, Carini C, Zilkha K. Food allergy in migraine: study of dietary exclusion and RAST. Lancet, 1980; 1–4.
196. Bentley D, Katchburian A, Brostoff J. Abdominal migraine and food sensitivity in children. Clin Allergy 1983; 14:499.
197. Hershey Foods Corporation. Hyperactivity: is candy causal? Topics Nutr Food Safety Winter 1993; 1.
198. Boris M, Mandel FS. Foods and additives are common causes of the attention deficit hyperactive disorder in children. Ann Allergy 1994; 72(5):462–468.
199. NIH Consensus Development Conference. Defined diets in childhood hyperactivity. Clin Pediatr 1982; 21(10):627–630.
200. Wilson N, Scott A. Alleged food-additive intolerance (asthma, eczema, urticaria, behavioral disturbance, abdominal pain) in 19 children. Clin Exp Allergy 1989; 19:267–272.
201. Kaplan BJ, McNicol J, Conte RA, Moghadam HK. Dietary replacement in preschool-aged hyperactive boys. Pediatrics 1989; 83(1):7–17.
202. Egger J, Carter CM, Soothill JF, Wilson J. Oligoantigenic diet treatment of children with epilepsy and migraine. J Pediatr 1989; 114(1):51–58.
203. Sandberg DH, Bernstein CW, McIntosh RM, Carr R, Strauss J. Severe steroid-responsive nephrosis associated with hypersensitivity. Lancet 1977; 388–391.
204. Laurent J, Rostoker G, Robeva R, Bruneau C, Lagrue G. Is adult idiopathic nephrotic syndrome food allergy? Value of oligoantigenic diets. Nephron 1987; 47(1):7–11.
205. Taino VM, Savilahti E. Value of immunologic tests in cow milk allergy. Allergy 1990; 45:189–196.
206. Rasanen L, Lehto M, Reunala T. Diagnostic value of skin and laboratory tests in cow's milk allergy/intolerance. Clin Exp Allergy 1992; 22(3):385–390.
207. Freed DLF. Laboratory diagnosis of food intolerance. In: Brostoff et al., pp 873–891.
208. Bindslev-Jensen C, Skov PS, Madsen F, Poulsen LK. Food allergy and food intolerance—what is the difference? Ann Allergy 1994; 72(4):317–320.
209. Bindsley-Jensen C. Some limitations in the use of specific IgG in the diagnosis of food hypersensitivity. Diagn Proc 1996; 32:216–220.
210. Hill DJ, Duke AM, Hosking CS, Hudson IL. Clinical manifestations of cow's milk allergy in childhood. II. The diagnostic value of skin tests and RAST. Clin Allergy 1988; 18(5):481–490
211. Walsh BJ, Hons, BS, Wrigley CW, Musk AW, Baldo BA. A comparison of the

binding of IgE in the sera of patients with bakers' asthma to soluble and insoluble wheat-grain proteins. J Allergy Clin Immunol 1985; 76(1):23–28.

212.   Pastorello E, Stocchi L, Bigi A, Pravettoni V, Schilke ML, Valente D, Zanussi C. Value and limits of diagnostic tests in food hypersensitivity. Allergy 1989; 44 (suppl 9):151–158

213.   Bock SA. Use of the term "false positive" in referring to results of food skin tests. J Allergy Clin Immunol 1985; 75(4):528–529.

214.   Iwasaki E, Yamaura M, Masuda K, Miyabayashi Y, Yamaguchi K, Zaitsu M, Fuji-maki K, Baba M. Diagnostic value of glass microfibre-based basophil histamine release test in food allergic children: Comparison with specific IgE antibody and skin scratch test. Arerugi 1994; 43(5):609–618

215.   Prahl P, Krasilnikof F, Stahl Skov P, Norn S. Basophil histamine release in children with adverse reactions to cow milk: comparison with RAST and skin prick test. Allergy 1988; 43(6):442–448.

216.   Yunginger JW. Proper application of available laboratory tests for reactions to foods and food additives.

217.   Mita H, Tadokoro K, Mishima T, Shida T. Clinical usefulness of histamine release test in determining allergens in food hypersensitivity. Arerugi 1993; 42(8):900–906

218.   Ohtsuka T, Matsumaru S, Uchida K, Onobori M, Matsumoto T, Kuwahata K, Arita M. Time course of plasma histamine and tryptase following food challenges in children with suspected food allergy. Ann Allergy 1993; 71:139–145

219.   Marinkovich V. Specific IgG antibodies as markers of adverse reactions to food. Monogr Allergy 1996; 32:221–225

220.   Rafei A, Peters SM, Harris N, Bellanti JA. Diagnostic value of IgG4 measurements in patients with food allergy. Ann Allergy 1989; 62:94–99

221.   Wuthrich B. Specific IgG antibodies as markers fo adverse reactions to food. Contra! Monogr Allergy 1996; 32:226–227

222.   Leary HL, Halsey JF. An assay to measure antigen-specific immune complexes in food-allergy patients. J Allergy Clin Immunol 1984; 74(2):190–195

223.   Bell JD, Potter PC. Milk whey-specific immune complexes in allergic and nonallergic subjects. Allergy 1988; 43:497–503.

224.   Breneman JC, Sweeney M, Robert A. Patch tests demonstrating immune (antibody and cell-mediated) reactions to foods. Ann Allergy 1989; 62(5):461–469

225.   Fisher AA. Dimethyl sulfoxide as a vehicle for food allergy patch tests. Cutis 1985;36(2):109–110.

226.   Frieri M, Martinez S, Agarwal K, Trotta P. A Preliminary study of interleukin 4 detection in atopic pediatric and adult patients: effect of dietary modification. Pediatr Asthma Allergy Immunol 1993; 7:27–35.

227.   Ford RPK, Barnes GL, Hill DJ. Gastrointestinal hypersensitivity to cow's milk protein: the diagnostic value of gut function tests. Aust Paediatr J 1986; 22: 37–42

228.   Andre C, Andre F, Colin L, Cavagna S. Measurement of intestinal permeability to mannitol and lactulose as a means of diagnosing food allergy and evaluating therapeutic effectiveness of disodium cromoglycate. Ann Allergy 1987; 59:127–130.

229. Tronocone R, Caputo N, Florio G, Finelli E. Increased intestinal sugar permeability after challenge in children with cow's milk allergy or intolerance. Allergy 1994; 49(3):142–146.

230. Pasula MJ. The ALCAT test: in vitro procedure for determining food sensitivities. Folia Med Cracov 1993; 34(1–4):153–157

231. Mylek D. ALCAT Test results in the treatment of respiratory and gastrointestinal symptoms, arthritis, skin and central nervous system. Rocz Akad Med Bialymst 1995; 40(3):625–629.

232. Bindsley-Jennsen C. What do we at present know about the ALCAT test and what is lacking? Monogr Allergy 1996; 32:228–232.

233. Bahna SL. Diagnostic tests for food allergy. Clin Rev Allergy 1988; 6(3): 259–284

234. David TJ. False allergic reactions in children with atopic eczema. Eur J Clin Nutr 1991; 45(suppl 1):47–51.

235. Pearson DJ. Clinical diagnosis in food allergy. Clin Exp Allergy 1989; 19(1):83–85.

236. Food allergy in childhood: hypersensitivity to cows' milk allergens. Clin Exp Allergy 1993; 23:481–483. Committee Report

237. Bahna SL. Blind food challenge testing with wide-open eyes. Ann Allergy 1994; 72(3):235–238.

238. Daul CB, Morgan JE, Hughes J, Lehrer SB. Provocation-challenge studies in shrimp-sensitive individuals. J Allergy Clin Immunol 1988;81(6):1180–1186.

239. Bock SA, Atkins FM. Patterns of food hypersensitivity during sixteen years of double-blind, placebo-controlled food challanges. J Pediatr 1990; 117(4):561–567

240. Bock SA. Double blind, placebo-controlled food challenge (DBPCFC) as an office procedure: a manual. Jaci 1988; 82:986–997

241. Huijbers GB, Colen AA, Jansen JJ, Kardinaal AF, Vlieg-Boerstra BJ, Martens BP. Masking foods for food challenge: practical aspects of masking foods for a double-blind, placebo-controlled food challenge. J Am Diet Assoc 1994; 94(6): 645–649.

242. Fukutomi O, Kondo N, Agata H, Shinoda S, Kuwabara N, Shinbara M, Orii T. Timing onset of allergic symptoms as a response to a double-blind, placebo-controlled food challenge in patients with food allergy combined with a radioallergosorbent test and the evaluation of proliferative lymphocyte responses. Int Arch Allergy Immunol 1994; 104(4):352–357.

243. Taylor SL, Bush RK, Busse WW. Avoidance diets—how selective should we be? New Engl Reg Allergy Proc 1986; 7(6):527–532.

244. Buisseret PD, Youlten LJ, Heinzelman D, Lessof MH. Prostaglandin synthetase inhibitors and food intolerance. Monogr Allergy 1979; 14:197–202.

245. Ciprandi G, Scordamaglia A, Banasco M, Canonica GW. Pharmacologic treatment of adverse reactions to foods: comparison of different protocols. Ann Allergy 1987; 58(5):341–343.

246. Kondo N, Fukutomi O, Kameyamam T, Nishida T, Li GP, Agata H, Shinbara M, Shinoda S, Yano M, Orii T. Suppression of proliferative responses of lymphocytes to food antigens by an anti-allergic drug, ketotifen fumarate, in patients with food-sensitive atopic dermatitis. Int Arch Allergy Immunol 1994; 103(3):234–238.

247. Paganelli R, Levinsky RJ, Brostoff J, Wraith DG. Immune complexes containing food proteins in normal and atopic subjects after oral challenge and effect of sodium cromoglycate on antigen absorption. Lancet 1979; 1270–1272.

248. Dahl R. Oral and inhaled sodium Cromoglycate in challenge test with food allergens or acetylsalicylic acid. Allergy 1981; 36:161–165.

249. Molkhou P. Waguet JC. Food allergy and atopic dermatitis is children: treatment with oral sodium cromoglycate. Ann Allergy 1981; 47:173–175.

250. Freeman GL. Oral corn pollen hypersensitivity in Arizona Native Americans: some sociologic aspects of allergy practice. Ann Allergy 1994; 72(5):415–417.

251. Paganell R. Prophylaxis and treatment of food allergy with disodium cromoglycate. Monogr Allergy 1996; 32:246–252.

252. Grazioli I, Melzi G, Balsamo V, Castellucci G, Castro M, Catassi C, Ratsch JM, Scotta S. Food intolerance and irritable bowel syndrome of childhood: clinical efficacy of oral sodium cromoglycate and elimination diet. Minerva Pediatr 1993; 45(6):253–258.

253. Van Dellen RG, Lewis JC. Oral administration of cromolyn in a patient with protein-losing enteropathy, food allergy, and eosinophilic gastroenteritis. Mayo Clin Proc 1994; 69(5):441–444.

254. Edwards AM. Oral sodium cromoglycate: its use in the management of food allergy. Clin Exp Allergy 1995; 25(suppl):31–33.

255. Overhulser PI, Inglefield Jr, Miller CS, Kniker WT. Utility of oral cromolyn in food associated disease. Annual meeting of the American College of Allergy, Asthma, and Immunology, San Antonio, Oct. 30, 1990.

256. Oelgoetz AW et al. The treatment of food allergy and indigestion of pancreatic origin with pancreatic enzymes. Am J Dig Dis Nutr 1935; 2:422–426

257. Oelgoetz AW et al. Pancreatic enzymes and food allergy. Med Rec 1939; 150: 276–279.

258. McCann ML, Bahna SL. Pancreatic enzyme supplements benefit food-allergic patients. 50th Anniversary Meeting of the American Academy of Allergy and Immunology, Chicago, March 12–17, 1993.

259. Brostoff J, Challacombe. Food Allergy and Intolerance. Eastbourne, England. Bailliere Tindall, 1987.

11

Cutaneous Manifestations of Hypersensitivity and Adverse Reactions to Food

VINCENT S. BELTRANI

College of Physicians and Surgeons, Columbia University, New York, New York

What is food to one man is bitter poison to others—Lucretius

INTRODUCTION

"Health consists in the moderate use of the air we breathe, of food and drink, activity and repose, sleep and waking, and of the passions of the soul" (School of Salerno, 1694). The word *diet* derives from Greek *diaita*, meaning "way of life." The science of dietetics has existed since Hippocrates. It was basically a form of preventative medicine—"the second part of medicine is called dietetics, which helps the sick by good health in life," said Ambroise Pare. Medieval cookery books combined recipes with dietary advice, since health depended on the proper use of food.

Skin is surely the most visible organ of the body, and the consumption of food is never far from the thoughts of humans. The basic physical law that "an event that causes an illness must occur prior to the illness" has almost naturally led to the association of nutrition and physical appearance. Subsequently, the association of food, health, and disease evolved.

Adverse reactions to foods are clinically abnormal responses attributed to the ingestion or exposure to a foodstuff. The mechanisms causing the adverse reactions are many and diverse. Labeling of all adverse reactions as "allergic" is naive and sophomoric. *True food allergy* (or immediate-type hypersensitivity) is an immunological reaction that involves an immunoglobulin E (IgE) mast cell (type I) immunological mechanism of which *anaphylaxis* is the classic example. Clinically similar symptoms of "anaphylaxis" can be seen when the mast cell degranulation is *not* initiated by an IgE antibody, but by other immunological and nonimmunological secretagogues, e.g., strawberries, and the term *anaphylactoid* is assigned to that event. Foods, however, have been associated with other immunological (and nonimmunological) reactions and with diseases. *Contact allergy* to food is a (type IV) delayed-type hypersensitivity, often seen in foodhandlers. There have been reports of allergic (leukocytoclastic) vasculitis resulting from an (type III) *immune complex reaction* [1]. More recently food-induced pemphigus (a type II or *cytotoxic type* of hypersensitivity) has been noted [2]. Recent evidence suggests that atopic dermatitis may represent the paradigm of an IgE- (type I)-mediated T cell (type IV) reaction [3].

Food intolerances are nonimmunological mechanisms of adverse reactions resulting from atypical physiological responses to an ingested foodstuff. These intolerances can include *idiosyncratic* (monosodium glutamate, [MSG], sulfites), *metabolic* (lactase or other enzyme deficiencies), *pharmacological* (insomnia from caffeine), or *toxic* (poisons released from foods or organisms contaminating the food) mechanisms.

In this chapter an attempt will be made to present the cutaneous manifestation of the adverse reactions mentioned, plus a review of the *facts and myths regarding food and the skin.*

SOME "BASIC" DERMATOLOGY (SKIN AND MUCOUS MEMBRANES)

Only a few millimeters thick, *the skin* is the body's largest organ, and although it has been always considered primarily a physical barrier to external insults, in the past 10 years it has also been recognized as the "peripheral arm of the immune system" and capable of expressing "visible" immunological reactions. The immunological components of the skin are identified in the epidermis (i e, the cytokine-laden *keratinocytes* and the *Langerhan's cell,* which have been noted to be the "professional antigen presenting cells") and the dermis. *Mast cells* of the tryptase–chymase type are found predominantly adjacent to blood and lymphatic vessals of the dermis (and gastrointestinal [GI] submucosa, thus the association of GI complaints that can precede and/or accompany food-induced episodes of acute urticaria [4]. "Normal" skin contains relatively few lymphocytes, but when present they are of the *T cell* type.

Hence, it is not surprising to identify cutaneous reactions, assignable to the Gell and Coombs' classification of immunological reactions. These "immunological" cutaneous reactions have, in fact, made us appreciate the overlapping dynamics of the varied immune mechanisms. The reactions are better understood when the clinical presentation is not assigned to a single type (I, II, III, or IV) reaction, but should be seen as a finely tuned orchestration of all four mechanisms, with one type usually predominating (at different times of their evolution). When these mechanisms are functioning properly, our good health is maintained. A down-regulation of the mechanisms results in immunodeficiencies; an up-regulation is referred to as an allergy. Examples will be presented in this text.

CUTANEOUS MANIFESTATIONS OF FOOD HYPERSENSITIVITY

Type I (Immediate-Type)Reactions

The up-regulated immunological type I response is implemented by the degranulation of mast cells (and basophils), induced by activation of a threshold number of IgE receptors on their surface, resulting in the release of preformed and then newly formed pharmacological mediators. Histamine, one of the preformed mediators, has been noted to be the predominant IgE-induced mediator released, accounting for the vasoactive (urticarial) cutaneous presentation seen minutes after the specific activation of IgE-sensitized mast cells by antigen in the skin [5]. Histamine in the skin *almost always* produces the *triple response of Lewis:* (a) erythema due to vasodilation; (b) a wheal due to extravasation of serum; and (c) pruritus. At lower concentrations, histamine may cause variable degrees of flushing, since the dose required to produce itching and whealing is higher than that needed to provoke the vasodilatory response [6].

Antigen can be presented to the dermal mast cells by the epidermal Langerhans' cells (resulting as a contact urticaria) or by antigen presenting cells of mucosal surfaces [7], which induce the B cells to produce IgE. This then enters the circulation possessing the ability to bind to receptors on tissue-fixed mast cells throughout the body, and to the "late-phase" circulating basophils [8].

These reactions were first called *food anaphylaxis* and remain the best understood aspect of food allergy [9]. Type I reactions usually occur within a few minutes to several hours after ingestion (or inhalation) of the offending antigen. However, as with all type I reactions, the presence of (a specific) IgE antibody on the surface of mast cells (and basophils) must precede the reaction-causing ingestion of the (spe-

cific) food. Reactions can only occur after prior sensitization, and they can only occur in an *antibody excess* milieu. Patients often mistakenly discount a food they
"have eaten before" as a cause of their reactions and pursue "something they
never ate before." Immunologically, a new food could never be a cause unless
that food cross-reacts with a known allergenic hapten. Allergenic cross-reactivities between certain food proteins and pollens or other nonfood protein sources
have been described [10]. However, although peanuts and soybean are among
the most common food allergens in the United States, most patients allergic to
one member of the legume family uncommonly have clinical reactivity to more
than one [11]. Cross-reactivity among fish species, on the other hand, is felt to be
very common [12]. Sampson has reported that skin test and radioallergosorbent
test (RAST) cross-reactivity among tree nuts is common, but too few patients
have been challenged to determine whether it constitutes symptomatic or asymptomatic sensitivity [13]. The association between pollen sensitivity and reactions
to various raw fruits and vegetables is seen primarily in patients with significant
allergic rhinitis. Typically these patients experience an itchy mouth, tongue, and
soft palate, now recognized as the *oral allergy syndrome* [14].

Although atopics do have the genetic predisposition to produce increased amounts of IgE antibodies upon exposure to haptenic antigens and are
more likely to have (type I) "food allergies," these "allergic" food reactions
are not restricted to atopics (it is suspected, however, that atopics are more
likely to have a serious anaphylactic reaction). A greater misconception is
that all patients who demonstrate IgE antibodies to a food are "allergic" to
that food when it is ingested. Positive skin or RAST test results for foods
are poor predictors of food allergy and are more an indicator of the atopic
diathesis than a threat to an adverse reaction. In atopics, a negative food test
finding, especially if the foodstuff itself is used, is more reliable in ruling out
food allergy.

The spectrum of cutaneous manifestations of type I food allergy always
itch and may also include (a) *urticaria,* usually acute, rarely chronic; and/or (b)
flushing; and/or (c) *angioedema;* and/or (d) *anaphylaxis.* It must be remembered that the skin's tryptase/chymase-type mast cells are also present in the
gastrointestinal submucosa and are often activated prior to and/or concomitant
with the skin mast cells, causing GI symptoms, i.e., cramps, diarrhea, nausea,
and vomiting.

In a single study to assess the occurrence of food hypersensitivity (type I)
in adults, based on suggestive history and positive skin pricktest and/or RAST
results, of 3034 patients over 14 years old, only 30 (0.98%) of the subjects had a
positive finding. The foods implicated were: fruit (46.8%), dried fruit (19.1%),
seafood (14.9%), vegetables (12.8%), fish (4.2%), and egg (2.1%) [15]. This
study, revealing an incidence of less than 1%, confirms the low prevalence of
food allergy in adulthood.

Urticaria

Urticaria is a common skin reaction, reported to occur at least once in up to 20% of the population. These usually intensely pruritic, well-demarcated, erythematous, raised, smooth-surfaced plaques can appear as discrete small (millimeters) papules (or "papular urticaria," resembling insect bites), or as giant (centimeters), confluent, arcuate, scalloped, pseudopodal, polymorphic configurations. The more sudden and explosive their appearance, the more aware one should be of a possible anaphylactic reaction. Each individual (IgE-induced) hive usually lasts 2–4 hr and rarely persists for more than 24 hr, as new hives are appearing concomitantly. Each acute episode can last from hours to days but resolves spontaneously upon the dissipation of the antigen. Foods are the second most common cause of *acute* urticaria (drugs are the most common cause!).

Recent reports have documented some interesting cross-reactions of foods and nonfoods when applied topically. Approximately half the patients, most of whom are atopic, with latex sensitivity have been found to have a sensitivity to avocado, bananas, celery, chestnuts, figs, grape, kiwi, melon, papaya, passion fruit, peach, potato, and tomato. [16–19]. Although phylogenetically dissimilar, the cross-reactivity between *Hevea brasiliensis* (the latex source) and these fruits suggests the presence of a common antigen or antigenic determinant. Since it is not known whether latex allergy is more common in patients allergic to these fruits, it would seem prudent to advise such patients of the potential latex reactivity.

A report from France suggested that 4% of mite-allergic patients were clinically allergic to snails [20]. There is also a report of anaphylaxis after ingestion of beignets contaminated with *Dermatophagoides farinae* [21].

Urticarial episodes that occur almost daily for more than 6 weeks are labeled *chronic*. They are almost always idiopathic and despite extensive (and expensive) work-ups, a specific cause is rarely (if ever) identified! I prefer to regard these patients as having a "twitchy mast cell" syndrome, and their management should be symptomatic, without steroids if possible [22].

Patients reporting *recurrent episodes* of urticaria can frequently identify the trigger of their hives (i.e., drug or food). These hives will appear from minutes (usually 10–20) to hours (rarely more than 24) after the antigen is ingested and disappear when the antigen is no longer available (sometimes as long as 48 hr). Foods have been reported to be the cause of "acute" urticaria in 20%–57% of patients, and but 1%–13% of patients with "chronic" urticaria [23]. The most common challenge-proven foods provoking urticaria are: *egg, peanut, milk, nuts, soy, wheat, fish, and shellfish;* however, it must be remembered that virtually any protein-containing food may be allergenic. In some individuals, the ingestion of a large quantity of foods containing histamine, e.g., *tuna, mackerel, mahimahi, parmesan* and/*or blue cheese, chianti,* may *pharmacologically* produce symptoms easily confused with IgE-type reaction including itching, flushing, and occasionally urticaria. (When skin or RAST tested these patients show no IgE reaction to those foods; see Figure 2.)

When a suspected food inconsistently produces urticaria, the method of preparation must be considered as a cause of the variable result: i.e., food allergens are denatured by heating (especially clams—raw versus cooked), or the cryptic addition of additives or spices may be the allergen.

Contact urticaria has been recognized for centuries. Physicians applied substances (rubefactants) to intact skin to induce erythema. More recently many substances that cause erythema, a wheal, and a flare, have been identified. These urticaria can be induced immunologically and nonimmunologically. The immunological reactions require prior sensitization, whereas the nonimmunological reactions. do not [24]. Some contactants affect normal (intact) skin, whereas others produce a reaction only on damaged (eczematized or fissured) skin [25].

Food-induced contact urticaria has been observed in children with atopic dermatitis. Urticaria develops within a few minutes at the site of contact with food, and often an eczematous reaction gradually develops [26].

In patients with contact urticaria, results of the classic "patch" tests are negative and require "prick" testing with the raw foods to prove the cause of this "immediate" type of contact food dermatitis [27].

Contact urticaria may be caused by a nonimmunological mechanism [28].

TABLE 1   Foods Capable of Causing Contact Urticaria

Dairy product	*Grains*	*Vegetables*
Cheese	Flour	Beans
Egg	Malt (beer)	Cabbage
Milk	Wheat bran	Carrot
Seafood	*Honey*	Celery
Cod	*Nuts*	Chives
Fish	Sesame seed	Cucumber
Prawns	Sunflower seed	Endive
Shrimp	*Meats*	Garlic
Fruits	Beef	Lettuce
Apple	Chicken	Onion
Apricot	Lamb	Parsley
Banana	Liver	Parsnip
Kiwi	Turkey	Potato
Mango	*Spices*	Rutabaga (swede)
Orange	*Flavorings*	Soybean
Peach	Benzoic acid	Tomato
Plum	Menthol	Legume
		Peanut

Fish and spices (thyme, capsaicin of cayenne pepper) are the most common foods to cause the release of other vasoactive mediators besides histamine. These hives are usually less responsive to the administration of antihistamines.

Strawberries are frequently blamed for "allergic" reactions, but I have yet to identify a patient with strawberry IgE antibodies (by prick test or RAST test) [29]. Strawberries are listed (with radiopaque dye and jellyfish) as *nonimmunological secretagogues* for mast cells [30]. Other berries are reported to have a high salicylate content, and they are always denied to patients who are aspirin (and nonsteroidal antiinflammatory drug–[NSAID])-sensitive, still, I have not found any of my aspirin-sensitive patients reacting to "berries." A possible explanation for the "rare" occurrence of the latter type reactions is due to the dose dependency of salicylate hypersensitivity.

Angioedema

Recognized as nonpruritic, nonpitting, asymmetrical swellings, usually grotesquelly disfiguring, involving areas of loose tissue, i.e., periorally, periorbitally, and genitally, angioedema can become life-threatening when the tongue, epiglottis, or uvula is affected. The vascular reaction is similar to that which occurs in urticaria, except the small venules and capillaries involved are in the deeper dermis and subcutaneous tissues.

Angioedema is most often seen with urticaria but can occur *without* hives, in which case always rule out angiotensin converting enzyme (ACE) inhibitors, aspirin, nonsteroidal antiinflammatory drugs (NSAIDs), or Hereditary Angioedema (HAE) as a cause. Like urticaria, angioedema may not have a definitive cause determined for most cases that are chronic, whereas the cause of most cases of acute angioedema can be traced. Food-induced angioedema (as with urticaria) is the result of an IgE-mediated mechanism, whereas food-additive-induced angioedema is not IgE-mediated. The same foods are most often the cause of both angioedema and urticaria, namely, crustaceans, fish, nuts, peanuts, berries, eggs, and milk [31]. The incidence of allergic reactions to food is significantly higher among atopic persons. In some highly allergic patients, mere contact with nuts, peanuts, and crustaceans can cause severe angioedema [28]. These patients should have an epinephrine inhaler (i.e. Primetene Mist or Medi-Epi Inhaler) in their possession at all times for immediate use (10–15 sprays to swollen airway structure) at the earliest suspicion of "swelling." Should symptoms worsen they should take a Doxepin 10–25 mgms (a mos effective H1 and H2 antagonist) plus be ready to administer a dose of EpiPen, and get to an emergency room.

Anaphylaxis

It has been estimated that a minimum of 1000 severe food-induced anaphylactic reactions occur in the United States each year [32]. The IgE-induced massive degranulation of mast cells may result in the multisystem signs and symptoms of anaphylaxis. *Anaphylactoid* reactions are clinically similar [33], but the mast cell degranulation is not IgE-induced. The prognosis is usually less ominous, and *not* caused by foods, except perhaps for the oddity of the food-dependent, exercise-induced anaphylaxis. These patients have an IgE-positive response to a wide panel of food allergens, including seasoning (e.g., garlic or parsley) [34], celery, or shrimp, peanut, or hazelnut, or wheat [35–37]. The latter reactions all occurred during or immediately after exercise; they included pruritus, urticaria, angioedema, abdominal cramps, wheezing, and dyspnea. The ingestion of sulfiting agents has been associated with bronchospasm predominantly in asthmatics [18]. Urticaria, angioedema, pruritus, and anaphylactoid reactions have been described in both atopic and nonatopic patients after the ingestion of sulfites and histamine-containing foods.

The "Chinese restaurant syndrome" i.e., monosodium glutamate (MSG), does not cause pruritus, urticaria, angioedema, nor anaphylactoid reactions. The cutaneous manifestations of this syndrome are "burning skin," especially along the back of the neck, and sweating [39].

Urticaria and angioedema have been reported to occur in 88% of a compilation of anaphylactic reactions (R deShazo 11/93). Flushing was noted in 46%, and pruritus without any "rash" in 5%! There is almost always some cutaneous manifestation, but relying on the presence of urticaria to diagnose anaphylaxis would be foolhardy. H. Sampson reported 11/13 food-induced anaphylactic deaths occurred without urticaria. The more sudden the onset of symptoms after ingestion especially when itchy palms, soles, scalp, and/or mouth are ignored as the "heralding" signs of impending anaphylaxis, the more probably a disaster is brewing. The fatal reactions usually occur after several (four to six) prior "warning" episodes. The inadvertent ingestion of the allergen (food), especially peanuts, is the cause of most "food allergy" deaths. Since it is most likely to occur when eating in a restaurant, I instruct all my food allergic patients to show the chef a red identification card, alerting them to a potentially dangerous reaction should the foodstuff be in the meal. I instruct all my food allergic patients to discontinue β-adrenergic blocking agents and ACE inhibitors (see Fig. 1). They also have a Doxepin 10 mg capsule (a most effective H_1 and H_2 antagonist) to ingest if they suspect the allergenic food has been ingested, plus an EpiPen to be administered if necessary. Although cromolyn (Gastrocrom 200 mg, dissolved in 8 ounces of water 1 hr prior to eating) makes some teleologic sense, its efficacy has not been documented, and while it cannot be routinely recommended for the management of IgE-mediated food allergy, there are anecdotal reports of it aborting a serious reaction.

Type II (Cytotoxic-Type) Reactions

In type II hypersensitivity, antibody directed against cell surface tissue antigens interacts with molecules of the complement pathways and a variety of effector cells to bring about damage to those cells and surrounding tissues. The

	NJC	JHU/DUKE	UCSD	MAYO	TULANE	NIH
No. Pts DBPCFC*	407	190	47	11	30	25
No. Pts + DBPCFC†	157	118	23	6	9	10
No. DBPCFC‡	826	539	59	24	125	38
No. + DBPCFC§	204	222	29	6	12	8
Foods producing a positive DBPCFC						
Peanut	48	34 (18)||	4	2		?
Egg	53	90 (5)	14	1		1
Milk	47	32 (3)	7	1		
Nuts	21			2		
Soy	14	17 (1)	1			
Wheat	5	9	2			
Fish	6	13 (4)				
Shellfish (crustacea)	2	2			12	5
Chicken	2	4				
Pea	2	2				
Turkey	1					
Banana	1	2				
Rye	1	3				
Squash	1	0				
Potato		3 (1)				
Rice		2				
Beef		4				
Corn		2	1			
Other		3				

NJC, National Jewish Center; *JHU/DUKE*, Johns Hopkins University/Duke University; *UCSD*, University of California—San Diego; Mayo Clinic; Tulane University; *NIH*, National Institutes of Health; +, positive.
This table represents the cumulative experience with the technique of DBPCFC from the various centers of the authors of this article.
*Number of patients undergoing DBPCFC.
†Number of patients with positive DBPCFC.
‡Number of DBPCFCs performed.
§Number of positive DBPCFCs.
||Number in parentheses depict number of reactions based on convincing history of life-threatening reactions after ingestion (not included in total of 222 positive DBPCFC).

FIGURE 1

dermatological diseases demonstrating cytotoxic phenomena are the group of blistering disorder: Pemphigus (vulgaris, vegetans, foliaceus, erythematosus), drug-induced pemphigus, bullous pemphigoid, benign mucus membrane pemphigoid, *Herpes* gestationis, IgA bullous dermatosis, chronic bullous disease of childhood, epidermolysis bullosa acquisita, and dermatitis herpetiformis. Of all these entities, only dermatitis herpetiformis has been associated with a food (or gluten hypersensitivity). Of interest is the fact that drugs (rifampin, penicillamine, and captopril) have been associated with the precipitation of a pemphiguslike disease [40] and until recently, foods have not. But recently garlic compounds (with stable disulfide and thiol groups) have been reported to induce acantholysis in vitro [41]. It has thus been suggested that nutritional factors (the *Allium* group, including onion, leek, and garlic) should be suspect as an exogenous agent capable of inducing pemphigus [42].

Dermatitis herpetiformis (DH) or Duhring's disease is a rare intensely pruritic, chronic, symmetrical papulovesicular eruption, occurring at any age, usually on extensor surfaces, with a predilection for the presacral area. Often presenting with extensive excoriation, it is frequently misdiagnosed as a "factitial" neurodermatitis. The diagnosis of DH is confirmed by the presence of IgA at the dermal–epidermal junction, seen by direct immunofluorescence, in both involved and uninvolved skin. In addition these patients often have an asymptomatic gluten-sensitive enteropathy, histologically indistinguishable from that of celiac disease. Remissions can be induced by the administration of sulfones and/or the avoidance of gluten (the proteins gliadin and prolamin) from the diet (wheat, rye oats, barley, some ice cream, malted milk, etc.). The association of dermatitis herpetiformis with gluten-sensitive enteropathy and cutaneous IgA deposits, as well as the response of the skin disease to a gluten-free diet, have led to the hypothesis that the mucosal immune response is a critical element in the pathogenesis of dermatitis herpetiformis. Iodides (from seafood), both topically and systemically, may provoke an exacerbation of blisters in some patients with DH. This disease is permanent and symptoms/damage will occur after consuming gluten and/or iodine. The Gluten Intolerance Group of North America (PO Box 23053, Seattle, WA 98102-0353) is an excellent nonprofit organization dedicated to providing information, education, and support to patients with DH.

Type III (Immune Complex–Type)

Leukocytoclastic vasculitis represents an immune complex reaction, almost always associated with infectious diseases, drugs, serum sickness, neoplasia, autoimmune diseases, cryoglobulinemia, and other stimuli [43]. The dermatological presentation of leukocytoclastic vasculitis is purpura, which can be "palpable" or result in hemorrhagic craterform, painful ulcers. There are several reported cases of food-induced vasculitis [44,45]. Immune complex deposits have been also found in lesions of *recurrent aphthostomatitis* [46].

It seems surprising that food is not reported to be a cause of immune complex diseases more often, especially since we are now appreciating that drugs (a potential source of antigens) not infrequently can produce serum sickness–type syndromes. The possible reason for not identifying a food as a cause of some "idiopathic" serum sickness reactions is the necessary prolonged latency period (7–10 days) required for the elicitation of the clinical picture after ingestion of the culpable food.

Type IV (Delayed-Type)

In sensitized individuals, contact with certain foods most often results in a classic *allergic contact dermatitis,* the prototypical dermatological manifestation of delayed hypersensitivity. Although this eczematous eruption is clinically indistinguishable from any other "eczema," its localization is confined almost exclusively to the site of contact. The spectrum of all histological spongiosis spans the spectrum from the large bulla of acute allergic contact dermatitis (as noted in "poison ivy") to the chronic lichenified thickened scaly plaques of long-standing atopic dermatitis. The T cell inflammatory mediators that produce the clinical eczema can be released by "triggers" introduced on contact or delivered to it systemically. Food haptens coming in contact with the skin can result in "allergic" contact dermatitis, but foodstuffs can also cause a nonimmunological activation of T cells, whereby it then produces an "irritant" contact dermatitis [47]. The two types of contact dermatitis often are indistinguishable, but the latter type tends to be less pruritic and more painful and more "angry-looking" than inflamed. Virtually any food can act as an irritant (even an allergen), depending on its concentration and the condition of the skin on contact. The "irritant" overhydration common to bartenders and food handlers or the xerosis of atopic or geriatric skin allows for greater accessibility of antigens to the skin. It is not unusual for patients to have more than a single "trigger" causing their eruption, especially when evaluating a hand, or facial, or eyelid dermatitis.

Allergic contact dermatitis (ACD) has been reported from many foods. The main food allergens, however, are garlic and onion [48] which cross-react with tulips and hyacinths [49]. The allergens in garlic are diallyl disulfide and allicin, the allergen in onions has not been identified. Contact reactions to citrus fruits may be reactions to the peel or to chemicals applied to the fruit. An allergic cheilitis from orange peel may develop in individuals who remove orange peels with their teeth. The volatile orange oils may also produce circumoral dermatitis and hyperpigmentation. The terpene limonene is the principal sensitizer in orange and lemon peel [50]; it may cross-react with turpentine and bergamot [51]. Carrots, parsnips, parsley, and celery can cause either an allergic contact dermatitis or a phytophotodermatitis. The "golden standard" for identifying an allergen responsible for ACD is the patch test. Anyone who is to be patch tested should be tested to the available standard patch test kit (Hermal Labs or the Glaxo T.R.U.E test), and since foods are not included in the standard patch test kits, "suspected" foods are to be applied "as is" to uninvolved skin [52]. The patient is then instructed to allow the patch tests and the food material to remain on the skin for 48 hr, after which the site of patch test application is evaluated. Correct interpretation of the test site is graded 0 if no reaction is noted, 1+, 2+, or 3+ as outlined by the American Contact Dermatitis Society. Positive nonstandard patch test material may require the application of the same antigen on a "control" subject.

Positive patch test–proven food causing contact dermatitis has been reported to lettuce [53,54], horseradish, cabbage, broccoli, and brussel sprouts [42]. Coffee has been the cause of a persistent cheilitis [55]. At least 60 spices have been reported to produce dermatitis; the 5 spices that most commonly produce dermatitis are capsicum, cinnamon, cloves, nutmeg, and vanilla [42]. There are many additives to foods that can produce contact dermatitis including preservatives, antioxidants, dyes, flavoring agents, "spoilage retarder," "flavor protectors," and "cloudiness preventatives." The most common food-additive dermatitis is a hand dermatitis, particularly in housewives, food handlers, bakers, and cooks.

Almost every food substance that has been noted to cause contact urticaria (see Table 1) has caused allergic contact dermatitis. Although the most common causes of contact urticaria are fish and crustacea, garlic and onion are the most common causes of allergic contact dermatitis [56]. As mentioned, patch testing with suspected foods (as is) can confirm all suspicions of ACD, but a prick test is required to confirm contact urticaria [57].

Contact allergens have been reported to cause skin symptoms when ingested. Dr. Joseph Fowler presented his experiences as director of the occupational dermatology and patch test clinic at the University of Louisville School of Medicine, at the Westwood Conference on Clinical Dermatology in 1996. He reported that in patients who are sensitized to nickel, chromate, cobalt, balsam of Peru, propylene glycol, parabens, sorbic acid, benzoates, and a variety of cross-reactors dermatitis may develop when they ingest them, even in trace amounts in food, drink, and condiments. The skin reaction occurs from several hours up to 2 days after ingestion, frequently "flaring" at the site of the earlier contact reaction. Nickel-sensitive patients may unknowingly ingest a sufficient amount of nickel in (canned) foods—especially green leafy vegetables and grain. Ingested nickel can be stored in tissues and thus perpetuate a chronic eczematous eruption. Recent trials of disulfiram, used for avoidance conditioning in alcoholism, shows that it chelates nickel and improves the dermatitis of sensitized individuals.

Cobalt is also a potent contact sensitizer, and it too is present in many foods that contain nickel. There is some cross-reactivity between ingested cobalt and ingested nickel, but a significant number of cobalt-sensitized individuals are not allergic to nickel but react only to cobalt.

Chromate is the third most common metal contact allergen. The widespread distribution of chromate may help explain why some patients have persistent hand eczema due to chromate that is very difficult to clear, despite chromate avoidance. Food sources of chromate include cocoa, tea, escargot, nuts, dates, apricots, and figs.

Cinnamon flavorings, particularly cinnamic aldehyde, are probably the most common cause of allergic stomatitis [58]; they are used in candies, bubble gum, lipstick, lozenges, and dentrifices [59]. These patients frequently present with a perioral dermatitis in addition to a burning mouth with or without a stomatitis [60]. Cross-sensitization to balsam of Peru may result from sensitization to cinnamon. [61] and patients allergic to balsam of Peru may react to ingested cinnamon-flavored foodstuffs (pastries, cakes, soft drinks, wines, and liquors).

Although benzocaine is considered a fairly weak sensitizer, its popularity as a medicament in hundreds of different products has resulted in widespread sensitization. Benzocaine-sensitive individuals may encounter it in sore throat sprays and lozenges, cough tablets, drops, and oral and gingival pain relieving products.

Perhaps the most interesting example of cross-sensitivity has been reported to occur in patients who are sensitive to "poison ivy" (urushiol) and ingest cashew nuts (oil from their shells is most antigenic). A poison ivy–like dermatitis can occur shortly after their consumption. In some patients blisters of the mouth and rectal itching develop. Reginella et al. have reported that workers who become "hardened" to cashew shell oil noticed a decreased sensitivity or no sensitivity to poison ivy/oak. Cashew shell oil contains cardol and anacrdic acid, which are immunochemically similar to the catechols found in poison ivy/oak [62]. Patients who are sensitized to poison ivy may also acquire an allergic cheilitis from eating mango, which contains a catechol related to poison ivy, oleoresin [63].

Phototoxic reactions have occurred after handling (the furocoumarins containing) lime, celery, parsley, figs [64], and parsnips. Bakers are exposed to flour, flour additives (ammonium persulfate and benzoyl peroxide), flavors (cinnamon), and dyes.

ATOPIC DERMATITIS

The role of food allergy in atopic dermatitis has been the source of more controversy than perhaps any other subject matter in dermatology. Overzealous advocates are avidly contradicted by a sect of skeptical adversaries. At times it seems that rationality succumbs to emotions. The disagreement oftentimes is one of semantics. The fact that *some patients* with atopic dermatitis respond adversely to *some foods* at *some time* in the history of their disease cannot be denied. The fact that exacerbations of atopic dermatitis can be caused by multiple and varied "triggers" confounds the objective evaluation of the role of any single trigger. Thus to focus on a single trigger is sophomoric. The complex variables involved in the absorption, processing, metabolism, and antigenicity following the ingestion of food, combined with the sundry pathways of immunological host responses, depreciate the conclusions drawn by investigators, especially when they are from the diverse disciplines [65].

Allergists, whose bias favors the protagonistic role of IgE, rely too much on the rather unreliable significance of skin and/or RAST testing to foods. Skin test reactivity presumably mirrors serum food specific IgE responses to specific food antigens, which comprise only the afferent limb of an immunological response. To complete the immunological reaction, the efferent limb, with a responsive shock organ, is essential. This was clinically demonstrated by Sampson when he noted that, in his select population, only one-third of patients with positive skin test results correlated with positive food challenge results [66]. Positive skin prick test or RAST results have been reported in 51% to 96% of patients with AD [67–70]. Unfortunately, the presence of specific IgE antibodies to foods is not useful in predicting clinically relevant reaction. (although negative skin test outcomes are very reliable to exclude IgE-mediated food allergies). Isolauri and Turjanmaa recently reported that combined prick and patch testing significantly enhanced the identification of food allergy in infants with AD [71]. Paralleling dust mite patch testing results of patients with AD [72], they noted no relationship between reactivity to skin prick tests and patch tests. Consistent with the recognized pathogenesis of AD, there are multiple triggered pathways that can trigger exacerbations, and foods may be one trigger in a subset of patients at some time in their disease.

Double-blind placebo-controlled food challenges (DBPCFCs) must be considered the most reliable technique for confirming the diagnosis of food hypersensitivity. From the many studies utilizing this technique, 33% to 63% of patients with AD tested developed a reaction when challenged [73]. DBPCFC has been reported to produce cutaneous reactions in 84% to 96% of patients tested. These reactions, however, develop within minutes up to 2 hr after the challenge and last only 30 to 120 minutes, a pattern of response that is not typical of the T cell–induced diseases! It is more appropriate to suspect that those clinical symptoms are caused by IgE-mediated cutaneous mast cell activations (which are accompanied by a rise in plasma histamine concentration [74]). Histamine can be delivered to the skin by both mast cells (within minutes) and basophils during the late phase. Histamine in the skin can produce flushing and pruritus without urticaria [6], and incites the scratching that may validate the dictum "AD is an itch that erupts, and not an eruption that itches"! It has also been reported that TH-2 cells (the characteristic T cells in the skin lesions of AD [75]) require an exogenous pulse of interleukin 4 (IL-4) to initiate their differentiation and synthesis of cytokines [76] altered cytokine production of IL-4 and (γ-IFN) have been repeated in AD. Mast cells upon degranulation release that needed IL-4, plus IL-5, the chemotactic mediator for eosinophil (another late-phase participant). Thus IgE activation of mast cells in AD can play a salutory role in its pathogenesis.

If food allergens are significantly contributing to clinical exacerbations of AD, then strict avoidance should result in clinical improvement. Although this may seem an easy task, especially since the great majority of children with food allergy react to only one or two foods, and only six foods are responsible for 90% of all food allergies (egg, peanut, milk, wheat, fish, soy) [77] (see Fig. 1), elimination diets conducted in the home rarely produce any benefit. [78] This may be due to (a) the difficulty of adhering to a strict elimination diet; (b) frequent inability of parents to identify correctly the allergens relevant to their children; (c) the hope that food allergy is the sole cause of the problem causes all the other "triggers" exacerbating AD to be overlooked.

It is virtually impossible to agree on a reliable estimate of the incidence of true food allergy in patients with AD. It is safe to assume that the great majority of patients studied are referred to tertiary centers because they were suspected of having food allergies and/or they had severe unresponsive AD. In Dr. Sampson's tertiary referral population, 80% of the children evaluated were found to be food allergic. [79] Hanifin (in 1986) estimated that 10% to 20% of patients with AD have clinically relevant food hypersensitivities [80]. At my Atopic Skin Symposium (New York, October 1994), when the distinguished faculty was queried on what they suspected was the true incidence of food allergy in AD, a more realistic figure of 5%–10% for *all* infants with AD and 1%–5% for older patients with AD was proposed! From my personal experience over a period of 30 years, as an allergist/dermatologist in private practice and at a tertiary referral center (Columbia-Presbyterian Medical Center, New York), I believe the lower suspected incidence might be slightly inflated, but it is not 0%! I do concur with the authors who conclude that the detection of food allergy in a child with AD is likely to predict a prognosis of severe disease [56]. Therefore, I seriously consider food allergy only in those patients whose dermatitis is generalized, is very pruritic (especially after meals), and does not improve despite compliance with my aggressive therapeutic regimen.

There is no scientific evidence to support the routine use of rotational diets or immunotherapy with food antigens in the treatment of food-induced AD. Empirical trials of elimination diets I have found to be of no value. Vivonex [81] alone has been too "distasteful" in the home setting. In one double-blind cross-over trial of patients with food hypersensitivity documented by DBPCFC, oral cromolyn was found to be no more beneficial than the placebo control [82] Although histamine is almost certainly involved to some extent (since histamine concentrations are increased in the skin of patients with AD), H_1 receptor antagonists have not been uniformly effective in relieving the itch of AD. However, tricyclic antidepressants have been most helpful in the management of chronic pruritic conditions, and I have found the administration of doxepin (10–25 mg) at bedtime helpful for the patient with resistant AD. Gupta et al. offer two possible theories for the role of tricyclic antidepressants in AD: (a) their very potent H_1 plus H_2 antagonism (779 times greater than that of diphenhydramine and 7 times more effective than cimetidine, respectively), and (b) their effective antidepressant properties (addressing the psychological result of itching for many years) [83].

Fortunately, food hypersensitivity in young patients is not always a lifelong affliction [84]. The Guillets reported that food sensitivity persisted in 67% of children 7 to 16 years of age with severe AD and was always associated with aeroallergen sensitivity. Sampson reports that the development of tolerance was food-dependent, with children allergic to peanut, nuts, and seafood almost never "outgrowing" their allergies, whereas children sensitive to soy, milk, eggs, and wheat frequently outgrew their clinical reactivity after several years of allergen avoidance. (There is no correlation between results of prick skin tests or total serum IgE concentration in predicting the development of tolerance [85].)

The conundrum of whether to breast feed in high-risk atopic families parallels the role of food allergy in AD. The number of positive reports [86–88] equals that of the equivocal and/or negative reports [89–91]. At best, the evidence indicates that prolonged breast feeding and delayed introduction of potential allergens may protect against the development of AD in a small number of patients, and the benefits appear to be limited to the first year of life.

Conclusions

Foods, as allergens (ingested, and/or applied to the skin), can trigger an exacerbation of eczema in a small (1% to 10%) number of atopics. Evaluating foods as a trigger should not be part of a routine examination. Emphasizing the avoidance of the more likely triggers (heat and perspiration, 96%; wool, 91%; emotional stress, 81%; alcohol, viral infections, and dust mites [92]), [93] plus the topical prevention of xerosis with lubricants and proper application of topical steroids should have the highest priority when managing AD. Only in the patient with persistent, generalized, moderately severe to severe AD, who has been compliant with the "standard" management, should food allergy be considered. Before skin testing, a careful dietary history, with emphasis on establishing a pattern for the exacerbations, must be obtained. My routine for skin food prick tests includes only the most commonly reported foodstuffs (eggs, peanut, milk, wheat, fish, and soy) and adds only those foods the parent (or patient) suspects. Rarely do I test for more than 10 foods! The most difficult task is differentiating the true positive results from the false positive results. It is essential that the patient not be denied a foodstuff merely because of a positive skin test.

Chinese Herbal Therapy in Atopic Dermatitis

The earliest pharmacopoeia of Chinese herbs, known as the *Herbal Classic of the Divine Plowman*, was written in approximately 100 B.C. Therapy is based upon the interpretation of signs and symptoms encompassing the philosophy of yin and yang and a realignment of those forces. Chinese herbal therapy seeks to eliminate hostile pathogens and to realign fundamental yin and yang balance. It is not unusual to prescribe 10 to 12 herbs at a time, to work synergistically directed at a target area. The details of the principles of Chinese herbal therapy are excellently described by Rustin and Poulter [94]. Those authors undertook a scientific evaluation of Chinese herbal therapy (a standardized concoction from a single supplier of medicinal herbs (OPTEC, Shangai, China) and concluded that it is an effective treatment for severe atopic dermatitis that is not exudative nor grossly infected or impetiginized. They found that 80% of their patients (31 adults and 18 children) may derive benefit. Side effects may be possible, i.e., hepatoxicity and interstitial renal fibrosis. A major complaint encountered in the clinical trials was the unpleasant taste and smell of the liquid that was produced by boiling the herbs. The effects of Chinese herbal therapy they believe are due to (a) modulation of cortisone/cortisol release by adrenocortical stimulation, (b) potentiation of endogenous corticosteroids, (c) the presence of compounds that nave corticosteroidlike activity, (d) possible interference with the generation of inflammatory mediators, (e) central and peripheral antipruritic action, (f) antibacterial activity, and (g) modulate immune activation through either a cellular or cytokinal action. Multicenter studies are continuing, and at present this form of therapy should be considered investigational [95].

Linoleic Acid Therapy

The principal essential fatty acids (EFAs) in skin are linoleic acid, derived entirely from dietary sources, and arachidonic acid, derived mainly from linoleic acid. *EFA deficiency* in animals has been known to cause scaliness of the skin; changes are rapidly reversed if the animals are fed linoleic acid. In humans made EFA-deficient by disease or surgery, similar skin changes are seen and topical application of sunflower seed oil (rich in linoleic acid) lowers the rate of transepidermal water loss [96] and improves the clinical condition (which may resemble atopic dermatitis). In 1982 S. Wright and J. L. Burton reported their success in improving atopic dermatitis in patients with the administration of evening primrose seed oil (containing linoleic acid) [97]. Although other investigators have reported similar results [98], most report little success.

ADVERSE FOOD REACTIONS IN THE SKIN

The general description adverse food reactions in the skin is applied to a clinically "abnormal" response attributed to an ingested food or food additive. These reactions exclude all the immunological reactions described and include pharmacological, metabolic, toxic, and idiosyncratic reactions, which may be ascribable to inherent properties of the food or an abnormality of the host's physiological processes.

Pharmacological reactions occur as a result of the physiological effect of a compound that is a component of the ingested food. Reactions resulting from direct humoral action on vascular smooth muscle produce a "dry" flush (without sweating); and reactions mediated by autonomic nerve action on vascular smooth muscle and eccrine glands result in "wet" flushes (with sweating) [99]. Ingestion of histamine-containing foods such as cheese (parmesan, blue, Roquefort, and Monterey Jack), vegetables (spinach, eggplant, tomatoes), meats (chicken, salami, sirloin, chicken liver), and red wines (Chianti, Burgundy, and Concord grape) can cause "dry" flushes (and produce histaminurea) [100], Persons with type I skin ("always burn; never tan") are more likely to experience this clinically noticeable vasodilatory effect. It can also "light up" an erythematous (rosacea, seborrheic dermatitis, etc) eruption (just as the temperature of a hot shower or bath can). Certain skin disorders have been associated with alcohol misuse, in particular psoriasis and eczema. The pattern and distribution of those diseases in alcoholics are different and tend to be more difficult to treat [101]. Rosacea, postadolescent acne, superficial infections, and porphyria cutanea tarda may also be markers of alcohol misuse. Hot soup or hot coffee can also elicit a vasodilatory reaction as a result of the temperature and not the ingredients. The erythema is usually short-lived when it is due to temperature but can be more sustained with foods, alcohol, or spices.

Alcohol reactions are more common in women than in men and may occur with less alcohol intake [102]. Racial differences in alcohol sensitivity between Oriental and Caucasian populations have been well documented [103–105]. The primary manifestation is a highly visible facial flushing (47%–85% in Orientals vs. 3%–29% in Caucasians) accompanied by other objective and subjective symptoms of discomfort. Although flushing does not "immunize" an individual against alcohol use, those susceptible tend to consume less alcohol [106]. The alcohol-induced flushing phenomenon is believed to be metabolic. Flushing subjects have a higher accumulation of acetaldehyde aldehylde dehydrogenase isozyme (ALDHI). A pharmacogenetic defect in ALDHI has been proposed to be responsible for the flushing [107]. Interestingly, the alcohol-induced flushing can be antagonized by combined (H_1 and H_2) antihistamine administration [108]. (The combined H_1 and H_2 antagonists also neutralize the systolic hypotension induced by alcohol.)

Vasodilatation in the skin physiologically causes an increased heat loss and lowering of the body temperature. Thus the misconception that a "hot toddy" helps you when you are chilled may in fact produce a shaking chill if the environmental temperature is significantly lower than the body temperature.

Large doses of niacin or nicotinic acid, which is prescribed to treat of hyperlipidemia or to elevate the high-density lipoprotein (HDI) level, can cause a bothersome cutaneous reaction consisting of burning, itching, and tingling, often limiting the patient acceptability and tolerability of the drug. Fortunately, the dose necessary to achieve the flush cannot be attained with the ingestion of foods (milk, eggs, organ meats, and peanuts) containing the vitamin. Interestingly, the administration of aspirin or another nonsteroidal antiinflammatory drug prior to ingestion of niacin will decrease the warmth and flushing [109] (but not the pruritus). This therapeutic regimen suggests that prostaglandin activity may be another mechanism of flushing [110].

Histamine intoxication follows the degradation of histidine contained in contaminated dark fish meat or in cheese by enzymatically active bacteria. These histamine-producing microbes are gastrointestinal bacteria of humans, domestic animals, and fish. The entry point for contamination of cheeses is raw milk [111]. Refrigeration of raw meat and milk is an essential preventative step. Cooking will not destroy fully formed histamine.

Scombrotoxins, which are high in histamine content, found in raw (usually spoiled) tuna, mackerel, western Australian salmon, and mahimahi, can cause a classic histamine (vasodilatory) toxicity reaction with flushing (Fig. 2), burning of the mouth and throat, throbbing severe headache, palpitations, abdominal cramps and diarrhea, generalized pruritus urticaria, and angioedema. Bronchospasm and severe respiratory distress have been reported in atopic patients. These symptoms can be severe and distressing, resembling an immunoglobulin

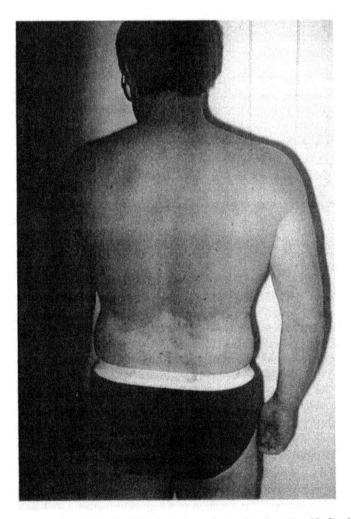

FIGURE 2 47 Year old male in whom "generalized" flushing developed within 30 minutes of ingesting "bad-tasting" bluefish. He became diaphoretic and had a throbbing headache. The episode lasted 3 hr after taking 50 mg Benadryl. The fish was not available for histamine analysis. (Photo courtesy of P. A. Schneiderman.)

TABLE 2 Differential Diagnosis of Flushing

Alcohol-related (e.g., fermented products)
Food additives (e.g., MSG, sulfites, nitrites)
Associated with eating (e.g., "dumping" syndrome, histamine-containing foods, scombroid poisoning)
Drugs (e.g., vasodilators, calcium channel blockers, nicotinic acid)
Neurological (e.g., anxiety, autonomic disorders)
Systemic diseases (e.g., carcinoid, mastocytosis)

E (IgE) reaction, but are rarely if ever severe. Recent investigators have established the fact that histamine ingestion alone will not produce the symptoms of scombroid poisoning. One hypothesis is that simultaneous intake of "saurine" is necessary. Onset of symptoms occurs within half an hour of ingestion of the affected fish [112]; this self-limited syndrome usually resolves spontaneously within 24 hr, but when symptoms are severe, antihistamines (H_1 antagonists may suffice, but adding H_2 antagonists may be more effective) should be administered. The diagnosis of scombroid "poisoning" can be confirmed by the presence of high histamine levels in the affected fish [113].

DERMATOLOGICAL DISEASES SUSPECTED OF BEING INFLUENCED BY FOODS

Acne vulgaris is the most common skin condition evaluated and managed by physicians in the United States [114] Although it is most prevalent in adolescents, 3% of 35–44 year olds have acne. Research has shown that acne is an inflammatory disease of the pilosebaceous unit, with a multifactorial pathogenesis. The primary lesion of acne vulgaris is the open ("blackhead") or closed ("whitehead") comedone. Other acneiform eruptions (rosacea; steroid-induced acne) lack comedones, suggesting a different pathogenesis. The pathogenesis of acne vulgaris includes excessive sebum production, abnormal desquamation of sebaceous-follicle epithelium, and a proliferation of *Propionibacterium acnes* resulting in inflammation. Hormones (and not foods) most notably androgens, which control the size and output of the sebaceous glands, play a key role. The excessive sebum production, a complex lipid mixture, is excreted onto the skin surface. The admixture of pure sebum with epidermally derived lipids forms the lipid film found on skin surfaces, the function of which is to maintain hydration of the skin and hair.

Although acne is not a life-threatening condition, it can have significant psychosocial effects on those who suffer with it. In 1948 Sulzberger and Zaidems noted that "there is no single disease which causes more psychic trauma, more maladjustment between parents and children, more general insecurity and feeling of inferiority and greater sums of psychic suffering than does Acne vulgaris" [115]

Except for starvation, diet rarely if ever plays an etiological role. Severe calorific restriction results in about a 40% decrease in sebum production, enough to be beneficial [116] For many years physicians told their patients to avoid certain fats, particularly those in pork, chocolate, and nuts. This suggestion was championed by some clinicians and attacked by others. A double-blind study by Fulton, Plewig, and Kligman clearly demonstrated that enriched chocolate did not affect the clinical severity of acne [117]. Despite ample negative supporting evidence some patients (and physicians) continue to associate exacerbations of acne with the ingestion of foods (especially pizza, soda, chocolate, and candies) [118]. The conviction that delicious foods are bad for acne is so entrenched that both parents and physicians do not rationally question the Calvinistic precept that "pimples" are a punishment for bad thoughts. Since the sebaceous glands are not an excretory pathway for ingested lipids, it is not surprising that the objective evidence does *not* support the belief that high carbohydrate and high fat intake increases sebum production or alters its composition [119].

In 1961 Hitch and Greenburg found a tenuous association between dietary iodides and the prevalence of cystic acne and scarring [120]. Oral iodides and bromides given over months in moderate doses have a well-deserved reputation for being able to cause acneiform eruptions (and topical application of potassium iodide can provoke papules and pustules) [121]. *Acneiform eruptions* resemble acne, but the initial lesion is inflammatory, and not comedonal. Typically the lesion is a papule or a pustule, and comedones are later, secondary lesions. Acneiform eruptions are often drug-induced (steroids, lithium, isoniazid [isonicotine hydrazine, (INH)] PUVA, thiourea, thiouracil, halogens, and paradoxically tetracyclines) [122]. *Chloracne* is a noninflammatory acneiform eruption associated with contamination of the skin with acneigenic (comedogenic) halogenated cutting oils, greases, tars, and other petroleum distillates.

Rosacea is incredibly common. The incidence has been reported to vary from 5% to 50% of Americans who have some degree of rosacea. This is the disease of patients who blush easily, but it is difficult to differentiate from a "ruddy" complexion. The vascular lability in rosacea, however, seems more pronounced in the middle third of the face, especially of the nose. As stated, any thing (or situation) that causes blood vessels to dilate will make a patient with rosacea appear redder. *Telangiectasias* or visibly dilated cutaneous blood vessels are another sequel of rosacea. *Acneiform papules* eventually appear with the blushing and telangectasia. These papules are less often pustular and involve the central face, especially the nose. Rosacea is not primarily a disease of sebaceous follicles (in contrast to acne vulgaris). Comedones are absent. In

TABLE 3 Foods and Beverages That Trigger Rosacea Flare-Ups

Foods

Liver	Eggplant
Yogurt	Avocado
Sour cream	Spinach
Cheese (except cottage cheese)	Broad-leaf beans and pods
Chocolate	Citrus fruits (including tomatoes
Vanilla	bananas, red plums, raisins, figs)
Soy sauce	Spicy and thermally hot foods
Yeast extracts (bread is OK)	Foods high in histamine
Vinegar	

Beverages

Alcohol, especially red wine, beer, bourbon, gin, vodka, champagne
Hot drinks, including hot cider, hot chocolate, coffee, and tea

young patients there may be a preceding history of acne leading to a hybrid status in which rosacea coexists with acne. Rosacea is considered by some to be a seborrheic disease; however, seborrhea is not a consistent cofeature. Eye involvement is surprisingly common in both rosacea and seborrheic dermatitis. The ophthalmic signs of rosacea are more variable, with blepharitis and conjunctivitis most common [123].

Rosacea is not curable but can be moderated with appropriate treatment. The most agreeable feature of rosacea is that it generally responds well to oral antibiotics. Rosacea patients have very irritable skin—stinging, burning, itchy, uncomfortable, easily irritated. All sources of topical local irritation such as soaps, alcoholic cleansers, tinctures and astringents, abrasives, and peeling agents must be avoided. Protection against sunlight is imperative. Although there is no specific rosacea diet, dietary limitations include all factors that provoke erythema, flushing, and blushing (Table 3).

Xanthomas [124] are tumors or skin infiltrations, varying from yellow (Greek *xanthos*) to brown or red–purple. They arise in a broad spectrum of conditions, the most important of which are those associated with specific defects in lipoprotein metabolism (dyslipoproteinemias). However, they also occur in normolipoproteinemic patients. A frequent clinical expression of hyperlipoproteinemias is the occurrence of xanthomas, which are deposits of lipoprotein components (including cholesterol, triglycerides, and phospholipids) in various parts of the skin [125]. The diseases represented are diverse, numerous, and of considerable importance, especially because of their relationship to cardiovascular disease (see Table 4).

The dyslipoproteinemias are associated with distinct clinical syndromes. History, physical examination, and laboratory evaluation all contribute to estab-

TABLE 4   Dyslipoproteinemias[a]

Type	Skin Manifestations	Other	Onset	Abnormalities
I	Eruptive xanthomas: extensor pressure surfaces, buttocks	Lipemia retinalis pancreatitis, xerostomia, dry eyes	Pre puberty	Chylomicro-nemia (Creamy plasma)
II	Tendon and tuberous xanthomas in digital webs, clefts Xanthelasma	Arcus juvenalis	Third or fourth decade	Hyperlipopro-teinemias Premature CV disease
III	Palmar creases Planar xanthomas Tuberous xanthomas on extremities	Premature CAD, PVD Abnormal GTT	Adulthood	Hyper(dysbet) liproteinemia
IV	None, or eruptive xanthomas	None, obesity, HSM	Adulthood	Hyperlipemia
V	Eruptive xanthomas	Same as type I	Fourth or fifth decade	

[a] CV, cardiovascular

lishing the diagnosis. The classification of lipoprotein disturbances by Fredrickson et al. [126] has been accepted as the standard for study.

In *chylomicronemia (type I and type V hyperlipoproteinemia)*, plasma triglyceride concentration is labile, depending primarily upon the time relationship of sampling to the intake of fat. Fasting plasma triglyceride levels >300 mg/dl are abnormal. Triglyceride levels >1500 mg/dl result in a distinct accumulation of chylomicrons, visible as a definite creamy layer on top of plasma. The clinical manifestations are eruptive xanthomas, lipemia retinalis, and other forms of system involvement. The majority of the symptoms are ameliorated with a reduction in plasma triglycerides.

Diabetic patients with eruptive xanthomas and chylomicronemia (combined with elevated very low density lipoprotein [VLDL] levels) are considered as having type V hyperlipoproteinemia. Eruptive xanthomas are usually asymptomatic, discrete papules with a yellow center and erythematous halo. They appear suddenly in showers and disappear with a drop in the plasma triglyceride level. Eruptive xanthomas have a predilection to form on pressure points on the extensor surfaces of the elbows, back, buttocks, and knees.

Therapy of chylomicronemia consists of dietary restriction of fats, but many also require drug therapy.

Type II hyperlipoproteinemias (with elevated LDL levels) are distinctive monogenetic and polygenetic diseases, e.g., familial hypercholesterolemia (FH), familial combined hyperlipidemia (FCH), and polygenetic ("common") hypercholesterolemia.

Familial hypercholesterolemia is one of the most important, relatively common codominant diseases. Heterozygote adults have plasma cholesterol levels usually in the 300 to 400 mg/dl range. Clinical manifestations typically do not appear until the third and fourth decades. Xanthomas are noted on the Achilles tendons and extensor tendons of the hands; xanthelasma palpebrarum may also be present. Homozygotes have markedly elevated cholesterol and LDL levels at birth, which gradually increase each decade to the 700–1200 mg/dl range. They develop unique xanthomas in the interdigital webs and in the cleft of the buttocks during childhood.

Treatment of familial hypercholesterolemia employs a low-fat, low-cholesterol diet used with combination drug therapy.

Familial combined hyperlipidemia may be one of the most common monogenetic disorders in humans. The clinical manifestations generally appear in the fourth or fifth decade. The diagnosis is presumptive and established only by analysis of the pattern of the dyslipoproteinemia. Most of these patients have no xanthomas, although tendon xanthomas and xanthelasma may be observed. The most frequent clinical manifestation is the development of premature cardiovascular disease.

Treatment of FCH is dependent upon the type of lipoprotein pattern. Because these patients have no xanthomas or other dermatological disease, they are not discussed further.

Clinical symptoms of Type III hyperlipoproteinemia (*familial dysbetalipoproteinemia*) develop in the fourth and fifth decades. Untreated patients have virtually pathognomonic yellow lines or infiltrations in the palmar creases and palmar xanthomas. Tuboeruptive xanthomas are also seen on the elbows, knees, and buttocks. Plasma concentrations of both triglycerides and cholesterol are elevated, with the principal elevation that of the plasma lipoprotein IDL.

Therapy requires appropriate management of aggravating factors including diabetes mellitus, systemic lupus erythematosus (SLE) paraproteinemias, and especially hypothyroidism. Modification of diet and caloric restriction are very effective in lowering plasma lipid levels. Additional lowering may be achieved by drug therapy with nicotinic acid or genfibrozil.

In type IV hyper-VLDL-emia or hyperlipemia the typical patient is obese and sensitive to carbohydrates. Oral contraceptives and alcohol excess cause exacerbation of their condition and may cause the appearance of eruptive xanthomas. When the serum triglyceride concentration rises above 2000 mg/dl, pancreatitis may occur [127].

Therapy in the form of a low-calorie, low carbohydrate diet with avoidance of alcohol generally gives excellent results.

Psoriasis is a common papulosquamous disease of unknown cause affecting up to 2% of the population. The disease can assume many morphological patterns: in some patients it is only a minor cosmetic disability, but in many cases it can cause lifelong misery and incapacity. The characteristic appearance of multiple well-demarcated large red patches covered with thick, silvery white scales is easy to recognize. The plaques are usually seen on elbows, knees, and scalp, but no part of the skin is spared.

Psoriasis is a disease in which there is an increase of the mitotic rate and deoxyribonucleic acid (DNA) synthesis in the epidermis [128,129]. The cell turnover time in normal viable epidermis is 28 days compared to 2 to 4 days in psoriatic epidermis. There are several explanations for the increased epidermal cell turnover in psoriasis, but the continued debate on the details of cell cycle change in psoriasis has not been resolved.

An observation that psoriasis defervesced in concentration camp victims instigated the consideration of the role of diet (starvation!) in psoriasis. That protein deprivation led to the search for a specific substance (amino acid) as a trigger for the overproduction of epidermal cells. Several amino acids (especially taurine) were incriminated, with the institution of elimination-type ("taurine-free") [130] diets. When each substance eliminated was subjected to scientific analysis, the success claims were not substantiated [131].

Fleisher et al. reported that in evaluating alternative medical treatments for psoriasis, psoriasis severity was worse in those who had tried herbal remedies, vitamin therapy, and dietary manipulation. They also noted that with the exception of vitamin therapy, there was no association between the intensity of conventional medical treatment and that of alternative treatment [132].

In some patients complaining of *fish-odor syndrome,* body malodor, a possible cause may be the autosomal recessive enzyme trimethylamine oxidase deficiency [133]. The "fishy odor" is caused by the massive excretion of a fragrant, volatile tertiary amine, trimethylamine (TMA)in the urine (the oxide form is odorless). The odor may also be present in the breath, in the sweat, or from the vagina [134] of affected individuals. TMA is of dietary origin, formed by intestinal bacterial degradation of the choline in egg yolk, liver, and soybeans (legumes) or by reduction of TMA oxide present in high concentrations in marine fish [135]. The diagnosis is established by measuring the percentage of total TMA in the patient's urine [136]. This syndrome has been associated with various psychosocial reactions including clinical depression. There is one report of clinical and biochemical response to treatment with metronidazole (250 mg po TID × 2 weeks) [113].

Pompholyx dyshidrotic eczema is a bilateral, roughly symmetrical recurrent eczematous reaction characterized in the acute phase by clear, dome-shaped vesicles (bubbles) on palms, soles, and the sides of the fingers and toes. During the eruptive phase, it is extremely pruritic and/or burning. Increased sweating is frequently reported. In the chronic phase, scaling, fissures, and erythema are present, often with secondary bacterial colonization. The association of "hand eczema" with atopy varies between 0% and 59%; the differences are due to the varied criteria used to identify atopy. This latter association has suggested an allergic cause to some clinicians. Although none was found, a dietary regimen of avoiding nickel in foods seems to have adherents. There are no double-blind studies to support the use of a nickel-free diet!

CUTANEOUS MANIFESTATIONS OF NUTRITIONAL DISORDERS

Nutritional disorders do occur in a number of settings, including congenital or postsurgical alterations of bowel anatomical features; wasting diseases such as metastatic cancer and renal and liver disease; anorexia nervosa; carcinoid syndrome; and Hartnup disease.

Fad diets, inappropriate management of food allergies, and psychiatric diseases such as anorexia nervosa may result in severe *protein deficiency*. With starvation (which in young children with total inanition is termed *marasmus*), the skin is dry, thin, wrinkly, pallid, cold, and inelastic, in addition to the obvious loss of subcutaneous fat. Follicular hyperkeratosis (small, hard elevated nodules around the hair follicles) is also associated with undernutrition [137]. *Kwashiokor,* which results from a diet low in protein and high in calories from sugar or starch, is associated with a dermatosis described as "flaky paint" but no edema.

Vitamin A deficiency is extremely prevalent and is a frequent cause of blindness and increased susceptibility to infection in underdeveloped countries. In affluent societies, overt deficiency is rare and occurs mostly as the result of disorders interfering with absorption, storage, or release of the vitamin: i.e., celiac disease, sprue, cyctic fibrosis, etc. Follicular hyperkeratosis is the most prominent cutaneous sign of vitamin A deficiency, however, other nutritional deficiencies are more probable causes of the disorder, such as deficiencies of essential fatty acids (discussed earlier) and B-complex vitamins [138].

In the 1920s epithelial changes were identified in vitamin A–deficient animals, and low levels of vitamin A were suspected of being related to dyskeratotic conditions [139]. Because the follicular keratoses observed in *Darier's disease* and *pityriasis rubra pilaris* resembled the skin lesions of vitamin A deficiency, systemic vitamin A was used clinically in the treatment of those disorders. Vitamin A therapy was reported as being beneficial for other hyperkeratotic conditions (e.g., *keratosis palmaris et plantaris*) [140].

Vitamin A therapy is now of historical interest. Vitamin A (retinol) is not a specific compound but describes the biological activity of a group of compounds identified today as *retinoids*. More than 1500 synthetic vitamin A derivatives have been synthesized in an effort to develop compounds of therapeutic use. Three synthetic retinoids have been widely studied and found to be efficacious therapeutic agents. Tretinoin is used as an effective keratolytic in acne vulgaris; isotretinoin (13-*cis*-retinoid acid) and etretinate are most effective in psoriasis and many of the disorders of keratinization previously treated with vitamin A.

Hypervitaminosis A (vitamin A toxicity) Recent media dissemination of information on the proposed anticancer effects of vitamin A has led some individuals to consume large amounts of the vitamin in the belief that is has anticancer-protection properties. Acute toxicity results in cutaneous exfoliation, dry scaly skin, hair loss, fissuring of the lips, and pruritus. These toxicities are caused by preformed vitamin A and do not occur with β-carotene [141]. Treatment involves discontinuing consumption of all vitamin A products and decreasing dietary intake of fish oil, liver, egg yolk, milk fat, green vegetables, and carrots.

Carotenoderma is usually not noticeable until the serum level of serum carotenoid is three or four times normal. The color of the skin is canary yellow, ochre, or golden. It never reaches the bronze, orange, or green tint of jaundice. Mucus membranes, including the sclera, are always spared. Hypercarotenosis does not cause itching, nor does it change the color of the urine. It is considered a harmless condition and slowly disappears when the intake is reduced to normal level [140].

CUTANEOUS SIGNS OF OTHER VITAMIN DEFICIENCIES

Whereas the causes of vitamin deficiencies may be generally understood, their recognition in clinical situations is usually delayed, often because there is a failure to understand the significance of the clinical signs. In this presentation we will only consider the morphological characteristics of the skin lesions and defer the etiological issues (Table 5).

Angular stomatitis is a nonspecific maceration and fissuring, with redness, superficial ulceration, and crusting that occur at the angles of the mouth and frequently extend onto the skin but not the buccal mucosa. In the majority of patients it is bilateral. In a single reported study, an infective agent was found in 54% of the 36 patients. *Candida* spp. and *Staphylococcus aureus* were the most common organisms identified [142]. Angular stomatitis may be due to a variety of causes, of which riboflavin (vitamin B$_2$) deficiency is only one. When due to ariboflavinosis, the angular cheilitis is associated with *cheilosis,* a characteristic thin, shiny, denuded, and linear redness along the line of lip closure. Angular stomatitis has been reported to respond to niacin, pyridoxine, pantothenic acid, ascorbic acid, folic acid, vitamin B$_{12}$, or iron, but there are no controlled studies substantiating these results [143].

TABLE 5   Cutaneous Signs of Vitamin Deficiency

Vitamin A	Vitamin B$_2$	Vitamin B$_6$
Follicular hyperkeratosis over extremities, shoulders (*phrynoderma,* toad skin) Dry, wrinkled, scaly skin	Angular stomatitis, cheilosis Glossitis, perleche Seborrheic dermatitis (midface) Inc. wrinkles around eyes, flexures	Seborrheic dermatitis (rare) "Hot foot" due to sensory neuritis
Niacin	**Biotin**	**Vitamin C**
Pellagra (photodermatosis) "pellagrin nose," cheilosis, glossitis, aphthous ulcers	Scaly dermatitis Xerosis Loss of lingual papilla Alopecia	Purpura Perifollicular hemorrhage Increased susceptibility to bruising
	Vitamin K	
	Ecchymosis	

ESSENTIAL ELEMENTS IN THE SKIN

Iron

Chronic iron deficiency causes a diagnostic spoon-shaped deformity (koilony-chia) of fingernails and toenails. Angular stomatitis and glossitis with atrophy of the lingual papilla are frequently seen in iron deficiency. Generalized pruritus has been reported less frequently [144]. Iron overload causes a generalized bronzing of the skin as seen in *hemochromatosis* and is a major factor in *porphyria cutanea tarda.*

Zinc

Acrodermatitis enteropathica is the prototypical zinc deficiency disease, most usually an autosomal recessive condition due to impaired absorption of zinc, but may be seen in any inadequate dietary zinc intake condition, e.g., anorexia nervosa. The cutaneous lesions of acrodermatitis enteropathica range from dry, scaly, eczematous (usually perioroficial) plaques to vesiculobullous, pustular, and erosive lesions (acrally). Secondary infection with bacteria and *Candida albicans* can occur. The skin findings are most responsive to zinc supplementation.

Copper

Nutritional copper deficiency is rare. *Menkes' kinky-hair syndrome* is a rare X-linked disorder resulting from a defect in intercellular copper transport. The dermatological manifestations of that syndrome include steely hair texture (pili torti) and depigmentation of hair and skin. There is no effective treatment for patients with Menkes' syndrome.

Selenium

In several patients on prolonged parenteral nutrition in the United States a syndrome developed that included a white appearance of the the fingernail beds and dyschromotrichia that were reversed by selenium [145]. The nail changes are reversible with intravenous selenium supplementation.

Although selenium is an essential trace element, it can be highly toxic when taken in excess. Symptoms of toxicity include nausea, vomiting, diarrhea, hair loss, and exfoliative dermatitis [146].

Nutrition and "Healthy" Skin

Entrepreneurs have been made very healthy by the promotion and sale of "natural" nostrums to the panacea-seeking gullible health-oriented consumer. Foodstuffs have been added to creams, lotions, soaps, and shampoos. Until recently scientific evidence to confirm their claims was wanting. The success of fruit-based "beauty" consumer products has been rationalized by the identification of glycolic acid—the "fruit-acid" that belongs to the family of chemicals known as alpha-hydroxy acids (AHAs). AHAs are not moisturizers. At certain concentrations they both stimulate and increase the rate of epidermal cell turnover and reduce corneocyte adhesion [147]. These latter attributes indirectly alleviate the signs of dry skin and are utilized by dermatologists performing chemical peels. They do not alleviate fine lines and wrinkles, clarify, nor retexturize the skin. At high concentrations and low (acid) pH they are irritating, and rarely they are phototoxic.

Hair and nail consumer products abound. Preparations containing iron, calcium, zinc, cystine, vitamin A, and gelatin are most popular but have not been proved effective when subjected to the scientific laws of verification. Colombo et al. have convincing evidence that splitting and brittle nails, in women, improve with oral administration of biotin [148].

CONCLUSIONS

S L. Parker et al. [149] reported that those patients referred to allergists for suspected adverse reactions to foods represent two distinctly different groups. The first group included patients with positive IgE food reactions; the second group were patients in whom symptoms and offending foods were incompatible with classic IgE-mediated food allergy and in whom results of food challenges were negative. Demographic characteristics of all reported cases consistently noted a preponderance of female subjects [116]. Patients in the second group are more likely to be influenced by accounts in the popular news media suggesting that commonly eaten foods often cause adverse reactions. They are also more likely to rely on lay sources for information related to adverse food reactions and to have consulted a nontraditional health practitioner. The emergence of alternative medicine and medical subcultures, such as clinical ecology and holistic and orthomolecular medicine, has introduced and popularized unconventional and often unfounded dietary modifications and nutritional therapies in the treatment and/or prevention of disease. It is important that clinicians assess patients carefully for such dietary manipulations.

ACKNOWLEDGMENTS

Special thanks to Janet Prystowsky, M.D. Ph.D., for her important suggestions in the preparation of this chapter.

REFERENCES

1. Michaelsson G, Petterson L, Juhlin L. Purpura caused by food and drug additives. Arch Dermatol 1974; 109:49–52.
2. Brenner S, Ruocco V, Wolf R et al. Pemphigus and dietary factors. Dermatology 1995; 190:197–202.
3. Bieber T. Role of Langerhans cells in the pathophysiology of atopic dermatitis. Pathol Biol (Paris) 1995; 43:871–875.
4. Sampson HA, Metcalfe DD. Food allergies. JAMA 1992; 268:2840–2844.
5. Phanuphak P, Schocket AL, Arroyave CM et al. Skin histamine in patients with urticaria. J Allergy Clin Immunol 1980; 65:371–374.
6. Hagermark O. Peripheral and central mediators of itch. Skin Pharmacol 1992; 5:1–8.
7. Braciale VL. Molecular aspects of antigen processing and presentation. In: Molecular and Cellular Biology of the Allergic Response. Levinson AI, Patterson Y, eds. New York: Marcel Dekker, 1994, p 179.
8. Roitt I, Brostoff J, Male D. Hypersensitivity—Type I. In ed. Immunology. Mosby 1987; 19:3.
9. The Scientific Status Summaries of the Institute of Food Technologists' Expert Panel on Food Safety & Nutrition; Institute of Food Technologists, 221 N. LaSalle St., Chicago, IL.
10. Ebner C, Hirshwehr R, Bauer L, Breiteneder H et al. Identification of allergens in fruits and vegetables: IgE cross-reactivities with the important birch pollen allergens Bet v 1 and Bet v 2. J Allergy Clin Immunol 1995; 95:962–969.
11. Bernhisel-Broadbent J. Allergenic cross-reactivity of foods and characterization of food allergens and extracts. Ann Allergy Asthma Immunol 1995; 75:295–303.
12. Bernhisel-Broadbent J, Scanlon SM, Sampson HA. Fish Hypersensitivity. I. In vitro and oral challenge results in fish-allergic patients. J Allergy Clin Immunol 1992; 89:730–737.

13. Sampson HA. Food cross-reactivity and its clinical relevance. American College Asthma Immunol 1996 Annual Meeting. Syllabus p 423–430.
14. Pastorello E, Ortolani C, Farioli L, Pravettoni V et al. Allergenic cross-reactivity among peach, apricot, plum, and cherry in patients with oral allergy syndrome: an in vivo and in vitro study. J Allergy Clin Immunol 1994; 94:699–707.
15. Joral A, Villas F, Garmendia J, Villareal O. Adverse reactions to foods in adults. J Investig Allergol Clin Immunol 1995; 5:47–49.
16. Fisher AA. Association of latex and food allergy. Cutis 1993; 52:70–71.
17. Blanco C, Carrillo T, Castillo R, Quiralte J, Cuevas M. Latex allergy: clinical features and cross-reactivity with fruits. Ann Allergy 1994; 73:309–314.
18. Crisi G, Belsito DV. Contact urticaria from latex in a patient with immediate hypersensitivity to bana, avocado and peach. Contact Dermatitis 1993; 28:247–248.
19. Hamann CP, Sullivan KM. Natural rubber latex hypersensitivities. In: Charlesworth EN, eds. Cutaneous Allergy. Oxford: Blackwell Science, 1997, p 186.
20. vanRee R, Antonicelli L, Akkerdaas JH, Pajno GB et al. Asthma after consumption of snails in house dust mite allergic patients: a case of IgE cross reactivity. Allergy 1996; 51:387–393.
21. Erbe A, Rodriquez JL, McCullogh J et al. Anaphylaxis after ingestion of beignets contaminated with *Dermatophagoides farinae*. J Allergy Clin Immunol 1993; 91:846–849.
22. Beltrani VS. Urticaria and angioedema: current therapy. 1996; 14:171–198.
23. Atkins FM: The diagnosis of food-induced urticaria. In: Metcalfe DD, Sampson HA, Simon RA, eds. Food Allergy: Adverse Reactions to Foods and Food Additives. Oxford: Blackwell Scientific, 1991, pp 129–138.
24. Fisher AA. Contact Urticaria. In: Fisher AA, ed. Contact Dermatitis. 3rd ed. Philadelphia: Lea & Febiger, 1986, pp 686–709.
25. Odom RB, Maibach HI. Contact urticaria: a different contact dermatitis in dermatotoxicology and pharmacology. In: Marzulli FN, Maibach HI, eds. Advances in Modern Toxicology. Vol 4. Washington, DC: Hemisphere, Publishing Corporation, 1977, pp 441–450.
26. Oranje AP, Van Gysel D, Mulder PG, Dieges PH. Food-induced contact urticaria syndrome (CUS) in atopic dermatitis: reproducibility of repeated and duplicate testing with a skin provocation test, the skin application food tes (SAFT). Contact Dermatitis 1994; 31:836–842.
27. Fisher AA. Contact urticaria. In: Fisher AA, ed. Contact Dermatitis. Philadelphia: Lea & Ferbiger, 1986, pp 686–709.
28. Burdick AE, Mathias CGT. The contact urticaria syndrome. Dermatol Clin 1985; 3:71–84.
29. Beltrani VS. Urtcaria and angioedema. Dermatol Clin 1996; 14:171–198.
30. Anderson JA, Sogn DD. Adverse food reactions that involve or are suspected of involving immune mechanisms: an anatomical categorization. In: American Academy of Allergy and Immunology Committee on Adverse Reactions to Foods. Washington DC: National Institute on Allergy and Infectious Diseases, 1984, pp 43–102.

31. Farnam J, Grant A. Angioedema. Dermatol Clin 1985; 3:85–95.
32. Bock SA. The incidence of severe adverse reactions to food in Colorado. J Allergy Clin Immunol 1992; 90:683–685.
33. Terr AI. Allergic diseases. In: Stites DP, Stobo JD, Wells JV, eds. Basic and Clinical Immunology. Norwalk, CT: Appleton & Lange.
34. Romano, A, DiFonso M, Giuffreda F, Quaratino D et al. Diagnostic work-up for food-dependent, exercise-induced anaphylaxis. Allergy 1995; 50:817–824.
35. Kidd JM, Cohen SH, Sosman AJ, Fink JN. Food-dependent exercise induced anaphylaxis. J Allergy Clin Immunol 1983; 71:407–411.
36. MartinMunoz F, Lopez Cazana JM, Villas F et al. Exercise-induced anaphylactic reaction to hazelnut. Allergy 1994; 49:314–316.
37. Guinnepain MT, Eloit C, Raffard M, Brunet-Moret MJ et al. Exercise-induced anaphylaxis: useful screening of food sensitization. Ann Allergy Asthma Immunol 1996; 77:491–496.
38. Taylor SL, Bush RK, Nordlee JA. Sulfites In: Metcalfe DD, Sampson HA, Simon RA, eds. Food Allergy: Adverse Reactions to Foods and Food Additives. Oxford: Blackwell Scientific,
39. Allen DH. Monosodium glutamate. In: Metcalfe DD, Sampson HA, Simon RA, eds Food Allergy: Adverse Reactions to Foods and Food Additives. Oxford: Blackwell Scientific,
40. Robledo MA, Diaz LA. Pathology of pemphigus. In: Soter NA, Baden HP, eds. Pathophysiology of Dermatologic Diseases. New York: McGraw-Hill,
41. Brenner S, Ruocco V et al. Pemphigus and dietary Factors. Dermatology 1995; 190:197–202.
42. Brenner S, Wolf R. Possible nutritional factors in induced pemphigus. Dermatology 1994; 337–339.
43. Wolff HH, Scherer R. Allergic Vasculitis. In: Ring J Burg G, eds. New Trends in Allergy. Berlin: Springer, 1981, p 140.
44. Ancona GR, Ellerhorn MJ, Falconer EH. Purpura due to food sensitivity. J Allergy 1951; 22:487–493.
45. Michaelsson G, Petterson L, Juhlin L. Purpura caused by food and drug additives. Arch Dermatol 1974; 109:49–52.
46. Ring J. Dermatologic diseases secondary to food allergy and pseudoallergy. In: Reinhardt D, Schmidt E eds. Food Allergy. New York: Raven Press, 1988, pp 271–89.
47. Beltrani, VS, Beltrani VP. Contact dermatitis: a review. Ann Allergy 1997; 78(2):160–195.
48. Marks JG, DeLeo VA. Occupational skin disease. In: Marks JG, DeLeo VA, eds. Contact and Occupational Dermatology. St Louis: Mosby Year Book, 1994, pp 281–283.
49. Burks JW. Classic aspects of onion and garlic dermatitis in housewives. Ann Allergy 1954; 12:592–595.
50. Puglisi V. Dermatoses caused by lemons. G Ital Dermatol 1951; 92:237–241.
51. Fisher AA. Contact dermatitis from foods and food additives. In: Fisher AA, ed. Contact Dermatitis. 3rd. ed. Philadelphia: Lea & Febiger, 1986.

52. Beltrani VS, Beltrani VP. Contact dermatitis: a review (CME article). Ann Allergy 1997; 78(2):160–175.
53. Rinkel HJ, Ballyeat RM. Occupational dermatitis due to lettuce. JAMA 1932; 98:137–140.
54. Closson JB. Oral allergy after lettuce ingestion. JAMA 1973; 230:113–118.
55. Lupton ES. Cheilitis due to coffee. Arch Dermatol 1961; 84:798–800.
56. Marks JG, DeLeo VA. Occupations commonly associated with contact dermatitis. In: Marks and DeLeo eds. Contact and Occupational Dermatology. St Louis: Mosby Year Book, 1992, pp 281–283.
57. Nethercott JR, Holness DL. Occupational dermatitis in food handlers and bakers. J Am Acad Dermatol 1989; 21:485–490.
58. Kern AN. Contact dermatitis from cinnamon. Arch Dermatol 1960; 81:599–603.
59. Fisher AA. Allergic contact dermatitis. Cutis 1975; 15:149.
60. Miller RL, Gould AR, Bernstein ML. Cinnamon-induced stomatitis venata. Oral Surg Oral Med Oral Pathol 1992; 73:708.
61. Fisher AA. Contact stomatitis and cheilitis. In: Fisher AA, ed. Contact Dermatitis. Lea & Febiger, Philadelphia: 1986, pp 773–800.
62. Reginella RF, Fairfield JC, Marks JG. Hyposensitization to poison iny after working in a cashew nut shell oil processing factory. Contact Dermatitis 1989; 20:274–279.
63. Fisher AA. Ibid Ref 61.
64. Watemberg N, Urkin Y, Witztum A. Phytophotodermatitis due to figs. Cutis 1991; 48:151–152.
65. Halbert AR, Weston WL, Morelli JG. Atopic dermatitis: is it an allergic disease? J Am Acad Dermatol 1995; 33:1008–1018.
66. Sampson HA. Eczema and food hypersensitivity. In: Metcalfe DD, Sampson HA, Simon RA, eds. Food Allergy: Adverse Reactions to Foods and Food Additives, Oxford: Blackwell Scientific Publications, 1992.
67. Sampson HA, McCaskill CC. Food hypersensitivity and atopic dermatitis: evaluation of 113 patients. J Pediatr 1985; 107:669–675.
68. Ogawa M, Berger PA, McIntyre R et al. IgE in atopic dermatitis. Arch Dermatol 1971; 103:575–580.
69. Burks AW, Mallory SB, Williams LW et al. Atopic dermatitis: clinical relevance of food hypersensitivity reactions. J Pediatr 1988; 113:447–451.
70. Guillet G, Guillet M-H. Natural history of sensitization in atopic dermatitis: a 3-year follow up in 250 children. Arch Dermatol 1992; 128:187–192.
71. Isolauri E, Turjanmaa K. Combined skin prick and patch testing enhances identification of food allergy in infants with atopic dermatitis. J Allergy Clin Immunol 1996; 97:9–15.
72. Imayama S, Hashizume T, Miyahara H, Tanahashi T et al. Combination of patch test and IgE for dust mite antigens differentiates 130 patients with atopic dermatitis into four groups. J Am Acad Dermatol 1992; 27:531–538.
73. Halbert AR, Weston WL, Morelli JG. Atopic dermatitis: is it an allergic disease? J Am Acad Dermatol 1995; 33:1008–1018.
74. Sampson HA, Jolie PL. Increased plasma histamine concentrations after food challenges in children with atopic dermatitis. N Engl J Med 1984; 311:372–376.

75. Piletta PA, Wirth S, Hommel L Sauret JH et al. Circulating skin-homing T cells in atopic dermatitis. Arch Dertmatol 1996; 132:1171–1176.
76. Horsmannheimo L, Harvima I, Jarvikallio A, Harvimo RJ et al. Mast cells are on major source of IL-4 in atopic dermatitis. Br J Dermatol 1994; 131(3)348–353.
77. Sampson HA. The role of food allergy and mediator release in atopic dermatitis. J Allergy Clin Immunol 1988; 81:635–645.
78. Webber SA, Graham-Brown RAC, Hutchinson PE et al. Dietary manipulation in childhood atopic dermatitis. Br J Dermatol 1986; 114:121:91–98.
79. Sampson HA. The Role of Food in Atopic Dermatitis. Plenary Session Presentation at the Clinical Cutaneous Allergy and Immunology Meeting, New York, October 1996.
80. Hanifin JM. Significance of food hypersensitivity in children with atopic dermatitis. Pediatr Dermatol 1986; 3:161–174.
81. Hill DJ, Lynch BC. Elemental diet in the management of severe eczema in childhood. Clin Allergy 1982; 12:313–315.
82. Juto P, Engberg S, Winberg J. Treatment of infantile atopic dermatitis with a strict elimination diet. Clin Allergy 1978; 8:493–500.
83. Gupta MA, Gupta AD, Ellis CN. Antidepressant drugs in dermatology. Arch Dermatol 1987; 113: 647–652.
84. Bock SA, Lee WY, Remigio LK, May CD. Studies of hypersensitivity reactions to foods in infants and children. J Allergy Clin Immunol 1978; 62:327–334.
85. Sampson HA, Scanlon SM. Natural history of food hypersensitivity in children with atopic dermatitis. J Pediatr 1989; 115:23–27.
86. Grulee CG, Sanford HN. The influence of breast feeding and artificial feeding in infantile eczema. J Pediatr 1936; 9:223–225.
87. Lucas A, Brooke O, Morley R, Cole T, Bamford M. Early diet of preterm infants and development of allergic or atopic disease: randomized prospective study. Br Med J 1990; 300:837–840.
88. Sigurs N, Hattevig G, Kjellman B. Maternal avoidance of eggs, cow's milk, and fish during lactation: effect on allergic manifestation, skin prick test, and specific IgE antibodies in children at age 4 years. Pediatrics 1992; 89:735–739.
89. Gustafsson D, Lowhagen T, Andersson K. Risk of developing atopic disease after early feeding with cow's milk based formula. Arch Dis Child 1992; 67:1008–1010.
90. Kay J Gawkrodger DJ, Mortimer MJ et al. The prevalence of childhood atopic eczema in a general population. J Am Acad Dermatol 1994; 30:35–39.
91. Zeiger RS, Heller S, Mellon MH et al. Effect of combined maternal and infant food-allergen avoidance on development of atopy in early infance: a randomized study. J Allergy Clin Immunol 1989; 84:72–89.
92. Beltrani VS. The role of dust mite in atopic dermatitis. Allergy Clin Immunol Int 1997; 9:37–40.
93. Wahlgren CF. Provokers of itch in atopic dermatitis. Acta Derm Venerol 1991.
94. Rustin MHA, Pooulter L. Chinese herbal therapy in atopic dermatitis. Dermatol Ther 1996; 1:83–93.
95. Brehler R, Hildebrand A, Luger TA. Recent developments in the treatment of atopic eczema. J Am Acad Dermatol 1997; 36:983–994.

96. Prottey C et al. J Invest Dermatol 1968; 64:228.
97. Wright S, burton JL. Oral evening primrose seed oil improves atopic eczema. Lancet 1982; 11:1120–1122.
98. Bordoni A Biagi PL, Masi M, Ricci G et al. Evening primrose oil (Efamol) in the treatment of children with atopic eczema. Drugs Exp Clin Res 1987; 14:291–297.
99. Wilkins JK. Flushing reactions. In: Rook AJ, Recent Advances in Dermatology. Vol. 6. Maibach H, eds. New York: Churchill-Livingstone, 1983; p 157.
100. Spencer DM, Wilkin JK. Parmesan cheese and vegetable-induced histaminurea in a thermal flusher. Cutis 1994; 54:185–186.
101. Higgins EM, du Vivier AW. Cutaneous disease and alcohol misuse. Br Med Bull 1994; 50:85–98.
102. Whitfield JB, Martin NG. Alcohol reactions in subjects of European descent: effects on alcohol use and on physical and psychomotor responses to alcohol. Alcohol Clin Exp Res 1996; 20:81–86.
103. Chan AW. Racial differences in alcohol sensitivity. Alcohol 1986; 21:93–104.
104. Newlin DB. The skin-flushing response: autonomic, self-report, and conditioned responses to repeated administrations of alcohol in Asian men. J Abnorm Psychol 1989; 98:421–425.
105. Yu PH, Fang, Dyck LE. Cutaneous vasomotor sensitivity to ethanol and acetaldehyde: subtypes of alcohol-flushing response among Chinese. Alcohol Clin Exp Res 1990; 14:932–936.
106. Slutske WS, Heath AC, Madden PA, Bucholz KK et al. Is alcohol-related flushing a protective factor for alcoholism in Caucasians. Alcohol Clin Exp Res 1995; 19:582–592.
107. Chan AW. Ibid.
108. Miller NS, Goodwin DW, Jopnes FC, Gabrieli WF et al. Antihistamine blockade of alcohol induced flushing in orientals. J Stud Alcohol 1988; 49:16–20.
109. Whelan AM, Price SO, Fowler SF, Hainer BL. The effect of aspirin on niacin-induced cutaneous reactions. J ??46??am Pract 1992; 34:165–168.
110. Fiedler P, Wolkin A, Rotrosen J. Niacin-induced flush as a measure of prostaglandin activity in alcoholics and schizophrenics. Biol Psychiatry 1986; 21:1347–1350.
111. Burnett JW. Histamine poisoning. Cutis 1994; 388.
112. Smart DR. Scombroid poisoning: a report of seven cases involving the Western Australian salmon, Arripis truttaceus. Med J Aust 1992; 157;748–751.
113. Gilchrist A. Foodborne diseases. In: Foodborne Diseases and Food Safety. Gilchrist, ed. American Medical Association Publisher, 1981, pp 1–40.
114. Bergfeld WF, Odom RB. New perspectives on acne. Clinician 1994; 12(2):4–30.
115. Sulzberger MB, Zaidems SH. Psychogenic factors in dermatological disorders. Med Clin North Am 1948; 32:669.
116. Pochi PE, Downing DT, Strauss JS. Sebaceous gland response in man to prolonged total caloric deprivation. J Invest Dermatol 1970; 55:303–309.
117. Fulton JE, Plewig G, Kligman AM. Effect of chocolate on acne vulgaris. JAMA 1969; 210:11–22.
118. Rasmussen JE. Diet and acne. Semin Dermatol 1982; 1:257–265.

119. Kligman AM. Acne - treatment: general statements. In: Acne and Rosacea. 2nd ed. Plewig G, Kligman AM, eds. Berlin: Springer-Verlag, 1993, pp 558–560.
120. Hitch JM, Greenburgh BG. Adolescent acne - dietary iodine. Arch Dermatol 1961; 84:898–902.
121. Plewig G. Acneiform Eruptions. In: Plewig G, Kligman AM, eds. Acne and Rosacea. 2nd ed. Berlin: Springer- Verlag, 1993, pp 406–409.
122. IBID.
123. Kligman AM. Ocular rosacea: current concepts. Arch Dermatol 1997; 133:89–90.
124. Polano MK, FreedbergIM. Xanthomatoses and Dyslipoproteinemias. In: Dermatology in General Medicine. 4th ed. Fitzpatrick TB, Eisen AZ, Wolff K, Freedberg IM, Austen KF, eds. New York: McGraw-Hill, 1993, pp 1901–1916.
125. Parker F. Xanthomas and hyperlipidemias. J Am Acad Dermatol 1985; 13:1–12.
126. Fredrickson DS et al. Fat transport in lipoproteins: an integrated approach to mechanism and disorders. N Engl J Med 1967; 267:34–41.
127. Keeling JH. Eruptive xanthomas: a cutaneous marker of hypertriglyceridemia. J Geriatr Dermatol 1996; 4:139–144.
128. Weinstein GD, Frost P. Abnormal cell proliferation in psoriasis. J Invest Derm 1958; 50:254–259.
129. Weinstein GD, VanScott EJ. Autoradiographic studies of normal and psoriatic epidermis. J Invest Dermatol 1965; 45:257–262.
130. Zacheim HS, Farber EM. Taurine and psoriasis. J Invest Dermatol 1968; 50:227–230.
131. Zacheim HS, Farber EM. Low protein diet and psoriasis: a hospital study. Arch Dermatol 1969;99:580–586.
132. Fleisher AB, Feldman SR, Rapp SR, Reboussin DM et al. Alternative therapies commonly used within population of patients with psoriasis. Cutis 1996; 58:216–220.
133. Treacy E, Johnson D, Pitt JJ, Danks DM. Trimethylaminuria, fish odor syndrome: a new method of detection and response to treatment with metronidazole. J Inherit Metab Dis 1995; 18:306–312.
134. Gordon N. Semen and vaginal fish odor. Am Fam Physician 1995; 52:374.
135. Sela BA, Trau H, Spira A. Trimethylaminuria: fish-odor syndrome. Harefuah 1993; 124:138–139.
136. Ayesh R, Mitchell SC, Zhang A, Smith RL. The fish odour syndrome: biochemical, familial, and clinical aspects. Br Med J 1993; 307:605–607.
137. McLaren DS. Cutaneous lesions in nutritional, metabolic, and heritable disorders. In: Fitzpatrick TB, Eisen AZ, Wolff K, Freedberg IM, Austen KF, Dermatology in General Medicine, 4th eds. New York: McGraw-Hill, 1993, pp 1815–1854.
138. Delahoussaye AR, Jorizzo JL. Cutaneous manifestations of nutritional disorders. Dermatol Clin 1989; 7:559–570.
139. Wolbach SB, Howe PR. Tissue changes following deprivation of fat-soluble A vitamin. J Exp Med 1925; 42:753–759.
140. Domonkos A. Some genodermatoses. In: Andrews GC, Domonkos AN, eds. Diseases of the skin. 5th ed. Philadelphia, WB Saunders, 1964, pp. 495–500.
141. Mathews-Roth MM, Pathak MA, Fitzpatrick TB et al. Carotene as an oral photoprotective agent in erythropoietic protoporphyria. JAMA 1974; 228:1004–1008.

142. Dias AP, Samaranayake LP. Clinical, microbiological and ultrastructural features of angular cheilitis lesions in southern chinese. Oral Dis 1995; 1:43–48.
143. Archard HO. Biology and pathology of the oral mucosa. In: Fitzpatrick TB, Eisen AZ, Wolff K, Freedberg IM, Austen KF. eds. Dermatology in General Medicine, 3rd ed. New York: McGraw-Hill, 1987, p 1202.
144. Valsecchi R, Cainelli T. Generalized pruritus: a manifestation of iron deficiency. Arch Dermatol 1983; 119:630–634.
145. Brown MR. Proximal muscle weakness and selenium deficiency associated with long term parenteral nutrition. Am J Clin Nutr 1986;43:549–554.
146. Food and Drug Administration. Toxicity with superpotent selenium. FDA Drug Bull 1984; 2:19–20.
147. Jackson EM. Review of FDA commissioned study on AHAs. Cosmetic Dermatol 1997; 10:23–26.
148. Colombo VE, Gerber F, Bronhofer M, Floersheim GL. Treatment of brittle fingernails and onychoschizia with biotin: scanning electron microscopy. J Am Acad Dermatol 1990; 23:1127–1132.
149. Parker SL, Leznoff A, Sussman GL, et al. Characteristics of patients with food-related complaints. J Allergy Clin Immunol 1990; 86:503–511.
150. Pearson DJ. Food allergy, hypersensitivity, and intolerance. J R Coll Physicians Lond 1985; 19:154–162.

12

Anaphylaxis

MICHAEL A. KALINER
Institute for Asthma and Allergy, George Washington University
School of Medicine, Washington, D.C.

Nothing can be as frightening to a patient as the experience of ingesting an ordinary food and suddenly having life-threatening anaphylaxis. Within minutes, an otherwise healthy individual may be suddenly prostrate, unconscious, gasping for breath, hypotensive, and in immediate danger of death.

Portier and Richet used the word *anaphylaxis* to describe the fatal reaction induced by the introduction of minute amounts of antigen into dogs that had been previously sensitized to that antigen. The dramatic and unexpected fatal response was the opposite (Greek *ana*, back, backward) of protection (Greek *phylax*, guard). *Anaphylaxis* is the syndrome elicited in a hypersensitive subject upon subsequent exposure to the sensitizing antigen. The components of the anaphylactic response are (a) a sensitizing antigen, usually administered parenterally; (b) an immunoglobulin E (IgE) class antibody response resulting in systemic sensitization of mast cells (and basophils); (c) reintroduction of the sensitizing antigen, usually systemically; (d) mast cell degranulation with mediator release and/or generation; and (e) production of a number of responses by the mast cell–derived mediators and manifested as anaphylaxis. Because the mediators that are released or generated by mast cells cause anaphylaxis, any event associated with mast cell activation may produce the same clinical disease. The term *anaphylaxis* usually refers to IgE-mediated, antigen-stimulated mast cell activation, whereas *anaphylactoid* reactions denote other, non-IgE-mediated responses, such as may be produced by chemical agents capable of causing mast cell degranulation (e.g., radiocontrast media or opiates).

CAUSES OF ANAPHYLAXIS

IgE-Mediated Anaphylaxis

IgE-mediated anaphylaxis has been implicated in untoward reactions elicited by many foods as well as drugs, chemicals, insect stings, preservatives, and environmental factors (see Table 1). Foods that commonly can cause anaphylaxis include peanuts, tree nuts, fish, shellfish, cow's milk, eggs, soy beans, and wheat and other cereal grains. Other IgE-mediated reactions can be elicited by aller-

TABLE 1   Causes of Anaphylaxis/Anaphylactoid Reactions

Immunoglobulin E– mediated reactions
Foods
Antibiotics and other drugs
Foreign proteins (insulin, seminal proteins, latex, chymopapain)
Immunotherapy
Hymenoptera stings
Exercise plus food ingestion
Complement-mediated reactions
Blood; blood products
Nonimmunological mast cell activators
Opiates (narcotics)
Radiocontrast media
Vancomycin (red man syndrome)
Dextran
Modulators of arachidonic acid metabolism
Nonsteroidal antiinflammatory agents
Tartrazine (possible)
Sulfiting agents
Idiopathic causes
Exercise
Catamenial anaphylaxis
Idiopathic recurrent anaphylaxis

genic extracts used for immunotherapy of allergic diseases, insulin, *Hymenoptera* venom, seminal plasma, L-asparaginase, chymopapain, and latex proteins. Ingestion of foods provides a rich source of antigens and may cause anaphylaxis in a sensitive individual. Some subjects exhibit such extreme sensitivity that even exposure limited to the opening of a jar of peanut butter or the odor of cooked fish may cause a systemic response. Other less frequently implicated foods include chocolate, fruits (especially in latex-sensitive individuals), seeds (sunflower, cottonseed, and others), teas (chamomile, especially in ragweed-sensitive individuals), and vegetables.

Sulfiting Agents

Sulfiting agents (sodium and potassium sulfites, bisulfites, metabisulfites, and gaseous sulfur dioxide) are added to foods as preservatives, to prevent discoloration. Before restrictions were placed on their use by the U.S. Food and Drug Administration (FDA), sulfites were added in high concentrations to leafy salad greens at salad-bar restaurants; they are still added to light-colored fruits and vegetables (particularly dried fruits like apples or golden raisins, and instant potatoes); wine, beer, dehydrated soups, fish, and shellfish (particularly shrimp); and rapidly perishable foods such as avocados. Sulfites are also used as preservatives in a variety of medications. Ingestion of sulfites may produce asthma and anaphylactoid reactions in susceptible persons. The mechanism involves conversion of the sulfites in the acid environment of the stomach to SO_2 and H_2SO_3, which are then inhaled. Asthmatics react with bronchospasm to concentrations of SO_2 below 1 ppm.

Exercise-Induced Anaphylaxis

Strenuous exercise may lead to anaphylaxis in susceptible subjects. This reaction can be differentiated from exercise-induced asthma by the frequency with which the responses follow exercise (in the asthmatic, exercise *regularly* causes asthma) and the symptom complex experienced. The response resembles anaphylaxis in every respect, including elevated urine and plasma histamine levels. The syndrome often requires both exercise and ingestion of foods to which the subject is sensitive. This reaction should be suspected in any subject who collapses after exercise, particularly if flushing, urticaria, and angioedema are evident. Most subjects are not aware of concomitant food sensitivity, as ingestion of the implicated food does not cause symptoms unless exercise occurs within 2–6 hr. Thus, it is important to skin test patients with exercise-related anaphylaxis to foods that are implicated by the history, even if the food can apparently be eaten safely (in the absence of exercise).

TABLE 2   Incidence of Reactions and Frequency of Anaphylactic Deaths

Agent	Mild Reactions	Severe Reactions	Deaths/year (U.S.)
Penicillin	1:100–200	1:2500	400–800
Hymenoptera stings	1:200	1:2000	40 or more
Contrast media	1:20	1:1000	250–1000

Idiopathic Recurrent Anaphylaxis

A group of subjects who recurrently experience anaphylaxis that has no recognized cause has been identified. This group commonly experiences flushing (100%), tachycardia (100%), angioedema (96%), upper airway obstruction (76%), urticaria (72%), bronchospasm (48%), gastrointestinal complaints (32%), and syncope or hypotension (28%). The diagnosis is based upon the spectrum of clinical signs and symptoms, evidence of elevated urine histamine level, and an exhaustive search for causative factors.

CLINICAL FINDINGS IN ANAPHYLAXIS

The primary anaphylactic shock organs in humans are the cutaneous, gastrointestinal, respiratory, and cardiovascular systems (Table 3). Characteristically, patients describe an immediate sense of impending doom, coincident with flushing, tachycardia, and often pruritus (either diffuse, localized to the palms and soles, and/or noted particularly in the genital and inner-thigh areas). The initial signs and symptoms rapidly evolve to urticaria, angioedema, rhinorrhea, bronchorrhea, nasal congestion, asthma, laryngeal edema, abdominal bloating, nausea, vomiting, cramps, arrhythmias, faintness, syncope, prostration, and death. The organ systems involved in these responses have two features in common: they are exposed to the external environment, and they contain the largest number of mast cells.

Involvement of the respiratory and cardiovascular systems is most significant as regards mortality. The most common causes of death are cardiovascular collapse and asphyxiation secondary to laryngeal edema. In most cases, laryngeal edema is preceded by a sensation of "a lump in the throat," hoarseness, changes in voice quality, and difficulty in breathing. Hypotension due to anaphylactic shock is usually preceded by diffuse flushing, urticaria, lightheadedness, faintness, and syncope. Anaphylactic deaths after immunotherapy are most commonly due to severe asthma, probably reflecting the specific predisposition of the population receiving immunotherapy for the development of asthma.

The usual progression of symptoms begins within minutes of exposure to

TABLE 3   Clinical Findings in Anaphylaxis and Anaphylactoid Reactions

System	Signs	Symptoms
Cutaneous	Flushing, urticaria, angioedema	Flushing, pruritus
Cardiovascular	Tachycardia, hypotension, shock, syncope, arrhythmias	Faintness, palpitations, weakness
Gastrointestinal	Abdominal distension, vomiting, diarrhea	Bloating, nausea, cramps, pain
Respiratory	Rhinorrhea, laryngeal edema, wheezing, bronchorrhea, asphyxiation	Nasal congestion, shortness of breath, difficulty in breathing, choking, cough, hoarseness, lump in throat
Other	Diaphoresis, fecal or urinary incontinence	Feeling of impending doom, conjucntivitis, genital burning, metallic taste

the inciting agent, peaks within 15 to 30 minutes, and is complete within hours. Some subjects have spontaneous recrudescence of anaphylaxis 8 to 24 hr later. For this reason, individuals who have experienced a significant episode of anaphylaxis may require hospital admission for overnight observation.

PATHOGENESIS

When mast cells degranulate, preformed and rapidly generated mediators are released into the connective tissue along with the molecules that constitute the granular matrix. Although many of these mediators induce dramatic local effects, few other than histamine are capable of entering the circulation in an active state. Thus, the symptoms of anaphylaxis can be attributed primarily to the local actions of the many mast cell mediators and the circulating effect of histamine. Infusion of histamine into normal subjects causes the following signs and symptoms, which can be diminished by antagonists of specific histamine receptors (as noted in parentheses): flushing (H_1 plus H_2), hypotension (H_1 plus H_2), headache (H_1 plus H_2), tachycardia (H_1), pruritus (H_1), rhinorrhea (H_1), and bronchospasm (H_1). Tryptase, an enzyme found in mast cell granules, can also be detected in the serum after generalized anaphylaxis. Since it persists for hours, plasma tryptase level may be a useful marker of mast cell–mediated reactions.

DIFFERENTIAL DIAGNOSIS

The diagnosis of anaphylaxis is not difficult, given the constellation of an acute exposure to a provocative condition followed within minutes by the evolution of multisystem manifestations, including flushing, urtication, pruritus, and angioedema (Table 4). Anaphylaxis is most easily confused with a vasovagal reaction. The clearest differential considerations are the presence in vasovagal reactions of pallor, extreme diaphoresis, and bradycardia or normal sinus rhythm, and the absence of tachycardia, flushing, urticaria, angioedema, pruritus, and asthma as seen in anaphylaxis.

The correct diagnosis is much more difficult to determine in a syncopal or sedated patient. The usual differential diagnoses include cardiac arrhythmias, myocardial infarction, pulmonary embolism, seizures, asphyxiation, hypoglycemia, and stroke. In analyzing the syncopal subject, anaphylaxis should be considered if flushing, urticaria, angioedema, or asthma is present or if the history suggests an acute exposure to conditions associated with anaphylaxis (e.g., *Hymenoptera* sting). If the reaction occurs during a medical procedure, it is important to consider a possible reaction to latex or anesthesia along with other drugs.

If laryngeal edema is the presenting problem, hereditary angioedema (HAE) must be considered. This disorder is usually inherited and is accompanied by painless (and pruritus-free) angioedema, gastrointestinal (GI) cramps and distension, recurrent attacks, and usually a family history of similar attacks and/or sudden death. HAE is not associated with flushing, asthma, or urticaria;

TABLE 4 Differential Diagnosis of
Anaphylaxis and Anaphylactoid
Reactions

Anaphylaxis
Immunoglobulin E–mediated
Complement-mediated
Nonimmunological mast cell degranulation
Idiopathic
Exercise-related
Sulfiting agents
Idiopathic causes
Nonsteroidal antiinflammatory drug reaction
Vasovagal collapse
Hereditary angioedema
Serum sickness
Systemic mastocytosis and urticaria pigmentosa
Pheochromocytoma
Carcinoid syndrome
Panic reactions
Munchausen's syndrome

is of slower onset; and, in the absence of severe airway obstruction, is not a cause of hypotension.

Serum sickness is characterized by fever, lymphadenopathy, maculopapular and urticarial rashes, arthralgias and arthritis, myalgias, and, less frequently, nephritis and neuritis. Serum sickness generally develops 5 to 10 days after exposure to antigens (usually medications or serum as in antilymphocytic serum for treatment of aplastic anemia) and may persist for 2 to 3 weeks. Hypotension and tachycardia are not features of this disease, and the symptoms are usually much less acute. The syndrome is usually self-limited and treated either symptomatically or with corticosteroids if nephritis develops.

Systemic mastocytosis is a generalized disease of mast cells, which may represent an isolated overgrowth of those cells. Urticaria pigmentosa is a generalized overgrowth of mast cells, which take on the form of salmon-colored frecklelike lesions. In either disease, it is possible for the mast cells to degranulate, generally producing local or systemic effects resembling those of anaphylaxis. Degranulation of mast cells can occur after exposure to NSAIDs, alcohol, narcotics, and other nonimmunological mast cell degranulating agents. The diagnosis should be suggested by the recognition of the classic reddish brown macular to low-papular skin lesions that urticate on trauma (Darier's sign), flushing attacks, evidence of bone involvement (pain, abnormal bone scan findings, abnormal x-rays results), gastrointestinal (GI) pain and peptic ulcers, histaminuria, histaminemia, and increased urinary prostaglandin D_2 (PGD_2) metabolites. Bone marrow or skin biopsy is usually diagnostic.

Other conditions within the differential diagnosis include overdoses of medications, cold urticaria, cholinergic urticaria, pheochromocytoma, carcinoid tumors, and sulfite or monosodium glutamate ingestion in sensitive subjects.

TREATMENT OF ACUTE ANAPHYLAXIS

Anaphylaxis is an acute medical emergency requiring prompt and appropriate attention (Table 5). If possible, remove the source of antigen or retard its systemic circulation. If a bee sting is responsible, carefully remove the stinger, apply a venous tourniquet to the extremity, and inject aqueous epinephrine (0.1–0.2 ml, 1:1000) directly into the antigen source in order to reduce the local circulation. Aqueous epinephrine (1:1000, 0.3–0.5 ml subcutaneously [SC]) is the mainstay of the treatment plan. This drug maintains the blood pressure, antagonizes many of the adverse actions of the mediators of anaphylaxis, and reduces the subsequent release of mediators.

In moderate to severe cases in which epinephrine alone is not adequate therapy, administer both H_1 and H_2 antihistamines, diphenhydramine, 25 to 50 mg intramuscularly (IM), and cimetidine, 300 mg, or ranitidine, 50 mg, *slowly* intravenously (IV) (over 3 to 5 minutes). If upper airway obstruction is evident

TABLE 5 Treatment of Acute Anaphylaxis (Adult)

1. When possible, apply a tourniquet to obstruct the draining blood flow from the source of the antigen or inciting medication. When possible, remove the stinger if an insect sting. Release the tourniquet every 15 minutes.
2. Place patient in recumbent position, elevate lower extremities, keep warm, provide O_2.
3. Epinephrine aqueous 1:1000, 0.3–0.5 ml SC; inject epinephrine 1:1000, 0.1–0.2ml 1:1000, mixed in 10 ml saline solution, slowly IV in cases of severe hypotension.
4. Diphenhydramine, 25–50 mg IM or IV.
5. Cimetidine, 300 mg IV, or ranitidine, 50 mg IV, over 3–5 minutes.
6. Establish and maintain airway; administer racemic epinephrine by metered dose inhaler or epinephrine 1:1000 by wall-driven nebulizer to closed airway if laryngeal edema is present.
7. Maintain blood pressure with fluids, volume expanders, or pressors: dopamine hydrochloride, 2–10 µg/kg/min, or norepinephrine bitartrate, 2–4 µg/min.
8. If wheezing is a problem, administer aminophylline, 5.6 mg/kg over 20 minutes, with maintenance dose of 0.9 mg/kg/hr thereafter.
9. For prolonged reactions, repeat epinephrine every 20 minutes × 3; give hydrocortisone, 100 mg IV, every 6 hr.

(lump in the throat, hoarseness, stridor), have the patient spray epinephrine from a metered-dose inhaler or wall-driven nebulizer against a closed glottis in order to try to reduce the local swelling. If the obstruction is progressing, *immediate* tracheal intubation or tracheostomy is indicated. Once laryngeal edema has developed, tracheal intubation may become impossible.

Blood pressure should be maintained with fluid, plasma expanders, and pressors, as needed. Asthma should be treated with aminophylline (loading dose = 5.6 mg/kg/20 min followed by 0.9–1.0 mg/kg/hr) and inhaled β_2-adrenergic agonists. Corticosteroids have no immediate effect but should be administered to prevent prolonged or recurrent sequelae. The usual dose is 100 mg hydrocortisone every 6 hr.

Treatment of anaphylaxis may be complicated by β-adrenergic blocking agents (e.g., for headaches, tremor, hypertension, cardiac arryhythmias, and glaucoma). In this setting, if initial treatment with epinephrine is ineffective, glucagon (5–15 µg/min IV) should be infused.

PREVENTION AND PROPHYLAXIS OF ANAPHYLAXIS

Subjects with known sensitivity to recognized foods should be cautioned to avoid reexposure. Foods prepared at home are relatively easy to control with regard to allergic exposure. The difficulty arises with prepared foods or eating away from home. Persistent queries about the contents of dishes, careful reading of labels, and cautious tasting of food are imperative precautions. It is important for any person who has had systemic anaphylaxis after eating to obtain an emergency treatment kit (an Epipen or other preparation of injectable epinephrine). It is equally important that such an individual be trained in how and when to use the injectable epinephrine, and many offices have such patients actually inject themselves in order to overcome any fear they may have about the effects of the injection.

The rule of thumb that food-sensitive patients have to be taught is that *no prepared food can be assumed to be safe*. Many anecdotal examples of foods contaminated with allergens have reinforced the need for being cautious, having emergency injectable epinephrine always at hand, and responding to the early symptoms of anaphylaxis promptly. It should also be required that such patients wear a MediAlert bracelet or necklace that states, "Food allergic; if found unconscious, inject with epinephrine (adrenalin)."

The Food Allergy Network is a useful resource for patients (1-800-929-4040).

13

Gastrointestinal Manifestations of Food Allergy

MICHAEL K. FARRELL

University of Cincinnati College of Medicine, Children's Hospital Medical Center, Cincinnati, Ohio

INTRODUCTION

Ingested foods obviously can affect the gastrointestinal tract; the mechanisms are either immunological or nonimmunological [1]. Immunological reactions may be immunoglobulin E–(IgE-) mediated immediate or delayed. Nonimmunological reactions may be permanent or transient after a primary insult to the gastrointestinal mucosa. Nonimmunological reactions may also be pharmacological, due to caffeine, or toxic, such as scromboid poisoning. The gastrointestinal tract responds in a limited manner to various stimuli including stress: nausea, vomiting, constipation, diarrhea, and abdominal pain. Noxious stimuli to the gastrointestinal tract are common, not limited to foods, and infectious agents and toxins are commonly encountered. Occasionally food may be contaminated with these environmental agents, further complicating the interpretation of cause and effect. It is easy to blame any gastrointestinal reaction occurring temporally after the ingestion of a specific food on that food, and it is important to recognize that even if an adverse reaction occurs, it may not be immunologically mediated.

There is a large gap between the public's perception of the frequency and seriousness of food allergy and the actual documented prevalence. Ingelfinger stated in 1949, "Gastrointestinal allergy is a diagnosis frequently entertained, occasionally evaluated and rarely established" [2]. Not much has changed since then. Severe reactions to food do occur and may be life-threatening (true immunological–IgE-mediated anaphylactic reactions); thus the possibility that particular symptoms are due to food allergy cannot be summarily dismissed [3]. However, the vast majority of gastrointestinal symptoms are not related to specific foods. Parents believe that 23%–28% of their children have experienced at least one adverse reaction to food. However, after challenge only one-third of the reactions can be confirmed, giving an overall incidence of 8% [4]. Several prospective studies have established that the incidence of cow's milk allergy in the first 3 years of life is between 2.2% and 2.8% [4,5]. Virtually all children in whom a cow's milk allergy develops allergy is manifested in the first year of life. Gastrointestinal and cutaneous symptoms predominate in children [6,7]. Tolerance develops with time: approximately 85% of children lose clinical reactivity to cow's milk by age 3 years. The prevalence of true food allergic reactions decreases with age, as do food allergy–related gastrointestinal reactions. Challenge studies in adults have confirmed that less than one-third of individuals reporting a food allergy actually have documented symptoms when exposed to that particular food. This suggests that the incidence of food allergy in adults is less than 2% in the general population [8].

Gastrointestinal symptoms from a variety of conditions are common, especially in children. Incomplete evaluation and indiscriminate testing result in overreaction and misdiagnosis. Standard skin or radioallergosorbent test (RAST) testing frequently produces false positive findings, as discussed elsewhere; hence positive reactions must be confirmed by history and proper challenge. If not, food allergy is overdiagnosed and important foods may be unnecessarily eliminated from the diet, resulting in poor growth or nutrient deficiencies [9,10]. There are a significant number of parents whose infants had formulas changed empirically for colic who later believed that their children had "illnesses" or "allergies" [11]. These beliefs may result in inappropriate treatment of the child and undue dietary restrictions, "the vulnerable child syndrome" The purpose of this chapter is to review the gastrointestinal manifestations of food allergy and suggest a rational approach to the evaluation of such patients. The most common gastrointestinal disorders that mimic food allergy in various age groups will also be discussed.

EVALUATION

The evaluation of the patient with gastrointestinal symptoms must begin with a comprehensive history and physical examination. A detailed history of the time and circumstances of the onset of symptoms as well as the frequency and duration is important; any suspected correlation with specific foods or other factors must be sought. Exposure to enteric pathogens must be excluded; in infants and children day care causes exposure to large number of pathogens [12].

The characteristics of the vomiting must be clarified. Projectile vomiting, particularly in the infant, suggests pyloric stenosis or other gastric outlet obstruction. Bilious vomiting must always be considered serious, and obstructive conditions such as malrotation with midgut volvulus excluded. The presence of blood suggests esophagitis, peptic disease, or a Mallory-Weiss tear. Effortless regurgitation after meals suggests gastroesophageal reflux (GER). Associated pulmonary symptoms suggest aspiration or GER-associated pulmonary disease. The child whose only symptom is vomiting, especially if it is protracted, deserves special attention. In this group conditions such as neurological abnormalities; gastrointestinal obstructions; renal, hepatic, and pancreatic disorders; as well as metabolic disturbances must be excluded [13] (Table 1).

The location, duration, and triggers of abdominal pain should be sought. Most functional abdominal pain is in the periumbilical region; the farther the pain from the midline, the more likely is an organic cause [14]. The relation of pain to eating in general and to specific foods should be examined. The relation of the pain to defecation and the pattern of defecation are important. The presence of nocturnal pain is uncommon and frequently an indicator of peptic disease. The presence or absence of systemic symptoms such as fever, rash, and arthralgia is important. Table 2 lists the differential diagnosis of abdominal pain. Table 3 lists indicators of an organic cause of pain.

The nature, duration, and frequency of diarrhea should be elicited. Acute onset usually implies an infectious cause. Systemic symptoms such as fever must be excluded. The pattern and nature of the diarrhea are important: alternating constipation and diarrhea suggest the irritable bowel syndrome or encopresis in the younger child. Watery diarrhea implies small bowel infection or osmotic diarrhea; bloody diarrhea suggests colonic involvement and a possible bacterial cause. Bulky, foul smelling stools may signify steatorrhea and pancreatic insufficiency such as seen in cystic fibrosis or severe mucosal injury.

The dietary history must be meticulously reviewed. When were solids introduced into the diet (celiac disease)? How much fluid and particularly fruit juice does the child consume in an average day (toddler's diarrhea)? The parents should be queried about the use of herbal preparations or other alternative medical approaches, which are more commonly being given to children and may have gastrotinestinal effects. Table 4 lists the differential diagnosis of acute and chronic diarrhea.

In the infant and child, determination of normal growth patterns is critical: serial height, weight, and head circumference measurements should be obtained and plotted on standardized charts. In adolescents, the progression through puberty should be recorded. Normal growth and progression through puberty are reassuring that significant gastrointestinal disease is not present;

TABLE 1 Differential Diagnosis of Vomiting

Anatomical
  Tracheoesophageal fistula
  Esophageal stricture
  Gastric web, duplication
  Malrotation with Ladd's bands
  Intestinal atresia, stenosis
  Abdominal tumors
  Annular pancreas
  Choledochal duct cyst
  Supermesentery artery syndrome
Central nervous system
  Anatomical, hydrocephalus
  Expanding intracranial lesion
  Meningitis, encephalitis
Metabolic disorders
  Carbohydrate metabolism
    Glycogen storage disease
    Hereditary fructose intolerance
    Lactic acidosis syndromes
  Amino acid metabolism
    Urea cycle defects
    Phenylketonuria
    Maple syrup urine disease
  Organic acidemias
  Fatty acid oxidation defects
    Carnitine deficiency syndromes
    Medium- and long-chain fatty acyl codehydrongenase
      deficiency
  Lysosomal storage diseases
  Peroixsomal disorders
  Congenital adrenal hyperplasia
Infectious and inflammatory disorders
  Esophagitis
  Pancreatitis
  Hepatitis
  Pertussis (posttussive emesis)
  Labyrinthitis
  Otitis media
Peptic disorders
Neuromuscular disorders
  Muscular dystrophies
  Hirschsprung's disease
  Intestinal pseudoobstruction
  Achalasia

TABLE 1 Continued

Miscellaneous

Chronic congestive heart failure
Psychiatric disorders (bulimia, rumination)
Munchausen's syndrome by proxy
Drug toxicity
Pregnancy
Foreign body
Food allergy
Conditioned or anticipatory emesis

Source: Adapted from Ref. 13.

conversely deviation from previously established growth percentiles demands an explanation. When caloric intake or utilization is insufficient, weight is affected first, then height velocity slows. The head circumference is affected last.

In the fully grown adolescent and adult, recent weight loss is a warning sign. Constitutional symptoms such as fever, arthralgia, rashes, and mouth ulcerations should be sought; their presence suggests inflammatory bowel disease. In the infant, the stooling pattern in early life should be examined. The onset of constipation in the first few weeks or a delay in passing meconium suggests Hirschsprung's disease. Family history of first-degree relatives with celiac disease or inflammatory bowel disease should raise suspicions.

The physical examination must be complete and thorough. Hydration and nutritional status must be evaluated; decreased muscle mass and subcutaneous fat, especially around the buttocks, suggest protein calorie malnutrition. Digital clubbing is seen in celiac disease and inflammatory bowel disease as well as chronic pulmonary disease. Erythema, especially around the mouth and perianal region, suggests acrodermatitis enteropathica, seen with primary or secondary zinc deficiency. Edema suggests hypoalbuminemia. Lymphadenopathy and hepatosplenomegaly must be excluded. Pallor, oral mucosal ulcerations, abdominal tenderness or mass, or the presence of perianal disease suggests the possibility of inflammatory bowel disease. Hemorrhoids and perianal fistulas are uncommon in children. Rectal examination excludes constipation as a cause of the symptoms and allows inspection of the perianal region and collection of stool for analysis.

The initial laboratory evaluation usually includes a complete blood count and sedimentation rate if inflammatory bowel disease is suspected. The presence or absence of blood in vomitus and/or stool must be confirmed. Upper gastrointestinal series should be performed to exclude obstruction; a small bowel follow-through should be performed at the same time to exclude small bowel involvement. If diarrhea is bloody or the child appears to have a toxic reaction,

TABLE 2 Causes of Acute
Abdominal Pain by Age

Neonate
  Necrotizing enterocolitis
  Spontaneous gastrointestinal perforation
  Hirschsprung's disease
  Meconium ileus
  Intestinal atresia/stenosis
Infant (< 2 years)
  Colic(< 3 months)
  Acute gastroenteritis
  Traumatic perforation
  Intussusception
  Incarcerated hernia
  Malrotation (volvulus)
  Sickling syndromes
School age (2–12 years)
  Acute gastroenteritis
  Urinary tract infection
  Appendicitis
  Trauma
  Constipation
  Pneumonia
  Pancreatitis
  Sickling syndromes
Adolescent
  Acute gastroenteritis
  Urinary tract infection
  Appendicitis
  Trauma
  Constipation
  Pelvic inflammatory disease
  Pneumonia
  Mittelschmerz

Source: Adapted from Ref. 55.

bacterial stool cultures should be obtained. If the diarrhea is chronic, stool should be examined for *Giardia lamblia* and *Cryptosproidia* antigens. If malabsorption is suspected, the stool should be examined for reducing substances to confirm carbohydrate malabsorption. Fecal α_1 antitrypsin may be measured if protein-losing enteropathy is suspected; fecal levels will be elevated [15]. Fat malabsorption can be confirmed by stool smears; a 72 hr quantitative fecal fat collection is the gold standard. Upper endoscopy and colonoscopy should be re-

TABLE 3 "Flags"
Suggesting Organic
Cause of Pain

Fever
Any gastrointestinal bleeding
Weight loss
Pain away from midline
Other systemic symptoms

served for situations in which direct visual inspection of the mucosa will be diagnostic or pathological diagnosis is necessary. Although gastrointestinal endoscopy can be safely performed on children of any age, it is expensive and invasive and should be used judiciously.

The usual treatment of food-related gastrointestinal reactions is avoidance of the food. It is vital that adequate nutrition be maintained. In patient with suspected multiple food-related symptoms, dietary consultation should be obtained to assure an adequate age-appropriate diet. Skin testing may help identify suspected foods but the reaction must be confirmed by appropriate challenge. If cow's milk protein is suspected in an infant, a soy formula may be substituted. However, soy formulas are antigenic and approximately 20% of children who react to cow's milk will react to soy [16]. In addition, changing to soy formulas changes both the protein and carbohydrate sources so it is difficult to tell what accounts for any response noted. Protein hydrolysate formulas are the main treatment of food allergy–related gastrointestinal symptoms in infants. Casein (Nutramagen, Pregestimil; Alimentum) and whey (Good Start) hydrolysates are available. Anaphylactic-type reactions have occurred in response to these formulas because they may contain immunogenically intact proteins, they should contain no peptides of greater than 1200 Da molecular weight [17,18]. Unfortunately, all do contain small amounts of higher-molecular-weight peptides. In those cases, amino acid–based formulas (Vivonex, Tolerex, Neocate) should be used [19].

Nonimmunological Food Reactions

Nonimmunological reactions to food are the most common encountered in clinical practice. Most are transient and may be related to a previous enteric infection. We will discuss the most common of these, the role food allergy may play, and the current thinking regarding cause, diagnosis, and treatment.

Colic

Colic is a poorly understood, poorly defined set of symptoms in otherwise healthy, well fed infants: paroxysms of inconsolable crying, lasting 3 hr or more a day and occurring on more than 3 days in any 1 week [20]. The crying is often accompanied by drawing up of the legs, abdominal distension, and excessive gas. In approximately 15% of infants colic develops; the vast majority are under 6 weeks of age [21]. The incidence is approximately the same in breast and bottle fed infants. Women who self-report themselves as type A personalities have infants who exhibit more coliclike behavior [22]. The symptoms usually subside spontaneously between 3 and 6 months of age.

Currently four theories regarding the cause predominate in the literature: (a) transmission of allergens in breast milk/the effect of foods or food components such as egg, cow's milk, or lactose; (b) abnormal intestinal peristalsis or excessive abdominal gas; (c) immature central nervous system; (d) parental anxiety/tension or sensitivity/response models [23]. Colicky infants have increased breath hydrogen, suggesting increased lactose load to the colon and/or lactose intolerance. Elimination of lactose has had variable results [24,25]. Nursing infants who in feeding change from breast to breast too soon may obtain relatively more of the lactose-rich, fat-poor foremilk rather than the calorically dense hindmilk. This results in more rapid gastric emptying and more lactose presented to the colon for fermentation [26]. Bovine whey protein has been shown to increase crying in colicky infants in a double-blind cross-over study [27]. Responses have been documented after both formula changes/maternal dietary manipulation and counseling [27,28]. In one randomized trial, counseling about infant crying and the parental response to it was superior to dietary changes [28]. Sampson has estimated that "food allergy or intolerance probably accounts for increased crying (and 'colic') in 10–15% of colicky infants and a 2–3 month trial of hypoallergenic formula may be warranted in some colicky infants, especially those from atopic families" [29]. A reasonable approach is to eliminate cow's milk from the breast-feeding mother's diet or to change the formula to a casein hydrolysate. If no response is noted, further dietary manipulations are not useful [30]. It is important to realize that colic is a distressing but self-limited process. Making numerous formula changes is not helpful and may be harmful [10]. Emphasis should be placed on helping the family cope with the stress of the crying infant.

Gastroesophageal Reflux

Vomiting is common in infancy and gastroesophageal reflux is the most common cause [31]. The vomiting of gastroesophageal reflux is effortless and occurs during and immediately after feedings; it is occasionally projectile but never bilious. The causes of the reflux are immaturity of the lower esophageal sphincter and inappropriate transient sphincter relaxation. The vast majority of infants improve by 12–18 months of age. Vomiting may also be the initial symptom of milk allergy so careful evaluation is necessary. Changing the formula once may be beneficial, but repeated changes are rarely helpful [11,30]. Evaluation begins with a detailed feeding history; overfeeding is a frequent cause of vomiting in infants.

If growth is normal and there are no associated pulmonary symptoms, no therapy besides reassurance is necessary. Small frequent feedings and positioning of the infant in the prone position help decrease postprandial vomiting.

If the vomiting is projectile or the infant is not gaining weight, upper gastrointestinal obstruction should be excluded by an upper gastrointestinal series, which will exclude anatomical abnormalities; it is not sensitive or specific for gastroesophageal reflux. Ultrasound will detect pyloric stenosis but will not detect other causes of obstruction such as malrotation. If there are symptoms suggestive of esophagitis (crying, irritability, guaiac-positive stools, poor feeding), a trial of a H_2 blocker such as ranitidine may be helpful. Endoscopy *with biopsy* is the most specific test for esophagitis but is expensive and invasive. Cisapride improves gastric emptying and increases lower esophageal sphincter tone and may be helpful but has potentially severe cardiac side effects [32]. However, the clinician must be careful not to turn a benign self-limited process into a "disease."

The role of cow's milk allergy in gastroesophageal reflux is controversial. Eosinophilic infiltration of the esophageal mucosa is commonly seen in esophagitis [33,34]. A recent study examined 204 infants confirmed to have gastroesophageal reflux by pH probe testing and biopsy. Nineteen had a history compatible with cow's milk allergy, and 93 had positive prick tests results. Elimination of cow's milk and two double-blind challenges confirmed cow's milk allergy in 85/204 infants. The infants with cow's milk allergy were more likely to have diarrhea and atopic dermatitis [35]. Elimination of cow's milk protein might be judicious in more severe cases of GER; response to withdrawal and rechallenge should be noted.

Chronic Diarrhea

Most infantile and childhood diarrhea is of acute onset, infectious (usually viral) in cause, and self-limited. Chronic diarrhea does develop in some patients. The most common causes of chronic diarrhea in children are (a) infection, (b) toddler's diarrhea, (c) postenteritis enteropathy [36]. The most likely infectious agent to cause chronic diarrhea is *Giardia lamblia,* which is especially common in children in day care centers. Some bacterial pathogens can cause protracted diarrhea (greater than 2 weeks). These include *Clostridium difficile, Yersinia, Salmonella, Aeromonas,* and *Cryptosporidium* spp., *and* enteropathogenic *Escherichia coli.* Closely related to those with prolonged infectious diarrhea are those infants who continue to have diarrhea after the disappearance of the pathogen; the cause is presumed to be transient mucosal damage and subsequent malabsorption (postenteritis enteropathy).

A common clinical patient is the healthy toddler with chronic diarrhea. The diarrhea is watery and occurs one to seven times a day. Physical examination findings are normal, as is growth. All laboratory evaluations have normal results. The usual cause of this "toddler's diarrhea" is excessive intake of carbohydrate containing fluids such as juices, tea, and sports drinks [37,38]. Food containing sorbitol as well as "sugar-free" gums and candies may also present large amounts of unabsorbed carbohydrate to the colon [39]. The diet consequently is high in carbohydrate and low in fat. The child usually responds to a normal diet [40].

A key determinant in deciding about the seriousness of chronic diarrhea is determining nutrient intake and weight gain. If caloric intake is normal and there is no weight loss, clinically significant malabsorption is unlikely. If the diet has been limited, a normal diet should be prescribed and the response noted. The causes of chronic diarrhea are listed in Table 4.

Infants less than 3 months of age are at particular risk for protracted diarrhea and subsequent malnutrition after an infectious episode [36]. Avery defined this group as infants with onset of diarrhea less than 3 months of age, having

TABLE 4 Differential Diagnosis of Chronic Diarrhea

Anatomical
    Short bowel syndrome
    Gastroschisis
    Intestinal obstruction, stenosis
    Malrotation
Metabolic
    Acrodermatitis enteropathica
    Abetalipoproteinemia
    Wolman's disease
    Hypoparathyroidism
    Hyperthyroidism
    Adrenal insufficiency
    Glucose–galactose malabsorption
    Sucrase–isomaltase deficiency
Pancreatic insufficiency
    Cystic fibrosis
    Schwachman-Diamond syndrome
Associated with villous injury
    Allergic enteropathy
    Postenteritis enteropathy
    Celiac disease
    Immunodeficiency
    Giardia lamblia
    Malnutrition
    Familial microvillus atrophy
    Autoimmune enteropathy

symptoms for 2 weeks or longer and having negative results of cultures [41]. There is marked mucosal injury; the resulting malabsorption causes further mucosal injury, thus initiating a viscous cycle. Young infants who have an episode of infectious diarrhea require close follow-up evaluation. Early recognition is critical; feeding with a semielemental formula should be begun immediately. Continuous nasogastric infusions and/or parenteral nutrition may be necessary [42]. Intact proteins may be absorbed across the denuded surface, resulting in sensitization; cow's milk and soy are usually withheld until age 1 year and reintroduced into the diet slowly.

Carbohydrate intolerance causes diarrhea, bloating, and abdominal pain in both children and adult [43]. The unabsorbed carbohydrate reaches the colon; bacterial fermentation produces gas and osmotically active products resulting in diarrhea (Table 4). Lactose intolerance is the most common carbohydrate intolerance; it develops as a result of a deficiency of lactase, the enzyme that hydrolyzes lactose. Lactase is produced in the mature enterocyte: the cell develops the capacity to make lactase as it matures; it is not inducible [44]. Any injury to the gastrointestinal mucosa can result in disaccharidase deficiency. The most common cause is transient mucosal injury after an infection. Another common form of lactose intolerance is that seen in most non-Caucasian populations; after infancy they are genetically programmed no longer to produce lactase; ingestion of lactose results in symptoms [45].

Carbohydrate intolerance can be diagnosed by finding reducing substances in the stool, elevated breath hydrogen after ingestion of the suspected sugar, or the response to elimination from the diet [46]. Milk is the major source of calcium in many diets; if it is restricted, an alternative source must be provided.

Frequent antibiotic use frequently results in diarrhea; some patients may be infected with *Clostridium difficile*. The patient who has repeated episodes of diarrhea may have an immune deficiency such as common variable immunedeficiency (CVI); both IgA deficiency and human immunodeficiency virus (HIV) infection may present with chronic diarrhea [47]. Occasionally, the cause of the chronic diarrhea may be factitious (Munchausen by proxy); phenolphthalein and other laxatives have been administered to provoke diarrhea [48].

Whole Cow's Milk Gastrointestinal Bleeding

The feeding of whole cow's milk to infants under 1 year of age results in mucosal injury, gastrointestinal bleeding, iron deficiency anemia, and hypoproteinemia [49,50]. The hypoproteinemia is due to protein leakage across the injured mucosa. In 40% of infants fed pasteurized cow's milk at 6 months of age fecal blood loss develops' heat treatment of the cow's milk prevents it [49]. Recent data confirm that infants age 6–12 months have similar fecal blood losses after ingestion of whole cow's milk [50]. Small bowel biopsies do not demonstrate an "immunological" injury but suggest a direct toxic injury. Respiratory symptoms may develop and are related to an associated pulmonary hemosiderosis (Heiner's syndrome) [51].

The best treatment is prevention; infants less than 12 months should not receive whole cow's milk but rather should receive breast milk or an iron-fortified formula. This recommendation has become more critical with the recognition that iron deficiency has profound and prolonged neurodevelopmental effects [51]. If an infant receiving whole cow's milk is noted to have anemia or iron deficiency, the cow's milk should be removed from the diet.

Protein-Losing Enteropathy

Hypoproteinemia and hypoalbuminemia may develop after any gastrointestinal injury; nongastrointestinal processes such as constrictive pericarditis, hepatic venous outflow obstruction, and lymphangiectasia may also result in enteric protein loss [53]. The complete differential diagnosis is listed in Table 5. Whether symptoms develop is determined by the balance between enteric protein loss and the hepatic protein synthetic rate. Common findings include edema, ascites, and pleural effusions. If there is extensive mucosal injury, steatorrhea may be present; malabsorption results in poor growth. However, actual gastrointestinal symptoms may be minimal. No other cause for the protein loss can be found. Dietary intake of calories and protein is adequate for age. No urinary or skin losses are present. Fecal protein loss can be confirmed by elevated fecal α-antitrypsin levels [15]. Findings of laboratory studies are consistent with hypoproteinemia; in lymphangiectasia there may be lymphopenia. Signs of protein calorie malnutrition and secondary nutrient deficiencies may be present. Protein-losing enteropathy can follow a food protein–induced enteropathy [54]. Therapy is the treatment of the underlying disorder. Protein hydrolyzed formulas may be helpful if there is extensive mucosal damage; if fat malabsorption is present a medium-chain triglyceride formula is indicated.

Chronic Abdominal Pain/Irritable Bowel Syndrome

Chronic abdominal pain in children is common, affecting 10%–15% of the school age population [14]. Three varieties have been described: (a) nonspecific periumbilical pain that is usually nonorganic in cause; (b) epigastric discomfort associated with nausea, bloating, and early satiety ("nonulcer dyspepsia"); and (c) abdominal pain associated with alterations in defecation: "irritable bowel syndrome" [55]. The current opinion is that these disorders are on a continuum and represent alterations in gastrointestinal motility, visceral hypersensitivity that may be aggravated by environmental factors including stress [56]. No data consistently suggest that any of these variations of abdominal pain is related to food allergy. Some symptoms may be related to the

TABLE 5 Causes of Protein-Losing
Enteropathy

Gastrointestinal disease without ulceration
 Hypertrophic gastritis (Menetrier's disease)
 Acute viral enteritis
 Parasitic infestations
 Intestinal bacterial overgrowth
 Allergic enteropathy
 Celiac disease
 Malrotation, chronic obstruction
 Polyposis syndromes
 Immunodeficiency states (agammaglobulinemia)
 Schönlein-Henoch purpura
Gastrointestinal disease with ulceration
 Erosive esophagitis
 Erosive gastritis
 Multiple ulcers
 Gastrointestinal lymphoma
 Crohn's disease
 Ulcerative colitis
 Pseudomembranous colitis
Lymphatic obstruction
 Intestinal lymphangiectasia
 Lymphoenteric fistula
 Mesenteric tuberculosis, sarcoidosis
 Intestinal lymphoma
 Chronic pancreatitis
 Pancreatitis
 Constrictive pericarditis
 Congestive heat failure
 Budd-Chiari syndrome
Disorders not limited to gastrointestinal tract
 Measles
 Lupus erythematosus
 Hereditary angioedema
 Iron deficiency
 Retroperitoneal fibrosis

pharamacological properties of food, e.g., caffeine, or to carbohydrate malabsorption, e.g., lactose. The clinician must recognize that parents are frequently concerned that food intolerance may be responsible for the symptoms; their concerns must be addressed.

 The diagnosis is confirmed by normal growth, normal physical examination findings, and normal screening laboratory study results. Several studies have suggested that increasing dietary fiber may relieve symptoms [57].

Inflammatory Bowel Disease

Crohn's disease and ulcerative colitis can affect any age child or adult. Crohn's disease involves any level of the gastrointestinal tract from mouth to anus; all layers are involved; the characteristic lesion is the granuloma [58]. Clinically Crohn's disease is characterized by abdominal pain and diarrhea; growth failure is present in 30% of children at diagnosis [59]. However, abdominal symptoms may be minimal or absent. Extraintestinal symptoms such as arthritis and arthralgia, episcleritis, erythema nodosum, and sclerosing cholangitis may be present before the abdominal symptoms [60]. The presence of any perianal abnormalities is a strong indication for evaluation for Crohn's disease [61]. Laboratory studies may reveal a microcytic, hypochromic anemia; elevated sedimentation rate; hypoalbuminemia; and evidence of malabsorption. Diagnosis is made by radiography; the small bowel must be examined since the ileum is very often involved. Endoscopy and the demonstration of granulomas in the mucosa are diagnostic.

Ulcerative colitis is a mucosal disease; onset is usually more abrupt. Bloody diarrhea is the initial symptom. Stool cultures for bacterial pathogens have negative results. Extraintestinal symptoms may be present. Endoscopy is usually superior to radiography in that direct visualization and biopsy of the mucosa are possible. The disease begins at the anal verge and any amount of the colon may be involved contiguously [58].

Treatment of the inflammatory bowel diseases is with steroids and other antiinflammatory agents. There are no data to suggest that a reaction to a specific food is involved in the cause. Patients must be advised to consume a balanced adequate diet; they should avoid any food that causes problems.

Immunologically Mediated Food Reactions

Oral Hypersensitivity Syndromes

A variety of symptoms related to the oral cavity develop in reaction to foods. In some patients edema develops at the site of contact with a dietary antigen. About 7% of patients with pollen allergy have oral pruritus after the ingestion of dietary antigens; swollen lips, pharyngeal pruritus, and aphthous ulcerations also occur [62]. Patients with both aphthous lesions and jejunal mucosal abnormalities have been reported and have responded to a gluten-free diet [63]. Chronic fissuring of the mouth has been seen in patients with eosinophilic gastroenteropathy; results of biopsies of the oral mucosa have shown eosinophilic infiltration [64].

Colitis

Food protein–induced colitis is characterized by inflammatory changes in the rectum and colon and represents an immune-mediated reaction to ingested foreign proteins [65]. It may be the most common cause of colitis in infancy [66]. Symptoms usually begin in the first few months of life; in one series the mean onset was at 66 days of age. Infants fed cow's milk formula tend to become symptomatic sooner (21 days) than those fed soy (36 days) or breast-fed (85 days) [67]. Onset is insidious; stools become loose, mucus filled, and then bloody. Constitutional symptoms are absent; the infants generally look well. The infant recovers promptly after removal of the offending antigen. Tolerance usually develops by age 1 year. Many foods have been associated with food protein–associated colitis; most common are cow's milk and soy. In exclusively breast-fed infants colitis may develop as a result of maternal consumption of immunogenic proteins that then are transferred into the breast milk [68]. Approximately 45% of allergic colitis occurs in exclusively breast-fed infants.

The differential diagnosis includes infectious causes of diarrhea (*Salmonella, Shigella, Campylobacter,* and *Aeromonas* spp. and *Escherichia coli* 0157), the enterocolitis of Hirschsprung's disease, Behçet's syndrome, necrotizing enterocolitis, hemolytic uremic syndrome, and inflammatory bowel disease (rare in infants). The perianal area must be closely examined for anal fissures. There is no specific test; peripheral eosinophilia suggests the diagnosis. Stool smears may show increased eosinophils. Sigmoidoscopy, if performed, reveals focal erythema, friable mucosa, and nodularity, suggesting lymphoid hyperplasia. Rectal biopsies show focal eosinophilic infiltrates, especially in the lamina propria. More than 60 eosinophils per high-power field is considered diagnostic [69]. Eosinophilic infiltration may be noted in the epithelium or muscularis mucosae; crypt abscesses, if present, contain a mixture of eosinophils and neutrophils. Histological features suggesting another diagnosis are absent. Diagnosis is confirmed by elimination of the antigen from the diet and then rechallenge of the patient. In most cases the use of hydrolyzed protein formulas or the elimination of cow's milk from the maternal diet is sufficient. Follow-up studies have not shown evidence of either food allergy or chronic colitis [70].

Food Protein Enterocolitis and Gastroenteropathy

Food-induced enterocolitis is an uncommon systemic reaction to ingested food antigens; the precise mechanisms remain unidentified. The syndrome usually affects infants, most often by 6 months of age. Symptoms appear shortly after the ingestion of the offending food. Both cow's milk and soy proteins have been implicated [54,71]. Infants appear ill: emesis and diarrhea are very common. Blood streaked stools may be present. Stool contains blood and white cells; there is also evidence of malabsorption, suggesting both colonic and small

bowel involvement. Poor growth may be noted. Laboratory studies reveal peripheral eosinophilia and hypoalbuminemia. Infants usually respond to withdrawal of the offending protein; casein hydrolysate formulas have been
successfully used. Mucosal injury may be so severe that a protracted recovery is
necessary so careful monitoring is prudent.

The acute nature of the injury suggests anaphylaxis but immunological
studies to date have been unrevealing. Immunoglobulin E (IgE) antibodies are
negative. Powell developed a challenge test to identify the suspected protein;
symptoms follow the ingestion of 0.6 g/kg of the suspected protein. A positive
response occurs within 12 hr; peripheral leukocytosis, fecal blood, and white
cells are noted. Gastrointestinal symptoms are also noted [54]. The reaction may
be severe and acute; the challenge is best performed in the hospital setting. Tolerance usually develops in infants by age 2 years and the offending protein can
be slowly introduced into the diet. Colonic strictures have been reported as a
long-term complication [72].

Food-induced enteropathy has been described after the ingestion of a variety of foods, including milk, soy, egg, chicken, rice, and fish [73–75]. Most infants experience symptoms by 9 months of age. The onset tends to be insidious;
it may mimic an acute enteritis; there are initial vomiting and anorexia, and protracted diarrhea. There has been speculation that an acute enteritis predisposes to
development of food-induced enteropathy by allowing absorption of intact proteins across an injured mucosa [76]. This may predispose to soy protein intolerance. However, any infant who has an acute illness with vomiting after exposure
to a soy formula must have fructose intolerance excluded since sucrose is a common sugar in soy formulas [77].

The clinical features are those of small bowel injury. Acute symptoms such
as vomiting and diarrhea are followed by delayed symptoms such as poor growth
and evidence of malabsorption. Anemia may be present, suggesting malabsorption of iron and folate; fecal blood loss is not increased. Disaccharide intolerance
is common secondary to the mucosal injury; monosaccharide intolerance occurs
but is rare. The diagnostic features are best seen on small bowel biopsy. The degree of intestinal injury varies from slight changes to subtotal villous atrophy.
Classic features are villous atrophy with hyperplasia of crypts, patches of
thinned mucosa, and increase in intraepithelial lymphocytes [78]. Because the
lesion may be "patchy," a single small histological specimen must be interpreted
cautiously [79]. Treatment is elimination of milk and soy protein; hydrolyzed
formulas are useful but occasionally amino acid–based formulas may be necessary. The offending agents can usually be reintroduced into the diet by age 2.

Eosinophilic Gastroenteropathy

Eosinophilic gastroenteritis or gastroenteropathy is an uncommon disorder
marked by eosinophilic infiltration of the gastrointestinal tract. Any level of the

gastrointestinal tract may be involved, but the stomach and small bowel are the most common [80]. The gastric antrum is frequently involved. Esophageal and colonic involvement is being recognized more frequently. The eosinophilic infiltration may involve the mucosa, muscularis, or serosa; this forms the basis for the classification of the disease. The peak incidence is in the third decade of life, but cases have been reported in patients as young as 10 days of age [81].

Symptoms are determined by the location and depth of the eosinophilic infiltration. The mucosal form is characterized by abdominal pain, nausea, vomiting, diarrhea, fecal blood loss, and poor growth; malabsorption is the major feature. The muscular form is characterized by abdominal pain, vomiting, and weight loss; obstructive symptoms are common. In several infants it may resemble pyloric stenosis [82]. The serosal variety is found in adults and is characterized by ascites and pleural effusions. The involved portion of the gastrointestinal tract is thickened and swollen with varying degrees of induration, edema, and nodularity. Small discrete ulcerations may be present. The most striking pathological features are edema and marked eosinophilic infiltration [83].

The cause in the pediatric population is most likely an allergical immunological reaction to food antigens [84]. Approximately 50% have a history of atopy; peripheral eosinophilia is common. In adults, it is associated with malignancy, connective tissue diseases, dermatitis herpetiformis, and gluten enteropathy. Common laboratory findings are peripheral eosinophilia, occult blood in the stool, and evidence of malabsorption.

Treatment consists of identifying and removing the causative agent; in children it is usually food antigens. The most common are milk, egg, and wheat. In older patients an identifying agent is not easily identified. Patients usually respond to steroid therapy; the response to cromolyn is variable and remains controversial.

Gluten-Sensitive Enteropathy (Celiac Disease)

Few topics seem to cause as much confusion as celiac disease. Celiac disease is a permanent, *lifelong* condition of gluten intolerance. Gluten is a protein found in the grain of wheat and some other cereals. Rye is also toxic; barley and oats are controversial. The working definition of the European Society for Pediatric Gastroenterology and Nutrition requires that the initial mucosal lesion be flat and recover when the patient is treated with a gluten-free diet; reintroduction of gluten produces histological relapse within 2 years [85]. Gluten intolerance is not the same as wheat allergy. Since it is a lifelong condition and arduous dietary restrictions are necessary, the diagnosis should be firmly established at the outset. Celiac disease is more common in people of European descent, especially those of Italian, Celtic, or Scandinavian origin. Patients with IgA deficiency, diabetes mellitus, and Down's syndrome are more prone to celiac disease [86,87]. First-degree relatives of patients diagnosed with celiac disease have a greater incidence than the general population [88].

Symptoms usually begin within months of the addition of gluten to the diet. In most children they appear between 9 and 18 months of age. If the diagnosis is missed in infancy, it can be diagnosed at any time up into adulthood. Symptoms in infancy are usually diarrhea, failure to thrive, and abdominal distension. Stools are loose, bulkier, and foul smelling; they are rarely greasy. Constipation is present in about 10% of infants [89]. Infants are pale, and irritable and have decreased weight and height. There are marked muscle wasting and loss of subcutaneous fat. Edema, rickets, and bleeding may occur; there may be other signs of fat-soluble-vitamin deficiencies. Vomiting occurs in about one-third of infants; anorexia may precede other symptoms. The older child may have isolated short stature [90]. Abdominal distension, dental enamel hypoplasia, microcytic anemia, and osteopenia are also potential initial problems. Megaloblastic anemia may develop as a consequence of folic acid deficiency [91–93]. Intracranial calcifications have been reported in celiac disease [94]. In adolescents depression and suicide attempts may be the initial presentation of celiac disease [95].

The development of reliable serological markers has improved the diagnosis of celiac disease. Antigliadin antibodies are of two classes, IgA and IgG. The IgA antibody is the more specific and sensitive but is not useful in patients with IgA deficiency. The combination of IgA and IgG antigliadin antibodies is 96%–100% sensitive and 96% sensitive [96]. IgA and IgG antireticulum antibodies are very specific for celiac disease; they are virtually never present in other childhood enteropathies. However, they are only 50%–60% sensitive, thus limiting their usefulness. Recently IgA antiendomysial antibodies have been evaluated and found to be 97% sensitive and 98% specific. They tend to be age-dependent and are only 80% sensitive before age 2 [97]. Serological markers are useful to screening; however, any suspected case must be confirmed by small bowel biopsy. The characteristic lesion is subtotal villus atrophy with epithelial lymphocytic infiltration. Crypt cells are hyperplastic with an increased mitotic index; the crypt/villous ratio is increased [98]. These findings are not diagnostic; similar lesions are noted in other enteropathies such as that due to cow's milk; hence confirmation of response to gluten withdrawal is mandatory. Rechallenge is necessary only when the diagnosis is suspects or there is not complete response to gluten withdrawal. Serum antibodies decline with improvement and are useful for monitoring the patient. IgA antigliadin antibodies fall to normal level within 2–3 months; IgA antibodies decline more slowly and level is normal after 6 months. IgA reticulum and endomysial antibody levels normalize in 2–3 months [99].

The current thought is that celiac disease is an immunological disorder. The genetic susceptibility arises from inheriting certain human leukocyte antigen (HLA) alleles. Initially an increased incidence of HLA-B8 was described; this is particularly common among the Irish [100]. However, not all persons with this phenotype have celiac disease. A stronger association was then found with DR3 and DR7 phenotypes [101]. The DQw2 antigen, a product of genes closely linked but separate from DR3 and DR7, has been suggested as being primarily involved in the susceptibility to celiac disease. In 35 children with celiac disease, 98% were found to be HLA-DQw2 [102]. Most recently, it has been suggested that celiac disease is associated primarily with a particular HLA-DQ heterodimer -DQA1*0501, -DQB1 *0201 [103]. The mucosal lesion appears to be the direct consequence of T cell responses to gluten in the lamina propria after an as yet unknown sensitizing process.

The only treatment for celiac disease is a strict lifetime gluten-free diet. Gluten is found in many foods; the assistance of a professional nutritionist is critical in counseling the family and designing an appropriate diet. There is increasing evidence that adhering strictly to a gluten-free diet decreases the risk of development of lymphoma [104].

REFERENCES

1. Dockhorn RJ. Atopic and non-atopic intolerance to foods. In: Hamburger RN, ed. Food Intolerance in Infancy. New York: Raven Press, 1989, pp 59–63.
2. Ingelfinger FJ, Lowell FC, Franklin W. Gastrointestinal allergy. N Engl J Med 1949; 241:303–340.
3. Sampson HA, Mendelson L, Rosen JP. Fatal and near-fatal anaphylactic reactions to food in children and adolescents. N Engl J Med 1992; 327:380–384.
4. Bock SA. Prospective appraisal of complaints of adverse reactions to foods in children during the first 3 years of life. Pediatrics 1987; 79:683–688.
5. Bishop JM, Hill DJ, Hosking CS. Natural history of cow milk allergy: clinical outcome. J Pediatr 1990; 116:862–867.
6. Alintas D, Guneser S, Evliyaoglu N et al. A prospective study of cow's milk allergy in Turkish infants. Acta Paediatr 1995; 84:1320–1321.
7. Jakobsson I, Lindberg T. A prospective study of cow's milk protein intolerance in Swedish infants. Acta Paediatr 1979; 68:853–859.
8. Joral A, Villas F, Germendia J, Villareal O. Adverse reactions to food in adults. J Invest Allergol Clin Immunol 1995; 5:47–49.
9. Dagnelie PC, VanStaveren WA, Hautvast JG. Stunting and nutrient deficiencies in children on alternative diets. Acta Paediatr 1991; 374:111–118.
10. Pugliese MT, Weyman-Daum M, Moses N, Lifshitz F. Parental health beliefs as a cause of nonorganic failure to thrive. Pediatrics 1987; 80:175–182.
11. Forsyth BWC, Canny PF. Perceptions of vulnerability 3 1/2 years after problems of feeding and crying behavior in early infancy. Pediatrics 1991; 88:757–763.
12. Pickering LK, Bartlett AV, Woodward WE. Acute infectious diarrhea among children in day care: epidemiology and control. Rev Infect Dis 1986; 8:539–547.
13. Sondheimer JM. Vomiting. *In:* Walker WA, Durie PR, Hamilton JR, Walker-Smith JA, Watkins JB, eds. Mosby, Pediatric Gastrointestinal Disease: Pathophysiology, Diagnosis, Management. St. Louis: 1996, pp 195–203.

14. Apley J, Naish N. Recurrent abdominal pains: a field survey of 1,000 school children. Arch Dis Child 1958; 33:165–170.
15. Thomas DW, Sinatra FR, Merritt RJ. Random fecal alpha-1-antitrypsin in children with gastrointestinal disease. Gastroenterology 1981; 80:776–782.
16. Businco L, Bruno G, Giampietro PG, Cantani A. Allergenicity and nutritional adequacy of soy protein formulas. J Pediatr 1992; 121:S21–S28.
17. Saylor JD, Bahna SL. Anaphylaxis to casein hydrolysate formula. J Pediatr 1991; 118:71–74.
18. Committee on Nutrition, American Academy of Pediatrics. Hypoallergenic infant formulas. Pediatrics 1989; 83:1068–1069.
19. Isolauri E, Sutas Y, Makinen-Kiljunen SM et al., Efficacy and safety of hydrolyzed cow milk and amino acid derived formulas in infants with cow milk allergy. J Pediatr 1995; 127:550–557.
20. Wessel MA, Cobb JC, Jackson EB et al. Paroxysmal fussing in infants, sometimes called "colic." Pediatrics 1954; 14:421–434.
21. Hide DW, Guyer BM. Prevalence of infantile colic. Arch Dis Child 1982; 57:559–560.
22. Parker SJ, Barrett DE. Maternal Type A behavior during pregnancy, neonatal crying, and early infant temperament: do type A women have type A babies? Pediatrics 1992; 89:474–479.
23. Barr RG. *In:* Walker WA, Durie PR, Hamilton JR, Walker-Smith JA, Watkins JB, eds. Pediatric Gastrointestinal Disease: Pathophysiology, Diagnosis, Management. St. Louis: Mosby, 1996, pp 241–250.
24. Miller JJ, McVeagh P, Fleet GH et al. Breath hydrogen excretion in infants with colic. Arch Dis Child 1989; 64:725–729.
25. Moore DJ, Robb TA, Davidson GP. Breath hydrogen response to milk containing lactose in colicky and noncolicky infants. J Pediatr 1988; 113:979–984.
26. Woolridge MW, Fisher C. Colic, "Overfeeding," and symptoms of lactose malabsorption in the breast fed baby: a possible artifact of feed management? Lancet 1988; 2:382–384.
27. Lothe L, Lindberg T. Cow's milk whey protein elicits symptoms of infantile colic in colicky formula fed infants: a double blind crossover study. Pediatrics 1989; 83:262–266.
28. Taubman B. Parental counseling compared with elimination of cow's milk or soy milk protein for the treatment of infant colic syndrome: a randomized trial. Pediatrics 1988; 81:756–761.
29. Sampson HC. In Oski FA, Stockman JA, eds. The Yearbook of Pediatrics 1991, St. Louis: Mosby Year Book, 1991, pp 99–101.
30. Forsyth BWC. Colic and the effect of changing formulas: a double blind, multiple crossover study. J Pediatr 1989; 115:521–526.
31. Vanderplas Y. Gastroesophageal reflux in children. Scand J Gastroenterol 1995; 30(suppl 213):31–38.
32. Vanderplas Y, de Roy C, Sacre I. Cisapride decreases prolonged episodes of reflux in infants. J Pediatr Gastroenterol Nutr 1991; 12:44–47.
33. Winter HS, Madara JL, Stafford RJ, Grand RJ, et al. Intraepithelial eosinophils: a

new diagnostic criterion for reflux esophagitis. Gastroenterology 1982; 83:818–823.

34. Shub MD, Ulshen MH, Hargrove CB, et al. Esophagitis: a frequent consequence of gastroesophageal reflux in infancy. J Pediatr 1985; 107:881–884.
35. Iacono G, Carroccio A, Cavataio F, et al. Gatroesophageal reflux and cow's milk allergy in infants: a prospective study. J Allergy Clin Immunol 1996; 97:822–827.
36. Laney DW, Cohen MB. Approach to the pediatric patient with diarrhea. Gastroenterol Clin 1993; 22:499–516.
37. Hyams JS, Etienne NL, Leichtner AM, et al. Carbohydrate malabsorption following fruit juice ingestion in young children. Pediatrics 1988; 82:64–68.
38. Ravry MJR: Dietetic food diarrhea. JAMA 1980; 244:270.
39. Greene HL, Ghishan FK: Excessive fluid intake as a cause of chronic diarrhea in young children. J Pediatr 1983; 102:836–840.
40. Boyne LJ, Kerzner B, McClung HJ: Chronic nonspecific diarrhea: the value of a preliminary observation period to assess diet therapy. Pediatrics 1985; 76:557–561.
41. Avery GB, Villavicencio O, Lilly JR, et al. Intractable diarrhea in early infancy. Pediatrics 1968; 41:712–722.
42. Orenstein SR: Enteral versus parenteral therapy for intractable diarrhea of infancy: a prospective, randomized trial. J Pediatr 1986; 109:277–286.
43. Gray GM: Carbohydrate digestion and absorption. Gastroenterology 1970; 58:96–107
44. Arola H, Tamm A: Metabolism of lactose in the human body. Scand J Gastroentrol 1994; 29(Suppl):21–25.
45. Simoons FJ, Johnson JD, Kretchner N: Perspective on milk-drinking and malabsorption of lactose. Pediatrics 1977; 59:98–108.
46. Hyams JS, Stafford RJ, Grand RJ, Watkins JB: Correlation of lactose breath hydrogen test, intestinal morphology, and lactase activity in young children. J Pediatr 1980; 97:609–612.
47. Levinsky RJ et al. Protracted diarrhea, immunodeficiency and viruses. Eur J Pediatr 1982; 138:271–272.
48. Zahavi I, Shaffer EA, Gall DG: Child abuse with laxatives. Can Med Assoc J 1982; 127:512–513.
49. Fomon SJ, Ziegler EE, Nelson EE, Edwards BB: Cow milk feeding in infancy: gastrointestinal blood loss and iron nutritional status. J Pediatr 1981; 98:540–545.
50. Ziegler EE, Fomon SJ, Nelson SE, et al. Cow milk feeding in infancy: further observations on blood loss from the gastrointestinal tract. J Pediatr 1990; 116:11–18.
51. Heiner DC, Sears JW, Kniker WT: Multiple precipitins to cow's milk in chronic respiratory disease. Am J Dis Child 1962; 103:40–46.
52. Lozoff B, Jimenez E, Wolf AW: Long-term developmental outcome of infants with iron deficiency. N Engl J Med 1991; 325:687–694.
53. Waldmann TA: Protein losing enteropathy. Gastroenterology 1966; 50:422–443.
54. Powell GK: Milk- and soy-induced enterocolitis of infancy. J Pediatr 1978; 93:553–560.
55. Boyle JT: *In:* Walker WA, Durie PR, Hamilton JR, Walker-Smith JA, Watkins JB,

eds. Pediatric Gastrointestinal Disease: Pathophysiology, Diagnosis, Management. St. Louis: Mosby, 1996, pp 205–215.

56. Zighelboim J, Talley NJ: What are functional disorders? Gastroenterology 1993; 104:1196–1201.

57. Feldman W, McGrath P, Hodgson C et al. The use of dietary fiber in the management of simple, childhood, idiopathic, recurrent, abdominal pain. Am J Dis Child 1985; 139:1216–1218.

58. Kirshner BS: Ulcerative colitis and Crohn's disease in children: diagnosis and management. Gastroenterol Clin 1995; 24:99–117.

59. Kirshner BS, Voinchet O, Rosenberg IH: Growth retardation in children with inflammatory bowel disease. Gastroenterology 1978; 75:504–510.

60. Greenstein AD, Janowitz HD, Sachar DB: The extra-intestinal complications of Crohn's disease and ulcerative colitis: a study of 700 patients. Medicine 1976; 55:401–412.

61. Markowitz J, Daum F, Aiges H, et al. Perianal disease in children and adolescents with Crohn's disease. Gastroenterology 1984; 829–833.

62. Anderson LB, Dreyfuss EM, Logan J, et al. Melon and banana sensitivity coincident with ragweed pollinosis. J Allergy 1970; 45:310–319.

63. Wray D: Gluten-sensitive recurrent aphthous stomatitis. Dig Dis Sci 1981; 26:737–740.

64. Huntley CC, Bowers GW, Vann GL: Allergic protein-losing gastroenteropathy: report of an unusual case. South Med J 1970; 63:917–920.

65. Odze RD, Wershil BK, Leichtner AM, Antonioli DA: Allergic colitis in infants. J Pediatr 1995; 126:163–170.

66. Jenkins HR, Pincott JR, Soothill JF, Milla PJ, Harries JT: Food allergy: the major cause of infantile colitis. Arch Dis Child 1984; 59:326–329.

67. Odze RD, Bines J, Leichtner AM, et al. Allergic proctocolitis in infants: a prospective clinicopathologic biopsy study. Hum Pathol 1993; 24:668–674.

68. Anvveden-Hertzberg L, Finkel Y, Sandstedt B, Karpe B. Proctocolitis in exclusively breast fed infants. Eur J Pediatr 1996; 155:464–467.

69. Winter HS, Antonioli DA, Fukagawa N et al. Allergy related proctocolitis in infants: diagnostic usefulness of rectal biopsy. Mod Pathol 1990; 3:5–10.

70. Lake AM: Food protein-induced gastroenteropathy in infants and children. In: Metcalfe DD, Sampson HA, Simon RA, eds. Food Allergy: Adverse Reactions to Foods and Food Additives. Boston: Blackwell Scientific Publications, 1991, pp 174–185.

71. Gryboski JD: Gastrointestinal milk allergy in infants. Pediatrics 1967; 40:354–362.

72. Schwarzenberg SJ, Whitington PF: Colonic stricture complicating formula protein intolerance enterocolitis. J Pediatr Gastroenterol Nutr 1983; 2:190–192.

73. Kuitunen P, Visakorpi JK, Savilahti E et al. Malabsorption defect with cow's milk intolerance: clinical findings and course in 54 cases. Arch Dis Child 1975; 50:351–356.

74. Vitoria JC, Camarero C, Sojo A, Ruiz A et al. Enteropathy related to fish, rice and chicken. Arch Dis Child 1982; 57:44–48.

75. Iyngkaran N, Abidin Z, Meng LL et al. Egg-protein-induced villous atrophy. J Pediatr Gatroenterol Nutr Child 1982; 1:29–33

76. Sanderson IR, Walker WA: Uptake and transport of macromolecules by the intestine: possible role in clinical disorders (an update). Gastroenterology 1993; 104:622–639.

77. Odievre M, Gentil C, Gauntier M, Alagille D. Hereditary fructose intolerance in childhood. Am J Dis Child 1978; 32:605–608.

78. Walker-Smith JA. Diagnostic criteria for gastrointestinal food allergy in childhood. Clin Exp Allergy 1995; 25:20–22.

79. Manuel PD, Walker-Smith JA, France NE. Patchy enteropathy in childhood. Gut 1979; 20:211–215.

80. Trounce JQ, Tanner MS. Eosinophilic gastroenteritis. Arch Dis Child 1985; 60:1186–1188.

81. Vanderplas Y, Quenon M, Renders F et al. Milk-sensitive eosinophilic gastroenteritis in a 10 day-old boy. Eur J Pediatr 1990; 149:244–245.

82. Snyder JD, Rosenblum N, Wershil B, et al. Pyloric stenosis and eosinophilic gastroenteritis in infants. J Pediatr Gastroenterol Nutr 1987; 6:543–547.

83. Katz AJ, Goldman H, Grand RJ. Gastric mucosal biopsy in eosinophilic (allergic) gastroenteritis. Gastroenterology 1977; 73:705–709.

84. Caldwell JH, Mekhjian HS, Hurtubise PE et al. Eosinophilic gastroenteritis with obstruction: immunological studies of seven patients. Gastroenterology 1978; 77:258–252.

85. Meeuwisse G: Diagnostic criteria in coeliac disease Acta Paediatr Scand 1970; 59:461–464.

86. Polanco I: Associated diseases in children with coeliac disease. *In:* Mearin ML, Maleder CM, eds. Coeliac disease 40 years gluten free. Dordecht: Kluwer, 1991.

87. Dias JA, Walker-Smith JA: Down's syndrome and coeliac disease. J Pediatr Gastroenterol Nutr 1990; 10:412–443.

88. Rolles CJ et al. Family study of coeliac disease. Gut 1974; 15:827–830.

89. Egan-Mitchell B, McNicholl B: Constipation in childhood coeliac disease. Arch Dis Child 1972; 47:238–240.

90. Groll A, Candy DC, Preece MA et al. Short stature as the primary manifestation of coeliac disease. Lancet 1980; 2:1097–1099.

91. Pittschieler K. Neutropenia, granulocytic hypersegmentation and coeliac disease. Acta Paediatr 1995; 84:705–706.

92. Mariana P, Mazzilli MC, Margutti G et al. Coeliac disease, enamel defects and HLA typing. Acta Paediatr 1994; 83:1272–1275.

93. Gibbons RA. The coeliac affliction in children. Edin Med J 1889; 35:321–345.

94. Gobbi G, Bouquet F, Greco L et al. Coeliac disease, epilepsy, and cerebral calcifications. Lancet 1992; 340:439–443.

95. Pellegrino M, D'Altilla MR, Germano M: Untreated coeliac disease and attempted suicide. Lancet 1995; 346:915.

96. Savilahti E, Viander M, Perkkio M et al. IgA anti-gliadin antibodies: a marker of mucosal damage in childhood coeliac disease. Lancet 1983; 1:320–322.

97. Cataldo F, Ventura A, Lazzari R et al. Antiendomyesium antibodies and coeliac disease: solved and unsolved questions: an Italian multicentre study. Acta Paediatr 1995; 84: 1125–1131.

98. Schmitz J: Coeliac disease in childhood. In: Marsh MN, ed. Coeliac Disease. Oxford: Blackwell Scientific, 1992, pp 17–48.

99. Burgin-Wolff A, Gaze H, Hadziselimovic F et al. Anti-gliadin and antienomysial antibody determination for coeliac disease. Arch Dis Child 1991; 66:941–947.

100. Stokes Pl: Histocompatibility antigens associated with adult coeliac disease. Lancet 1972; 2:162.

101. Keuning JJ et al. HLA-DW3 associated with coeliac disease. Lancet 1976; 1:506.

102. Tosi R et al. Evidence that coeliac disease is associated with a DC locus allelic specificity. Clin Immunol Immunopathol 1983; 28:359–404.

103. Sollid LM et al. Evidence for a primary association of coeliac disease to a particular HLA-DQ/hetrodimer. J Exp Med 1989; 169:345–350.

104. Holmes GKT, Prior P, Lane MR et al. Malignancy in coeliac disease—effect of a gluten free diet. Gut 1989; 30:333–338.

14

Neurological Manifestations of Adverse Food Reactions

LYNDON E. MANSFIELD

El Paso Institute for Medical Research and Development and
University of Texas at El Paso, El Paso, Texas

INTRODUCTION

The notion that food causes neurological illness or behavioral change is distinguished by the amount of passion this concept evokes. No other set of disorders involving adverse reactions to foods or additives is characterized by so many devoted believers and dedicated nonbelievers.

There are understandable reasons for these positions. Neurological disorders, of themselves, are extremely complex, being perturbations of complex systems. The tools to measure objective neurological change are not easily accessible or familiar to allergy specialists. Often the neurology specialist is unfamiliar with the clinical pathophysiological features of hypersensitivity disorders. Many times, the end point of a challenge relies on the subjective response and cooperation of the patient. For example, investigators must depend on the subject to tell them whether a headache occurs and how great is the pain.

Other barriers interfere with clear evaluation. These include the incomplete understanding of the epithelial blood–brain barrier in humans and which factors lead to its disruption [1–3]. There is also variability in the nervous system's generation of neurotransmitter, which can be influenced by diet, immune responses, and psychological factors [4]. Recent demonstrations of cytokine generation in the nervous system and cytokine receptors on neural cells are adding another set of factors to consider [5,6].

Nevertheless, there are sufficient observations in the medical literature to allow the reader to form an opinion about the relevancy and importance of food triggered disorders of the nervous system. Some of the works cited are from the earlier literature, which emphasize description rather than the testing of hypotheses and have no *P* values. These studies remain as valuable clinical insights. Time has proved them to be correct, even if the initial methods are not up to the standards of the recent modern medical literature.

PATHOPHYSIOLOGY OF FOOD DERIVED NEUROLOGIC DISORDERS

Mechanism of the Reactions

Toxic Reactions

Foods may contain substances that are directly toxic to the nervous system. These are a natural component of the food or a result of microbial or human contamination. Members of the mushroom family contain powerful muscarinic agents. Fortunately, with commercial mushroom farming, toxic reactions from mushroom are uncommon. Contamination of food with *C. botulina* toxin causes an often fatal neurological disease. A product of a wheat smut is a recognized source of the hallucinogen lysergic acid diethylamide (LSD), which causes serious disorganization of cerebral nervous system function.

Intolerant Reactions

Foods can contain substances with desirable pharmacological activities. Chocolate is capable of uplifting moods, containing phenylethylamine, caffeine, and theobromine. Alcoholic beverages in moderate amounts have pleasant effects for humans. For people who have diminished activity of the respective catabolic enzymes, chocolate can cause excessive stimulation and modest amounts of alcohol cause inebriation and "hangover." Caffeine in a cup of coffee has a mild stimulant effect for most people, but others experience anxiety or insomnia with this same drink. Red wine–induced headaches occur in people who are deficient in the enzyme phenylsulfone transferase or monamine oxidase.

Food Hypersensitivity

An immune-mediated reaction implies a specific sensitization to a food antigen and similar cross-reacting antigens. Perturbation of the nervous system results from the activity of biological modifiers generated by the immune response. Both the more classic mediators and more recently described cytokines can influence nervous system function [7,8]. There is evidence that a nearby local allergic response can alter function of the peripheral nerves [8a].

Food Idiosyncracy

Food idiosyncracy is a proposed mechanism for the role of dyes and preservatives in attention deficit hyperreactivity disorder. It may explain the Chinese restaurant syndrome associated with monosodium glutamate. Headaches have been described on challenge of patients with these sensitivities. It has been suggested that the reactions may be mediated through NO, increasingly recognized as an important inflammatory mediator [9].

ACTIONS OF ALLERGY-RELATED MEDIATORS IN THE NERVOUS SYSTEM

Most of the information about the actions of neurotransmitters in the nervous system is based on studies in animals or in human brain slices. Interpretations of the results and their meaning for human illness must consider this. The animal species used for models do not always share similar patterns of nervous system reactions with humans. For example, a neurotransmitter may be stimulatory in one species and inhibitory in another. Interpreting results of studies in isolated human brain slices also must be cautious. With these caveats, the results to be described do give us a conceptual basis to explain how allergic reactions could affect the nervous system.

Histamine

Histamine serves a critical role in activation and regulation of the central and peripheral nervous systems. Three differing pharmacological receptors for histamine, H_1, H_2, H_3, have been described, with the use of different antagonists [10]. Central nervous system histamine is synthesized from histidine by neurons in the hypothalamus. Pyridoxal phosphate is a key cofactor in histamine synthesis. The brain contains two systems for degrading histamine, the enzymes diamine oxidase and imidazole N-methyl transferase. Under normal circumstances, peripheral histamine appears not to cross the blood–brain barrier [11]. However, during food triggered allergic reactions, plasma histamine levels can increase more than 10-fold to 100-fold. These levels may overcome the capacity of the blood–brain barrier. Higher concentrations of peripheral histamine break down the endothelial blood–brain barrier [12]. Release from perivascular mast cells found in the brain may contribute to histamine levels, after an antigen–antibody reaction.

Histamine, acting through its H_1 receptor, increases reuptake of norepinephrine (noradrenalin) and serotonin in brain slice experiments [13]. Histamine stimulates alertness in rodents, cats, and probably in humans by the H_1 receptor [14]. This may explain the sedating effect of the classic H_1 antagonists. The H_2 and H_3 receptors are important in the autoregulation of histamine synthesis [15]. All three histamine receptors are found on cerebral blood vessels. Blocking H_1 and H_2 receptors has not proved to be clinically effective in migraine therapy or prophylaxis. Animal studies suggest blockade of the H_3 receptor may have potential value in preventing vascular headaches [16]. Histamine applied to the brain causes electroencephalographic (EEG) abnormalities, increasing the frequency of electrical spikes [17].

Adding histidine the precursor to histamine to the diet increases the histamine concentration in the central nervous system of rats and in peripheral basophils. Pyridoxine added to the diet also raises the central nervous system (CNS) histamine content. The combination increases CNS histamine levels more than either agent alone [18].

Serotonin

Only 2% of the body's serotonin is found in the central nervous system, 8% is bound to platelets, and 90% is in the enterochromafin cells of the intestine [19]. Serotonin is synthesized by cells in the hypothalamus. Increases in dietary tryptophan and vitamin B_6 will increase the concentration of serotonin in the brain [18]. It is possible that the massive release of serotonin from platelets during a migraine attack may transiently increase brain serotonin level. Serotonin is important in regulating mood, appetite, and sleep [20]. It is a spasmogenic mediator, constricting the external carotid system arteries. Serotonin release in migraine may represent an attempt to reverse the vasodilatation of a migraine. If serotonin is depleted, then migraine frequency and intensity increase [21].

Prostaglandins and Leukotrienes

Prostaglandin D perturbs the effectiveness of the epithelial blood–brain barrier, with resultant increased permeability and acute cerebral edema in animals [22]. Cerebral edema has been described in immune complex–mediated serum sickness affecting the central nervous system [23].

Prostaglandin E2 causes hypalgesia and is an antagonist of natural and synthetic opioids [24]. When injected peripherally, prostaglandin E2 causes a short-lived migraine attack [25].

Leukotrienes also can cause cerebral edema, by perturbing the blood–brain barrier They also cause recruitment of inflammatory cells into the brain [26]. Leukotrienes and prostaglandins are synthesized by a number of different cell types in the nervous system, including the microglial cells, epithelial cells, and astrocytes.

Bradykinin

When it is injected subcutaneously, bradykinin causes pain and erythema. If it is applied to the central nervous system, bradykinin excites the sensory neurons mediating the pain response. The application leads to peripheral hypalgesia [27]. Intracerebral bradykinin also magnifies the inflammatory reaction of carrageenan-induced paw edema in rats [28]. Bradykinin is yet another mediator capable of disrupting the integrity of the endothelial blood–brain barrier, allowing for passage of other molecules and cerebral edema [29].

Platelet Activating Factor

The mediator platelet activating factor (PAF) has a number of actions, many of which are associated with the late-phase allergic response. PAF has dramatic effects in the nervous system. It causes increased vascular permeability and breakdown of the blood–brain barrier [30]. In disorders such as migraine, there is evidence of increased platelet activation. The platelets of migraine patients demonstrate decreased responses when treated with exogenous PAF, suggesting they are already in an up-regulated state [31].

Neuropeptides

Neuropeptides are a group of peptide hormone–like molecules, which include substance P (SP), neuropeptide Y (NP-Y), calcitonin gene-related peptide (CGRP), and vasoactive intestinal peptide (VIP). Neurokinin is a presumed cause of the pain of migraine. Neuropeptides have a wide range of activities. They are released during peripheral allergic reactions and can affect the nervous system through this mechanism. SP, VIP, and CGRP are potent vasodilators. NPY is a vasoconstrictor found in a network of sympathetic fibers in arteries, arterioles, and veins [32]. Neuropeptides can be responsible for some of the pain described in certain allergic reactions. They also cause vasospasm of the cranial vessels. Levels of VIP and CGRP are elevated in cluster headaches, but only CGRP level is elevated during a migraine Neuropeptides are important neuroregulators [33].

Complement

Various components of the complement cascade are synthesized by astrocytes, ependymal cells, microglia, and neurons. These cells also express receptors for complement fractions. The synthesis of complement and its receptors on membranes is regulated by both proinflammatory and antiinflammatory cytokines. Complement components participate in immune reactions of antigen and antibody in the nervous system. It has been suggested that complement may have additional nonimmune functions in the central nervous system [34].

Cytokines

There is strong evidence that cytokines act as bidirectional messengers between the immune system and nervous system [35]. The ever increasing number of recognized cytokines indicates that it may be some time before the exact pathways and interactions will be understood. Interleukin 1 (IL-1) generated from peripheral immune reactions stimulates release of corticotropin releasing factor in the brain. IL-1 also increases the levels of norepinephrine in the central nervous system [36]. Nerve growth factor (NGF) synthesis is increased by tumor necrosis factor α (TNF-α) and IL-1. NGF is synthesized peripherally and will pass into the brain only when there is an inflammatory process that perturbs the blood–brain barrier [37]. Patients with common migraine demonstrate the spontaneous release of TNF-α from mononuclear cells at a rate greater than that of nonmigrainous control subjects [38]. Cytokines found in the nervous system result from local production but also are derived from peripheral cell synthesis. This allows peripheral immune responses to influence the activities of the nervous system [39].

ALLERGY IN THE NERVOUS SYSTEM

Do significant allergic responses occur in the nervous system, or are the reported clinical allergic disorders of the nervous system the result of peripheral mediator overflow into the nervous system? There is insufficient evidence to answer this question in humans; animal models may be unsuited to answer it. Large macromolecules are normally able to penetrate the brain of the rat [40]. In humans, such permeability has been reported only in autoimmune disease, such as CNS lupus erythematosus [41]. Animal experiments show breakdown of the epithelial blood–brain barrier by the common allergic mediators. It is unknown whether these effects occur in humans, but it appears reasonable to consider this disturbance of the blood–brain barrier in humans probable.

Although there is a relative paucity of perivascular mast cells in the CNS, an attenuated immunoglobulin E (IgE) antigen-mediated response can likely occur. Circulating basophils also move through the CNS with the potential for further interaction and mediator release. How much these components can contribute to central nervous system derangement is unclear. At present it appears both local and peripheral sensitivity reactions are involved in human disorders.

CLINICAL NERVOUS SYSTEM DISORDERS ASSOCIATED WITH ADVERSE FOOD REACTIONS

Migraine

Food induced or dietary migraine has been extensively studied. The association between migraine and diet is better established than any other aspect of food related neurological disease. More recent studies, utilizing double-blind placebo-controlled studies, have demonstrated that food or additives can trigger migraine. Some of these studies also have provided evidence for the involvement of mast cells and basophils (see below, Refs. 64–66).

There are several references in the Talmud that describe a hemicranial throbbing headache associated with eating certain foods. In the nineteenth century, migraine was considered one of the atopic disorders, along with eczema, rhinitis, and asthma. At the beginning of the twentieth century, pioneers in allergy research, including Richet, classified migraine as an anaphylactic disorder [42].

Surprisingly, after all this time, the exact relationship between migraine and the atopic disorders is not resolved. This difficulty may be overcome, at some future date, as the important mechanistic differences between classic and common migraine are considered in the analysis. Food- and foodstuff-provoked head aches are typically common migraines without any aura. In some patients, a throbbing unilateral or bilateral headache without the characteristic nausea and vomiting occurs. These are simple vascular headaches. In both cases food related headaches seem to arise from disturbance in vessels predominantly of the external carotid system. In classic migraine with aura, there are defects in intracerebral electrical activity or blood flow [43].

Older Clinical Reports

Brunton in 1883 reported that milk and eggs caused migraine attacks in his patients. Brown almost 40 years later found that food hypersensitivity was one of the four commonly recognized precipitants of migraine attacks [44].

Vaughan, in one of the most insightful early reports, described his experience with food related migraines. His study involved 33 patients, 12 of whom had relief of migraines using dietary avoidance He noted that the foods triggering migraine caused a late-phase response when he performed allergy skin testing [45].

De Gowin reported that 78% of migraine patients could obtain complete or partial relief from dietary manipulations based on history and intradermal food skin tests [46]. Eyermann evaluated 63 patients with allergic headaches, which were characterized as unilateral and throbbing. Often the headache was preceded by unilateral nasal congestion, clear nasal discharge, abdominal discomfort, and nausea. Over a third of the patients improved with elimination diets [47].

Nonallergic Mechanisms

Besides allergic mechanisms, other dietary factors provoking migraine have been reported. These include a number of monamines (tyramine, phenylethylamine), which are vasoactive and can enter the central nervous system. Other food additives or chemical components of foods can trigger migraine, including sodium metabisulfite, monosodium glutamate, sodium nitrite, sodium nitrate, and histamine. [48,49]. Many patients with migraine experience a typical attack or an unusual bitemporal pulsatile headache after eating smoked meats, sausages, and flavored cheeses. Nitrates and nitrites are potent vasodilators, and the amount tolerable to the general population, which is estimated and approved as up to 500 µg/g, has deleterious effects in migrainers. This is an example of the nonspecific vascular hyperreactivity in migraine analogous to the bronchial hyperreactivity of asthma. Migraine patients demonstrate a shift to the left in the dose–response curve to the nonspecific cerebral vasodilatation caused by carbon dioxide or histamine [50].

Alcoholic beverages, particularly red wines, are common precipitants of migraine. Red wine contains alcohol, histamine, and many phenylsulfones, all of which individually can trigger migraine attacks. Ethanol is a peripheral vasodilator, does not affect intracerebral blood vessels. It can, however, affect branches of the external carotid. In a very interesting study, the ability of equivalent amounts of ethanol provided as vodka or red wine to provoke a migraine in patients was tested. The amount of ethanol in the volume of red wine that triggered a migraine was dispensed in the form of vodka and did not cause a migraine. The conclusion was that the phenolic monamines in the wine were the significant precipitants [51].

Reports of challenge provocation of migraine headaches by aspartame, monosodium glutamate, and metabisulfite have appeared in the medical literature [52]. On the other hand, studies attempting to define the value of routine avoidance of these food components have shown disappointing clinical results. There was little change in migraine frequency or intensity. This is particularly true of diets avoiding the monamines such as tyramine, in spite of the fact that tyramine appeared capable of altering EEG patterns of migraine patients [53].

Later Clinical Reports

Unger and Unger described an extensive experience in the diagnosis and treatment of migraine. They reported achieving good clinical results using a combination of therapies including elimination diets. Thirty-five of 55 patients had complete relief of migraines, and another 9 had a 75% improvement. They observed that foods seem to trigger attacks directly or can serve as facilitators of migraines triggered by other factors such as fatigue, stress, or hormonal events [54]. This aspect of food induced disease, that is, facilitation, has been more recently reported and confirmed by blind challenges in disorders such as food related exercise induced ana-phylaxis and delayed pressure urticaria. There is a need for a careful study evaluat-ing the same relationship of two stimuli in triggering migraines.

With the advent of radioallergo sorbent test (RAST) technology, Monro asked whether this new tool could help predict an successful avoidance diet for migraine patients. Twenty-three of 36 subjects with migraine who were placed on an extensive elimination diet trial with reintroduction had decreased migraine attacks. Unblinded rechallenges triggered attacks. Monro discovered that a per-forming a panel of 25 in vitro RAST food tests for specific IgE predicted the foods that were the triggers of migraine in the patients who obtained relief. In general the RAST values at foods provoking migraine were highly positive [55].

In an earlier report, Grant, a neurologist, used a lengthy strict elimination diet beginning with lamb and pear and then single food introductions after 5 days, to evaluate the role of diet in migraine subjects. With this meticulous and laborious approach, of 60 patients, 51 became migraine-free, and 9 improved. From 1 to 30 foods appeared to provoke attacks of migraine (average number was 10 foods). No double-blind challenges were performed. Grant used a pulse test to determine whether the subject was sensitive to a food. This test is gener-ally considered invalid. Some of the remarkable results may have been placebo effects [56].

Double-Blind Placebo-Controlled Studies of Food Related Migraine

A series of double-blind placebo-controlled studies have been performed in the last two decade (Table 1). These studies have provided double-blind placebo controlled evidence that ingesting certain foods would reproducibly provoke a migraine. In general, the rate of migraine during placebo challenges was less than 15%. Active foods suspected of causing migraine administered in a double-blind fashion triggered migraine in 70% of the challenges.

Egger et al. reported on 99 migrainous children, who were placed on an oligoantigenic diet consisting of one meat (chicken or lamb), one starch (rice or potato), one fruit (apple or banana), one vegetable (brassica), water, and vitamin supplements. Children who improved then had foods reintroduced to determine which may have precipitated migraine. Eighty-eight children completed the diet trial. Seventy-eight children became free of migraine, 4 improved, and 6 showed no benefit. Upon reintroduction of foods, 74 children had one or more foods that seemed to trigger migraines.

Forty children underwent double-blind placebo-controlled challenges, us-ing masked whole foods. Migraine responses occurred in 6 of 40 placebo chal-lenges (15%) and in 26 of 40 active challenges (65%). If allergy skin testing had been used to plan the diet, only 3 children would have had all the dietary precip-itants of migraine eliminated [57].

TABLE 1   Double-Blind Placebo-Controlled Challenges in Migraine[a]

Author [Ref.]	Number subjects	Placebo positive	Placebo negative	Active positive	Active negative	Mediator changes
Egger [57]	40	6	34	30	10	No
Mansfield [58]	10	0	10	8	2	Histamine
Vaughan [59]	23	3	20	16	7	No
Olsen [60]	5	0	5	5	0	Histamine PGD$_2$
Steinberg [61]	1	0	1	1	0	Histamine PGF$_2$
Total	79	9 (11.4%)	70 (88.6%)	60 (75.9%)	19 (24.1%)	

[a] See text for references; in all cases in which mediators were measured, they increased during a migraine-producing challenge. PG = prostaglandin.

Mansfield, Vaughn, and colleagues studied 43 adults with at least four common migraine episodes per month. The subjects were diagnosed and referred from the neurology service. The patients were placed on an elimination diet trial, based on the patient's history and food allergy skin testing. If there were no positive skin test, results, then the subjects were placed on a milk, egg, wheat, corn-free diet.

Thirteen of the 43 subjects had a 66% or greater reduction in migraine attacks during the diet trial. Double-blind placebo-controlled challenges were performed in seven subjects with opaque capsules containing 8 g of freeze dried foods or the equivalent number of placebo capsules. No placebo responses occurred, whereas five of seven active challenges led to migraines. In 3 subjects who agreed to another blind challenge, plasma histamine levels rose during the active food challenge, that induced migraine, while staying unchanged in the placebo challenges (Fig. 1). The plasma histamine level peaked just before or at the onset of the migraine. Overall dramatic improvement occurred in 30% of the study subjects, with a confirmation rate of 70% by double-blind placebo-controlled challenges. This study also provided the first demonstration of mediator elevations during a blind food challenge triggering migraine.

In accord with Egger's findings, prick skin testing read at 15 minutes was not useful to determine the foods involved in provoking migraine. However, patients with any allergic sensitization were more likely to have food triggered migraines than nonallergic subjects [58].

Vaughn, in a follow-up study, reported a series of 104 subjects with at least three migraines per month. They were all placed on a milk; egg; wheat; corn-free

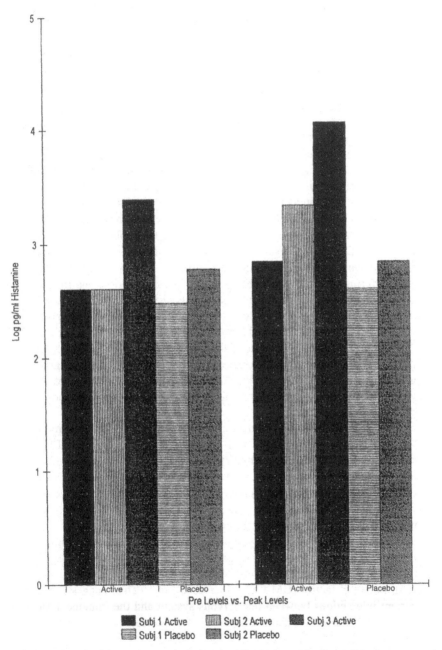

FIGURE 1 Challenge pre and peak Histamine. Active-migraine-caused placebo. No migraine occurred.

diet along with avoidance of foods suggested by history, or skin test–positive foods. Forty of the 104 subjects had at least a 50% reduction in migraines during the diet trial. Eight became headache-free.

Subsequently, 27 of 36 subjects who underwent open food reintroduction could identify one to four foods that precipitated migraine. Twenty-three patients underwent a double-blind challenge phase that consisted of 2 days of placebo capsules alternating with 2 days of active food capsules. A positive response was a migraine on either the first or second active challenge day without a headache on the placebo days.

In 3 of the subjects, migraine occurred during the placebo days; active challenge triggered migraines in 15 subjects, with 4 subjects not having migraines on either day. In this study, there did not appear any benefit of immediate allergy food skin tests in identifying migraine provoking foods [59].

Olsen studied five subjects from the study group with repeat double-blind placebo-controlled challenges. He measured changes in plasma histamine and prostaglandin D_2 (PGD_2) levels. The placebo challenges did not trigger migraines or changes in the levels of the mediators. Histamine levels increased markedly during the food provoked migraine just before or at the time of migraine. PGD_2 level increased at the same time as histamine level, and also 4 to 6 hours after challenge. Histamine did not increase at the later time. The investigators suggested that lack of elevated histamine level made the role of the basophil less important in the pathogenesis of the migraine attack [60]. This finding if confirmed would greatly alter the concepts of basophil dynamics in migraine. In contrast, in a single case example, a woman with beef induced migraines showed elevations of histamine and PGF_{2a} levels during active challenge but not during placebo challenge [61].

Guarisco and colleagues studied 22 adolescents with at least two migraines per month. Twenty one teenagers with migraine served as controls. The study group ate an oligoantigenic diet while the controls ate their usual diets. If a study subject improved, then foods were introduced in a open fashion. Foods thought to cause migraine were retested with a modified blind challenge. Twelve patients completed the oligoantigenic diet phase. Six became migraine free, five improved. There were no changes in the control diet group [62].

Marteletti discovered that cytokines in plasma were altered during a food challenge–induced migraine. The levels of Il-4 and Il-6 decreased after a positive challenge result, whereas levels of IFN-γ and granulocyte macrophage colary stimulating factor (GM-CSF) increased [63]. This suggests possibly important interactions between the nervous system and the immune system in dietary migraine at a level distinct from hypotheses offered prior to the recognition of the cytokines.

The foods that have been commonly associated with migraine and for which there is double-blind confirmation are shown in Table 2.

TABLE 2 Foods and Additives Commonly Reported to Cause Migraine or Headaches Confirmed by Blinded Challenges[a]

Possible enzyme deficiency
Red wine
Monosodium glutamate
Sodium metabisulfite
Aged cheeses
Aspartame sweetened foods
Vasoactive agents
Alcoholic beverages—ethanol, aromatic compounds
Chocolate—phenylethylamine, theobromine
Coffee—caffeine
Coca-Cola
Allergic mechanisms
Cow's Milk
Wheat
Corn
Legumes—peas, beans. peanuts
Cinnamon
Pork
Eggs
Coffee
Shrimp

[a] Any food appears capable of causing allergic migraine. In general allergy is a response to foods commonly eaten and unrecognized.

Laboratory Evidence of the Relationship Between Allergy Food and Migraine

There are a number of abnormalities described in migraine patients that are shared with other recognized food allergic subjects. The serum or plasma histamine level at baseline is generally higher in migraine patients than normal individuals [64]. Spontaneous release of histamine from basophils is increased in migraine [65]. Basophil degranulation occurs during migraine attacks including release of heparin [66].

Platelets in migraine are activated and demonstrate increased aggregation in nonstimulated and epinephrine stimulated studies [67]. Releasable platelet serotonin level decreases during a migraine attack, whereas serum levels of serotonin and its metabolites increase [68].

Recently, it was reported that release of TNF_α was higher from cells of migraine patients than normal individuals [38].

Common migraine subjects have evidence of nonspecific vascular hyperactivity, which may even be unilateral on the side where headaches most often occur. Migraine patients have a lower threshold to the vasodilating effects of carbon dioxide and histamine [69]. Intravenous histamine given to normal individuals causes a bilateral throbbing headache, with the same response occurring in migraine patients at lower concentrations. Interestingly, the side where the patient usually suffered the migraine attack often demonstrated a response at an even lower histamine dose. The contralateral side did not start pulsating until a higher histamine or carbon dioxide concentration was used [70]. These results are analagous to the nonspecific hyperactivity that occurs in the nose of rhinitics and the lungs of asthmatics.

At present, the bulk of migraine therapy is either symptomatic relief or prophylaxis based on neurovascular mechanisms. The approach is similar to using bronchodilators to treat asthma. The finding of nonspecific hyperreactivity and the clinical benefit of corticosteroids in migraine suggest that attention to inflammatory mechanisms would be worthwhile for migraine. One might expect a increase in histamine and carbon dioxide tolerance after a period of successful allergen avoidance. Presumably these changes would be associated with clinical improvement. Recently developed oral agents that affect the arachidonic acid, lipoxygenase pathways, or agents such as azelastine may also benefit such patients.

Cluster Headaches

Cluster headache shares many metabolic and pathological abnormalities with migraine; however, it clearly has a number of important differences. Except for dietary agents that are vasodilators, there is no evidence to support an important role for food and foodstuff in the provocation of the clusters. The headaches are usually unlateral, described as boring or piercing, and can be accompanied by ipsilateral nasal symptoms and Horner's syndrome. They occur in groups or clusters of headache and relief and headache and relief, with several or groups during any given day. Elevations of plasma histamine level during the clusters are much greater than those found in common migraine during an attack. Elevations of levels of urinary serotonin metabolites are also found in cluster headache attacks, suggesting release and physiological activity as seen in migraine. The cluster headaches respond to corticosteroids, sumatriptan, calcium channel blockers, oxygen, and intranasal lidocaine. There is a beneficial response to the combination of H_1 and H_2 antagonists, not reported in migraine. This may reflect a difference in pathogenesis. Platelet abnormalities are found in cluster headaches comparable to those of migraine headaches. Serotonin is released during clusters comparable to those of migraine. Similar but not exact perturbations of neuropeptides and cytokines have been found in cluster headache patients and in migraine patients [71,72].

Epilepsy

A link between migraine and epilepsy has been suggested by many authors [73,74]. Epileptics were reported to have the same spasmogenic substance in their blood as asthmatics, migrainer patients, and atopic eczema patients [75]. Pioneer neurologists such as Foster Kennedy described convulsions presumed caused by food allergy [76]. Dr. Kennedy personally observed acute transient edema of the optic nerve and retina caused by food allergy.

Ward and Patterson evaluated 1000 epileptics in two long-term residential facilities. They used 100 normal individuals and 100 mentally retarded patients as their control population. They tested all subjects with 64 to 72 scratch food skin tests. The incidence of at least one positive test result was 57% in the epileptics, 38% percent in the mentally retarded controls, and 8% in the normal patients [78].

Wallis et al. reported 38% of epileptic subjects reacted to one or more food allergens with only 4% of the control population reacting [79]. These pioneer investigators thought that allergy sensitization provoked some seizures and that allergic management could decrease seizure frequency and severity.

Dr. Susan Dees tested this hypothesis by treating 22 epileptic patients with a combination of desensitization, avoidance measures, and antiallergic medications. Epileptic problems decreased in 18 of 22 epileptic children. Nine of the 20 treated patients taking anticonvulsants were able to stop the medications. In a control group of 15 nonallergic epileptic children, only 1 of 15 was able to discontinue anticonvulsant drug therapy during the study. There were only minimal changes in the comparison patients' clinical status [80].

Egger more recently reported that an oligoantigenic diet decreased seizures in 63 epileptic children. Forty-five of the epileptic children also suffered from migraine or hyperactivity. Epilepsy by itself occurred in only 18 children. Twenty-five subjects became seizure-free, and 11 others improved. All of the subjects who improved had epilepsy plus migraine or hyperactivity. The 18 patients who had epilepsy as a single problem did not improve on the diet [81].

The diet was followed by a reintroduction phase, with certain foods being associated with the return of seizures. On the basis of the responses during the reintroduction phase, 16 subjects underwent placebo-controlled blinded food challenges. Eight children out of 16 had seizures with one or more food challenges. No seizures occurred during the placebo challenges [81].

Attention Deficit Disorder Hyperactivity Syndrome

In 1922 Shannon reported that food sensitivity affected learning ability and activity. [82] Differing food allergy problems have been suggested as triggers of attention deficit disorder hyperactivity (ADHD) syndrome. These include sucrose and preservatives, pharmacologically active foods (caffeine), and immunological food reactions.

Sugar (Sucrose) Sensitivity

There is a popular idea that sucrose is an important cause of behavior problems. Studies of sucrose's effects on behavior and attention have shown that even relatively large amounts of sucrose did not adversely affect behavior, except perhaps in some preschool children [83–90]. There may be local cerebral dysfunction in glucose metabolism among adults who had been hyperactive in childhood [91].

Dyes and Preservatives

Dr. Ben Feingold wrote a book to the lay community proposing that dyes, preservatives, and salicylates from the diet caused attention deficit hyperreactivity disorder [92]. The hypothesis was not tested in scientific study before being proclaimed to the public. Testimonials to the diet's effectiveness abounded.

After an enthusiastic public response, investigators evaluated the hypothesis that dye, preservative, and salicylate caused ADHD with blinded placebo-controlled methods. In no study did the diet control symptoms better rhan stimulants In fact, only one subgroup of patients appeared to benefit from the diet. This was the group of younger preschool children [93]. Table 3 summarizes some of these studies [94–99].

It soon became apparent that the Feingold diet did not remove salicylates and these components now appear of less concern.

Blind Controlled Studies

Besides the study by Egger, other investigators have reported experience with food related ADHD. In a recent study by Carter with a double-blind placebo-controlled challenge phase with 16 children with ADHD, the children were more symptomatic on food dye and preservative challenge days, compared to placebo days. They were less symptomatic on the days off dyes and preservatives [100].

Boris and Mandel reported a similar study confirming a benefit of removing dyes and preservatives from the diet of ADHD children. Sixteen of 26 children showed lessened symptoms on the dye- and preservative-free diet. Complete symptom relief was not obtained [101].

Egger, using the same type of oligoantigenic diet described, noted improved behavior in 62 of the 76 children with ADHD he studied. Many children appeared to be adversely affected by benzoic acid and tartrazine. However, there were no children identified as solely reactive to one or the other or both of these agents. Forty-six different food sources provoked hyperactivity. During the oligoantigenic diet trial, 21 children's behavior became completely normal. Dur-

TABLE 3 Trials of Feingold Hypothesis in Attention Deficit Hyperactivity Disorder

First author	[Reference] year	Subjects, Number	Blinded	Results	Raters	Comments
Cook	[94] 1976	15	No	Improved on diet	P	Order effect
Conners	[95] 1976	15	Yes	Improved on diet	P and T	Younger better
Harley	[96] 1978	36 nine challenges	Yes	Diet was Superior Challenges 1/9 worse	P and T	Younger children
Goyotte	[97] 1978	16 >= 6Yr 13<= 5yr	Yes	Challenges d> 6 yr no effect <5 yr worsen	Authors	All had responded to diet
Williams	[98] 1978	26	Yes	8 improve on diet	P and T	Modest effect Medication superior
Egger	[99] 1985	76	Part I = no Part 2 = yes	Improved = 62 Normal = 21 28 have rechallenge return to hyperactive	P and N and Psy	No effect on psychological testing

P, parents; T, teachers; N, neurologists; Psy, psychologists.

ing the double-blind challenge diets, suspected foods more often were associated with behavioral changes than were the placebos [99].

Kittler and Baldwin reported normalization of EEG result abnormalities in 9 of 20 children with behavior disorders while they were on an elimination diet. No blinded challenges were performed. No performance changes occurred in tests of intellectual function, even when the EEG result improved [102].

Diet may stimulate hyperactive behavior as a result of pharmacological activity such as that of caffeine in cola drinks or coffe, and phenylethylamine in chocolate. There is marked variation in the catabolism of these agents.

Insomnia and increased activity, with a letdown and lethargic phase, can occur. Aspartame and monosodium glutamate can show an excitogenic effect on EEG of animal models. In larger doses, they also lower the seizure potential of the animals [103,104].

Food or foodstuffs presumably acting on an allergic basis may aggravate attention deficit syndrome. The group most likely to benefit from diet control are preschool children. Studies have tested the hypothesis that food or food additives affect behavior and learning in children. There is an effect of diet on affected children. Children with the milder behavioral changes appear to benefit from diet changes alone, making this approach sufficient for their care. Severely affected children still require the other recognized means of treatment. However, we believe dietary factors should be explored in these patients also.

Tension Fatigue Syndrome: Allergic Toxemia

In 1930, Rowe described a syndrome of "allergic toxemia" caused by food allergy [105]. The symptoms of this syndrome were (a) drowsiness; (b) mental confusion, (c) lack of initiative, (d) slowness of thought, (e) fatigue, (f) weakness, (g) bodily aches, (h) irritability; (i) and a feeling of being poisoned. The patients often had gastrointestinal complaints. The average age of these patients was 45 years. They were most often female. These types of patients are presently diagnosed as having chronic fatigue syndrome. Rowe reported great benefit with diets. There were no double-blind challenges or controls in his studies.

The symptom complex was renamed the *allergic tension–fatigue syndrome* by Speer [106], who added the important concept of fatigue, which was not relieved by rest. He stressed the occurrence of insomnia in some patients and an uncomfortable, nonphysiological fatigue. He and others, such as Crook, believed that food allergy was an important provoker of this symptom [106]. Recent work suggests that allergic reactions of the tension–fatigue syndrome may be mediated through cell sensitization [107].

One controlled study of patients confirming that food allergy provocation of the syndrome occurs has been performed [108]. This study is only partially accepted by the general medical community. The described symptoms are common to patients seen by physicians in all specialties.

A recent study of patients who described food related fatigue symptoms discovered a large percentage with depressive disorders [109].

At present there is a clear need for additional studies of food and foodstuff in the diverse group of patients who present the symptoms of chronic fatigue. At present there is no clear support for a prominent role of food allergy in the pathogenesis of chronic fatigue syndrome.

Meniere's Syndrome, Vertigo, and Fluctuating Hearing Loss

Duke placed five patients with Meniere's syndrome on elimination diets that allowed long-term relief [110]. That food allergies trigger vertigo, along with more classic Meniere's syndrome symptoms, is a well accepted idea among otolaryngological allergists [111,112].

Some infants and young children suffer from benign paroxysmal vertigo with fluctuating hearing loss. They improve on an avoidance diet. Challenges with cow's milk provoke the symptoms. This is the best demonstration that foods can affect the vestibular and auditory organs [113].

Paralytic Syndromes

Stafferi reported that hemiplegia and allergic symptoms routinely followed ingestion of certain foods in a patient [114]. Although the authors stated similar cases had ben described, they cited no references, so that this statement is not verifiable. At this present time, there is no support for this association.

Insomnia

Kahn observed infants who were fitful sleepers or insomniacs in a pediatric sleep laboratory. When the infants drank cow's milk or cow's milk–derived formulas, the symptoms were present. If cow's milk or cow's milk formula was replaced in the diet, the infants slept normally. Upon reintroduction of cow's milk, the sleep disturbance returned. The infants did not demonstrate specific anti–cow's milk immmunoglobulin E (IgE) antibodies [115].

Metabolic Psychiatrict Disease

Dohan, a psychiatrist, noted that the incidence of schizophrenia was decreased among the populations of the Nazi occupied countries during World War II. The populations had a restricted diet. Normal dietary items such as wheat were expropriated for use by the German army and civilians. He subsequently theorized that gluten was a factor in the pathogenesis of schizophrenia. In a series of articles, Dohan reported resolution of schizophrenic episodes was more rapid on a wheat-free diet and specified the medication requirements for successful treatment [116]. There is a blind challenge study that supports Dohan's conclusions [117].

A rather interesting case report described a nurse who repeatedly suffered depressive symptoms after blinded challenges with cow's milk but not placebo [118]. Investigators in Norway provided evidence that autisitic children fare better on a milk-free and gluten-free diet. The excretion of abnormal urinary peptides by autistic patients was decreased. The change in peptide excretion was associated with improved autistic symptoms [119].

Special Considerations in the Evaluation of Food Triggered Neurological Disorders

Details of the general approach to the evaluation of food related illness are discussed in other chapters. As stated in the Introduction to this chapter, there remains a great deal of controversy about neurological, neuromuscular, emotional or psychiatric disease that is caused by dietary factors [120] (in spite of the well recognized effects of things humans eat and drink on their physical health, performance, and mood.)

It is important to understanding the role of unique hypersensitivy to dietary factors as a possible cause of neurological disease for the evaluating physician to think about other recently described mediators such as the cytokines that change during immune hypersensitivy responses. There is evidence for the activation of sensitized mononuclear cells which can participate in these reactions. The modification by peripheral immune responses in nervous system function has been described [8]. The metabolic disturbances demonstrated in serum during certain illnesses such as migraine suggest that we need to reexamine concepts about mediator exclusion from the central nervous system by the blood–brain barrier. The previously described evidence from animal models suggests high concentrations of these mediators will disrupt the epithelial blood–brain barrier.

There are some special issues relating to neurological disease possibly caused by food or foodstuff. The first step is taking a detailed history of the problem from the patient or parent. The second step is providing for a period of symptom diet diary recording by the patient. It is important to be candid with the patient about the present state of knowledge and disagreement. However, for each patient a careful evaluation can lead to an accurate evaluation of dietary effects on the medical condition of concern.

1. The evaluation may take place over a long period of observation, sometimes involving months, with careful well planned recording of food symptom diaries. The patient should be aware of the importance of this recording during a baseline period, during the elimination diet trial, and during a reintroduction phase. Figure 2 is a modified milk, egg-, corn-, and wheat-free diet that we have found useful to begin the evaluation.

2. Foods or foodstuffs that seem to be incriminated during the open trial should be confirmed by blind challenges if at all possible. This may not al-

Please Note :

1. *For this diet, all fruit and vegetables except for lettuce and melons must be cooked.*
2. *All foods should be either fresh or frozen*
3. *Avoid foods containing preservatives or colorants, dry cereals, dried fruits*
4. *Avoid smoked meats or cheeses, hot dogs, sausages, ham, bacon*
5. *It is best to avoid alcohol or keep intake to a minimum (less good), you must avoid red or rose wines*
6. *Try to limit the use of cokes, coffee, tea, chocolate. Use decaffeinated drinks whenever possible.*
7. *Avoid chewing gums, thickened salad dressings*
8. *Avoid any foods which you have found cause headaches*

FOODS YOU MAY EAT

Tapioca	Beef	Asparagus
White Potato	Chicken	Spinach
Rice	Pork (Not ham or smoked)	Carrots
Sweet Potato	Squash	Cranberries
Lettuce	Chard	Apricots
Maple Syrup	Peaches	Pears
Beets	Gelatin (plain)	Pineapple
Artichoke	Apples	Grapes
Avocado	Melons	Sorghum
Water	Club Soda	Coffee
Tea	Vegetable Oil	Vegetable (100%) Shortening
Vinegar	Salt, Pepper, Garlic, Onion	

FIGURE 2   Migraine diet: a modified milk-, egg-, wheat-, and corn-free diet.

ways be possible in today's medical environment. However, if the food or foodstuff is very difficult to avoid or a major diet constituent, approval can be usually obtained.

3.   An analog scale can be helpful to determine degrees of pain or increases in subjective discomfort. Figure 3 is an example of a recording device for migraine. This device can be used during the trial as well as the challenges.

4.   With respect to laboratory testing, skin tests, that allow for evaluation of late-phase responses as well as early responses may be of greater utility than simple immediate skin tests. However, this area needs further study before it will be clear how much additional benefit late-phase testing will offer.

Radioallergosorbent testing (RAST), perhaps because it is less sensitive than usual skin testing, may actually be superior in diagnosing IgE-mediated food reactions affecting the nervous system. Additional studies like Monro's are required to confirm whether this is true [55].

Please complete this record as soon as you can. Accurate information will help us better understand how to help relieve your migraines.

Migraine Headache Record   Patient Name
Date

What time did the attack start ?:   am/pm   date
What time did it stop?:   am/pm   date
Did you have any sensations before this attack? yes   no
If yes, what were they?:

Where was the headache?   Right Side   Left Side   Both Sides
What was the pain like?:   Constant   Throbbing   Pulsating   Sharp   Pressure
How much did it hurt at the peak of the pain ?:
a little   mild   moderate   severe   very severe   excruciating
(1)   (2)   (3)   (4)   (5)   (6)

Place a mark on the line which best describes your pain.
Did you also have?:   Nausea   Vomiting   Abdominal Pain   Light Sensitivity
Did you take any medications?   Yes   No
What medicines in what doses and when did you take them?

medication name	dose used	time taken
1		
2		
3		
4		
5		
6		

Comments

FIGURE 3   Example of a recording device for a migraine.

REFERENCES

1. Wald M, Unterberg U, Baethmann A, Schilling L. Mediators of blood brain barrier dysfunction and formation of vasogenic brain edema. J Cereb Blood Flow Metab 1988; 8:621–633.
2. Betz AL, Goldstein GW, Katzman R. Blood-brain cerebrospinal fluid barriers. In: Siegel G, Agrano FF, Albers RW, eds. Basic Neurochemistry: Molecular, Cellular and Medical Aspects: 4th ed. New York: Raven Press, 1989.

3. Lassmann H, Rossler K, Zimprich F, Vass K. Expression of adhesion molecules and histocompatibility antigens at the blood-brain barrier. Brain Pathol 1991; 1(2):115–123

4. Benveniste EN. Inflammatory cytokines within the central nervous system: sources, function, and mechanism of action. Am J Physiol 1992; 263 (1):1–16.

5. Suzumura A. Cytokine network in the central nervous system. Nippon Rinsho 1994; 52(11):2887–2893.

6. Otten U, Gadient RA. Neurotrophins and cytokines—intermediaries between the immune and nervous systems. Int J Dev Neurosci 1995; 13(3–4):147–151.

7. Rivest S, Lacroix S. Influence of cytokines on neuroendocrine functions during immune response: mechanisms involved and neuronal pathways. Ann Endocrinol (Paris) 1995; 56(3):159–167.

8. Press GD, Green JP. Histamine as a neuroregulator. Rev Neurosci 9:209–222.

8a. Undem BJ, Myers AC, Weinreich D. Angtigen-induced modulation of autonomic and sensory neurons in vitro. Int Arch Allergy Appl Immunol 1991; 94(1–4):319–324.

9. Scher W, Scher BM. A possible role for nitric oxide in glutamate (MSG)-induced Chinese restaurant syndrome, glutamate-induced asthma, "hot dog headache," pugilistic Alzheimer's disease, and other disorders. Med Hypotheses 1992; 38(3):185–188.

10. Arrang JM. Pharmacological properities of histamine receptor subtypes. Cell Mol Biol 1994; 40(3):275–281.

11. Nowak JZ. Histamine in the central nervous system: its role in circadian rhythmicity. Acta Neurobiol Exp (Warsz) 1994; 54 (suppl):65–82.

12. Schilling L, Wahl M. Effects of antihistamines on experimental brain edema. Acta Neurochir Suppl (Wien) 1994; 60:79–82.

13. Young CS, Mason R, Hill SJ. Inhibition by H1 antihistamines of the uptake of noradrenaline and 5-HT into rat brain synaptosomes. Biomed Pharmacol 1988; 37(5):978–981.

14. Monnier M, Sauer R, Hatt AM. The activating effect of histamine on the central nervous system. Int Rev Neurobiol 1970; 12:265–305.

15. Arrang JM, Devaux B, Chodkiewicz JP, Swartz TC. H_3 receptors controle histamine release in human braine. Neurochem 1988; 81(1):105–108.

16. Onodera K, Watanae T. Possible roles of brain histamine H_3 receptors and the pharmacology of its ligands. Nihon Shinkei Seishin Yakurigaku Zasshi 1995; 15(2):87–102.

17. Kostopoulos G, Psarropoulos C, Hass HL. Membrane properties, response to amines and retanic stimulation of hypocampal neurons in the genetically mutant epileptic tolering mouse. Exp Brain Res 1988; 72:43–50.

18. Lee NS, Muhs G, Wagner GC, Reynolds RD, Fisher H. Dietary pyridoxine interaction with tryptophan or histadine on brain serotonin and histamine metabolism. Pharmacol Biochem Behav 1988; 29: 559–564.

19. Clark WG, Brater DC, Johnson AR. Serotonin, kinins, and miscellaneous autacoids. In: Goth's Medical Pharmacology. 12th ed. St. Louis: Mosby, 1988, pp 214–226.

20. Chase TN, Murphy DL. Serotinin and central nervous system function. Annu Rev Pharmacol 1973; 13:181–197.

21. Sjaastad O. The significance of blood serotonin levels in migraine: a critical review. Acta Neurol Scand 1975; 51(3):200–210.
22. Harper AM, MacKenzie ET, McCulloch J, Pickard JD. Migraine and the blood-brain barrier. Lancet 1977 May 14; 1(8020):1034–1036.
23. Anthony M. Plasma free fatty acids and prostaglandin E1 in migraine and stress. Headache 1976; 16(2):58–63.
24. Taiwo YO, Levine JD. Prostaglandins inhibit endogenous pain control mechanisms by blocking transmission at spinal noradrenergic synapses. J Neurosci 1988; 8(4):1346–1349.
25. Bogucki A. Prostaglandins: their effect on cerebral blood vessels and role in the pathogenesis of migraine. Neurol Neurochir Pol 1981; 15(2):213–218.
26. Schurer L, Corvin S, Rohrich F, Abels C, Baethmann A. Leukocyte/endothelial interactions and blood-brain barrier permeability in rats during cerebral superfusion with LTB4. Acta Neurchir Suppl (Wien) 1994; 60:51–54.
27. Davis KD, Dostrovsky JO. Cerebrovascular application of bradykinin excites central sensory neurons. Brain Res 1988; 446:401–406.
28. Bhattacharya S, Mohanraq PJR, Neetadas G. Intracerebroventricularly administered bradykinin augments carrageenan-induced paw oedema in rats. J Pharm Pharmacol 198; 40:367–369.
29. Unterberg A, Dauterman C, Baethman A, Muller-Esterl W. The kallikrein-kinin system as mediator in vasogenic brain edema. J Neurosurg 1986; 64:269–273.
29a. Wahl M, Schilling L, Unterberg A, Baethmann A. Mediators of vascular and parenchymal mechanisms in secondary brain damage. Acta Neurochir Suppl (Wien) 1993; 57:64–72.
30. Page CP, Archer CB, Paul W. Paf-acether. A mediator of inflammation and asthma. Trends Pharmacol Sci 1984; 5:239.
31. Hanington E, Jones RJ, Arness JA et al. Migraine: A platelet disorder. Lancet 1981; 2:720.
32. Edvinsson L, Goadsby PJ. Neuropeptides in migraine and cluster headache. Cephalalgia 1994; 14(5):320–327.
33. Hanley MR. Peptide regulatory factors in the nervous system. Lancet 1989 June 17; 1(8651):1373–1376.
34. Barnum SR. Complement biosynthesis in the central nervous system. Crit Rev Oral Biol Med 1995; 6(2):132–146.
35. Benavides J, Toulmond S. Role of cytokines in the central nervous system. Therapie 1993; 48(6):575–584.
36. Benvfeniste EN, Benos DJ. TNF-alpha-and IFN-gamma-mediated signal transduction pathways: effects on glial cell gene expression and function. FASEB J 1995; 9(15):1577–1584.
37. Friden PM, Walus LR, Watson P, Doctrow SR, Kozarich JW, Backman C, Berman H, Hoffer B, Bloom F, Granholm AC. Blood-brain barrier penetration and in vivo activity of an NGF conjugate. Science 1993; 259:373–377.
38. Covelli V, Munno I, Pellegrino NM, Altamura M, Decandia P, Marcuccio C, Di-

Venere A, Jirillo E. Are TNF-alpha and IL-1 beta relevant in the pathogenesis of migraine without aura? Acta Neurol (Napoli) 1991; 13(2):205–211.

39. Villiger PM. Interactions between the nervous and the immune system. Schweiz Med Wochenschr 1994; 21 124(20):857–866.

40. Hemmings WA. The entry into the brain of large molecules derived from dietary protein. Proc R Soc Lond (Biol) 1978; 200:175–192.

41. Cochrane GC, Koffler D. Immune complex disease in experimental animal and man. Adv Immunol 1973; 16:185–264.

42. Vaughan WT, Black JH. Migraine. In: Practice of Allergy. St. Louis: CV Mosby, 1948, pp 1027–1039.

43. Olesen J, Larsen B, Lauritzen M. Focal hyperemia followed by spreading oligemia and impaired activation of rCBF in classic migraine. Ann Neurol 1981; 9:344–352.

44. Brown TR. Role of diet in etiology and treatment of migraine and other types of headache. JAMA 1921; 77:1396.

45. Vaughn WT. Allergic migraine. JAMA 1927; 88:1383.

46. DeGowin EL. Allergic migraine a review of sixty cases. J Allergy 1932; 3:557.

47. Eyermann CH. Allergic headache. J Allergy 1931; 2:106.

48. Sandler M, Youdim MBH, Hanington E. A phenylethylamine oxidising defect in migraine. Nature 1974; 250:335.

49. Koehler SM, Glaros A. The effect of aspartame on migraine headache. Headache 1988; 28:10–13.

50. Spierings LH. Craniovascular accompaniments of the vascular headache of the migraine type. Headache 1979; 19(7):397–399.

51. Littlewood JT, Glover V, Davies PTG, Gibb C, Sandler M, Rose FC. Red wine as a cause of migraine. Lancet 1988 Mar 12; 1(8585):558–559.

52. Perkin JE, Hartje J. Diet and migraine: a review of the literature. J Am Diet Assoc 1983; 83:459–463.

53. Medina JL, Diamond S. The role of diet in migraine. Headache J 1978; 18(1):31–34.

53a. Moffett A, Swash M, Scott DF. Effect of tyramine in migraine: a double-blind study. J Neurol Neurosurg Psychiatry 1972; 35:496–499.

54. Unger AH, Unger L. Migraine is an allergic disease. J Allergy 1952; 23:429.

54a. Fukutomi O, Kondo N, Agata H, Shinoda S, Shinbara M, Orii T. Abnormal responses of the autonomic nervous system in food-dependent excercise-induced anaphylaxis. Ann Allergy 1992; 68(5):438–445.

55. Monro J, Carini C, Brostoff J, Zilkha, K. Food allergy in migraine: study of dietary exclusion and RAST. Lancet 1980; 2:1–3.

56. Grant ECG. Food allergies and migraine. Lancet: 1979 May 5; 1(8123):966–967.

57. Egger J, Carter CM, Wilson J, Turner MW, Soothhill JF. Is migraine food allergy? A double-blind controlled trial of oligoantigenic diet treatment. Lancet 1983; 2:865–867.

58. Mansfield, LE, Vaughn TR, Waller SF, Haverly RW, Ting S. Food allergy and adult migraine. Double-blind and mediator confirmation of an allergic etiology. Ann Allergy 1985; 55:126–130.

59. Vaughn TR, Stafford WW, Miller BT, Nelson HS. Food and migraine headache (MIG):a controlled study (abstr). Ann Allergy 1988; 56:522.

60. Olson GC, Vaughn TR, Ledoux RA. Food induced migraine:search for immunologic mechansims (abstr). J Allergy Clin Immunol 1989; 83:238.

61. Steinberg M, Page R, Wolfson S. Food induced late phase headache (abstr). J Allergy Clin Immunol 1988; 81:185.

62. Guariso G, Bertoli S, Cernetti R, Battistella PA, Setari M, Zacchello F. Migraine and food intolerance: a controlled study in pediatric patients. Pediatr Med Chir 1993 Jan–Feb 15; (1):57–61.

63. Martelletti P, Stirparo G, Rinaldi C, Frati L, Giacovazzo M. Disruption of the immunopeptidergic network in dietary migraine. Headache 1993; 33(10):524–527.

64. Heatley RV, Dengurg JA, Bayer N. Increased plasma histamine levels in migraine patients. Clin Allergy 1982; 12:145–149.

65. Sanders WM, Zimmerman AW, Mahoney MA, Ballow M. Leukocyte histamine release in migraine. Headache 1978; 20:307–310.

66. Thonnard-Neumann E, Neckers LM. Immunity in migraine: the effect of heparin. Ann Allergy 1981; 47:328–332.

67. Hanington E. Migraine: the platelet hypothesis after 10 years. Biomed Pharmacother 1989; 43:719–726.

68. D'Andrea G, Welch KMA, Grunfeld MS, Joseph R, Nagel-Leiby S. Platelet norepinephrine and serotonin balance in migraine. Headache 1989; 29:657–659.

68a. Waldenlind E, Ross SB, Saaf J, Ekbon K, Wetterberg L. Concentration and uptake of 5-hydroxytryptamine in platelets from cluster headache and migraine patients. Cephalalgia 1985; 5:45–54.

69. Engel D. Studies on headache produced by carbon dioxide, histamine and adrenalin. Acta Neurochir (Wien) 1969; 21(4):263–283.

70. Sakai F, Meyer JS. Abnormal cerebrovascular reactivity in patients with migraine and cluster headache. Headache 1979; 19(5):257–266.

70a. Harer C, Von Kummer R. Cerebrovascular CO_2 reactivity in migraine: assessment by transcranial doppler ultrasound. J Neurol 1991; 238:23–26.

71. Connors MJ. Cluster headache: a review. J Am Osteopath Assoc 1995; 95(9):533–539.

72. Kittrelle JP, Grouse DS, Seybold ME. Cluster headache. Arch Neurol 1985; 42:496–498.

73. Dewar DC. The allergic approach to epilepsy, a critical review. Practitioner 1941; 147:776–778.

74. Pardee L. Two cases demonstrating allergic reactions in epilepsy. J Nerv Ment Dis 1938; 88:89–91.

75. Van Leeuwen S, Zeydner W. On the occurence of a toxic substance in the blood of cases with bronchial asthma, urticaria, epilepsy and migraine. Br J Exp Pathol 1922; 3:282–288.

76. Kennedy F. Cerebral symptoms induced by angioneurotic edema. Arch Neurol Psychiatry 1926; 15:28–33.

77. Pagniez P, Lietaud P. Phenomena of the anaphylactic type in the pathogenesis of certain epileptic attacks. Presse Med 1919; 27:693–696.

78. Ward JF, Patterson HY. Protein sensitization in epilepsy, a study one thousand cases and one hundred controls. Arch Neurol Psychiatry 1927; 17(8):427–443.
79. Wallis RM, Nicol WD, Craig M. The importance of protein hypersensitivity in the diagnosis and treatment of a special group of epileptics. Lancet 1923; 1:741–743.
80. Dees SC, Lowenback H. Allergic epilepsy. Ann Allergy 1951; 8:446–458.
81. Egger J, Carter CM, Soothill JF, Wilson J. Oligoantigenic diet treatment of children with epilepsy and migraine. J Pediatr 1989; 114(1):51–58.
82. Shannon WR. Neuropathic manifestations in infants and children as a result of anaphylactic reaction to foods contained in their diet. Am J Dis Child 1922; 24:89–94.
83. Rapoport JL, Kruesi MJ. Behavior and nutrition: a mini review. ASCD J Dent Child 1984; 51(6):451–454.
84. Hendley ED, Conti LH, Wessel DJ, Horton ES, Musty RE. Behavioral and metabolic effects of sucrose-supplemented feeding in hyperactive rats. Am J Physiol 1987; 253(3 pt 2):R434–R443.
85. Kruesi MJ, Rapoport JL, Cummings EM, Berg CJ, Ismond DR, Flament M, Yarrow M, Zahn-Waxler C. Effects of sugar and aspartame on aggression and activity in children. Am J Psychiatry 1987; 144(11):1487–1490.
86. Brenner A. Sugar and behavior. Md Med J 1987; 36(5):409–410.
87. Kanarek RB. Does sucrose or aspartame cause hyperactivity in children? Nutr Rev 1994; 52(5):173–175.
88. White JW, Wolraich M. Effect of sugar on behavior and mental performance. Am J Clin Nutr 1995; 62(suppl 1):242S–274S; discussion 247S–249S.
89. Wolraich ML, Wilson DB, White JW. The effect of sugar on behavior or cognition in children: a meta-analysis. JAMA 1995; 274(20):1617–1621.
90. Conners CK, Blouin AG. Nutritional effects on behavior of children. J Psychiatr Res 1982–83; 17(2):L193–L201.
91. Zamethetkin AJ, Nordahl TE, Gross M, King AC, Sekmple WE, Runsey J, Hamburger S, Cohen RM. Cerebral glucose metabolism adults with hyperactivity of childhood onset. N Engl J Med 1990; 323:1361–1366.
92. Feingold BF. The role of diet in behavior. Ecol Dis 1982; 1(2–3): 153–165.
93. Taylor E. Food additives, allergy and hyperkinesis. J Child Psychol Psychiatry 1979; 20:357–363.
94. Cook PS, Woodhill JM. The Feingold dictary treatment of the hyperkinetic syndrome. Med J Aust 1976; 2:85–90.
95. Conners CK, Goyette CH, Southwick MA, Lees JM, Andrulonis PA. Food additives and hyperkinesis. Pediatrics 1976; 58:154–166.
96. Harley JP, Ray RS, Tomasi L, Eichman PL, Mathews CG, Chun R, Cleeland CS, Traisman E. Hyperkinesis and food additives: testing the Feingold hypothesis. Pediatrics 1978; 61:818–828.
97. Goyette CH, Conners CK, Pettita, Curtiss LE. Effects of artificial colors on hyperactive children. A double blind challenge study. Psychol Pharm Bull; 1978; 14:39–40.
98. Williams JI, Cram DM, Tausing FT, Webster MB. Relative effects of drugs and

diet on hyperactive behaviors: an experimental study. Pediatrics 1978; 61:811–817.

99. Egger J, Carter CM, Graham PF, Grumely D. Controlled trial of oligoantigenic treatment in the hyperkinetic syndrome. Lancet 1985 Mar 9; 1(8428):540–545.

100. Carter CM, Urbanowiez M, Hemsley R, Mantilla L, Strobel S, Graham PF, Taylor E. Effects of a few food diet in attention deficit disorder. Arch Dis Child 1993; 69(5):564–568.

101. Boris M, Mandel FS. Food and additives are common causes of attention deficit hyperactive disorder in children. Ann Allergy 1994; 72(3):462–468.

102. Kittler FJ, Baldwin DC. The role of allergic factors in the child with minimal brain dysfunction. Ann Allergy 1970; 28:203–206.

103. Ting B, Knott MD, Mansfield LE, Ting S. Effects of oral cromolyn (C) on food-induced headaches and behavioral changes. Presented at the XII International Congress of Allergology and Clinical Immunology, Washington DC, Oct. 1985.

104. Maher TJ, Wartman RJ. Possible neurologic effects of aspartame, a widely used food additive. Environ Health Perspect 1987; 75:53–57.

105. Rowe H. Allergic toxemia and migraine due to food allergy. Cal West Med 1939; 33:785–793.

106. Speer F. The allergic tension-fatigue syndrome. Pediatr Clin North Am 1954;1019–1028.

107. Kendo N, Shinoda S, Ayala H. Fuji H. Lymphocyte responses to food antigens in food senstiive patients with allergic tension fatigue syndrome. Biotherapy 1992; 5:281–284.

108. Crook WG, Harrison WW, Crawford SE, Emmerson BS. Systemic manifestations due to allergy. Pediatrics 1961; 27:710–799.

109. Hickie I, Lloyd A, Wakefield D. Immunological and psychological dysfunction in patients receiving immunmotherapy for chronic fatigue syndrome. Aust NZ J Psychiatry 1992; 26:249–256.

110. Duke WW. Meniere's syndrome caused by allergy. JAMA 1923; 81:2179–2181.

111. Clemis JD. Medical management of Meniere's disease. Arch Otolaryngol 1969; 89:116–119.

112. Derebery MJ. Allergic and immunologic aspects of Meniere's disease. Otolaryngol Head Neck Surg 1996; 114:360–365.

113. Dunn DW, Snyder CH. Benign paroxysmal vertigo of childhood. Am J Dis Child 1976; 130:1099–1100.

114. Staffieri D, Bentolila L, Levit L. Hemiplegia and allergic symptoms following ingestion of certain foods: a case report. Ann Allergy 1952:38–39.

115. Kahn A, Rebufatt E, Blum D, Casimir G, Duchateau J, Mozin MJ, Jost R. Difficulty in initiating and maintaining sleep associated with cow's milk allergy in infants. Sleep 1987; 10(2):116–121.

116. Dohan FC. Cereals and schizophrenia: data and hypothesis. Acta Psychiatr Scand 1966; 25:125–132.

117. Vlissides DN, Venulet A, Jenner FA. A double blind gluten free/gluten load controlled trial in a secure ward population. Br J Psychiatry 1986; 148:447–452.

118. Mills N. Depression and food intolerance: a single case study. Hum Nutr 1986; 40(2):141–145.
119. Knivsberg DM, Wiig K, Und G, Nodland M, Rerchelt KL. Dietary intervention in autistic syndromes. Brain Dysfunc 1990; 3:315–327.
120. Frieri M. A consideration of the controversial relationships of attention deficit disorder, autism, and chronic fatigue with allergy and immunity. NCMC Proc 1996:16–19.

15

Exercise-Induced Anaphylaxis

MANDAKOLATHUR R. MURALI
Williston Park, New York

The human anaphylactic response results from the activation of a variety
of potent mediator systems, involving both immunoglobulin E– (IgE-) and
non-IgE-dependent pathways, and manifests as an immediate systemic response to a variety of stimuli. Recruitment and activation of the mast cell appear important in the causation of this syndrome [1]. The clinical spectrum
encompasses many organ systems, ranging from cutaneous flushing and
hives, in its mildest form, to cardiorespiratory distress, shock, and death in its
extreme manifestation.

Exercise-induced anaphylaxis (EIA) is a syndrome in which symptoms
similar to those of anaphylactic reaction to foreign substance occur, but in association with exercise. Awareness and recognition of this entity are increasing,
perhaps as a result of the surge in interest in and commitment to physical fitness
regimens that incorporate a variety of physical exercise programs.

Of the various physical allergies, EIA is the most dramatic clinical entity.
However, its true incidence and natural history are yet to be defined. This review
will highlight the clinical features, pathophysiological characteristics, differential diagnoses, and management of EIA.

CLINICAL FEATURES OF EIA

In 1970 Matthews and Pan reported on the clinical syndrome of EIA [2]. Sheffer and Austen in 1980 described the spectrum and clinical features of EIA in a group of 16 patients and related EIA to exercise [3]. These authors described 16 patients with EIA, 11 of whom were males and 5 who were females. Their ages ranged from 12 to 54 years of age with a mean of 24 years. These patients were accomplished athletes, and the episodes of EIA had occurred in association with running, sprinting, playing tennis or soccer, etc. The frequency of occurrence of these episodes varied from a single attack to several attacks a year and had spanned a period as long as 16 years. Their exercise regimens varied considerably. Although most of them exercise daily, two athletes exercised three times a week and two once a week. The striking clinical feature highlighted in that series, which still proves to be an enigma as well as a characteristic, is the inconsistency in the exercise threshold among different athletes and even in the same individual at different times. This contrasts with other forms of physical allergies, in which the physical stimuli consistently reproduce the evolution of the symptoms. This inconsistency led to the speculation that other factors (or cofactors) are contributory. In this series, these included exercise in a postprandial state, exercise after ingestion of aspirin or caffeine, and even meteorological variations such as higher ambient temperature and rain. Although these cofactors are intriguing in terms of pathophysiology, they emphasize the need for clinicians to identify them, with a view to eliminating or mitigating them in the therapeutic approach.

A comprehensive questionnaire analysis of 199 individuals diagnosed to have EIA on a clinical basis was conducted by Wade et al.; the study comprised 134 females and 65 males [4]. Their mean age of onset of symptoms was 24.7 years (range 4–74 years), and their mean age at time of survey was 32.8 years (range 9–80 years). The precipitating events included bicycling, walking, playing racquet sports, skiing, doing aerobic exercise, and jogging. Jogging was the most common activity reported in this series and might reflect that this modality is an increasingly popular form of physical fitness regimen. The evolution and spectrum of clinical features were similar to those described in the original series of Sheffer and Austen [3]. Premonitory symptoms include fatigue, flushing, warmth, and generalized erythema. Urticarial eruptions occur and coalesce, and angioedema of the face, palms, and soles is seen. Symptoms persist during the attack and subside in about 30 minutes to a few hours after cessation of exercise. Vascular collapse and transient loss of consciousness are not uncommon (ranging from 30% to 66% of subjects) and can occur during or after cessation of exercise. Features of upper airway obstruction such as choking and stridor have been recorded in as many as 59% of subjects. Generally wheezing is not a feature of EIA. Gastrointestinal symptoms such as nausea, vomiting, and colic were noted in a third of patients. Almost all of these features resolve in 2 hr after cessation of exercise and rarely do they last beyond 12 hr. The noticeable exception is headache, which can occur late in the sequelae of clinical features of EIA and can persist for up to 72 hr [4].

As in the initial series of Sheffer and Austen [3], the questionnaire series of Wade et al. [4] highlighted the importance of cofactors besides exercise in this entity. These include ingestion of alcohol, exercise, and other medications. Environmental factors contributing to the expression of EIA included a warm environment, cold weather, and humidity. About a fifth of women felt that the phase of the menstrual cycle affected the emergence of the syndrome [5].

An interesting and unique feature of EIA is the relationship of this entity to antecedent ingestion of specific foods. The role of specific foods varies from patient to patient and is often reflected by positive prick test responses to the food in question. Ingestion of food alone or exercise in the absence of food does not provoke an attack of EIA. This differentiates this entity from food allergy causing anaphylaxis. The list of incriminated foods varies from series to series and includes shellfish, celery, peach, wheat, chicken, cereal grains [5–10]. This entity of food-associated and exercise-induced anaphylaxis is now recognized as a distinct syndrome [11,12].

Equally important is the recognition that in some subjects exercise in the postprandial state (without a requirement for ingestion of specific foods) either was a prerequisite for the occurrence of EIA or increased the odds of development of EIA. Such an association was first noted in 3 of 16 patients described by Sheffer and Austen [3]. Later in the epidemiological survey conducted by Wade et al. in 1989 more than half of the respondents with EIA felt ingestion of food within 3 to 4 hr before exercise was an important factor in the emergence of their clinical presentation [4]. Ingestion of alcohol or aspirin prior to exercise resulted in EIA, suggesting that alcohol and aspirin act as cofactors.

The presence of atopy or family history of atopy is more common in subjects with EIA [13,14], implicating the role of mast cells and genetic predisposition.

PATHOPHYSIOLOGICAL CHARACTERISTICS

The sequence of biochemical events, mediator release, and cellular and neurohumoral pathways in the development of EIA is unknown. On the basis of the similarity of clinical presentation to that seen in IgE-mediated anaphylaxis it has been suggested that EIA invokes recruitment of mast cells, basophils, or both. Evidence for mast cell involvement includes experimental challenge studies as well as morphological evidence of mast cell degranulation.

Experimental exercise challenge or food-associated EIA have documented an increase in serum histamine levels in several studies [15,16]. Other mast cell mediators such as prostaglandin D_2 (PGD_2), leukotrienes, and platelet activating factor (PAF) have not been studied in this entity.

Morphological evidence of cutaneous mast cell involvement has been demonstrated [1]. Before exercise challenge the ultrastructural evaluation of cutaneous mast cells showed no abnormalities among patients with EIA compared with normal controls. After exercise challenge and the clinical expression of EIA numerous changes in the skin mast cells have been documented. These include loss of electron density and decrease in intact mast cell granules. Also noted was fusion of granule membranes with membranes of adjacent granules and mast cell membranes. These features are reminiscent of IgE–FcER-dependent activation of mast cells seen in vivo or in vitro on dispersed human mast cells.

No consistent abnormalities of complement activation have been demonstrated in EIA [17] though some reports have described isolated complement activation in individual patients [18,19].

It appears that a variety of physiological factors operative in exercise can induce mast cell degranulation or alter the threshold for degranulation. Such factors might include neuropeptides, endogenous opiates (endorphins), chemokines, and histamine releasing factors. Dimsdale and his colleagues have shown that although both norepinephrine and epinephrine levels are increased consequent to exercise, the response is significantly more marked for norepinephrine [20]. This norepinephrine-induced α-adrenergic response on mast cell mediator release may play a role in EIA. Fukutomi et al. have demonstrated increased parasympathetic nervous activity and reduced sympathetic nervous system response [21]. Collectively, these autonomic influences enhance mast cell release of mediators and therefore contribute to the pathogenesis of EIA. Fluxes in electrolyte gradients and alterations in cutaneous blood flow may also be contributory. Subjects in whom postprandial state is either prerequisite or contributory to the development of EIA may have either abnormal autonomic neuroregulation of vasomotor tone or aberrant neuropeptide homeostasis. It is important to note that neurokines influence mast cell function and gastrin has been shown to stimulate mediator release from human cutaneous mast cells [22].

Kivity et al. have suggested that in the development of food-associated EIA the interaction of food antigen and IgE might represent a subthreshold stimulus. This is augmented by the physiological alterations seen in exercise, and together they decrease the mast cell threshold for mediator release and consequent emergence of the clinical picture [23]. These authors performed skin testing using compound 48/80 (a direct mast cell degranulator) in subjects with food-associated (and skin prick test–positive) exercise-induced anaphylaxis. Food or exercise alone did not affect the dermal mast cell 48/80 wheal-and-flare response. However, an augmented wheal-and-flare response was observed with food intake plus exercise. These data suggest increased mast cell releasability caused by the combination of food plus exercise.

Thus, the pathogenesis of EIA is multifactorial, encompassing autonomic and neurohumoral vascular tone responses, abnormal mast cell mediator releasability potentiated in some patients by IgE-mediated reaction, as well as exercise-associated neurovascular responses.

DIFFERENTIAL DIAGNOSIS

The syndrome of exercise-associated characteristics such as cutaneous erythema, warmth, pruritus, and urticaria in conjunction with predominantly upper airway distress, and gastrointestinal colic with or without vascular collapse has been called EIA because of its similarity to classical features of IgE-mediated and mast cell–triggered anaphylaxis. Cardiac syndromes resulting from exercise cause angina, syncope, arrhythmias, palpitations, and even features of left ventricular failure but not pruritus, urticaria, angioedema, true airway obstruction, or gastrointestinal colic.

Exercise-induced asthma is characterized by cough (often in paroxysms), prominent wheezing, and clear evidence of airway obstruction on spirometry. These subjects do not manifest cutaneous warmth, erythema, urticaria, gastrointestinal colic, or vascular collapse. Though an occasional patient with EIA may demonstrate minimal alteration of the forced expiratory volume (FEV), these changes are minimal, transient, and not consistent.

Cholinergic urticaria needs to be differentiated from EIA as they both represent physical allergies, are temporally related to exercise, and have cutaneous manifestation. Table 1 highlights the differences between cholinergic urticaria and EIA.

Exercise challenge on a treadmill while wearing a plastic occlusive suit has been utilized for diagnostic purposes as well as for study of the mediator release phenomenon. One can use this technique to study and document the role of cofactors such as food-associated, postprandial, or medication-associated EIA [16].

Management of EIA

Emergency management of EIA is based on the same principles of therapy as are utilized for the treatment of anaphylaxis of any cause [24]: maintenance of patent airways, adequate oxygenation, ensuring of adequate and continued circulatory state, and tissue perfusion especially to the brain in states of shock, ensuring of adequate intravascular volume, and inhibition or antagonization of the effect of mediators at the tissue level. At the same time one should make sure that the offending stimuli are eliminated. The therapeutic measures in-

TABLE 1 The Difference Between Cholinergic Urticaria and Exercise-Induced Anaphylaxis

Clinical Features	Cholinergic Urticaria	Exercise-Induced Anaphylaxis
Characteristics of hives	Small, 1 to 3 mm punctate wheals, with surrounding erythematous flares; intensely pruritic	Larger initial hives, often coalesce
Lacrimation and salivation	May occur with hives	Not a feature
Headaches	Not a feature	Often present and protracted
Effect of elevation of core body temp., e.g., fever, hot bath, hot shower, or hyperthermic blanket	Consistently provokes hives and symptoms	Does not provoke hives or clinical features of EIA
Effect of stress/anxiety	May provoke hives	No effect
Effect of active exercise	Causes hives predictably; anaphylaxis extremely rare	Causes anaphylaxis but is variable; may require presence of cofactors
Upper airway involvement	Rare	Common
Lower airway involvement	Not uncommon	Exceedingly rare
Lung function test	May show mild to moderate and consistent airway obstruction	Rarely noted, transient, and inconsistent airway obstruction
Vascular collapse	Rarely seen and not a feature of syndrome	Commonly seen and a major feature of EIA
Role of food allergy	Not a factor	Food allergy possibly a cofactor
Type of mast cell degranulation	Zonal degranulation	Anaphylactic degranulation
Value of prophylactic H_1 and H_2 antagonists	Effective and valuable therapeutic modality	Inconsistent, ineffective, and not recommended as a routine

clude subcutaneous administration of epinephrine, intravenous fluid replacement, maintenance of airway patency even if it requires endotracheal intubation or tracheostomy, and oxygen therapy. Bronchospasm should be countered with inhaled β_2 agonist, antihistaminics help in blunting the severity of attacks. A bolus of intravenous steroid is mandatory to inhibit the effect of lipid mediators, promote microvascular integrity, and decrease effect of cytokines such as tumor necrosis factor α (TNF-α), which induce microvascular damage. Even though the occurrence of the late-phase reaction in human anaphylaxis is disputed, it is prudent to observe individuals closely for at least 12 hr or until such time as their circulatory status is stable, tissue perfusion is adequate, and there is no airway compromise [24].

Long-term management of EIA requires the delineation of the risk factors and cofactors in the causation of the syndrome and their avoidance. These include the following:

1. A thorough historical review and assessment of the chronological sequence of events. Particular attention is to be paid to evolution of hives, airway and gastrointestinal symptoms, and the precipitating situation such as hot showers, exercise, or ingestion of foods.
2. Antecedent use of alcohol, aspirin, or other medications such as beta blockers.
3. Environmental factors such as temperature and humidity.
4. Possible relationship to foods such as seafood, celery, wheat and other grains, nuts, and fruits. If indicated, prick skin tests are to be done to corroborate food allergy.
5. Relationship of EIA to the postprandial state.
6. In women any specific influence of the menstrual period on the emergence of EIA.

Since antihistamines do not appear to prevent EIA fully, their routine prophylactic use is not recommended. Occasionally antihistamines ameliorate the clinical picture, but this is a rarity. It is of utmost importance to educate patients on their prodromal symptoms so that exercise can be discontinued at the earliest warning sign. Modification of the affected individual's exercise regimen by reducing its duration or intensity may be required to prevent future episodes of EIA.

Individuals affected by EIA should be educated on the need to discontinue exercise at the earliest symptoms of pruritus or flushing. It will be ideal for these subjects to be accompanied by a companion or relative who is aware of the condition and capable of providing emergency assistance. Individuals with EIA should have a kit for self-administration of subcutaneous epinephrine at all times during exercise. They should wear a medical alert bracelet clearly defining a treatment protocol as well as depicting their diagnosis.

Once the trigger factors and conditions are well delineated and therapeutic strategies outlined, subjects with EIA should be able to exercise within the limits of their exercise-related mast cell degranulation.

REFERENCES

1. Sheffer AL, Tong AK, Murphy GF et al. Exercise-induced anaphylaxis: a serious form of physical allergy associated with mast cell degranulation. J Allergy Clin Immunol 1985; 75:4.
2. Matthews KP, Pan P. Post exercise hyperhistaminemia, dermographia and wheezing. Ann Intern Med 1970; 72:241.
3. Sheffer AL, Austen KF. Exercise-induced anaphylaxis. J Allergy Clin Immunol 1980; 66:106.
4. Wade JP, Liang MH, Sheffer AL. Exercise-induced anaphylaxis: epidemiologic observations. Prog Clin Biol Res 1989; 297:175.
5. Dohi M, Suko M, Sugiyama H et al. Food-dependent exercise-induced anaphylaxis: a study of 11 Japanese cases. J Allergy Clin Immunol 1991; 87:34.
6. Akutsu I, Motojima S, Ikeda Y et al. Three cases of food-dependent exercise-induced anaphylaxis. Arerugi 1989; 38:277.
7. Armentia A, Martin-Santos JM, Bianco M et al. Exercise-induced anaphylactic reaction to grain flours. Ann Allergy 1990; 65:149.
8. Buchbinder EM, Bloch KJ, Moss J et al. Food-dependent exercise-induced anaphylaxis. JAMA 1983; 250:2973.
9. McNeil D, Strauss RH. Exercise-induced anaphylaxis related to food intake. Ann Allergy 1988; 61:440.
10. Silverstein SR, Frommer DA, Dobozin B et al. Celery-dependent exercise-induced anaphylaxis. J Emerg Med 1986; 4:195.
11. Fink JN. Food plus exercise plus anaphylaxis: theories and challenge. Allergy Asthma Proc 1997; 18:249.
12. Caffarelli C, Cataldi R, Giordano S, Cavagni G. Anaphylaxis induced by exercise and related to multiple food intake. Allergy Asthma Proc 1997; 18:245.
13. Grant JA, Farnam J, Lord RA et al. Familial exercise-induced anaphylaxis. Ann Allergy 1985; 54:35.
14. Longley S, Panush RS. Familial exercise-induced anaphylaxis. Ann Allergy 1987; 58:287.
15. Casale TB, Keahey TM, Kaliner M. Exercise-induced anaphylactic syndromes: insights into diagnostic and pathophysiologic features. JAMA 1986; 255:2049.
16. Sheffer AL, Soter NA, McFadden ER, Jr. et al. Exercise-induced anaphylaxis: a serious form of physical allergy. J Allergy Clin Immunol 1983; 71:311.
17. Novey HS, Fairshter RD, Salness K et al. Postprandial exercise-induced anaphylaxis. J Allergy Clin Immunol 1983; 71:98.
18. Lewis J, Lieberman P, Treadwell G et al. Exercise-induced urticaria, angioedema and anaphylactoid episodes. J Allergy Clin Immunol 1981: 68:432.

19. Sheffer AL, Austen KF. Exercise-induced anaphylaxis: J Allergy Clin Immunol 1984; 73:69.
20. Dimsdale JE, Hartley LH, Guiney T et al. Post exercise peril: plasma cate-cholamines and exercise. JAMA 1984; 251:630.
21. Fukutomi O, Kondo N, Agata H et al. Abnormal responses of the autonomic nervous system in food-dependent exercise-induced anaphylaxis. Ann Allergy 1992; 68:438.
22. Tharp MD, Thirlby R, Sullivan TJ. Gastrin induces histamine release from human cutaneous mast cells. J Allergy Clin Imunnol 1984; 75:159.
23. Kivity S, Sneh E, Greif J et al. The effect of food and exercise on the skin response to compound 48/80 in patients with food-associated exercise-induced urticaria-angioedema. J Allergy Clin Immunol 1988; 81:1155.
24. Herrera AH, deShazo RD. Current concepts in anaphylaxis: pathophysiology, diagnosis and treatment. Immunol Allergy Clin North Am 1992; 12 (3):517.

16

Unusual Presentations

JOHN J. CONDEMI
University of Rochester, Rochester, New York

INTRODUCTION

Unusual presentation of food allergies can entail unexpected or hidden presentation of foods or unusual symptoms. This chapter deals with unusual symptoms; *unusual* is a relative term and can refer to the nature or frequency of symptoms. This chapter does not discuss mast cell–mediated symptoms such as urticaria, asthma, rhinitis, eczema, or gastrointestinal (GI) symptoms, which most allergists consider within their areas of expertise, but considers nonatopic symptoms. The techniques of food elimination and challenges with which these unusual symptoms are evaluated, however, are techniques with which allergists are familiar, and so the allergist may be called upon to evaluate or assist in the evaluation of symptoms or signs that normally are evaluated by other specialists. For allergists it is an opportunity to bring the scientific principles of food challenges to the attention of the medical community and may broaden the patient base. An example has been the acceptance of neurological symptoms, as exemplified by the inclusion of migraine in books dealing with adverse reactions to foods. The term *food* in this chapter includes both food and food additives.

Symptoms referable to every organ in the body have been attributed to foods. The public has an enormous interest in this subject and unfortunately is often driving by orthodox physicians to seek help from unqualified practitioners who may exploit their interest in this subject [1–4]. This chapter is not meant to be comprehensive, but to promote awareness of selected syndromes and the information that supports a relationship to foods so that you may be receptive to evaluating symptoms that patients suspect are food related.

In evaluating patients, one has to determine goals. In patients who have acute intermittent symptoms, one is more likely to effect a cure by finding a relationship to food than in chronic symptoms. Patients with chronic symptoms may have a preexisting disease in which foods are among the factors responsible for symptoms. An example would be aspirin-sensitive asthma. These patients continue to have symptoms from an underlying disease that may be aggravated by aspirin or nonsteroidal antiinflammatory agents. Patients are not interested in mechanisms but in the relationship of foods to symptoms. The techniques of food elimination to improve symptoms followed by double-blind, provocative food challenge can be applied to understand the relationship between food ingestion and symptoms, no matter what the mechanism.

SYSTEMIC LUPUS ERYTHEMATOSUS

In a study performed to determine whether alfalfa seed ingestion would be able to lower serum cholesterol level in humans, it was noted that in a previously healthy 59 year old man ingesting 80–160 g of ground alfalfa seeds daily after 5 months signs and laboratory abnormalities suggestive of systemic lupus erythematous (SLE) developed [5]. This patient experienced anemia, leukopenia, thrombocytopenia, and splenomegaly. Laboratory studies revealed direct and indirect micro-Coombs' and a positive antinuclear antibody (ANA) test results. Levels of antibodies to double-stranded deoxyribonucleic acid (DNA) were slightly elevated, and the total hemolytic complement assay was depressed. When alfalfa seeds were no longer ingested, the spleen size decreased to normal and results of serological and complement studies reverted to normal, with no recurrence of abnormal signs of laboratory tests. A relationship between alfalfa seed ingestion and SLE is further supported by the reports of two patients with SLE who noted reactivation of their systemic disease with both clinical and serological manifestations after the ingestion of 8–15 alfalfa tablets for a period of 9 months to $2\frac{1}{2}$ years [6].

Animal studies have also supported the ability of alfalfa sprouts to induce SLE [7]. In a blinded study in which alfalfa seeds or a normal diet was fed to 12 cynomolgus macaque monkeys, 2 of the 6 monkeys fed alfalfa seeds demonstrated a high-titer ANA result with a SLE-like illness, and a third had a high-titer ANA result without symptoms. The abnormalities that developed included hemolytic anemia, antinuclear antibodies, anti-DNA antibodies, positive LE cells, hypocomplementemia, immune complex–mediated glomerulonephritis, and deposition of immunoglobulin and complement in kidneys and skin at the epidermodermal junction. When the alfalfa sprouts were discontinued the clinical and serological abnormalities resolved. A year after the alfalfa sprouts were discontinued the 3 monkeys that had reacted were fed L-canavanine sulfate, a constituent of alfalfa sprouts, and the syndrome was reactivated [8]. On this occasion all the monkeys had symptoms and serological abnormalities of SLE that included splenomegaly and lymphadenopathy.

To explore further the significance of these observations in humans, sera from 35 patients with SLE, 28 with non-SLE rheumatic disorders, and 39 normal individuals were studied by immunodiffusion for antibodies to alfalfa seed extract, native DNA, denatured DNA, and rabbit thymus extract [9]. Of the 35 SLE sera, 11 (31%) and 1 of 39 (3%) normal individuals had precipitins demonstrating an immunoglobulin G antibody to the alfalfa extract. No precipitins were seen in patients with other rheumatic disorders. This precipitating antibody to alfalfa seed extract revealed lines of identity to both native DNA and thymus extract. These studies, therefore, support immunological identity among a component. present in alfalfa seeds, native DNA, and a thymus extract. This shared antigen may be L-canavanine, which is found in large concentrations in alfalfa seeds and germinating alfalfa seeds. It is one of the numerous nonprotein amino acids that occur in higher plants with structural similarities to components of mammalian proteins. The autoimmune phenomenon observed on eating alfalfa sprouts may therefore be the result of L-canavanine substituting for arginine in histone and thereby altering the DNA–nucleohistone complex to make it immunogenic. Another possibility is that there may be substitution of L-canavanine in the genome of certain cells in the immune system, thereby altering function and allowing autoantibody production. Although the mechanism by which the SLE syndrome is induced or activated is not known, it seems prudent that, at the present time, patients with SLE should not ingest large amounts of alfalfa tablets or bean sprouts. The degree of susceptibility, however, remains unknown, and whether this is a unique or a general phenomenon that is important in causing SLE is also unknown. Other food substances of concern in patients with SLE are psoralens, which increase photosensitivity, and hydrazines, which are felt to be responsible for drug-induced lupus. Foods containing these substances however, have not been associated with flares or induction of symptoms [10].

RHEUMATOID ARTHRITIS

Medical folklore has long suggested that there may be a relationship between foods and rheumatoid arthritis (RA). There are also a number of older medical articles that suggest that foods may exacerbate symptoms in patients with chronic arthritis [11–20]. These early reports, however, did not pay sufficient attention to classification of disease, appropriate controls, or blinded challenge techniques. In addition, the evaluation of symptoms was most often subjective, with no direct measurements and no serological data to classify the patients or to determine the effect of diet on serological characteristics. These preliminary reports have therefore had little credence in the medical community. Recently, however, reports have appeared that correct these deficiencies.

There are two case reports of patients in whom joint symptoms were documented in double-blind challenges to be related to food ingestion [21,22]. There are additional series in which symptoms improve when fasting or on diets [23–26]. Panush et al. studied a group of 26 patients with long-standing rheumatoid arthritis [25]. Of the 26 patients, 2, when placed on an experimental hypoallergenic diet for 10 weeks in a controlled, double-blinded randomized trial, improved sufficiently so that they elected to remain on the diet. This study, however, failed to provide evidence of overall clinical benefit in the remaining 24 patients. Further support that fasting is beneficial to patients with rheumatic disease comes from Sweden, where 16 patients with classic RA fasted for 7–10 days and were then placed on a special vegetarian diet for 9 weeks [24]. In this study, 10 RA patients acted as controls, taking a normal diet. Pain, stiffness, medication, and serological characteristics were measured before and during fasting and on the special diet. While fasting, 10 of 16 patients noted relief of pain, and 5 of these 10 had objective improvement. In the controls who did not fast, only 1 of 10 noted relief of pain. Of the fasting patients 2 dropped out of the study, and the remaining 14 continued on the special vegetarian diet. While on the diet, only 1 of the 14 patients had continued significant improvement in both subjective and objective parameters. None of the controls had objective improvement. The authors conclude that "although the special diet may be of benefit to a few patients with RA, they were unable to select parameters that would allow identification of these exceptional patients." To evaluate further the role of special diets Haugen studied an unselected group of patients with rheumatoid factor–positive RA [26]. Ten received an elemental diet and 7 a control soup containing milk, meat, fish, shellfish, orange, pineapple, tomatoes, peas, wheat, and corn. Improvement was noted in all the measured disease variables in 3 on the elemental and 2 on the control diet.

Double-blind placebo-controlled challenges were performed in a patient who fulfilled the criteria for RA, and because of side effects of gold, penicillamine, and azathioprine and a poor response to salicylates required 10 mg prednisone daily with only partial control of her arthritis [21]. She consumed large amounts of cheese daily and was not aware of any relationship of symptoms to the ingestion of milk or milk products. After discontinuation of milk and milk products for 3 weeks, definite improvement was noted in grip strength, morning stiffness, and walking time. Improvement was noted for 10 months on the milk-free diet with discontinuation of prednisone when she was challenged with milk. At 12 to 24 hr after the challenge, enlargement of joint size, decreased grip strength, and increased pain developed. Laboratory tests revealed a leukocytosis, presence of circulating immune complexes, and a positive radioallergosorbent test (RAST) result for immunoglobulin E (IgE) antibody to milk and cheese. The clearance of heat-damaged red blood cells was normal while avoiding dairy products but became considerably prolonged when tested 2 and 14 days after the challenge. This observation is noted when large amounts of immune complexes are believed to saturate the phagocytic system, thereby preventing the further removal of immune complexes and antibody-coated or heat-damaged red blood cells.

In a highly selective group of 43 patients alleging food-related symptoms, with classic rheumatoid arthritis studied in three hospital centers, a water fast under controlled environmental conditions improved seven parameters of arthritis activity [27,28]. These patients noted improvement in joint tenderness, joint swelling, grip strength, dolorimeter pain index, proximal interphalangeal joint circumference, functional activity index, and sedimentation rate. Of these patients, 27 were subsequently challenged with foods, and a statistically significant loss of grip strength, increased joint measurement, and pain was noted in 22 patients with selected foods [28]. In this study, corn, wheat, and animal proteins reacted more frequently and intensely than fruits and vegetables. To confirm food-related rheumatic symptoms Panush identified 16 patients who alleged food-related arthritis [29]. Nineteen double-blind controlled food challenges were performed and 3 subjects demonstrated subjective and objective rheumatic symptoms. The three were asymptomatic when receiving elemental nutrition or avoiding the offending food. The incriminated foods were milk, shrimp, and nitrates. One was a previously reported milk-sensitive patient [22]. All 3 were seronegative with nonerosive disease and palindromic symptoms. IgG, IgG_4, A, M, and E levels; Ig food immune complexes; food skin tests; and in vitro cellular reactivity to foods were not able to distinguish these patients from challenge-negative or other patients with rheumatic diseases who did not suspect food-related arthritis.

In a larger study Van-de-Laar studied 94 patients utilizing an elemental allergen-free or allergen-restricted liquid supplement diet containing lactoproteins and yellow dyes [30]. Subjective and objective improvement was noted in 9 (3 allergy-restricted, 6 allergen-free group) followed by disease exacerbation during rechallenge.

It is obvious that at the present time further studies are necessary to clarify the role of foods in arthritis. It appears that less than 5% of patients have food-related symptoms so that studying unselected cases is not cost-effective and may cause patients to emphasize diet and ignore medical treatment. In selected rheumatoid factor– (RF)-positive patients who suspect foods as a cause of the disorder it appears that starvation or severe diet manipulation is more important than the type of diet. These diet manipulations are severe in that patients are limited to liquids as the only food source. From the limited studies by Panush there may be an even smaller subset of patients who have intermittent symptoms, are rheumatoid factor–negative, and have nonerosive arthritis [29]. These patients appear to have symptoms related to a limited number of specific foods. At present there are no other markers except history to select patients for diet manipulation. It is important that orthodox practitioners be prepared to evaluate and advise patients so as to prevent discontinuation of necessary medicines and severe life-style changes often recommended by unorthodox health practitioners.

In addition to these clinical studies, animal studies have reported that ingested food is capable of producing RA-like joint lesions [31]. In three of six rabbits drinking cow's milk, clinical arthritis and synovitis developed. Histological examination of the synovium revealed a mononuclear cell infiltration. In another animal model, 8 week old pigs were fed a protein-rich diet [32]. In the first week after the diet there were disturbance of movement and swollen peripheral joints. During the second week an elevation of the sedimentation rate and hypergammaglobulinemia were present. Joint deformities similar to those of RA were observed after several months. The examination of joints revealed pannis formation with joint cartilage erosion and a lymphocytic infiltrate. In some animals subcutaneous rheumatoid nodules, abnormal urine sediment, and a proliferative glomerulonephritis also developed. The authors concluded that the protein-rich diet resulted in an abnormal intestinal flora consisting of *Clostridium perfringens* and that these pigs had an immune complex–mediated disease with the antigen being the bowel *Clostridium* species.

It is my belief that there are a few patients in whom diet manipulation will offer significant improvement in the underlying disease. In none of the studies demonstrating efficacy was it suggested that the food was the only cause or a cause of the chronic synovitis. In those studies in which there was improvement of symptoms, it was noted that the effect of diet can be demonstrated best in patients with milder disease. In patients with severe deforming arthritis it was less helpful. The cause of RA remains unknown. It is assumed that the pathophysiological characteristics of RA relate to a persistent immunological response of a genetically susceptible host to relevant antigens. An infectious agent seems most probable, but a food may be important in some individuals. The inflammatory response is felt to be T cell–driven with immune complex formation and activation of the complement cascade contributing to tissue injury. Immune complexes have been demonstrated in the serum in response to dietary materials in atopic and IgA-deficient patients [33–35]. Immune complexes have also been demonstrated in the serum of patients having intestinal bypass surgery for malignant obesity [36]. The immune complexes noted in these patients have been demonstrated to contain bacterial rather than food antigens. Other mechanisms that may induce an exacerbation of an inflammatory arthritis include the activation of prostaglandins by food materials and the release of serotonin from platelets [37]. It should be emphasized that there is more evidence for a beneficial role of fasting or severe diet manipulations in RA than for specific foods' inducing symptoms. In the fasting state many physiological events occur that may decrease inflammation and are independent of the ability of foods to induce symptoms. These same physiological events may occur with the liquid food formulas used in some studies. One should therefore not accept improvement in any symptoms that occurs with fasting to mean that a patient is food-"allergic." The proof of food-related symptoms necessitates the production of symptoms with eating specific foods administered blindly to the patient. As noted, in some studies, improvement continues even when patients have resumed their normal diet.

SCLERODERMALIKE SYNDROME (TOXIC OIL SYNDROME)

An epidemic of an illness involving multiple organ systems began in Spain in May 1981 with 19,828 cases and 315 deaths reported by June 1, 1982. An epidemiological investigation has linked the occurrence of the illness with ingestion of an unlabeled, illegally marketed cooking oil [38,39]. The clinical manifestations following the ingestion of this cooking oil involved multiple organs at different times after ingestion. The variety of clinical features underscores the role that environmental factors may play in the causation of human disease.

Early Phase

During the week following ingestion, patients experienced fever, chills, headache, tachycardia, cough, chest pain, and pruritus. On physical examination, various types of skin exanthema, splenomegaly, and generalized adenopathy were noted. The most common laboratory abnormality was pulmonary infiltrates, which were reported in 84% of the patients. Infiltrates were characterized as either interstitial or alveolar. The acute lung disorder of this phase was thought to be due to increased capillary permeability as a result of an endothelial lesion induced by something in the cooking oil.

Intermediate Phase

The intermediate phase began about the second week and persisted through the eighth week. This phase of the illness was characterized by the predominance of gastrointestinal symptoms and a marked eosinophilia in 42% of patients. The patients complained of abdominal pain, nausea, diarrhea, odynophagia, and dysphagia; physical examination often revealed hepatomegaly. Other abnormal laboratory results included high IgE levels, thrombocytopenia, and abnormal results of coagulation studies. In addition, some of the patients had evidence of hepatic dysfunction with abnormal enzymes, and a few became jaundiced.

Late Phase

The late phase occurred in 23% of cases and developed after 2 months of illness. This phase was characterized initially by neuromuscular and joint involvement but later by vasculitis and a sclerodermalike syndrome [40,41]. During this phase, patients complained of intense muscular pain, edema, and progressive muscular weakness that was more severe distally. In some of the patients who had severe atrophy of the proximal muscle groups, contractures developed as well. Neurological involvement included depressed or absent deep tendon reflexes, anesthesia, and dysesthesia. Ventilatory insufficiency occurred as a result of neuromuscular weakness. Late pulmonary manifestations included pulmonary hypertension and thromboembolic phenomena. The sclerodermalike manifestations included Raynaud's phenomenon, sicca syndrome, dysphagia, and contractures due to thickening of collagen in the skin. Pathological studies in this group revealed an eosinophilic fibrositis with vasculitis-type lesions. These vascular lesions were found in all organs of the body at postmortem studies. The predominant reasons for vascular obstruction, however, were endothelial proliferation and thrombosis rather than a necrotizing vasculitis. The muscular lesions of the late phase were characterized as due to atrophy caused by denervation with an intense fibrosis of the muscle. All patients in the late group had antinuclear antibody, and about half of the group had antibodies against smooth muscle and skeletal muscle [42]. Synovial biopsy revealed a lymphocytic plasma cell infiltration that was predominantly perivascular with thickening of the synovial membrane. The pathological and clinical features were compatible with those of such autoimmune diseases as graft-versus-host disease and systemic sclerosis. The development of glomerulonephritis was evidence for a role of immune complexes. Electron microscopy studies demonstrated a "lumpy bumpy" electron-dense deposit with glomerular basement membranes. These findings suggest that the late phase of the disease may be the result of autoimmune phenomena.

Cause

There is almost conclusive epidemiological evidence that this syndrome was due to oil purchased from itinerant vendors. Female patients with HLA-DR-3 and DR-4 antigens seem to be at an increased risk [43]. This oil contained oils from both plant and animal sources, but present evidence would indicate that the major toxin either was present in rapeseed oil or was rapeseed aniline that was not removed by treatment. The identity of the substances causing the disease, however, is unknown [44]. Unfortunately, feeding this oil to animals did not induce the disease so no experimental model exists. We therefore do not know the source or the identity of the substances causing the disease. The prevailing theory is that free radicals from aniline derivatives react with fatty acids, resulting in endothelial and vascular damage. The role of the elevated levels of IgE, circulating immune complexes, and antinuclear antibodies in the late phase is unclear but suggests that this phase may be related to an autoimmune phenomenon. As long as the precise cause of the disease remains undiscovered, no assurance can be given that it will not happen again or that this toxin, if present in small amounts in our oils, may be producing or aggravating such syndromes as scleroderma or vasculitis. Discovering this material may therefore have much broader implications than the prevention of further epidemics.

Vasculitis

Food hypersensitivity has been implicated as causing vasculitis in several anecdotal reports. Syndromes resembling Schönlein-Henoch purpura were first reported by Osler in 1914 [45]. Since Osler these have been reports of single cases due to crab and fish and larger series of 6 and 23 patients implicating egg, milk, chocolate, wheat, and beans [46–49].

Other authors have reported vasculitis manifesting as urticaria, erythema multiforme, or palpable petechia with positive skin biopsy results for leukocytoclastic vasculitis in relation to foods or food additives [51–53]. Panush and Bahna reported a 23 month old girl with arthritis, fever, skin vasculitis, and rectal bleeding in whom symptoms appeared to be related to ingestion of chocolate. Skin testing with foods including chocolate had negative results, [54]. Wuthrich reported 1 case of urticarial vasculitis provoked by sodium metabisulfite and petechiael vasculitis provoked by 500 mg of benzoic acid and 35 mg of tartrazine yellow. Both cases had positive biopsy results for leukocytoclastic vasculitis [53].

In order to determine whether a food or food additive is the cause of vasculitis one must first obtain a biopsy sample to confirm the diagnosis of vasculitis. Suspicion of the relationship to food or food additives can be aroused by history but requires confirmation by either a single- or double-blind placebo-controlled oral provocation test when the vasculitis has resolved by avoiding the food. It should be noted that although the number of foods reported is large, in an individual case, only one or two at the most have been associated with symptoms. The ultimate proof of the relationship between foods and vasculitis awaits the demonstration of the food antigen in the immune complexes that have been demonstrated in vessel walls. These types of studies have been performed in hepatitis B–induced and bacteria-induced vasculitis. From the information we have available to us, it seems that food-related vasculitis is rare and until the definitive studies concerning localization of antigen are performed there will be skepticism among physicians.

COW'S MILK

Other sections in this chapter are related to symptoms; the variety of manifestations resulting from the ingestion of cow's milk warrant separate discussion of this food. The first report of an adverse reaction to cow's milk was that by Hippocrates (460–370 B.C.), who described gastric upset and urticaria due to the ingestion of cow's milk [51]. Reports remained sporadic until the introduction of infant formulas made of cow's milk in the twentieth century. With that event, there have appeared a large number of articles relating adverse reactions to milk. In this section I deal with reactions that are unusual but reasonably well documented in order to expand the reader's views concerning adverse reactions to food.

Dermatitis Herpetiformis

The ingestion of cow's milk appeared to be the cause of dermatitis herpetiformis in a 30 year old women who experienced an idiopathic malabsorption syndrome for 3 years [56]. When the patient was placed on a gluten-free and milk-free diet, both the malabsorption and skin improved. After ingestion of milk, gastrointestinal symptoms recurred with typical dermatitis herpetiformis skin lesions. The syndrome could be repeatedly improved with avoidance and precipitated by the introduction of milk. No immunological studies were performed on this patient, but in view of the evidence for antibody-mediated injury in gluten-induced enteropathy and dermatitis herpetiformis, it is not unreasonable to suspect the same mechanism when milk is the food capable of inducing the syndrome [57].

Thrombocytopenia

There are three cases of thrombocytopenia related to milk ingestion: two cases of thrombocytopenia occurring in the newborn [58,59] and the third in an adult [60]. Purpura was the presenting symptom in one newborn and the other had bloody diarrhea. In both cases platelet counts returned to normal on a nonmilk formula, and the thrombocytopenia could be produced by the introduction of cow's milk. In one case the milk could be reinstituted without thrombocytopenia after 9 months of age. Thrombocytopenia has also been reported in an older individual in whom the platelet count returned to normal on a milk-free diet and symptoms and signs of thrombocytopenia could be induced by the introduction of milk into the diet. Food as an inducer of thrombocytopenia was suspected in only 0.7% of 433 cases [61]. This manifestation as a result of an adverse reaction to food must therefore be considered a rare event. When the reaction occurs with quinine-induced thrombocytopenia, the mechanism is thought to be an innocent bystander reaction. The immune complex formed by quinine and antiquinine antibodies adheres to platelets, resulting in immune elimination [62]. The mechanism by which milk induces thrombocytopenia is unknown.

Renal Involvement

Matsumura et al. demonstrated in 16 cases that orthostatic albuminuria could result from hypersensitivity to foods, and in 12 of these patients cow's milk was the incriminated allergen [63]. Sandburgh et al. studied six patients with idiopathic nephrotic syndrome in childhood whose renal disease was steroid-responsive [64]. Of the six, five had a positive history for asthma and/or eczema, and all patients had positive intradermal reactions to milk. In all patients, proteinuria was significantly reduced without corticosteroid on a milk-free diet. With an open oral challenge with 1 ounce of cow's milk, there are a significant increase in proteinuria and a decrease in urine output. During the challenge, four patients had a decrease in serum IgG level and in all six patients there was evidence for complement activation with a decrease in the total C_3 levels. When milk was eliminated from the diet, remissions occurred in 3–10 days. Siemawska evaluated milk protein intolerance in 17 steroid-resistant children with nephrotic syndrome [65]. Six patients with minimal change or mesangial proliferation went into remission after eliminating cow's milk. These patients had coexisting allergic symptoms and the three who were skin tested to cow's milk protein had negative findings, I have observed an additional case of proteinuria aggravated by milk ingestion in a patient with IgA antibody to milk proteins. This patient had diabetic renal disease as the primary cause of her proteinuria, but the proteinuria decreased from 4 to 1 g per 24 hr on a milk-free diet and increased with milk challenges. The suspected mechanism in these cases is most likely the production of immune complexes, although Siemawska felt there was a cellular mechanism in his patients because of a positive leukocyte migration inhibition test finding. To investigate whether patients with IgA nephropathy have an exaggerated serum IgA response to food antigens, Fornasieri measured serum IgA antibodies to gliadin ovalbumin, bovine serum albumin (BSA), β-lactoglobulin, and casein in 170 patients and 53 normal controls [66]. No significant differences were observed between patients and controls in serum Ig antibodies or IgG immune complexes. Nine patients but no controls had IgA antibodies to two or more food antigens and all had IgA immune complexes versus 24% in the controls. This subgroup of patients had anti-bodies to BSA, suggesting that these antibodies are involved in the formation of the immune complex. No dietary manipulations were performed to determine whether BSA is a clinically relevant antigen. One wonders whether these cases are extremely rare and why nephrologists have not considered the role of food ingestion in more patients with proteinuria.

Diabetes

The cause of insulin-dependent diabetes mellitus (IDDM) is multifactorial. The final cause is the destruction of the islet beta cells by autoimmune processes that operate in individuals of certain genetic backgrounds in response to external trig-gering factors such as virus infections and dietary factors. Among the latter, cow's milk protein, particularly BSA, may be important. Elevated levels of IgG anti-BSA antibodies were found in children from Finland and France with new onset of diabetes [63]. Finland has the highest incidence in the world and France a low incidence of diabetes and cow's milk consumption. A relation between di-abetes and consumption of cow's milk is also supported by animal studies. Elim-ination of intact cow's milk proteins from the diet significantly reduced the incidence of IDDM in the spontaneously diabetic rat. In addition there are in-creased levels of antibodies to cow's milk protein in newly discovered diabetic rats when compared to nondiabetic controls. In both rats and children the rele-vant antibody appears to be directed against BSA. Antibodies to BSA cross-react with a 69K beta cell membrane protein. At the molecular level a region of the BSA has distinct homology to the 69K beta cell membrane protein [68]. These studies support an immunological role of BSA in diabetic autoimmunity and may offer unique treatment opportunities by techniques capable of inducing tol-erance to peptides.

CONCLUSION

It is hoped that there are sufficient examples in this chapter to emphasize how lit-tle is known concerning the mechanism of food-induced signs or symptoms. In view of this ignorance, it behooves the physician to listen to the patient who is concerned about the relationship of foods to symptoms and attempt to assist the patient by appropriate testing to determine whether the symptom is due to the in-gestion of food. Although the mechanism of the reaction is of prime importance to the physician, to the patient, improvement of symptoms indicates that the physician has performed his or her role as a healer. It also should be recognized that in most situations, there will be no relationship of symptoms to foods, but the patient will appreciate this information as much as a positive correlation with food ingestion.

REFERENCES

1. Altman DR, Chiaramonte LT. Public perception of food allergy. J Allergy Clin Immunol 1996; 97:1247–1251.
2. Young E, Patel S, Stoneham M et al. The prevalence of reaction to food additives in a survey population. J R Coll Physicians London 1987; 21:241–247.
3. Mandell M, Waller-Scanlon L. Dr. Mandell's Five Day Allergy Relief System. New York: Thomas Y. Crowell, 1979.
4. Crook WG. The Yeast Connection. Jackson, TN: Tennessee Professional Books, 1984.
5. Malinow MR, Bardana EJ, Goodnight SH. Pancytopenia during ingestion of alfalfa seeds. Lancet 1981; 1:615.
6. Roberts, J.L., and Hayashi, J.A. Exacerbation of SLE associated with alfalfa (letter to the editor). N Engl J Med 1983; 308:1361.
7. Malinow MR, Bardana EJ, Pirofsky B. Systemic lupus erythematosus-like syndrome induced by diet in monkeys. Clin Res 1981; 29:6–6a.
8. Bardana EJ, Pirofsky B, Craig S. Systemic lupus erythematosus-like syndrome in monkeys fed alfalfa sprouts: role of a non-protein amino acid. Science 1982; 216:415–417.
9. Bardana EJ, Malinow B, Craig S, McLaughlin P. Cross-reacting antibody to alfalfa seed and desoxyribonucleic acid in SLE part 2. J Allergy Clin Immunol 1983; 71:102.
10. Steinberg AD, moderator. Systemic lupus erythematosus. Ann Intern Med 1991; 115:548–559.
11. Joseffson E, Landahl DE, Myvnerts R. Dietary treatment of rheumatoid arthritis. Excerpta Medica, 299, 13th International Congress of Rheumatology (suppl 39):10, 1973.
12. Cook RA. Hay fever and asthma. NY Med J 1918; 107:477–583.
13. Talbot EB. Role of food idiosyncrasies in practice. NY State J Med 1917; 17:419–425.
14. Tornbull JA. The relationship of anaphylactic disturbances to arthritis. JAMA 1924; 18:1757–1759.
15. Tornbull JA. Changes in sensitivity to allergenic foods in arthritis. J Dig Dis 1944; 15:182–190.
16. Pottenger RT. Constitutional factors in arthritis with special reference to incidents and role of allergic disease. Ann Intern Med 1928; 12:323–333.
17. Zeller M. Rheumatoid arthritis: food allergy as a factor. Ann Allergy 1949; 7:200–239.
18. Kaufman W. Food-induced allergic musculoskeletal syndromes. Ann Allergy 1953; 11:179–184.
19. Sussman BM. Food hypersensitivity stimulating rheumatoid arthritis. South Med J 1966. 59:935–939.
20. Millman M. An allergic concept of the etiology of rheumatoid arthritis. Ann Allergy 1972. 30:135–141.
21. Parke AL, Hughes GRV. Rheumatoid arthritis and food: a case study. Br Med J 1981; 282:2027–2029.

22. Panush RS, Stroud RM, Webster EM. Food induced (allergic) arthritis. Arthritis Rheum 1986; 29:220.

23. Panush RS, Stroud RM, Webster EM. Food induced (allergic) arthritis: clinical and serologic studies. Arthritis Rheum 1986; 29 (suppl):5–33.

24. Skoldstan L, Larsson L, Lindstrom FD. Effects of fasting and lacto vegetarian diet on rheumatoid arthritis. Scand. J. Rheum. 1979; 8:249–255.

25. Panush RS, Carter RL, Katz P, Kowsari B, Longley S, Finne S. Diet therapy for rheumatoid arthritis. Arthritis Rheum 1983; 26:462–471.

26. Au Haugen MA, Kjeldsen-Kragh J, Forre O. A Pilot study of the effect of an elemental diet in the management of rheumatoid arthritis. Clin Exp Rheumatol 1994; 12:275–279.

27. Marshall RT, Stroud RM, Kroker GF. The effects of food challenges on rheumatoid arthritis after fasting. 3rd International Food Allergy Symposium, Boston, Massachusetts, 1980.

28. Stroud RM. The effect of fasting followed by specific food challenge on rheumatoid arthritis. Current Topics in Rheumatology. Hahn BH, Arnett FC, Zizic TM, Hochberg MC, eds. Upjohn, 1983, pp 145–157.

29. Panush RS. Food induced "allergic" arthritis: clinical and serologic studies. J Rheumatol 1990; 17:291–294.

30. Van-de-Laar MA, Aalbers M, Bruin SF et al. Food intolerance in rheumatoid arthritis. Ann Rheum Dis 1992; 5:303–306.

31. Coombs RA, Oldham G. Early rheumatoid-like joint lesion in rabbits drinking cow's milk. Int Arch Appl Immunol 1981; 64:287–292.

32. Norberg G, Mansson R, Olhagen B, Bjorklund NE. Arthritis in pigs induced by dietary factors. J Exp Med 1971; 9:677–693.

33. Laphnelli R, Levinsky RJ, Brostoff J, Wraith DG. Immune complexes containing food proteins in normal and atopic subjects after oral challenge and effect of sodium chromoglycate on antigen absorption. Lancet 1979; 1:1270–1272.

34. Brostoff J, Carini C, Wraith DG, Johns P. Production of IgE complexes by allergen challenge in atopic patients and the effect of sodium chromoglycate. Lancet 1979; 1:268–270.

35. Cunningham-Rundels C, Brandeis WE, Good RA, Day NK. Milk precipitins, circulating immune complexes and IgA deficiency. Proc Natl Acad Sci USA 1978; 75:3387–3389.

36. Hallberg D, Nilsson BS, Blackman L. Immunologic function in patients operated on with small intestinal shunts for morbid obesity. Scand J Gastroimmunol 1976; 11:41–48.

37. Little CH, Stewart AG, Fennessy MR. Platelet serotonin release in rheumatoid arthritis: a study in food intolerant patients. Lancet 1983; 1:297–299.

38. Kilbourne EM, Rigau-Perez JG, Heath CW, Jr., Zack MN, Falk H, Martin-Marcos M, DeCarlos A. Clinical epidemiology of toxic oil syndrome: manifestations of a new illness. N Engl J Med 1983; 309:1408–1414.

39. Noriega AR, Gomez-Reino J, Lopez-Encuentra AL. Toxic epidemic syndrome, Spain 1981. Lancet 1982; 2:697–702.

40. Gilsan ZV. Late features of toxic syndrome due to denatured rapeseed oil. Lancet 1982; 1:335–336.
41. Isquierdo M, Fernandez-Dapica MP, Navas J, Cabello A, Gomez-Reino JL. Toxic epidemic syndrome musculoskeletal manifestations. J Rheum 1984; 2:333–338.
42. Rodriguez M, Nogura AE, DelVillaras S, Vegazo S, Mulero J, Cruz J, Larrea A. Toxic synovitis from denatured rapeseed oil. Arthritis Rheum 1982; 25:1477–1480.
43. Vicaro JL, Serrano-Rios M, San Andres F. HLA DR3, DR4 increase in chronic stage of toxic oil syndrome. Lancet 1982; 1:276.
44. Tabuenca JM. Toxic oil syndrome. Lancet 1983; 1:1257–1258.
45. Osler W. The visceral lesions of purpura and allied conditions. Br Med J 1914; 1:517–525.
46. Alexander HL, Eyermann CH. Allergic purpura. JAMA 1929; 92:2092–2094.
47. Ancona GR, Ellenhorn MJ, Falconer EH. Purpura due to food sensitivity: use of skin testing in etiological diagnosis. J Allergy 1951; 22:487–493.
48. Jensen B. Schonlein-Henoch's purpura. Acta Med Scand 1955; 152:61–70.
49. Ackroyd JF. Allergic purpura including purpura due to foods, drugs and infections, Am J Med 1953; 14:605–632.
50. Robinson BWS. Schonlein-Henoch purpura due to food sensitivity. Br Med J 1977; 1:510–511.
51. Harkavy J. Vascular Allergy and Its Systemic Manifestations. Washington, DC: Butterworth's, 1963.
52. Lunardi C, Bombara LM, Biasi D et al. Elimination diet in the treatment of selected patients with hypersensitivity vasculitis. Clin Exp Rheumatol 1992; 10:131–135.
53. Wuthrich B. Adverse reactions to food additives. Ann Allergy 1993; 71:379–384.
54. Panush RS, Bahna SL. Connective tissue reactions to foods. In MetcalFe Food Sampson Simon eds. Allergy. Boston: Blackwell Scientific, 382–391, 1991.
55. Chabot R. Pediatric Allergy. New York: McGraw-Hill, 1951.
56. Pock-Stein OC, Niordso AN. Milk sensitivity in dermatitis herpetiformis. Br J Dermatol 1970; 83:614–619.
57. Strober W, Falchuk SM, Rogentine GN, Nelson D, Kleasvemen HL. The pathogenesis of gluten sensitivity enteropathy. Ann Intern Med 1975; 83:242–256.
58. Whitfield MF, Barr DGD. Cow's milk allergy in the syndrome of thrombocytopenia with absent radius. Arch Dis Child 1976; 51:337–343.
59. Jones RHT. Congenital thrombocytopenia with milk allergy. Arch Dis Child 1977; 52:744–745.
60. Caffrey EA, Sladen GE, Isaacs PET, Clark KGA. Thrombocytopenia caused by cow's milk. Lancet 1981; 2:316.
61. Cohn J. Thrombocytopenia in childhood: an evaluation of 433 patients. Scand J Hematol 1976; 16:226–240.
62. Ackroyd JF. The immunologic basis of purpura due to drug hypersensitivity. Proc R Soc Med 1962; 55:30–36.
63. Matsumura T, Kuroume T, Matsuian L. Therapy of the nephrotic syndrome by and elimination diets. Proceedings of the 13th International Congress of Pediatrics 1971; 41:56.

64. Sandberg DH, Bernstein CW, McIntosh RM, Carr R. Severe steroid responsive nephroses associated with hypersensitivity. Lancet 1977; 1:388–399.
65. Siemawska M, Szymanik-Grzelak H, Kowalewska M. The role of cow's milk protein intolerance in steroid resistant nephrotic syndrome. Acta Paediatr 1992; 81:1007–1012.
66. Fornasieri A, Sinico RA, Maldifassi P et al. Nephrol Transplant 1988; 3:738–743.
67. Levy-Marchal C, Karjalainen J, Dubois F et al. Antibodies against bovine albumin and other diabetic markers in French children. Diabetic Care 1995; 18: 1089–1094.
68. Martin JM, Trink B, Daneman D et al. Milk proteins in the etiology of insulin dependent diabetes mellitus. Ann Med 1991; 23:447–452.

17

Psychological Manifestations in Idiopathic Environmental Intolerance (Foods)

HERMAN STAUDENMAYER
Behavioral Medicine & Biofeedback Clinic of Denver, Denver, Colorado

JOHN C. SELNER
University of Colorado Health Sciences Center, Denver, Colorado

INTRODUCTION

Idiopathic food intolerances are commonly presented as explanations for a variety of multisystem, general malaise symptoms. The attribution of these symptoms to foods has underlying issues and considerations parallel to the general problem of unsubstantiated complaints attributed to environmental intolerances. In February 1996, a World Health Organization (WHO) Workshop, Multiple Chemical Sensitivities, was conducted in Berlin, there, invited experts exchanged ideas, arrived at conclusions, and made recommendations to WHO and the International Program on Chemical Safety (IPCS) [1]. Although the conclusions and recommendations of the IPCS/WHO Workshop represent the opinions of the experts and not necessarily the decisions or the stated policy of WHO or any other international organization, they are germane to this chapter.

Unexplained Phenomena

The members of the ICPS/WHO Workshop drew the following conclusions:

> The term "Multiple Chemical Sensitivities (MCS)" should be discontinued because it makes an unsupported judgement on causation. A more appropriate descriptor is Idiopathic Environmental Intolerances (IEI). This term incorporates a number of disorders sharing similar symptomatologies, including what is described as "MCS". To reflect the diversity of unsubstantiated attributions to low-level environmental agents including foods, chemicals, and electromagnetic forces, the panel concluded that the descriptor may be modified by the putative origin of the disorder, e.g., IEI (food). A working definition of IEI is that it is:
>
> An acquired disorder with multiple recurrent symptoms
> Associated with diverse environmental factors tolerated by the majority of people
> Not explained by any known medical or psychiatric/psychological disorder
>
> Clinical assessment should be designed to rule out conditions requiring specific therapy. Appropriate evaluation should be based on a biopsychosocial understanding of the patient. This involves history, physical examination, psychological/psychiatric assessment, and laboratory testing designed to identify explanatory conditions. This is essential to avoid misdiagnosis of conditions that require specific treatments.

Double-Blind Placebo-Controlled Studies

The members of the IPCS/WHO workshop also drew other conclusions:

> Human research is urgently needed to determine the nature (e.g. psychogenic, toxicogenic) of IEI since the outcome will influence public policy and clinical practice for IEI prevention and treatment, respectively. The key question is whether subjects with IEI are able to discriminate in double-blind placebo-controlled studies between reported environmental (e.g., chemical [food]) triggers and placebos. Ability to discriminate suggests a toxicological (i.e., chemical-receptor) mechanism. Inability to discrimi-

nate would suggest a psychogenic (e.g., conditioned or other learned) mechanism.

The history of food allergy/sensitivity and the scientific literature on provocation challenges with foods serve as valuable sources to illustrate the issues and considerations of the members of the ICPS/WHO Workshop, [2], as illustrated by the following case study.

Case Report

The patient was a middle-aged woman who complained of IEI (foods) and reported multisystem, general malaise complaints including cognitive dysfunction and incapacitating fatigue. The severity of her illness was such that she could not function on the job and was granted disability leave. Her belief system was centered on her illness, the cause and exacerbation of which were attributed to food intolerances, leaving her incapacitated for days after a "reaction." Among the foods she reported intolerance to was soy, which was selected for a double-blind placebo-controlled study.

In addition to the symptom report, neurophysiological measurements were recorded, including galvanic skin response, peripheral finger temperature, and a 19 channel quantitative electroencephalogram (QEEG; Neurolex-24 system), which was monitored under eyes closed conditions throughout the study. At all other times, the patient had her eyes open. Baseline physiological measurements and QEEG recordings of 20 seconds duration were taken 20 minutes and immediately before food ingestion. On the first trial, placebo capsules filled with inert Fuller's earth were ingested at 9:50 A.M. For the first 3 hr after ingestion, symptom self-report was recorded every 20 minutes, and 20 second samples of QEEG were recorded. After that, symptoms and QEEG were recorded at 1 hr intervals for an additional 2 hr.

The results indicated that the patient reported a "reaction" with increased symptoms at 60 minutes post ingestion consisting of postnasal drip, lightheadedness, and nausea. She showed overt behavior indicating pain and requested a blanket and a pail in the event she might vomit (she did not vomit). Symptoms reached a maximum rating at 80 minutes and returned to baseline levels at 140 minutes. The QEEGs during baseline and all but one of the recordings throughout the 5 hour study showed consistent bimodal alpha frequencies with peaks in bands of 7.0–9.5 Hz and 9.6–12.0 Hz, symmetrical across hemispheres. The one exception occurred at 60 minutes after ingestion, during the time she reported symptoms, when the QEEG showed a suppression of alpha magnitude in the posterior regions. Alpha suppression reflects neurophysiological activation, which may be associated with increased attentional hyperactivity.

The galvanic skin response was extremely active during baseline, reflecting sympathetic nervous system arousal associated with anxiety. The galvanic skin response remained active up to 2 hr into the study, at which time it reached home-ostatic levels more characteristic of relaxation. The peripheral finger temperature was cool throughout the initial 3 hr of the study, starting at 75°F, consistent with a stress response. At the 3 hr mark, the temperature reached a maximum level of 89°F, which is in the homeostatic range and consistent with relaxation. There appeared to be no systematic relationship in either measure that correlated with symptoms. Rather, the patterns are consistent with an initial state characteristic of anticipatory anxiety and arousal, even before the challenge commenced, followed by relaxation after she had the "reaction."

This double-blind placebo trial was interpreted as a false-positive response and the results were presented to the patient along with an explanation of learned sensitivity. Before proceeding with further challenges, it was recommended that she enter a biofeedback assisted behavioral therapy program to learn to cope with her symptom amplification responses. She accepted our recommendation, learned to control her "reactions," and was able to eat a normal diet after the be-havioral program. Subsequently, she expressed interest in the psychological cause of her somatization and entered into psychotherapy.

Her family history revealed psychologically abusive parents and an inces-tuous rape by an older brother when she was in early adolescence that was ig-nored by her parents. She married at an early age, had one child, but lost it to a husband who kidnapped it and disappeared never to be seen again. After some difficulty in adjustment to the loss, including depression and anxiety, she re-turned to school and earned a professional degree. She worked successfully in her profession until she became involved in a clandestine relationship with a married supervisor, that triggered many of her unresolved issues. In addition, she faced social conflict in a stressful work environment. Progressively, she became more ill and eventually totally incapacitated with IEI, at which time her physi-cian referred her across the country to our facility.

Upon follow-up study, which continues after a 5 year period, this woman re-turned to her stressful profession and is coping quite well. Periodically, she returned for medical assessment of a recurrence of food intolerances, at times when her anx-iety overwhelmed her and she reverted to her beliefs about food sensitivities. After careful medical assessment and supportive interaction, the allergist (JCS) referred her to the psychologist (HS), the specific stressful situation was addressed, and the symptoms resolved. This patient represents successful treatment of an individual who was incapacitated and disabled with a false belief of food intolerance.

MISATTRIBUTION OF DIAGNOSES

There are numerous medical and psychiatric/psychological conditions that have been incorrectly attributed to foods. Epidemiological research has confirmed the large discrepancy between self-perception of food allergy among the public and its detection by objective methods [3]. For example, in one epidemiology study 30,000 people were asked to complete a mailed questionnaire in High Wycombe, a municipality in Britain [4]. Of the 18,582 (61.9%) responders, 7.4% stated that they had a problem (including behavioral/mood changes) they attributed to food additives, foods, and aspirin. Of these, 132 whose symptoms were regarded as sufficiently suggestive to warrant investigation were approached to participate in double-blind placebo-controlled studies utilizing capsules. There were 81 re-sponders, 3 of whom showed consistent responses to low and high doses of food additives. The first reactor was a 50 year old atopic male who reported a 5 year history of headaches after ingestion of colorants within 12 hr of ingestion. He re-acted to annatto, but he also reacted to placebo on one occasion. The second was a 31 year old nonatopic female who reported upper abdominal pain, which she attributed to ingestion of preservatives and antioxidants. She reported symptoms in response to challenge with annatto. The third was a 5 year old atopic child with eczema and a family history of hay fever who showed a change in mood 1 to 2 hr after azo dye challenge, but also after placebo on two occasions. The in-vestigators expressed some doubt about this last case. The estimated prevalence based on 132 was 4.9, for a population rate of 0.026%. To put this percentage into perspective, the prevalence rate established under controlled studies was 285 times less than that estimated from self-perceived food allergy or sensitivity.

This section of the chapter reviews three diagnoses that have been causally linked to foods, attention deficit/hyperactivity disorder, food allergies said to cause psychiatric conditions, and *Candida* hypersensitivity syndrome.

Attention Deficit Hyperactivity Disorder

Although scientific opinion favors a neurological explanation of genetic origin for most cases of attention deficit hyperactivity disorder, this explanation does not necessarily exclude alternative causes or precipitating factors, such as com-mon dietary components to which some persons are thought to be hypersensitive [5]. Cultural biases to environmental and life-style factors may have influenced parents' reports that their children become restless, irritable, hyperactive, and in-tractable in reaction to certain foods and additives. Clinical, unblinded provoca-tion challenges were supportive, but blinded studies were not.

Feingold's Diet: Salicylates and Food Additives

Beginning in the 1960s, foods and food additives became the focus as causes for attentional deficit disorders and hyperactivity, childhood dysfunctions that were receiving more media and social attention with the raised consciousness of the times. The relationship to foods was entrenched in the lay public with Feingold's best-seller *Why Your Child Is Hyperactive* [6], largely a book of opinions and testimonials. Feingold claimed that 50% of children placed on a salicylate-free diet showed improvement in hyperactivity behavior and learning disabilities. He further suggested that hyperactivity was a relatively recent phenomenon associated with the increased use of food additives in the American diet. In fact, hyperactivity in children was described in the medical literature at the turn of the century [7], and the incidence of the condition in the classroom based on the judgment of some schoolteachers has remained constant at about 3% [8].

Feingold, in an unfounded leap of logic, recommended the elimination of all food dyes and subsequently extended the restriction to preservatives and all food additives, which had an array of quite different chemical structures. The basis of his recommendation was allusion to other reputable scientific studies that demonstrated sensitivities to food coloring in some aspirin-sensitive asthma patients leading to bronchoconstriction, but not hyperactivity. In double-blind, placebo-controlled studies reactions to food dyes and preservatives are an uncommon cause of clinically significant bronchoconstriction even in moderately severe perennial asthmatics [9].

Abba Terr [10] noted several ironic occurrences about the Feingold diet. First, the salicylates that were the original culprits in Feingold's speculations are in fact found in virtually all plants. Second, with the shift in emphasis to food additives of all kinds, adherents to the Feingold diet in practice concentrated their efforts on the additives and ignored the presence of salicylates in their diet, the issue that had originally prompted the diet.

Consumer advocates, aided by media publications in the *Wall Street Journal* and *Readers Digest,* requested dietary advice from their physicians for children with attention deficit hyperactivity disorder as well as learning disabilities and conduct disorders. This represents yet another historical example of projection of attribution to an external cause for a problem. Scientific skepticism and caution and outright challenge of these unsubstantiated practices in a poignant critique [11] could not stem the tide of a populist movement. In 1982, in response to this confusion, the National Institutes of Health's Office of Medical Applications for Research published a consensus report based on the scientific evidence available and concluded that there was no evidence to date that toxicity, idiosyncrasy, or allergic hypersensitivity from food additives causes direct effects on the central nervous system; in short, Feingold's theory was not supported [12]. Although Feingold's claims of epidemic proportions were deemed unreasonable, the possibility that a very few children may be shown to have attentional disorders resulting from food additives was left to further study.

The Feingold diet in some small way may have contributed to the treatment of attention deficit disorder in that it offered hope to distraught parents, and the rigors of adhering to the strict diet cannot help but change the family dynamics. Most importantly, the child must surely believe that the parents and others have a greater commitment to his or her well-being [8].

Sugar: Sucrose and Aspartame

In 1975, an open challenge study reported results that supported parental observations that sugar "sets their children off" [13]. Behavioral disorders were suspected to result from ingestion of sugar in its natural form, sucrose, as well as the artificial sweetener aspartame, commonly found in diet carbonated beverages in the early 1980s [14]. By the mid-1980s, hundreds of anecdotal accounts of seizures associated with aspartame were reported to the Food and Drug Administration (FDA), prompting at least two controlled studies. A double-blind, placebo-controlled cross-over study of seizure activity in children with well-documented seizures demonstrated that aspartame does not provoke seizures or increase epileptiform discharges; the companion study with adults showed the same negative results [15]. The extensive literature evaluating the effects of sugar on hyperactivity and other behavioral problems consistently shows that open (nonblinded) studies affirm the relationship [13,16], but double-blind, placebo-controlled studies do not [17–20]. Those studies that have reported negative findings have been criticized for methodological flaws by proponents of the "sugar connection."

However, Wolraich and colleagues subsequently conducted a definitive double-blind, placebo-controlled study of the effects of diets high in sucrose or aspartame on the behavior and cognitive performance of children described to be sensitive to sugar [21]. The experimental group consisted of 23 school-age children described by their parents as sensitive to sugar; the controls were 25 preschool children without complaints related to sugar. In a double-blind cross-over design, three diets were compared. One diet was high in sucrose, another contained aspartame as a sweetener, and the placebo diet contained saccharin as a sweetener. All diets were essentially free of additives, artificial food coloring, and preservatives, and the amount of sweetener was regulated and plasma glucose levels were monitored. Psychological assessment was conducted at baseline. Thirty-nine behavioral and cognitive measures were evaluated. These had been proved sensitive to hyperactivity, attention deficits, and the effects of medications and foods in earlier research [22]. The measures included attention, impulsivity, hyperactivity, aggression, oppositional behavior, mood, cognition, motor performance, academic performance, activity level, and somatic symptoms. Results showed that for the children described as sugar-sensitive, there were no significant differences among the three diets. There were some differences among the diets for the control subjects, but the few differences associated with the ingestion of sucrose were more consistent with a slight calming effect than with hyperactivity. There were no adverse responses to sucrose or aspartame in either group. The investigators concluded that even when intake exceeds typical dietary levels, neither sucrose nor aspartame affects children's behavior or cognitive function. It had been recognized that there is no evidence that sugar alone or aspartame can turn a child with normal attention into a hyperactive child [5]. The Wolraich study has extended this conclusion to children judged to have attention deficit hyperactive disorder.

Candida albicans Hypersensitivity: The Yeast Connection

Candida hypersensitivity syndrome originated in the observations of Truss, who postulated that colonization of the organism *Candida albicans,* which normally exists in the gastrointestinal tract and vagina, results in the release of a toxin that leads to immune reactions including immune suppression, autoimmunity, and food allergy [23]. These events were hypothesized to cause systemic illness and multisystem symptoms characteristic of IEI, potentially spreading to other environmental triggers such as nonfood chemicals. The proponents list systemic and psychological symptoms such as fatigue, depression, loss of libido, premenstrual syndrome, muscle aches, constipation, and diarrhea as signals that one may have *Candida* hypersensitivity syndrome, or the label that was popularized with the publication of Crook's book, *The Yeast Connection* [24]. A recent printing of this book is advertised with the entrepreneurial assertion "If you feel sick all over, this book could change your life." The book is a collection of testimonial case histories but lacks any scientific data or clinical trials to differentiate the claimed effects of treatment from placebo or spontaneous recovery with the passage of time.

Like so many other unsubstantiated phenomena, it alludes to a real disease, systemic candidiasis or chronic mucocutaneous candidiasis, which is associated with immune irregularities that manifest as opportunistic infections [25]. By comparison, proponents of the yeast connection say that there are no diagnostic physical abnormalities, no laboratory test abnormalities, and no evidence of overgrowth of *Candida albicans* either locally or systemically. Nevertheless, it is postulated that the "yeast connection" is a predisposing factor for a host of diseases including multiple sclerosis, arthritis, psoriasis, schizophrenia, cancer, acquired immune deficiency syndrome (AIDS), depression, and various emotional and behavioral problems. This is a blatant distortion of the scientific evidence. Candidiasis does indeed exist and the populations reported to be susceptible include individuals undergoing cancer chemotherapy or prolonged antibiotic therapy, drug addicts; those suffering from conditions such as AIDS, chronic alcoholism, or diabetes mellitus; and individuals who are otherwise immunocompromised [26]. The proponents of *Candida* hypersensitivity syndrome would have the causality reversed, implying that such diseases somehow result from it.

The recommended treatment for the yeast overgrowth syndrome includes diet restrictions on intake of sugar, yeast, and foods containing molds, nutritional supplements of vitamins and minerals, and the use of certain medications including oral antifungal agents such as nystatin and ketaconazole. To date there have been no clinical trials evaluating the effectiveness of diet or nutritional supplements [10]. For lack of such evidence, a study to evaluate the effects of nystatin treatment alone seemed warranted.

Double-Blind Study of Nystatin Treatment

Dismukes and colleagues conducted a randomized, double-blind cross-over study with 42 premenopausal women diagnosed to be suffering from *Candida* hypersensitivity syndrome, comparing oral nystatin, vaginal nystatin, or a combination of the two to placebo [27]. As expected, the active nystatin therapies were significantly more effective than placebo in relieving vaginal symptoms. But both nystatin and placebo therapies reduced psychological symptoms and global indexes of distress equally, arguing against the proponent's hypothesis that depression and fatigue are alleviated by nystatin therapy. The investigators concluded that long-term nystatin therapy for women with complaints of *Candida* hypersensitivity syndrome appears to be unwarranted.

Controversy Continues

As was pointed out in an editorial accompanying the Dismukes publication [28], this study will not end the controversy. Negative outcomes invariably prompt criticism about how the study might have been better designed or assertions that the "key" catalyst variables necessary to realize the effect of the intervention were not included. For one, proponents who argue for the existence of chronic *Candida* hypersensitivity syndrome will contend that diet was not controlled in the trial of nystatin, despite any evidence that diet has an effect. Also, since there is no clear definition of the syndrome, any study of it will be subject to the criticism that the wrong subjects were studied. In short, the syndrome is not subject to scientific evaluation and nonfalsifiable.

However, a logical argument can be made to place doubt on the postulate that a diet high in sugar is a specific mechanism that aggravates *Candida* hypersensitivity syndrome. A diet free of sugar has not been shown to be effective in treating patients with well-characterized candidiasis [10]. The postulate of a low-sugar diet to treat *Candida* hypersensitivity syndrome lacks predictive validity in the sense that it does not respond to a specific treatment. Dismukes and colleagues have demonstrated that the same is true for nystatin therapy. Last, from a psychological perspective, the most absurd claim about the "yeast connection" is that it is an etiological mechanism for schizophrenia. Schizophrenia is a devastating disease of unknown cause and has a prevalence of 1% in the United States with an annual financial impact estimated at $10 to $20 billion. Its protean symptoms range from pervasive blunting of affect, thought, and socialization to florid hallucinations and delusions. Despite the history of speculation about the role of toxins and neurotransmitters in the biological processes of schizophrenia, there is currently no proof that either a neurotoxin or an abnormality of neurotransmission is a primary feature of schizophrenia [29].

The *Candida* hypersensitivity syndrome has created animosity between the medical community and a segment of the lay public who claim to suffer from it as well as from other manifestations of IEI. In 1986, a popular women's magazine, *Redbook,* featured an article, "The Newest Mystery Illness," wherein chronic *Candida* hypersensitivity was portrayed as a widespread condition affecting 10% of women in the United States that had an effective method of treatment even though there was no method of diagnosis [30]. In the same issue of the magazine, Cantrol's manufacturer ran an ad instructing consumers to purchase their product from their local health food store; according to a company official, more than 100,000 people responded [31]. Proponents of the syndrome have accused the medical community of being insensitive to the complaints of these patients, implying that the subjective complaints in and of themselves validate the syndrome, an argument that has been made repeatedly for IEI [32]. Further charges are that the medical community refuses to study chronic candidiasis even though there is an extensive medical literature on the subject [25]. These accusatory vignettes may have to be reconsidered in light of the argument of the potential harmful effects of unsubstantiated diagnostic and treatment methods imposed on a psychologically vulnerable population. The *American Academy of Allergy and Immunology* Position Statement on the *Candida* hypersensitivity syndrome states that the concept is speculative and unproven and elements of the proposed treatment program are potentially dangerous [33]. This reserved statement is consistent with conduct expected of the scientific community as well as the legal quicksand of liability of antitrust, restraint of trade, etc. Others living in less encumbered climates have referred to these practices in more poignant terms such as quackery [34] or an epidemic of nonsense [31]. Stephen Barrett, a board member of the National Council against Health Fraud, notes that under federal law, any product intended for the prevention or treatment of disease is a drug, and it is illegal to market new drugs that do not have FDA approval. The health food industry manufacturers claimed that their products were not medical treatments, but rather "dietary supplements," including products labeled CandiCare, Candida-Guard, Candida Cleanse, Candistat, Cantrol, Yeast Fighters, Yeast Guard, Yeaststop, Yeasterol, and Yeast-Trol. The FDA did not agree and in 1989 issued a letter indicating that it is illegal to market vitamin concoctions intended for the treatment of yeast infections. The courts upheld the FDA's position, and in 1990 a federal judge ruled that Yeaststop was a drug and ordered its manufacturer to pay for the seizure and destruction of Yeaststop initiated by the FDA, as well as legal costs. Additional legal cases in which manufactures were assessed penalties for illegally marketing their "yeast connection" products may be found in Barrett's review [31].

Food Sensitivity and Psychiatric Illness

Through media attention and the response of consumers to books and articles containing sensational testimonials of patients and physicians regarding food and behavior, it has been deemed "common sense" that food allergy or hypersensitivity can cause a variety of problems including migraines, depression, and hyperactivity in children. One survey study of college students [35] found that most (90%) believed that foods caused adverse behavioral effects, and the same number of students surveyed reported that they themselves reacted to sugar on occasion. At the extreme end of this propaganda continuum, proponents of toxicogenic explanations of IEI have argued that food allergies account for symptoms in well-characterized psychiatric conditions [16,36–42], theories that remain controversial and unaccepted by the medical community.

Somatic Effects of Foods

What is the scientific evidence to support hypotheses that foods cause somatic symptoms? There is ample evidence to confirm the role of organic adverse reactions to foods in several syndromes including atopic disease (allergy, asthma, eczema, urticaria, and rhinitis) and in gastrointestinal disturbances, which has been reviewed in the literature [43–45] and is also presented in other chapters of this book. Some of these reactions are due to immunoglobulin E– (IgE)-mediated allergy; others can be attributed to enzyme defects or metabolic or pharmacological idiosyncrasies. These must be differentiated from those with a psychogenic cause, mediated through psychophysiological responses. One example is in the area of migraines, where many studies have shown that effects are best explained by a placebo response, but a few suggest the possibility of organic effects due to foods [46]. In one study, double-blind, placebo-controlled challenges with an individual's suspected food found a significant increase in plasma histamine level [47].

Psychological Effects of Foods: Wheat and Schizophrenia

A provocative hypothesis about the psychological effects of foods is that wheat is associated with the exacerbation of idiopathic schizophrenia, mediated by opioid peptides (exorphins) produced by enzymatic action on gluten in cereal grains [48,49]. The hypothesis has generated strong editorial position statements in support [50,51] and in opposition [52].

The evidence to support this hypothesis comes largely from one study by Dohan and Grasberger of male veterans hospitalized for schizophrenia [53]. This study has been held up as most convincing because of the large number of subjects studied, which gave it a high level of statistical power, whereas some studies with negative findings [54] have been criticized for having much lower levels of statistical power [55]. Since the publication of this study over 20 years ago, there have been others who have taken up the hypothesis, largely following a model of celiac disease [56]. Recently, one cohort-controlled study of 48 schizophrenic patients found elevated IgA antibody levels [57]. However, most studies have failed to show a link between celiac disease and the majority of schizophrenia cases [58–60]. In a review of gluten-sensitive enteropathy (celiac disease), schizophrenia is not mentioned as either a definite or even a probable related disorder [60a].

Dohan's hypothesis about enzyme abnormalities suggested specific mechanisms (vasoactive monoamines [61]) by which the gluten exorphins would pass from the gut to the brain, where they cause dopaminergic and cholinergic dysfunction, neurotransmitter systems hypothesized to be related to schizophrenia. However, in a study of Swedish celiac patients, the notable psychiatric disorder was depression and no cases of schizophrenia were identified [62], suggesting that other neurotransmitter systems were dysfunctional. These patients showed elevated scale scores on depression on the Minnesota Multiphasic Personality Inventory (MMPI) [63], which were inversely correlated with levels of central monoamine metabolites in the cerebrospinal fluid of the celiac patients [64]. The finding of reduced central monoamine metabolism in untreated celiac patients is opposite that predicted by a celiac model for schizophrenia and may provide evidence against a genetic linkage between celiac disease and schizophrenia because schizophrenics show high levels of serotonin and dopamine metabolites in the cerebral spinal fluid [65].

In light of these findings and their theoretical implications, we reexamined the original study by Dohan and Grasberger [53]. Schizophrenics were randomly assigned upon admission to a diet free of cereal grains and milk while on a locked psychiatric ward. The authors concluded that the results of their study showed that these patients were discharged from the locked ward onto the open wards in the hospital about twice as rapidly as control patients assigned to a high-cereal diet. There are two serious flaws in this study, one methodological and the other statistical. In terms of the information presented in their paper, it appears that decisions about discharge and readmittance to the locked ward were made by the same staff who conducted the study: that is, the experimenters do not appear to have been blinded to the hypothesis as claimed. This is a serious methodological flaw for a variable such as ward privileges that is often based on subjective, clinical judgment.

But the more serious flaw of the study is that the discharge data were incorrectly analyzed. Of the 59 patients who received the cereal- and milk-free (CFMF) diet, 30 were discharged from the locked ward throughout the course of the 1 year study. Of the 56 control subjects who ate an unrestricted diet high in cereal, 22 were discharged during the same period. Statistical analysis was by the Fisher's exact test, with test results reported for each of the six categories, representing 30 day intervals from day of admission up to 180 days for the first half year, and a seventh category representing the next 180 days up to 1 year post admission. For each test, the probability that the difference in the cumulative number of patients discharged in each period is due to chance is reported, as reproduced in Table 1. The conceptual error in statistical analysis is that cumulative frequency rather than actual frequency was used, making the analyses of successive time intervals nonindependent, and therefore biased [66, p. 104].

Most puzzling about the data presented in Table 1 is that both the first (30 days) and last (360 days) cumulative categories are nonsignificant at an alpha level of 0.05. This result indicates that after 1 year, the likelihood of an early discharge any time during that year is not statistically different for the diet and control groups. However, it is still possible that the pattern of discharge across the different periods is suggestive of a benefit of the wheat-free diet, if the experimental group was discharged earlier in the course of the year than the control group, as is suggested by a plot of the trends in the data. But are these trends statistically reliable as suggested by the investigators? To address this question, we reanalyzed the original data by a 2 × 7 chi-square test of the observed frequency data in all seven categories for the two groups, added in parentheses in Table 1. The chi-square test yielded a value of 9.32, which is less than the value of 12.59 required for statistical significance at the .05 level with 6 degrees of freedom [67].

Assuming that the original data presented by Dohan and Grasberger [53] were inappropriately analyzed, the high level of statistical power in their study design, which was noted to be a strength [55], further weakens the hypothesis that wheat sensitivity affects the course of clinical manifestation of symptoms in schizophrenics.

TABLE 1 Cumulative Frequency Data from the Original Article for Effects on Time to Discharge for a Cereal-Free and Milk-Free (CFMF) Diet Compared with a High-Cereal Diet (HC) in Two Groups of Schizophrenics with Observed Frequency from the Corrected Statistical Analysis in Parentheses

Days after difference, Admission Chance	CFMF diet (N = 59) Number Discharged, Cumulative (Obs.)		HC diet (N = 56) Number Discharged, Cumulative (Obs.)		Prob. by
30	6	(6)	2	(2)	.15
60	17	(11)	7	(5)	.026
90	22	(5)	9	(2)	.009
120	24	(2)	12	(3)	.021
150	26	(2)	12	(0)	.008
180	27	(1)	15	(3)	.027
360	30	(3)	22	(7)	.145

Source: Ref. 53.

Psychological Effects of Foods: Autonomic Arousal

We should not be embarrassed to say "so what?" when confronted with an observation that an isolated finding of "statistical significance," without independent confirmation or a theoretical framework, might have a high clinical correlation but make no common sense. [68]

There is one notable study by King suggesting that sublingual provocation with foods could elicit psychiatric symptoms in "chemically sensitive individuals" [69]. Food sensitivity has been hypothesized to be mediated by such mechanisms as the kinin system, a class of peptide hormones that may produce certain psychosomatic symptoms, e.g., fatigue and irritability, by their ability to alter levels of neurotransmitters in the brain [36]. In King's study conducted at a clinical ecology diagnostic unit, 24 of 26 patients showed abnormal MMPI profiles, with elevations on scales of hypochondriasis, depression, hysteria, and schizophrenia most notable. The investigator claimed to have conducted double-blind sublingual provocation challenges with drops of diluent containing suspected foods on these patients. The results showed that there was a significant increase in reported cognitive and emotional symptoms. There was also a significant increase in the variance of the heart rate for active challenge compared to that of placebo controls, a finding described as "a serendipitous *post hoc* finding." Other dependent measures, specifically mean heart rate and neurobehavioral measures of cognitive function, were not affected by the allergens and placebos. These negative findings are noteworthy because the subjects were selected on the criterion of at least one psychological presenting symptom, including confusion or difficulty in concentrating. The study raised some criticism about the procedure to ensure blinding of taste as well as statistical design. Taste discrimination was not adequately controlled in the study in that the subjects learned to discriminate the tasteless placebo, making it an open rather than a blind challenge. Analysis of this study also revealed a flaw in design because twice as many "allergy" as placebo challenges were performed, thus creating a bias in favor of a positive reaction.

King subsequently reported a similar sublingual provocation study [35] with hyperactive children whose symptoms were attributed to food intolerance by their parents. In this study he found small changes in pulse rate (mean increase of 1.6 beats/minute) that were statistically significant. The conclusion from the second study by King [35] had a different flavor, as follows:

Nevertheless, the effects obtained in this study, although statistically significant, were of no clinical importance because of their subtlety. That is, effects of the magnitude we observed cannot account for hyperactivity, emotional disturbance, or other clinically relevant symptoms sometimes attributed to foods. In addition, the small differences in ratings and other dependent measures between test-food and placebo challenges raise serious questions about the use of sublingual testing for individual diagnosis under conditions similar to ours.

There remains an unanswered question about the psychological findings reported in King's original study [69]. If the psychiatric conditions assessed with the MMPI cannot be attributed to the effects of foods, what are we to make of them? In the discussion, King stated, "The pervasiveness of psychopathology on the MMPI could be due to psychogenic illness, to allergically induced symptoms, or to a combination of the two." In light of King's subsequent research, and that of others, it seems that psychogenic illness may be the only viable explanation for the findings. The elevations of the first three clinical scales on the MMPI (hysteria, depression, hypochondriasis) are reliable correlates of somatoform disorders.

Food Aversion and Eating Disorders

There is a distinction between food allergy/sensitivity and food aversion. Food aversion comprises both psychological avoidance and psychological intolerance. Psychological avoidance may result from taste preference or fears about natural carcinogens in foods, fears that are highly exaggerated [70,71]. Psychological intolerance is an unpleasant somatic reaction caused by emotions associated with food intake, often stemming from unpleasant experience with food in childhood. This distinction was recently demonstrated in the differential diagnosis of adverse reactions to cow's milk in two clinical cases [72]. In the first case, an 18 year old female showed IgE-mediated anaphylactic reactions to unprocessed cow's milk under double-blind challenges, and an elimination diet resulted in complete clinical remission. In the second case, a 35 year old male with a history of severe symptom reaction, including complete collapse after ingestion of cow's milk, showed no objective signs of milk allergy. Psychological evaluation revealed an early disturbance of the mother–child relationship with a hysterical conversion reaction. After 3 weeks of psychotherapy the patient reintroduced milk into his diet without any further symptoms.

In another study, the psychological characteristics of 45 patients with reported adverse reactions to foods were assessed by standardized psychological testing including the MMPI and the SCL-90R [73]. In a companion study, patients were clinically evaluated by means of medical history, physical examination, skin testing, and, if necessary, double-blind placebo-controlled food challenges [74]. Those with unconfirmed reactions ($n = 23$) scored higher than did the confirmed group ($n = 22$) on the MMPI scales of hypochondriasis and hysteria, and higher on the SCL-90R somatization scale and the positive symptom distress index. In another study of six patients with a long history of multiple food allergies, subjective symptoms were not typical of allergy, and purported association of food and symptoms was not reproducible [75]. In these cases long-standing abnormal eating behavior and weight problems preceded the purported food allergies, leading the investigator to suggest that clinicians be alert to an underlying eating disorder or weight control problem.

In conclusion, no satisfactory objective evidence has yet been presented to confirm the role of food allergy in the direct generation of psychological symptoms [76]. Under double-blind placebo-controlled challenges these appraisals can be reliably tested and the differential effects of biologically caused sensitivity can be discriminated from learned sensitivity [2,76]. The classical studies by Pearson and his colleagues deserve to be discussed in detail and are presented in the following material.

LEARNED SENSITIVITY: BIOLOGICAL MECHANISMS

> Although inborn reflexes and fixed action patterns play some role in human behavior, they are over-shadowed by learning as a basis for guiding action. Through symbolic, associative processes, stimuli that are inherently meaningless come to exert profound influences over the emotional systems of the brain. [77, p. 430].

Psychoneuroimmunology

Learned sensitivity is a term that describes expressions of environmental intolerances that are centrally mediated and were hypothesized to have immunological mechanisms [78]. The term *learned sensitivity* is used to allow for cognitively mediated learning (thinking), which does not strictly fall in the Pavlovian conditioning paradigm. The neuronal encoding of Pavlovian conditioned learning has been shown to be different from that of associative learning [79–81].

Conditioned Immunomodulation

Conditioned immunomodulation is recognized as an important line of evidence for the involvement of psychological and psychophysiological factors in what was traditionally believed to be a domain of immunology proper [82,83]. A review of animal conditioning studies shows that the central nervous system (CNS) affects immune system responses at virtually every level, including antibody production, lymphocyte proliferation, delayed hypersensitivity, natural killer cell activity, graft-versus-host response, total white blood cell count, T helper/T suppressor ratio, arthritic inflammation, and systemic lupus erythematosus [84]. Histamine release, a mechanism of hypersensitivity, can be centrally mediated. In one series of animal studies, Pavlovian conditioning experiments showed increased plasma histamine levels in response to a conditioned stimulus [85]. Since histamine is produced by many tissues and cells other than mast cells, additional studies were needed to link histamine specifically to mast cells to show conditioning of a hypersensitivity response. In one particularly elegant study, Bienenstock and colleagues showed conditioned increase of rat mast cell protease II (RMCP II), the enzyme that is restricted to mucosal mast cells unique to the immune system [86]. This study was summarized by Bienenstock [84] as follows:

> In this study rats were sensitized to egg albumin. Exposure to audiovisual cues (CS) was followed by a subcutaneous antigen challenge (UCS). Eleven days after 3 weekly CS–UCS pairings a test trial was performed. Exposure to audiovisual cues followed by an injection of saline [placebo] (presentation of CS alone) resulted in an increase of serum RMCP II that was comparable to the increase observed in the group of animals challenged with antigen, but significantly higher than the levels of RMCP II found in the appropriate control groups, as shown in Figure 1. The finding of conditioned mast cell degranulation implicates a functional relationship between the elements of the central nervous system and the elements of the immune system that are involved in immediate hypersensitivity. The information that was processed and stored by the central nervous system was used by the organism in order to modulate mast cell function.

Human Learning

In humans, the association of the CNS with mast cells suggests that psychoneurological mechanisms could produce non-IgE-mediated mast cell mediator release [87] consistent with the clinical experience reported by MacKenzie in 1886 as a case of "rose allergy" [88]. In humans, conditioned effects have been demonstrated in modulation of immunity such that a delayed hypersensitivity reaction to tuberculin is curtailed [89], although a conditioned false-positive reaction to saline solution was not achieved [90]. This study extended earlier findings in which four tuberculin-positive subjects showed inhibited delayed-type hypersensitivity reactions after direct hypnotic suggestion not to react to the skin test [91].

To place *learned sensitivity* in the context of the reactions of IEI patients, consider the following: Odor is usually identified as a significant trigger for a response. What the odor is associated with is not clear. Is it the actual toxic chemical, as in the case of a Pavlovian conditioned response to a documented exposure of low-level neurotoxins [92]? Or is it a fear response associated with the belief that this chemical will induce symptoms? Where does the fear come from in the labyrinth of memory networks? Could it be associated with a fragmented memory of a sensory or emotional sensation triggered by the stress response after the

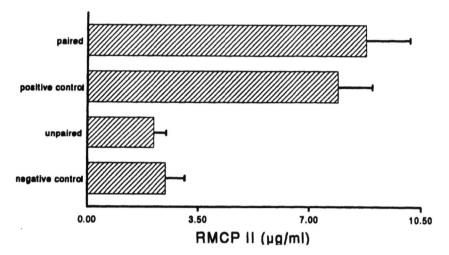

FIGURE 1 Results of the conditioning experiment [86]. The positive control group was challenged with antigen and the conditioning stimulus. The unpaired group consisted of animals in which the conditioning stimulus was separated from unconditioned stimulus by a period of 24 hr in order to prevent conditioning. The negative control group was presented with the conditioning stimulus together with saline solution injection to control for the injections themselves. The paired group received only the conditioning stimulus without antigen (but with saline solution injection). RMCP II was measured in serum radioimmunoassay. Mast cells from paired groups of animals released mediators in response to the CS. RMCP II, rat-mast cell protease II; CS, conditioned stimulus. (From Ref. 84.)

stimulus is perceived to be harmful [93]? Is the reaction a reenactment of emotional and sensorimotor schema in memory that lack links to contextual knowledge referents and are accessed out of context? In evaluating the effects of *learned sensitivity* on the reactions of IEI patients, we must take into account not only the stimuli associated with the environmental agent, but also the mediating psychological and psychophysiological processes [78].

The history of the study of asthma shows that similar questions were asked about conditioning as an explanation for emotionally triggered asthma attacks. Clinical histories of asthmatics often contain examples of asthmatic attacks after emotional events. In the 1950s, behavioral explanations were investigated as alternatives to the prevailing psychoanalytical explanations [94] offered to explain the psychogenic effects of asthma.

In the 1950s, Dekker and colleagues conducted several studies of classical Pavlovian conditioning with asthmatic patients using emotional stimuli from individual patient histories as the conditioned stimulus. In one study of 12 asthmatics, 6 did not react at all, 3 reacted only with transient decrease in breathing capacity, but 3 did respond with frank asthma attacks. The great individual differences did not fit well with their expected conditioning effects. In a related study of two patients who reacted to an emotional stimulus and who were studied in detail, the authors concluded that although there were some learning effects that seemed in line with a conditioning mechanism, they did not represent classical examples of such a mechanism [95]. In the discussion of the results of the patients who reacted with asthma attacks in the earlier study, a rather revealing observation was presented [96]:

> Consequent to the provocation tests these patients related traumatic life experiences, emotional phantasies, and disturbing dreams. No attempt will be made to give a psychiatric interpretation of these observations, but in a number of instances it was quite obvious that the environmental asthmatogenic stimulus was associatively related to former traumatic life experiences. The clinical picture of the patients during these psychogenic attacks was indistinguishable from "spontaneous" attacks or from attacks provoked by the inhalation of allergens. They could be aborted by the administration of thiacinamine or isoprenaline.

Food Intolerances: Physiological and Immunological Characteristics

Intolerance to foods was one of the earlier manifestations of IEI, dating to the turn of the century with the autointoxication phenomenon. Foods were also a focal point in the clinical ecological manifestations that began with Theron Randolph in the 1940s. Although there was a great deal of speculation and false attribution about the ill-health effects of foods, there were also systematic research programs that discriminated immune-mediated food intolerances from psychogenic intolerances. Two research programs that deserve recognition as exemplary are those of Harold Wolff and David Pearson and their respective colleagues.

Harold Wolff's Pioneering Work

Shortly after World War II, Harold Wolff and his associates conducted studies to test the beliefs people had about the adverse effects of foods by using double-blind, placebo-controlled provocation challenges in both normal controls and patients with psychological disorders [97]. One such study was conducted on four physicians who believed they could provoke migraine headaches in themselves by eating chocolate in any form and in minimal amounts [98]. They were each given envelopes containing 8 g of powdered chocolate or lactose (placebo-control) in eight black capsules that were indistinguishable. A within-subject, cross-over design was employed over a 4 month period, with the subjects carefully logging their symptoms daily and also noting when they ingested the capsules. Most migraine attacks occurred without reference to the ingestion of capsules. Migraines followed the ingestion of lactose just as frequently as they did the ingestion of chocolate.

In another demonstration, Wolff and associates showed how symptoms commonly seen in allergy could be manipulated with emotional material and suggestion. In one patient it was possible to alter the response of the skin to histamine and pilocarpine from negative to positive, and then to reverse it again, by changing the topic of discussion. Mention of the patient's sister triggered a physiological response, as shown in Figure 2.

In a single-blind demonstration, Wolff and associates showed how symptoms of gastric and duodenal activity responded to suggestion in a 50 year old woman with multisystem complaints including pressure in her head, poor thinking and memory, unclear vision, dizziness, abdominal cramps, nausea, hives, and abdominal bloating. The symptoms occurred within 10–20 minutes after ingesting low doses of milk. She claimed that 4 drops of milk in a glass of water induced symptoms. The onset of attacks was dated to 11 years prior after she had had a cesarean section. The patient had never liked milk but had ingested a great deal during the pregnancy, gaining 60 pounds. In the experiment, balloons were introduced into the stomach and duodenum. After establishing a baseline, under single-blinded conditions 50 cm^3 of whole milk (substantially more than the minimal 4 drops) was introduced into the stomach via a feeding tube. She was told she was being given water as a preliminary testing procedure. There was no significant change in the duodenal motility pattern and the patient exhibited no symptoms. Two weeks later the experiment was repeated, but this time she was given 50 cm^3 of water and was told that milk was being introduced. She had nausea and abdominal discomfort after this suggestion, associated with change in the duodenal motility pattern as shown in Figure 3.

The investigators concluded:

> Unless the circumstances of administration of the agent preclude all opportunity for conditioning factors to operate, it may not be inferred that such reactions are allergic in nature.

Pearson's Controlled Studies for IEI (Food)

With the influence of clinical ecology on IEI, there was a shift in symptom emphasis to cognitive effects, e.g., confusion, difficulty in concentrating, and poor memory [40,42]. In Britain, David Pearson and associates studied the effects of foods on psychological and cognitive symptoms [99]. In their study of 23 patients presenting to a allergy clinic, only 4 had objective food sensitivity based

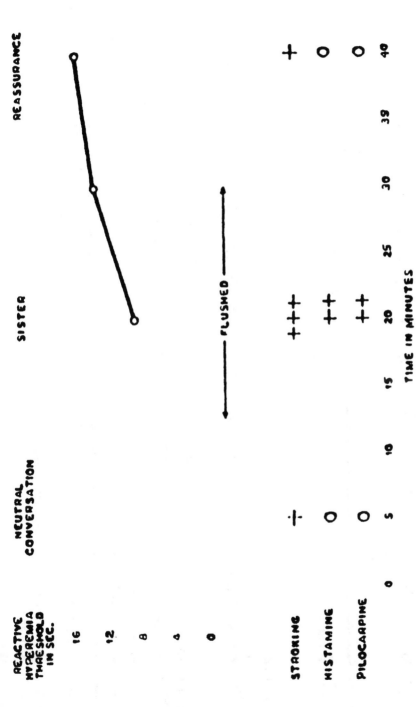

FIGURE 2 Simultaneous changes in the response of the skin to histamine, to pilocarpine, and to stroking during a stressful interview with a woman patient with hives (histamine acid phosphate 0.001% and pilocarpine hydrochloride 1% at 10 μA for 2 minutes over 1 cm²). There was no response to isotonic sodium chloride solution applied in the same way before, during, or after the period of stress. (Ref. 98.)

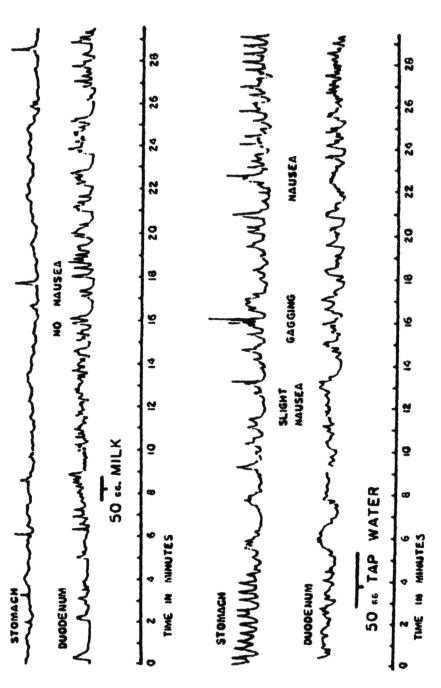

FIGURE 3 Changes in symptoms and gastric and duodenal activity in the patient after the administration of milk and of tap water. (Ref. 98.)

on double-blind, placebo-controlled challenges [100]. Pearson's group also demonstrated how patients with nonallergic food intolerances report false-positive responses during open food challenges. With open challenges, a middle-aged woman reported significant psychological symptoms in response to a multitude of foods to which she believed she was sensitive. Double-blind, placebo-controlled studies showed that her coffee and sugar intolerances were not organic.

The investigators concluded:

> It is no longer adequate to accept the presence of an organic basis for such symptoms without the demonstration of repeatability under double-blind conditions.

This position had long been held by the scientific allergy community for the assessment of food sensitivities in the general population [43,44].

DISTORTED BELIEFS: ADVANTAGES AND EXPLOITATION

> A person in distress wants action—rational action if possible, of course, but irrational action, if necessary, rather than none at all. [101]

Why would someone believe in IEI? The anxiety reduction process suggested by Findley does not necessarily imply a motive for psychological gain from being ill. The authors have seen many IEI patients with stress response symptoms who had been influenced by physicians in which these patients' symptoms of IEI were purely iatrogenic. Often, an explanation to the patient of the unsubstantiated theory and practice of some physicians is sufficient to dispel misconceptions about the appraisal of symptoms. Other motivations must be considered when the IEI patient has something to gain from being ill and often remains ill despite appropriate medical intervention. This is referred to as adopting the *sick role*.

Patient Motivation: Secondary Gain

If viewed as a disease, IEI legitimizes withdrawal from responsibility of work, obligation, and interpersonal relations. Like one of its historical predecessors, neurasthenia, IEI sanctions isolation, depression, anxiety, and demoralization. Although secondary gain can be conscious and function in the same way as malingering, clinical experience suggests that, more often than not, it is unconscious in IEI patients. Self-deception is often mediated by psychological defenses, motivated by anxiety reduction. Because the beliefs are irrational from

TABLE 2 Motivations and Reinforcements
Associated with Secondary Gain

Interpersonal
    Sympathy, attention
    Affection from family and friends
    Assurance of importance (Durkheim's "nobility")
    Rationalization of failure (avoid humiliation)
    Protection from criticism
    Explanation for not trying
    Avoidance of difficult relations
Monetary
    Disability insurance
    Workman's compensation
    Medical insurance
    Litigation
Exemption
    Responsibility
    Work and employment
    Achievement
    Interaction with the outside world
Power
    Manipulation and control in relationships
    Employee empowerment
    Community problems
    Political cause

a medical standpoint, many doctors underestimate the resistance this unconscious motivation can muster. There are several manifestations of secondary gain that can occur alone or in combination in any one clinical case, as shown in Table 2.

Secondary gain as a social and economic dynamic is a powerful influence on some patients presenting with IEI [102,103]. However, the most difficult clinical cases that the authors have encountered involved unconscious, unintentional symptom exacerbation, which is the result of primary gain [104,105].

Patient Motivation: Primary Gain

In the psychodynamic tradition, primary gain is defined as intrapsychic conflict; in the cognitive–behavioral psychology approach, it is defined in terms of overload of coping resources. Several hypotheses have been offered as to the cause of primary gain, including (a) trauma and resulting posttraumatic stress disorder (PTSD), (b) cultural or economic deprivation, (c) social alienation, (d) demoralization, and (e) unbearable loss [106]. In IEI patients who have a history of trauma, their beliefs and associated behavior about IEI serve as defenses against awareness of the trauma, which, if brought into conscious awareness, would create extreme anxiety or overload coping resources. IEI patients have been found to report grotesque memories of early childhood physical and sexual abuse experiences [104]. Intrafamilial trauma invariably has associated psychological abuse that contributes to the disruption of personality development [107] and undermines the formulation of a healthy, cohesive, and integrated concept of self [108]. Sexual and physical trauma in childhood can also create permanent biological and physiological effects that alter and compromise coping resources [109,110]. The basis for the overload of coping resources in other IEI patients may also be found in stressful life events less traumatic than those associated with PTSD such as divorce, loss of job, job stress, or self-imposed unrealistic expectations. These reactions can often be traced to beliefs originating in childhood that have become self-defeating in adulthood, beliefs imposed by controlling parents or a puritanical moral influence. Beliefs about chemical sensitivities serve the psychological defense mechanism of *projection,* such that factors external to the psyche are held responsible for the illness, and the core psychological conflicts and anxieties remain constrained in the unconscious [111]. The character trait of projecting blame has been identified as a common characteristic in individuals who are diagnosed with any kind of personality disorder [112]. According to psychodynamic theory, projection often interacts with another defense mechanism, *conversion reaction,* which diverts underlying anxiety into somatization. These two psychodynamic defense mechanisms are often seen in IEI patients who are diagnosed as having a somatoform disorder, or a variety of comorbid personality disorders [113].

In psychology, similar ideas are discussed in terms of attribution of causality [114]. The link between individual differences and the attribution of causality and responsibility was made by Rotter [115], who defined *locus of control* as a personality trait. Individuals with an internal *locus of control* tend to attribute both favorable and unfavorable experiences and life events to their own efforts, or the lack thereof, or to personal traits. Individuals with an external *locus of control* tend to project responsibility outward and attribute life events primarily to external factors such as fate, chance, the actions of other people, or environmental agents. One difference between the psychodynamic and psychological formulations of mechanisms of displacement seems to be the degree to which the avoidance of deep-seated conflicts is postulated as a motivational factor.

CONCLUSION: THE MYTH OF PHYSICAL ILLNESS

In many cultures, including our own, functional illness is often misconstrued as lacking biological correlates: "It's all in your head," and the stigma of malingering is attached to it. The discovery of the biological and physiological effects of the stress response has helped to curtail these misconceptions and dampened some of the associated stigma, but unfortunately some long-standing attitudes about psychological dysfunction are hard to overcome. Depending on the prevailing cultural ethics and morality of any historical period, psychological illness has been portrayed in stereotypes reflecting demonic influence, wrong political thinking, malingering, a bad attitude, weak character, or simply the badness or undesirability of the person. Throughout history, few societies have been willing to face the horrifying reality of the cause and personal suffering associated with mental illness, and ours is no exception. Under many liability, compensation, and disability laws in the United States, it is necessary to demonstrate that a physical injury has been inflicted in order to claim secondary psychological harm and suffering. Ironically, most IEI patients claiming disability on the basis of chemical sensitivities resist any suggestion of disability on the basis of psychiatric disorders even in those circumstances in which it is allowed.

Throughout history, societies have usually been unwilling to take responsibility for the mentally ill, often incarcerating them as unfortunate chattel to be mistreated and subjected to psychiatric experimentation in institutions [116]. In recent times, they have also been discarded into the streets to swell the ranks of the homeless under misguided regulations purporting to protect their civil rights. For these and other more personal reasons, having a functional illness has been associated with loss of face. It has also sensitized some who have lost their ability to cope to the frightening possibilities they believe could result from a disability for a mental disorder.

In contrast, most societies offer sanctions to individuals who are physically ill or disabled. There are sanctioned relief from the responsibility of daily life and permission to be passive (e.g., bed rest) or indecisive (e.g., catered care). The ill person is not expected to engage in difficult interpersonal or social interactions. Physical illness is accepted as involuntary, and therefore the individual is personally absolved of responsibility for the sickness. But there are also responsibilities to having a physical illness. Society supposes that the sick patient is motivated to get well and expects the patient to cooperate with medical treatment and function at a level of maximal medical improvement. Rejection of efficacious treatment and nonadherence to a medication regimen are not sanctioned. The disabled are expected to maximize their functional abilities through rehabilitation. In summary, society expects the ill and the disabled to relinquish the *sick role,* not to elaborate it [117].

Calling IEI a toxicogenic illness fosters the myth that it is an objective, validated physical disease. To date, IEI does not meet the criteria to be labeled a disease, or even a medical syndrome, because no plausible mechanism other than psychological has been identified [118]. Neither is the behavior of many IEI patients consistent with what is expected of those with a physical illness.

Instead, it can be argued that the basis of the illness claimed by IEI patients lies in their failure to cope with problems of living, whether these be biological, economic, political, social, or psychological in nature, and related to premorbid trauma or not. The allusion that IEI is a disease creates the illusion that there is an impersonal "thing" to blame. But, unlike so many physical illnesses, problems of living cannot be treated or cured impersonally. Rather, the "frightening psychological therapies" that IEI patients dread and avoid are often directed at painful self-reflection. Psychotherapy with IEI patients should be directed to identify and resolve conflicts that have generated demoralization and undermined self-esteem, and to replace distorted beliefs and false defenses with effective coping processes to facilitate functioning in the real world [119].

REFERENCES

1. Smith E. Conclusions and recommendations of a workshop on "Multiple Chemical Sensitivities (MCS)." Sponsored by the International Program on Chemical Safety of the World Health Organization (IPCS/WHO), Berlin, Germany, February, 21–23, 1996.
2. Selner JC, Staudenmayer H. Food allergy: Psychological considerations. In: Metcalfe DD, Sampson HA, Simon RA, eds. Food Allergy: Adverse Reactions to Foods and Food Additives. Boston: Blackwell Scientific, 1991:370–381.
3. Howard LM, Wessely S. The psychology of multiple allergy. Br Med J 1993; 307:747–748.
4. Young E, Patel S, Stoneham M, Rona R, Wilkinson JD. The prevalence of reaction to food additives in a survey population. J R Coll Physicians Lond 1987; 21(4):241–247.
5. Kinsbourne M. Sugar and the hyperactive child (letter to editor). N Engl J Med 1994; 330(5):355–356.
6. Feingold BF. Why Your Child is Hyperactive. New York: Random House, 1975.
7. Still GF. Some abnormal psychical conditions in children. (The Goulstonian lectures). Lancet 1902; 1:1008–1012, 1077–1082, 1163–1168.
8. Forbes GB. Nutrition and hyperactivity (editorial). JAMA 1982; 248(3):355–356.
9. Weber RW, Hoffman M, Raine DA, Jr., Nelson HS. Incidence of bronchoconstriction due to aspirin, azo dyes, non-azo dyes, and preservatives in a population of perennial asthmatics. J Allergy Clin Immunol 1979; 64(1):32–37.
10. Terr AI. Unconventional theories and unproven methods in allergy. In: Middleton E, Jr., Reed CE, Ellis EF, Adkinson NF, Jr., Yunginger JW, Busse WW, eds. Allergy: Principles and Practice. Vol 2. 4th ed. St. Louis: Mosby-Year Book, 1993, pp 1767–1793.
11. Werry JS. Food additives and hyperactivity (editorial). Med J Aust 1976; 2(8):281–282.
12. Consensus Conference: Defined diets and childhood hyperactivity. JAMA 1982; 248(3):290–292.

13. Crook WG. Food allergy: the great masquerader. Pediatr Clin North Am 1975; 22:227–238.

14. Wurtman RJ. Neurochemical changes following high-dose aspartame with dietary carbohydrates (correspondence). N Engl J Med 1983; 309:429–430.

15. Tollefson L. Multiple chemical sensitivity: controlled scientific studies as proof of causation. Regul Toxicol Pharmacol 1993; 18(1):32–43.

16. Rapp DJ. Does diet affect hyperactivity? J Learn Disabil 1978; 11(6):383–389.

17. Behar D, Rapaport JL, Adams AJ, Berg CJ, Cornblath M. Sugar challenge testing with children considered behaviorally 'sugar reactive.' J Nutrition Behavior 1984; 1:277.

18. Milich R, Pelham WE. Effects of sugar ingestion on classroom and playground behavior of attention deficit disordered boys. J Consult Clin Psychol 1986; 54(5):714–718.

19. Milich R, Wolraich ML, Lindgren SD. Sugar and hyperactivity: a critical review of empirical findings. Clin Psychol Rev 1986; 6:493–513.

20. Wolraich M, Milich R, Stumbo P, Schultz F. Effects of sucrose ingestion on the behavior of hyperactive boys. J Pediatr 1985; 106:675–682.

21. Wolraich ML, Lindgren SD, Stumbo PJ, Stegink LD, Appelbaum MI, Kiritsy MC. Effects of diets high in sucrose or aspartame on the behavior and cognitive performance of children. N Engl J Med 1994; 330(5):301–307.

22. Barkley RA. Attention Deficit Hyperactivity Disorder: A Handbook for Diagnosis and Treatment. New York: Guilford Press, 1990.

23. Truss CO. The Missing Diagnosis. Birmingham, AL: Missing Diagnosis, 1983.

24. Crook WG. The Yeast Connection: A Medical Breakthrough. 3rd ed. Jackson, TN: Professional Books, 1986.

25. Kirkpatrick CH. Chronic mucocutaneous candidiasis. Eur J Clin Microbiol Infect Dis 1989; 8:448–456.

26. Blonz ER. Is there an epidemic of chronic candidiasis in our midst? (commentary). JAMA 1986; 256(22):3138–3139.

27. Dismukes WE, Wade JS, Lee JY, Dockery BK, Hain JD. A randomized, double-blind trial of nystatin therapy for the candidiasis hypersensitivity syndrome. N Engl J Med 1990; 323(25):1717–1723.

28. Bennett JE. Searching for the yeast connection (editorial). N Engl J Med 1990; 323(25): 1766–1767.

29. Mesulam MM. Schizophrenia and the brain (editorial). N Engl J Med 1990; 322(12):842–844.

30. Thomas DC. The newest mystery illness. Redbook 1986; 166:120–121, 152–153.

31. Barrett S. Unproven 'Allergies': An Epidemic of Nonsense. New York: American Council on Science and Health, 1993.

32. Rosenthal NE. Multiple chemical sensitivity: lessons from seasonal affective disorder. Toxicol Ind Health 1994; 10(4/5):623–632.

33. American Academy of Allergy and Immunology. Position statement: candidiasis hypersensitivity syndrome. J Allergy Clin Immunol 1986; 78:271–273.

34. Pearson DJ. Food allergy, hypersensitivity and intolerance. J R Coll Physicians Lond 1985; 19(3):154–162.

35. King DS. Biological and social factors in food sensitivities. Toxicol Ind Health 1992; 8(4):137–144.
36. Bell IR. A kinin model of mediation for food and chemical sensitivities: biobehavioral implications. Ann Allergy 1975; 35(Oct):206–215.
37. Bell IR. Clinical Ecology: A New Medical Approach to Environmental Illness. Bolinas, CA: Common Knowledge Press, 1982.
38. Crayton JW. Immunologically mediated behavioral reactions to foods. Food Technol 1986; 40:153–157.
39. Philpott WH. Allergy and ecology in orthomolecular psychiatry. In: Dickey LD, ed. Clinical Ecology. Springfield, IL: Charles C. Thomas, 1976:729–737.
40. Philpott WH, Kalita D. Brain Allergies: The Psychonutrient Connection. New Canaan, CT: Keats, 1980.
41. Randolph TG. Allergy as a causative factor in fatigue, irritability, and behavior problems of children. J Pediatr 1947; 31:560–572.
42. Randolph TG, Moss RW. An Alternative Approach to Allergies. New York: Lippincott & Crowell, 1980.
43. Lessof MH, Wraith DG, Merrett TG, Merrett J, Buisseret PD. Food allergy and intolerance in 100 patients: local and systemic effect. Q J Med 1980; 49: 259–271.
44. May CD. Objective clinical and laboratory studies of immediate hypersensitivity reactions to food in asthmatic children. J Allergy Clin Immunol 1976; 58(4):500–515.
45. Metcalfe DD, Sampson HA, Simon RA, eds. Food Allergy: Adverse Reactions to Foods and Food Additives. Boston: Blackwell Scientific, 1991.
46. Vaughn TR, Mansfield LE. Neurologic reactions to foods and food additives. In: Metcalfe DD, Sampson HA, Simon RA, eds. Food Allergy: Adverse Reactions to Food and Food Additives. Oxford: Blackwell Scientific, 1991, pp 355–369.
47. Mansfield LE, Vaughn TR, Waller SF, Haverly RW, Ting S. Food allergy and adult migraine: double-blind and mediator confirmation of an allergic etiology. Ann Allergy 1985; 55:126–129.
48. Dohan FC. Cereals and schizophrenia: data and hypothesis. Acta Psychiatr Scandinavica 1966; 42:125–152.
49. Dohan FC. Genetic hypothesis of idiopathic schizophrenia: its exorphin connection. Schizophr Bull 1988; 14:489–494.
50. Dohan FC. Genetics and idiopathic schizophrenia (letter). Am J Psychiatry 1989; 146(11):1522–1523.
51. Hemmings GP. Is schizophrenia a G-I disease (letter). Br J Psychiatr 1990; 156:448.
52. Pardes H, Kaufmann CA, Pincus HA, West A. Reply to Dr. Dohan (letter). Am J Psychiatry 1989; 146(11):1523.
53. Dohan FC, Grasberger JC. Relapsed schizophrenics: earlier discharge from the hospital after cereal-free, milk-free diet. Am J Psychiatr 1973; 130(6):685–688.
54. Storms LH, Clopton JM, Wright, C. Effects of gluten on schizophrenics. Arch Gen Psychiatry 1982; 39:323–327.

55. King DS. Statistical power of the controlled research on wheat gluten and schizophrenia (comment). Biol Psychiatry 1985; 20:785–787.
56. Singh MM, Kay SR. Wheat gluten as a pathogenic factor in schizophrenia. Science 1976; 191:401–402.
57. Reichelt KL, Landmark J. Specific IgA antibody increases in schizophrenia. Biol Psychiatry 1995; 37:410–413.
58. Dean G, Hanniffy L, Stevens F. Schizophrenia and coeliac disease. J Irish Med Assoc 1975; 685:545–546.
59. Lambert MT, Bjarnason I, Connelly J, Crow TJ, Johnstone EC, Peters TJ, Smethurst P. Small intestine permeability in schizophrenia. Br J Psychiatry 1989; 155:619–622.
60. Stevens FM, Lloyd RS, Gerachty SM, Reynolds MTG, Sarsfield MJ, McNicholl B, Fottrell PF, Wright X, McCarthy CF. Schizophrenia and coeliac disease: the nature of the relationship. Psychol Med 1977; 7:259–263.
60a. O'Mahony S, Ferguson A. Gluten-sensitive enteropathy (celiac disease). In: Metcalfe DD, Sampson HA, Simon RA, eds. Food Allergy; Adverse Reactions to Foods and Food Additives. Boston: Blackwell Scientific, 1991: 186–198.
61. Zeitz HJ. Pharmacologic properties of foods. In: Metcalfe DD, Sampson HA, Simon RA, eds. Food Allergy: Adverse Reactions to Foods and Food Additives. Boston: Blackwell Scientific, 1991:311–318.
62. Hallert C, Derefeldt T. Psychic disturbances in adult coeliac disease. I. Clinical observations. Scand J Gastroenterol 1982; 17:17–19.
63. Hallert C, Astrom J. Psychic disturbances in adult coeliac disease. II. Psychological findings. Scand J Gastroenterol 1982; 17:21–24.
64. Hallert C, Astrom J, Sedvall G. Psychic disturbances in adult coeliac disease. III. Reduced central monoamine metabolism and signs of depression. Scand J Gastroenterol 1982; 17:25–28.
65. Hallert C. Psychiatric illness, gluten, and celiac disease (letter). Biol Psychiatry 1982; 17(9):959–961.
66. Siegel S. Nonparametric Statistics For the Behavioral Sciences. New York: McGraw-Hill, 1956, p 104.
67. Siegel S. Nonparametric Statistics for the Behavioral Sciences. New York: McGraw-Hill, 1956, Appendix, Table C.
68. Brodie JD. Imaging for the clinical psychiatrist: facts, fantasies, and other musings (editorial). Am J Psychiatry 1996; 153(2):145–149.
69. King DS. Can allergic exposure provoke psychological symptoms? A double-blind test. Biol Psychiatry 1981; 16(1):3–19.
70. Coon JM. Natural toxicants in foods. J Am Diet Assoc 1975;67:213–218.
71. Havender WR, Flynn LT. Does Nature Know Best? Natural Carcinogens in American Food. New York: American Council on Science and Health, 1992.
72. Traenckner I, Wehrmann J, Vieluf D, Abeck D, Ring J. Differential diagnosis of adverse reaction to cow's milk: Allergy versus psychological aversion (abstr). American Academy of Allergy and Immunology, 51st Annual Meeting, New York, March 1, 1995.
73. Parker SL, Garner DM, Leznoff A, Sussman GL, Tarlo SM, Krondl M. Psycholog-

ical characteristics of patients with reported adverse reactions to foods. Int J Eat Disord 1990; 10(4):433–439.

74. Parker SL, Leznoff A, Sussman GL, Tarlo SM, Krondl M. Characteristics of patients with food-related complaints. J Allergy Clin Immunol 1990; 86(4):503–511.

75. Terr AI. Food allergy: a manifestation of eating disorder? Int J Eat Disord 1986; 5(3):575–579.

76. Rix KJB, Pearson DJ, Bentley, SJ. A psychiatric study of patients with supposed food allergy. Br J Psychiatry 1984; 145:121–126.

77. LeDoux JE. Emotion. In: Mountcastle VB, section ed., Blum F, vol. ed., Geiger SR, exec. ed. Handbook of Physiology. Section 1. The Nervous System. Bethesda, MD: American Physiological Society, 1987, p 430.

78. Selner JC, Staudenmayer H. Psychological factors complicating the diagnosis of work-related chemical illness. Immunol Allergy Clin North Am 1992; 12(4):909–919.

79. Bailey CH, Kandel ER. Structural changes accompanying memory storage. Annu Rev Physiol 1993; 55:397–426.

80. Kandel ER, Hawkins RD. The biological basis of learning and individuality. Sci Am 1992; 267 (Sept):79–86.

81. McNaughton BL. The mechanism of expression of long-term enhancement of hippocampal synapses: Current issues and theoretical implications. Annu Rev Physiol 1993; 55:375–396.

82. Ader R, ed. Psychoneuroimmunology. New York: Academic Press, 1981.

83. Ader R, Felten DL, Cohen N, eds. Psychoneuroimmunology. 2nd ed. New York: Academic Press, 1991.

84. Djuric VJ, Bienenstock J. Learned sensitivity. Ann Allergy 1993; 71:5–14.

85. Russell M, Dark KA, Cummins RW, Ellman G, Callaway E, Peeke HV. Learned histamine release. Science 1984; 225:733–734.

86. MacQueen G, Marshall J, Perdue M, Siegel S, Bienenstock J. Pavlovian conditioning of rat mucosal mast cells to secrete rat mast cell protease. II. Science 1989; 243:83–85.

87. Bienenstock J. Nerves, neuropeptides and mast cells. Prog Immunol 1989;7:709–715.

88. Mackenzie JN. The production of the so-called "rose cold" by means of an artificial rose. Am J Med Sci 1886; 91:45–57.

89. Frankenhaeuser M. Experimental approaches to the study of catecholamines and emotions. In: Levi L, ed. Emotions: Their Parameters and Measurement. New York: Raven Press, 1975, pp 209–234.

90. Smith GR, Jr., McDaniel SM. Psychologically mediated effect on the delayed hypersensitivity reaction to tuberculin in humans. Psychosom Med 1983; 45:65–70.

91. Black S, Humphrey JH, Niven JS. Inhibition of Mantoux reaction by direct suggestion under hypnosis. Br Med J 1963; 1:1649–1652.

92. Bolla-Wilson K, Wilson RJ, Bleeker ML. Conditioning of physical symptoms after neurotoxic exposure. J Occup Med 1988; 30:684–686.

93. Miller NE. Learnable drives and rewards. In: Stevens SS, ed. Handbook of Experimental Psychology. New York: Wiley, 1951, pp 435–472.

94. French TM, Alexander F. Psychogenic factors in bronchial asthma. Psychosom Med 1941; monograph 4.
95. Dekker E, Pelser HE, Groen J. Conditioning as a cause of asthmatic attacks: a laboratory study. J Psychosom Res 1957; 2:97–108.
96. Dekker E, Groen J. Reproducible psychogenic attacks of asthma: a laboratory study. J Psychosom Res 1956; 1:58–67.
97. Wolff HG. Life stress and bodily disease—a formulation: The nature of stress in man. Proceedings of the Association for Research in Nervous and Mental Disease. Baltimore: Williams & Wilkins, 1950, pp 1059–1094.
98. Graham DT, Wolf S, Wolff HG. Changes in tissue sensitivity associated with varying life situations and emotions; their relevance to allergy. J Allergy 1950; 21:478–486.
99. Pearson DJ, Rix KJB. Psychological effects of food allergy. In: Brostoff J, Challacombe SJ, eds. Food Allergy and Intolerance. East Sussex, England: Baillieres Tindall, 1987, pp 688–708.
100. Pearson DJ, Rix KJB, Bentley SJ. Food allergy: how much in the mind? A clinical and psychiatric study of suspected food hypersensitivity. Lancet 1983; 8336:1259–1261.
101. Findley T. The placebo and the physician. Med Clin North Am 1953; 37:1821–1826.
102. Brodsky CM. "Allergic to everything": a medical subculture. Psychosomatics 1983; 24(8):731–742.
103. Brodsky CM. The psychiatric epidemic in the American workplace. Occup Med State Art Rev 1`988; 3(4):653–662.
104. Staudenmayer H, Selner ME, Selner JC. Adult sequelae of childhood abuse presenting as environmental illness. Ann Allergy 1993; 71(6):538–546.
105. Selner JC, Staudenmayer H. The relationship of the environment and food to allergic and psychiatric illness. In: Young SH, Rubin JM, Daman HR, eds. Psychophysiological Aspects of Allergic Disorders. New York: Praeger, 1986, pp 102–146.
106. Frank JD, Frank JB. Persuasion and Healing: A Comparative Study of Psychotherapy, 3rd ed. Baltimore: Johns Hopkins Press, 1991.
107. Bowlby J. Attachment and Loss. Vol. III. Loss: Sadness and Depression. New York: Basic Books, 1980.
108. Kohut H. The Analysis of the Self. New York: International Universities Press, 1971.
109. Schwarz ED, Perry BD. The post-traumatic response in children and adolescents. Psychiatr Clin North Am 1994; 17(2):311–326.
110. van der Kolk BA. The body keeps the score: memory and the evolving psychobiology of posttraumatic stress. Harvard Rev Psychiatry 1994;1(5):253–265.
111. Staudenmayer H, Camazine M. Sensing type personality, projection and universal "allergic" reactivity. J Psychol Type 1989; 18:59–62.
112. Cloninger CR, Svrakic DM, Przybeck TR. A psychobiological model of temperament and character. Arch Gen Psychiatry 1993; 50:975–990.

113. Black DW, Rathe A, Goldstein RB. Measures of Distress in 26 "environmentally ill" subjects. Psychosomatics 1993; 34(2):131–138.
114. Kelley HH. Attribution theory in social psychology. In: Levine D, ed. Nebraska Symposium on Motivation. Lincoln: University of Nebraska Press, 1967:192–238.
115. Rotter JB. Generalized expectancies for internal versus external control of reinforcement. Psychol Monographs 1966; 80:suppl 1.
116. Gilman SL. Seeing the Insane. New York: Wiley, 1982.
117. Alexander L. Illness maintenance and the new American sick role. In: Chrisman NJ, Maretzki TW, eds. Clinically Applied Anthropology. Boston: Reidel, 1982, pp 351–367.
118. Gots RE, Tamar DH, Flamm WG, Carr CJ. Multiple chemical sensitivities: a symposium on the state of the science. Regul Toxicol Pharmacol 1993; 18:61–78.
119. Staudenmayer, H. Clinical consequences of the EI/MCS 'diagnosis': two paths. Regul Toxicol Pharmacol 1996; 24:596–5110.

18

Challenge Procedures for the Diagnosis of Adverse Food Reactions

AMAL HALIM ASSA'AD
Children's Hospital Medical Center, Cincinnati, Ohio

Adverse reactions to foods are any untoward reactions both nonimmunological and immunological, that follow food ingestion. Nonimmunological reactions are due to either a host factor or a food factor; whereas immunological reactions, referred to as food sensitivity, are either non–immunoglobulin E- (non-IgE-) or IgE-mediated. The IgE-mediated food reactions are referred to as food allergy [1,2]. This chapter will discuss the challenge procedures used to confirm and characterize adverse reactions to foods and their interpretation.

The diagnosis of adverse reactions to foods has three basic components. The first is to elicit from the history an accurate description of the reaction, including timing and severity, and the food(s) suspected of causing the reaction. The second is to define the underlying mechanism, whether nonimmunological or immunological, and in the latter, whether it is IgE- or non-IgE-mediated. The third component is to document whether the reaction occurs reproducibly upon ingestion of the same food.

DEFINING THE ADVERSE FOOD REACTION: HISTORY

The history should aim at identifying the following elements, which will describe the reaction in detail and which are also needed to plan a subsequent food challenge:

1. The suspected food: If a single food ingredient had been ingested and was followed by an adverse reaction, the diagnosis would be simple. However, a meal with several food items is usually ingested, and even single food items are usually composed of several ingredients. In that case, looking for a food item or ingredient common to several meals that were followed by reactions can be helpful. Obtaining food labels is essential in identifying the food ingredients. Frequently, contacting the manufacturer is necessary to elicit a complete list.

2. The amount of food that causes a reaction: It is important to specify the least amount of the food item to cause a reaction. In planning the food challenge, the starting amount will be less than the amount known to elicit reactions.

3. The form of the food that causes a reaction: Different patients react to foods in different forms or to different parts of the same food. For example, since cooking can denature some food allergens, the form of the food, whether raw or cooked, should be determined. This will determine the form of the food that will be used for the challenge.

4. The timing of the reaction: The time of onset of a reaction after food ingestion has to be identified, since this will determine the interval between subsequent doses during the food challenge. It can also be used as a clue in identifying the mechanism of the food reaction, since IgE-mediated reactions are more immediate in onset than nonimmunological reactions, most occurring from 2 minutes to 2 hr.

5. The reproducibility of the reaction: More weight can be given to the history if the same reaction occurs reproducibly upon ingestion of the same food and if the reaction occurs every time the food is ingested.

6. The most recent occurrence of an adverse food reaction: Patients who have had an adverse reaction to a food in the past but have later tolerated the food in a different form may not need to be challenged.

7. An accurate description of the symptoms and the severity of the reaction: If the patient had been examined by a medical personnel, or treated in an emergency room, then written records should be actively sought. The records should be examined carefully for evidence of an anaphylactic reaction, for example, hypotension or loss of consciousness, since well documented anaphylaxis to an identified food is a contraindication for food challenge.

8. Any other medical or psychiatric condition that would preclude performing a food challenge.

9. The current diet: Reviewing the current diet is important to ascertain that it is nutritionally adequate for growth and development. It can also be of diagnostic importance if the patients who report a reaction to a food ingredient are found to be consuming the food regularly without knowing it. It is quite common for parents to report that their child had an untoward reaction to cow's milk and that they have eliminated it from their diet. However, on detailed questioning, one finds that the child has been consuming cow's milk in various foods, for example, yogurt, ice cream, or cheese. Also, if the patient or the parents have not been reading labels, it is most likely that the patient is exposed to the food ingredient hidden under various names in commercially prepared foods.

DEFINING THE MECHANISM OF THE FOOD REACTION: PRICK SKIN TEST AND IN VITRO METHODS

In vitro methods of measuring antigen-specific IgE, for example, by the radioallergosorbent test (RAST), only demonstrate that antigen-specific IgE is present in the circulation. Skin tests have the added advantage of demonstrating that the antigen-specific IgE is bound to the mast cells in the skin and that bridging the IgE receptor with antigen leads to mast cell degranulation. This means that the patient is immunologically sensitized to the food allergen, but does not necessarily predict a clinical reaction when the food is ingested. Immunological diagnosis of food reactions is discussed in detail in Chapter 19, but in the diagnostic scheme, a negative prick skin test result or failure to detect antigen-specific IgE in the circulation has greater than 95% negative predictive accuracy for a clinically significant reaction on challenge [3]. Negative skin tests or negative in vitro test results to a food(s) can be used as a guide to help determine which food(s) is less likely to cause an IgE-mediated reaction to a food challenge when multiple foods are suspected. The tests, however, do not exclude a non-IgE-mediated reaction or nonimmunological reaction. On the other hand, the positive predictive value of those tests in detecting a clinical reaction is rather low, less than 50% [3]. Therefore, evidence of IgE sensitization by prick skin tests or by in vitro tests, which is sometimes obtained when screening panels of skin tests or RAST is used, should not be the sole basis for the diagnosis of adverse food reactions. It should not be a substitute for diagnostic challenge procedures in the presence of a suggestive clinical history.

ESTABLISHING THE REPRODUCIBILITY OF THE FOOD REACTION: FOOD CHALLENGES

Types of Food Challenges

Open Challenge

Open challenges are an easy way to limit the number of blinded challenges performed. In a prospective study of 480 children from birth to 3 years of age, 133 of whom had a history of an adverse food reaction, Bock [4] found that an open challenge failed to reproduce the symptoms in 96 children and was a successful indication to reintroduce the food in the diet. An open challenge performed in a physician's office under monitored conditions usually lessens patient anxiety and the accompanying subjective complaints. It is also an easy way to document objective symptoms, such as urticaria. A positive open challenge result, with adequate documentation of objective symptoms, is diagnostic of adverse food reactions, and a negative challenge result excludes the diagnosis. A challenge that only results in subjective symptoms should be confirmed by a blind challenge. Open challenges are particularly useful in infants and small children since the procedure time is markedly shortened.

In a preliminary study in six adults during an open food challenge, assessment of plasma histamine along with serum and food-stimulated mononuclear cell interleukin 4 levels appeared to be useful objective data [5].

Blind Challenge

Single Blind Challenge

A single-blind challenge will remove the element of patient bias but will not remove observer bias. Bahna [6] has advocated that the procedure be used to screen the foods that are least suspected to cause reactions in a patient who reports adverse reactions to numerous foods. There are no studies that compare the results of single-blind challenges to those of double-blind placebo-controlled challenges, and therefore the validity of this technique has not been established. In practice, when a placebo is included in the challenge, a single-blind challenge does not save any time or effort over a double-blind placebo-controlled challenge.

Double-Blind, Placebo-Controlled Challenge

The procedure of double-blind, placebo-controlled food challenge (DBPCFC) was introduced by May [7] in 1976. As a research tool, it has become the gold standard to which other methods of evaluating adverse reactions to foods are compared. In clinical practice, it has become the clinician's most reliable procedure in making the diagnosis of an adverse food reaction and the basis for prescribing a food-specific elimination diet. It is also the procedure by which the clinician can confidently dismiss the role of foods as the causative agents in the patient's symptoms.

Results of Food Challenges in Various Patient Populations

Food challenges have had various results with regard to patterns of reactions and their timing depending on the patient population examined. It is therefore crucial for the clinician to be aware of these findings in order to interpret the results of a challenge correctly. The following section will discuss the most prominent features of adverse reactions to foods in the patient populations in which the diagnosis is commonly entertained. This will include the general pediatric population and a selected adult population. It will also include patients with asthma and atopic dermatitis.

The General Pediatric Population

Children under 3 Years of Age

Bock et al. [8] studied 25 children 5 months to 3 years of age who had a history of an adverse reaction to one or more foods. An unspecified number of the children had a diagnosis of bronchial asthma. The food challenges were done in a double-blinded fashion, but a placebo challenge was used only when the reactions were equivocal. Thirteen children (50%) manifested 20 adverse reactions in 49 challenges. Of 14 foods studied, adverse reactions occurred only with milk and egg in 7 challenges each, and with peanut and soy in 3 challenges each. Although wheezing was a symptom by history in 7 of the 13 patients and in 11 reactions, it was reproduced in only 2 patients during the challenge. Sneezing and rhinitis occurred in 3 reactions. The majority of symptoms produced during the challenge were gastrointestinal (12/20 reactions), mainly nausea, vomiting, diarrhea, and abdominal pain; and cutaneous (10/20 reactions), in the form of eczema, urticaria, and periorbital angioedema. The reactions occurred in less than 2 hrs in 9 of the 13 children. The delayed reactions, diarrhea and a contact dermatitis–like rash, occurred up to 3 days after the challenge and the reintroduction of the food in the diet. All children with immediate reactions had evidence of IgE sensitization by prick skin tests. However, the prick skin test result was also positive in a third of the subjects who had no reactions to the food challenges. The prick skin test result was positive in only 1 of the 4 subjects who exhibited a delayed reaction.

In a larger, prospective trial Bock [4] studied an unselected population of 480 children less than 3 years of age. In the 133 children in whom an adverse reaction to food was suspected, the food was first eliminated from the diet until the symptoms improved. On open challenge, 21 children (16%) had objective reactions, e.g., skin rashes, prompt vomiting, and diarrhea. Sixteen children (12%) had subjective findings on open challenge that were confirmed by a blind challenge. Although many foods were implicated in the history, only milk, soy, peanut, and egg caused symptoms on challenge. Symptoms given in the history included gastrointestinal and respiratory symptoms, skin rashes, and behavioral changes. Symptoms reproduced by challenges were confined to vomiting, colic, urticaria, erythematous rash, angioedema, and nasal congestion.

In a prospective study of the incidence and natural history of adverse reactions to cow's milk in an unselected population of Danish children during the first 3 years of life, Høst and Halken [9] used challenge procedures to confirm and classify the reactions. They used open challenges and confirmed equivocal results by DBPCFC. In 117 children with symptoms suggestive of adverse reactions to cow's milk, the diagnosis was confirmed in 39 (33%). Nineteen children were immediate reactors, with symptoms occurring within 1 hr, and 20 were late reactors. In the later reactors, symptoms developed in 12 more than 24 hr after beginning the milk challenge and after an intake of more than 8 g of milk protein. The symptoms were cutaneous in 64%, gastrointestinal in 59%, and respiratory in 33%. Most children (92%) with reactions to milk had more than one symptom. This study, compared to the previously cited study by Bock [4], showed a higher prevalence of adverse food reactions in this age group. Noting that the reactions were only to cow's milk highlights the fact that the prevalence of reactions precipitated by food challenges will vary with the food tested.

Repeated food challenges have also been used in this age group in the determination of the natural history of adverse food reactions and as an indicator for a suitable time to reintroduce the food in the diet safely. Bock [4] repeated the challenges at 1 to 3 month intervals until ingestion of the food caused no symptoms. The majority of the food reactions resolved by each child's third birthday. Høst and Halken [9] showed that the combination of testing for IgE sensitization and the challenge procedure gives prognostic indicators of recovery by 3 years of age. The group who demonstrated IgE sensitization at 12 months had a low remission rate of 76% by 3 years compared to the group without evidence of IgE sensitization, who had a 100% remission rate by 3 years of age. Bock [10] used very cautious food challenges under controlled conditions in the hospital to determine the natural history of severe food reactions in nine children less than 2 years of age. Over a period of time, three of the children could tolerate the food in usual portions, and four could tolerate only small amounts.

An interesting group of children in whom DBPCFC was used to confirm the diagnosis are those with a history of adverse reactions to several foods who are found on skin testing to have positive skin test reactions to foods they had never ingested. Cafarelli et al. [11] studied 21 children who had an history of adverse reactions to some foods, had never ingested eggs, but had a positive skin test response to egg. DBPCFC to egg had a positive result in 13 (61%) children. The challenge reactions were positive in only 1 of 12 children with a similar history of adverse reactions to some foods excluding eggs, but with negative skin test responses to egg. Therefore, despite the lack of a history of an adverse reaction to a food, in children with a history of adverse reactions to foods, a positive skin test reaction to a known common food allergen should be followed by a food challenge before introducing that food into the diet.

In children less than 3 years of age with suspected adverse reactions to foods, challenge procedures were shown to have multiple uses:

1. To exclude the diagnosis in the majority of children whose symptoms were attributed by the parents or physicians to be due to foods: this prevents the deleterious nutritional effects of unnecessary food elimination and the social and financial burdens that may ensue.

2. To confirm the diagnosis in children who truly have an adverse reaction to a food: this convinces the parents and the physicians of the need to adhere to the only proven therapy we have to date, a strict elimination of the offending food in all forms.

3. To prevent prolonged food elimination: knowing the natural history of adverse reactions to individual food in this age group, repeated challenges at 3 to 6 month intervals are indicated to identify the time when the food can be tolerated and safely reintroduced into the diet.

Children Older than 3 Years of Age

Bock and Atkins [12] used the DBPCFC to evaluate 315 children 3 years and older. Of 669 food challenges 133 (20%) produced symptoms in 111 (35%) children. The foods commonly causing symptoms in order of frequency were peanut, egg, nuts, and milk. Other foods, including fish, soy, peas, wheat, shrimp, chicken, turkey, and banana, provoked symptoms in fewer challenges. Interestingly, in this age group, positive skin test responses occurred in 98% of the positive challenge outcomes and no patients had delayed reactions to the DBPCFC.

The Adult Population

Young et al. [13] used the DBPCFC procedure in conjunction with a questionnaire to identify the prevalence of reactions to eight foods commonly perceived to cause sensitivity in the United Kingdom. The eight foods in question were cow's milk; hen's egg; wheat; soybean; citrus fruit; fish/shellfish; nuts, including peanuts; and chocolate. Approximately 50% of 20,000 individuals surveyed responded to a questionnaire about a perceived connection between food ingestion and itching, eczema, urticaria, angioedema, asthma, rhinitis, intestinal symptoms, joint symptoms, behavioral or mood changes, and headache. Of the population surveyed, 20% stated a problem related to food ingestion. Of 93 subjects tested by DBPCFC 18 subjects (19.4%) had a positive challenge response. The symptoms precipitated, in order of descending frequency, were joint symptoms, intestinal symptoms, headache, behavioral symptoms, urticaria, and asthma. Their results gave a prevalence of intolerance for the eight test foods studied of 1.4% to 1.8%.

In another population study, Niestijl et al. [14] used a questionnaire, screening tests, and DBPCFC to determine the prevalence of food allergy and intolerance in the adult Dutch population. Of 1483 subjects chosen by random sampling for the survey, 12.4% reported an adverse reaction to a food. Of the subjects available for clinical evaluation, a more detailed history and skin prick tests excluded the diagnosis in one-third. Of 37 subjects available for food elimination and challenge procedures, lack of improvement of symptoms after food elimination excluded the diagnosis in 4 subjects, a negative open challenge result excluded the diagnosis in 8 subjects, and a negative DBPCFC response excluded the diagnosis in 13 subjects. The foods that precipitated symptoms on DBPCFC were pork, fish and shrimp, kiwi fruit, menthol, white wine, preservatives, and histamine containing foods. Apart from urticaria and skin rashes, the other symptoms were vague symptoms of dizziness, blurred vision, perspiration, and flushing. Only the reaction to kiwi fruit could be confirmed to be IgE-mediated by a positive skin test finding. The authors estimated the minimum prevalence of food intolerance in the study population to be 0.8%, and in the general population to be 2.4%.

In a study by Bernstein et al. [15] of adult patients, ages 18 to 67 years, who were selected because of a history of apparent food sensitivity to one or more foods, DBPCFC findings were positive to at least one food in 9 of 22 patients and positive to placebo in 1 patient. Close examination of the presenting symptoms, which were the same symptoms precipitated by the challenges, reveals that they were mostly subjective symptoms of stomatitis, sore throat, pruritus, shortness of breath, nausea, abdominal pain, and headache. Few patients had objective symptoms of urticaria, rhinorrhea, conjunctivitis, and diarrhea. The total amount of 14 g of dried food was consumed before a reaction was elicited. The foods producing symptoms were tomato, milk, chocolate, shrimp, coconut, pork, sunflower, and oat. Skin test reactions were positive to only 4 of 19 foods tested.

Nørgaard and Blindslev-Jensen [16] confined their study to the examination of egg and milk allergy in the adult population. DBPCFC responses were positive in 10 of 19 patients. All patients exhibited gastrointestinal symptoms, and 80% had accompanying respiratory or skin symptoms. The dose eliciting reactions varied from 0.005 to 50 g of fresh egg and 5 to 250 g of fresh milk. All reactions were immediate, within 10–40 minutes. There was no concordance between skin prick test and DBPCFC results in their patient population.

The previous studies indicate that in the adult population reporting adverse reactions to foods, DBPCFC is the only method to substantiate the reactions. In a population selected for a history of adverse reaction to foods, DBPCFC will confirm the reaction in only a third to a half of the patients. The food antigens eliciting reactions are more varied, and the concordance of skin test findings and challenges is low.

Patients with Atopic Dermatitis

Sampson [17] challenged 320 patients aged 6 months to 25 years with moderate to severe atopic dermatitis to foods suspected as a result of history, by skin test results, or by in vitro IgE test responses. The challenges were done after the skin was cleared with intensive topical therapy in the hospital. The reactions were cutaneous in 75% of positive challenge outcomes. The skin symptoms provoked by DBPCFC usually consisted of a markedly pruritic, erythematous, morbilliform rash that developed at patient's predilection site for eczema. Four to eight hours after the primary reaction, diffuse pruritus and an erythematous macular rash developed in many patients. Urticarial lesions were not reported after the first challenge, but were seen in follow-up challenges a year later in patients whose eczema had resolved with a food specific elimination diet. Although not suggested by history, gastrointestinal symptoms occurred in 53% of challenges, respiratory symptoms in 46%, with wheezing in 10%. The foods that caused positive challenge responses were eggs in 30%, milk in 22%, peanut in 15%, soy in 9%, wheat in 5%, and fish in 3%. Food challenges were also used to evaluate the natural history of the sensitization to food in this population, and the results of repeated challenges showed that only 25% lost food reactivity after 2 years, and an additional 11% after 3 years.

Patients with Asthma

In children with asthma, the role of foods as a trigger has been difficult to establish. May [6] used the food challenge procedure in 38 children with severe asthma, in whom the parents or the physician suspected foods to be a trigger for asthma exacerbations. When tested by double-blind (without a placebo control) challenge, 28% of the children were found to have confirmed food reactions. However, the symptoms were confined to the gastrointestinal tract and the skin, and no respiratory symptoms could be documented. Novembre et al. [18] used food challenges in 140 patients with either asthma alone or asthma and atopic dermatitis. Only patients with both asthma and atopic dermatitis exhibited respiratory symptoms after food challenges in 20 of 48 challenges. Among these, immediate or delayed wheezing occurred in 5.7%. James et al. [19] found that even in the absence of a measurable bronchospastic response, this population can respond to a food challenge by an increase in bronchial hyperreactivity, manifested by an increased sensitivity to methacholine.

The Challenge Procedure

The Elimination Period

Challenges are preceded by a total elimination of the food that will be used for a period that ranges in various published studies from 1 to 6 weeks. The longer elimination periods have been used in patients with atopic dermatitis or behavioral symptoms. The elimination period should not be too long since the longer the period before a challenge, the more likely the challenge result would be negative. Sloper et al. [20] found that in patients with atopic dermatitis, negative challenge results were associated with a median time of avoidance of the particular food of 7.5 months, whereas positive challenge results were associated with a median time of avoidance of 3.5 months.

The elimination period is meant to show that definite resolution of the symptoms occurs when the food(s) is removed from the diet. It also is necessary so that the patient is free of symptoms at the beginning of the challenge procedure. The improvement in symptoms may be relative rather than complete when the symptom investigated is atopic dermatitis. It may be necessary in those patients to design a symptom score that will allow an objective evaluation of the symptoms at baseline and after the period of elimination. Sloper et al. [20], in their study of the clinical response of children with atopic dermatitis to food elimination, assessed the extent of skin involvement by scoring the presence or absence of erythema, vesiculation, excoriation, and lichenification in 20 body areas, making a total possible eczema score of 80. Using an arbitrary criterion of a fall in total skin score of at least 3 as an indication of improvement, they found that atopic dermatitis improved in 49 of 66 patients (74%) after elimination of cow's milk, egg, and other foods. The median skin score change from the initial visit to the visit after food elimination was −6 with a range of −36 to +10. These scores indicate that the improvement in symptoms after elimination of the suspected food(s) in each individual patient is rather subtle and should be evaluated with objective measurements.

Concomitant Medications

Prior to a challenge patients should have restricted medications with antihistamines for an appropriate period according to the half-life of the drug used. Patients should not use beta agonists for 12 to 24 hr.

The Challenge Design

The challenge procedure should be flexible and designed in a way that will best reproduce the exposure and the symptoms, whether immediate reactions, e.g., urticaria, or delayed chronic symptoms, e.g., atopic dermatitis.

The challenge focuses on one food item at a time. A challenge for immediate reactions can be done in 1 day, randomizing the food and the placebo to the morning and afternoon. Alternatively, it can be performed on 2 consecutive days, again randomizing the food and the placebo to either day.

A challenge procedure can also be designed in a manner that allows the effect of chronic repeated exposure to be tested, as in the study by Young et al. [13]. The challenges, with either the food or the placebo, were conducted on two 7 day periods consisting of an initial 3 day challenge followed by a 4 day rest period. For patients with behavioral symptoms or eczema, the procedure was conducted over two 14 day periods, with a 7 day challenge and a 7 day rest period.

In exclusively breast-fed infants, the procedure can be done by elimination of the food, e.g., cow's milk, from the maternal diet, and the challenge can be done by renewed ingestion by the mother of at least 0.5 liter of cow's milk per day.

In patients with a history of reactions to multiple foods, a practical approach is to challenge foods that have elicited a positive skin prick test result. Of those, one can also prioritize the challenges to the foods that are known to be frequent allergens and that are ubiquitous in a normal diet, e.g., cow's milk, egg, soy, and peanut in children. Foods that are easier to avoid and that are not important as nutritional sources can be given a lower priority in the challenges.

The Food, the Placebo, and the Vehicle

The preparation of the foods for a DBPCFC has been reviewed in detail in several publications [21–23]. The food is prepared in a way that will help mask its taste, smell, texture, and consistency in the vehicle used. The following are options:

1. To use the foods in a powder form that can be stirred or dissolved in a liquid vehicle or can be placed in capsules: Grains can be obtained as flour; nuts can be ground; fruits, vegetables, and some meats can be lyophilized; milk and egg can be obtained as dry powder.

2. To homogenize the fresh food in a blender with a liquid vehicle. In this method, a food that the patient is known to tolerate and that has the same texture and consistency as the food in question can be added to the vehicle and used as a placebo.

The vehicle has to be convenient for the patient's age; for example, for patients who cannot swallow capsules, particularly young children, the fresh food or the food in a powder form can be disguised in a drink or a food the patient would consume readily. The vehicle also has to suit the purpose of the challenge. If the challenge is to reproduce oral symptoms or if the oral symptoms are according to the patient's history the first warning of a reaction, then similarly disguising the food in question in a liquid or in another food will assure contact with the oral mucosa. The liquid vehicles most commonly used are elemental formulas that are made of amino acids and do not have intact proteins. Otherwise, the most convenient manner for performing a DBPCFC is to place the powdered food in question in gelatin capsules. For placebo, the capsules are filled with dextrose.

There are no studies that directly compare the results of DBPCFC using dried or dehydrated food to those using fresh food. Vatn et al. [24] compared the protein content of commercially available lyophilized food in capsules and fresh food from the grocery store by SDS-polyacrylamide gel electrophoresis and Coomassie brilliant blue R staining. The constituents of the corresponding preparations of cow's milk, egg, hazelnut, wheat, and cod were found to be identical.

Of the patients' serum that had immunoglobulin G (IgG) and IgA to milk and wheat, Western blots using protein from the lyophilized food or the fresh food gave similar results. If one can extrapolate from the results of other studies that compared the allergenicity of fresh foods to that of commercial extracts or foods denatured by heat or enzymatic digestion, the use of fresh foods gives a small advantage. Norgaard et al [25] compared fresh food extracts and commercial extracts in skin prick tests and measurements of histamine release from basophils. In testing for cow's milk and egg allergy, the fresh extracts significantly improved the specificity of the skin prick test and histamine release over the results obtained using commercial extracts. Another study by Burks et al [26] determined the allergenicity of peanut and soybean extracts after thermal denaturation using temperatures up to 100°C for 60 minutes and after enzymatic denaturation using a system that simulates gastric and small intestinal hydrolysis. The thermal denaturation did not change the allergenicity of both extracts, whereas the enzymatic denaturation decreased the allergenicity of the peanut extract 100-fold, and that of the soybean extract 10-fold.

The Monitoring

On the day of the challenge, a complete history and physical exam should precede challenge. It should be ascertained once again that the patient has not had previous anaphylaxis to the food to be challenged that day. Special attention should be directed to the target organs of the adverse food reaction given in the history of the patient and the known target organs of allergic reactions, for example, the skin, nose, and lungs. Whether the challenge is conducted in the office or in the hospital, medications to treat possible severe or anaphylactic reactions, namely, epinephrine, diphenhydramine, and prednisone, in the correct dose for the patient's age and weight should be available at the bedside. Vital signs should be recorded prior to the challenge. Vital signs, inspection of the skin, and auscultation of the lungs should be done before each dose given during the challenge. A form can be designed to note the timing and the nature of patient's subjective symptoms and the examiner's objective findings [22,27]. The challenge continues until the patient's symptoms or signs of a reaction are documented, or until the full dose is given. If the full challenge has been tolerated without reactions, the patient should be given the food in an open form, in an amount usually consumed during a meal. The patient is then monitored for another hour, or longer if suggested by the history.

CONCLUSION

The diagnosis of adverse reactions to foods using the food challenge procedures requires accurate evaluation of the patient's history, thoughtful planning of the procedure, and careful administration of the challenge. Knowing the published results of food challenges in various patient populations should provide the physician with a realistic expectation of the outcome of the challenge with regard to the percentage of positive challenge results, the reactions to be expected, and the foods causing them. The goal of the challenges is to establish the diagnosis of adverse reaction to a food in order to eliminate it from the diet, and to reintroduce into the diet foods that are safely tolerated in order to prevent unnecessary dietary elimination.

REFERENCES

1. Anderson JA, Sogn DD, eds. Adverse Reactions to Foods. AAAI and NIAID NIH publication No 84-2442, 1984.
2. Bruijzeel-Koomen C, Ortolani C, Aas K, Bindslev-Jensen C, Bjorksten B, Moneret-Vautrin D, B. Wuthrich Adverse reactions to food. Eur Acad Allergolo Clin Immunol Subcommittee *Allergy 1995; 50(8):*623.
3. Burks AW, Sampson HA. Diagnostic approaches to the patient with suspected food allergies. *J Pediatr 1992; 121:*S64.
4. Bock SA. Prospective appraisal of complaints of adverse reactions to foods in children during the first 3 years of life. *Pediatrics 1987; 79:*683.
5. Chavarria V, Young RM, Zitt M, Karnik A, Kurpad C, Fitzgerald D, Frieri M. Interleukin-4 and plasma histamine levels in challenged food hypersensitive patients. Ann Allergy 1994; 72:57a.
6. Bahna SL. Blind food challenge testing with wide-open eyes. *Ann Allergy 1994;* 72:235.
7. May CD. Objective clinical and laboratory studies of immediate hypersensitivity reactions to foods in asthmatic children. *J Allergy Clin Immunol 1976; 58:*500.
8. Bock A, Lee W, Remigio L, May C. Studies of hypersensitivity reactions to foods in infants and children. *J Allergy Clin Immunol 1978; 62:*327.
9. Høst A, Halken S. A prospective study of cow milk allergy in Danish infants during the first three years of life. *Allergy 1990; 45(8):*587.
10. Bock A. Natural history of severe reactions to foods in young children. *J Pediatr 1985; 107:*676.
11. Caffarelli C, Cavagni G, Giordano S, Stapane I, Rossi C. Relationship between oral challenges with previously uningested egg, and egg-specific IgE antibodies and skin prick tests in infants with food allergy. *J Allergy Clin Immunol 1995; 95:*1215.
12. Bock SA, Atkins FM. Patterns of food hypersensitivity during sixteen years of double-blind, placebo-controlled food challenges. *J Pediatr 1990; 117:*561.
13. Young E, Stoneham MD, Petruckevitch A, Barton J, Rona R. A population study of food intolerance. *Lancet 1994; 343:*1127.
14. Niestijl Jansen JJ, Kardinaal AFM, Huijbers G, Vlieg-Boerstra BJ, Martens BPM, Ockhuizen T. Prevalence of food allergy and intolerance in the adult Dutch population. *J Allergy Clin Immunol 1994; 93:*446.
15. Bernstein M, Day JH, Welsh A. Double-blind food challenge in the diagnosis of food sensitivity in the adult. *J Allergy Clin Immunol 1982; 70:*205.

16. Norgaard A, Binslev-Jensen C. Egg and milk allergy in adults: diagnosis and characterization. *Allergy 1992; 47:*503.

17. Sampson HA. The immunopathogenic role of food hypersensitivity in atopic dermatitis. *Acta Derm Venereol (Stockh) 1992; 176:*71.

18. Novembre E, Martino M, Vierucci A. Foods and respiratory allergy. *J Allergy Clin Immunol 1988; 81(2):*1059.

19. James J, Eigenmann P, Eggleston P, Sampson H, Airway reactivity changes in asthmatic patients undergoing blinded food challenges. *Am J Respir Crit Care Med 1996; 153:*597.

20. Sloper S, Wadsworth J, Brostoff J. Children with atopic eczema: the clinical response to food elimination and subsequent double-blind food challenge, *Q J Med New Series* 1991. *80L:*677.

21. Leinhas JL, McCaskill CC, HA Sampson. Food allergy challenges: guidelines and implications. *J Am Diet Assoc 1987; 87:*604.

22. Bock SA, Sampson JA, Atkins FM, Zieger RS, Lehrer S, Sachs M, Bush RK, Metcalfe DD. Double-blind, placebo-controlled food challenge (DBPCFC) as an office procedure: a manual. *J Allergy Clin Immunol 1988; 82:*986.

23. Huijbers GB, Colen AAM, Niestijl Jansen JJ, Kardinaal EFM, Vlieg-Boerstra BJ, Martens BPM. Masking foods for food challenge: practical aspects of masking foods for a double-blind, placebo-controlled food challenge. *J Am Diet Assoc 1994; 94:*645.

24. Vatn M, Grimstad I, Thorsen L, Kittang E, Refnin I, Malt U, Løvik A, Langeland T, Naalsund A. Adverse reactions to food: assessment by double-blind placebo-controlled food challenge and clinical, psychosomatic and immunologic analysis. *Digestion 1995; 56:*421.

25. Norgaard A, Skov PS, Bindslev-Jensen C. Egg and milk allergy in adults: comparison between fresh foods and commercial allergen extracts in skin prick test and histamine release from basophils, *Clin Exp Allergy 1992; 22:*940.

26. Burks W, Williams L, Thresher W, Connaughton C, Cockrell G, Helm R. Allergenicity of peanut and soybean extracts altered by chemical or thermal denaturation in patients with atopic dermatitis and positive food challenges. *J Allergy Clin Immunol 1992; 90:889.*

27. Bahna S. Practical considerations in food challenge testing. *Immunol Allergy Clin North Am 1991; 11(4):*843.

19

Laboratory Diagnosis of Food Allergy

MANDAKOLATHUR R. MURALI
Williston Park, New York

Adverse reactions to foods have varied clinical spectrums resulting from diverse mechanisms. This heterogeneity constitutes a challenge to clinicians when evaluating a patient with an adverse reaction consequent to the ingestion of a food.

Adverse reaction to a food incorporates any syndrome directly attributable to the ingestion of an identifiable food. It can be food hypersensitivity (allergy) or food intolerance [1]. *Food allergy* is defined as an abnormal immune response resulting from the ingestion of a food or food additive. It includes the classical immunoglobulin E– (IgE-) mediated reaction with immediate symptoms provoked by degranulation of mast cells/basophils induced by specific food antigens as well as immune mechanisms involving lymphocytes cytokine networks, or other effector cells and/or mediators. Food intolerance is the result of nonimmune mechanisms and can be due to toxic contaminants in ingested food (e.g., *Escherichia coli* endotoxin or *Staphylococcus* exotoxin sp.), enzyme deficiencies (e.g., lactose intolerance), pharmacological properties of an ingested beverage (e.g., caffeine, cola), idiosyncratic reactions (e.g., sensitivity to tyramine in aged cheese), or a psychogenic reaction or poorly understood reaction such as those involving sulfites, tartrazine, or yellow dyes (F.D &C #5).

This chapter describes the immunological tests used to evaluate patients suspected of having food allergy and critically examines their clinical utility in corroborating the diagnosis. It must be stated at the outset that the laboratory tests detect or confirm immune sensitivity to food antigens, but their relevance to the patients' manifestations need to be corroborated by meticulous clinical evaluation. The ultimate gold standard for establishing the diagnosis of the allergy is the double-blind placebo-controlled food challenge (DBPCFC). The appearance of symptoms after following such a challenge undeniably proves the existence of allergy or intolerance to some antigens or ingredients in the food material used for the challenge [2].

The various tests used to diagnose food allergy can be divided into in vivo tests and in vitro tests.

A. *In Vivo Tests*
  1. Passive transfer tests
    a. Prausnitz-Kustner (P-K) reaction
    b. Passive cutaneous anaphylaxis (PCA)
  2. Skin tests
  3. Gastrointestinal procedures
    a. Endoscopy and/or radiology after food challenge
    b. Eosinophils/mediators in stools
    c. Intestinal permeability studies
    d. Rectal mucosal imprints/biopsy
  4. Bronchial reactivity after food challenge
  5. Elimination diet
  6. DBPCFC
B. *In Vitro Tests*
  7. Radioallergosorbent test (RAST), enzyme-linked immunosorbent assay (ELISA), etc.
  8. RAST inhibition tests
  9. Precipitins or gel diffusion tests
  10. Mediators from basophils/mast cells and biological fluids
  11. Lymphocyte proliferation assays/cytofluorometry
  12. Leukocyte migration inhibition
  13. Complement activation
  14. Cytokine assay/in situ polymerase chain reaction (PCR)

IN VIVO TESTS

Passive Transfer Tests

Prausnitz-Kustner Reaction

Historically the P–K reaction (1921) was the earliest test used to diagnose ingestant or food allergy [3]. It involved the intradermal transfer of serum from the fish allergic individual (Prausnitz) to the skin of nonallergic Kustner. When the passively sensitized Kustner ingested fish a day later, local itching, erythema, and swelling (urticaria) or wheel and flare developed at the injection site. Not only was the P–K reaction utilized to diagnose allergy, but it also proved that the serum contained a factor that mediated allergic reaction. Years later the factor or reagin was discovered to be IgE by Ishizaka [4]. In the past P–K tests were used to evaluate allergic diseases in subjects whose skin or other conditions precluded skin testing [5]. These conditions included dermatographism, chronic urticaria, and extensive dermatitis; young infants and highly sensitive individuals were at risk of anaphylaxis caused by direct skin tests. Passive transfer tests are less sensitive than direct skin tests, but results generally correlate well with clinical symptoms. Presently, this test is relegated to medical history as it is time consuming and is hazardous as a result of risk of transmitting hepatitis, retroviruses, or slow viruses. Further, newer, more sensitive and rapid in vitro techniques for measuring specific IgE are available for routine clinical use.

Passive Cutaneous Anaphylaxis

Passive cutaneous anaphylaxis is used only for animal research. It involves intradermal injection of serum from a sensitive patient to a nonsensitized animal (usually a monkey). After 24 hr the relevant antigen and Evans blue are injected intravenously into the monkey. The resulting interaction of specific antigen with skin fixing antibody (IgE or IgG) causes local release of mediators of immediate hypersensitivity, which in turn increases vascular permeability and results in the extravasation of blue dye and plasma, manifested as a blue spot [6]. Although this test is useful in animal studies it has no clinical role. Further, it has been replaced by more sensitive in vitro sensitization studies using basophils/mast cells in culture.

Skin Tests

Skin testing remains the basic, cost-effective, and clinically valuable modality in the evaluation of allergic diseases. Skin tests provide a quick bedside answer to biological responses consisting of antigen–IgE interaction, mast cell activation, release of mediators, and their effect on the target organ response—components that define the basis of allergic inflammation [7].

Skin tests include scratch, prick, and puncture and intradermal techniques. Scratch tests are poorly reproducible, are less quantitative, and are not always used in clinical practice. In the evaluation of food allergy intradermal skin tests do not provide more clinically relevant improvement in sensitivity than prick tests. On the contrary, intradermal skin tests contribute to greater false positive test results, which are due to the lack of specificity. Further, intradermal skin tests carry an increased risk of adverse systemic reactions; with food antigens, are therefore, they are not utilized for diagnostic purposes.

The most useful clinical skin test is the prick test. Glycerinated food extracts are utilized for skin testing and they are commercially available from many laboratories. It is to be noted that lack of standardized extracts leads to variability of results when diverse sources are used. Nevertheless, when they are done carefully with both appropriate negative (glycerol–saline solution) and positive (histamine) controls, prick skin tests, in conjunction with a detailed temporal evaluation of the clinical presentation, constitute an extremely valuable diagnostic modality [7].

Recently significant advances have been made in the identification and characterization of the antigenic determinants of common food allergens. For example, the most abundant egg white protein is ovalbumin, but the most predominant antigenic moiety is ovomucoid. The peanut, a legume, is one of the most prevalent food allergens and also one that has been incriminated in many anaphylactic reactions. Even though there are 16 protein fractions on sodium dodecyl sulfate polyacrylamide gel electrophoresis (SDS-PAGE), two of these, Ara h I and Ara h II, are the major allergens [8]. Sera from more than 90% of peanut-allergic patients have been shown to have specific IgE to these two fractions. It is to be noted that by utilizing SDS-PAGE and Western blot many important food allergens are being identified and cross-reactivates defined. Examples include cross-reactivity between apple and birch, and between latex and banana [9,10]. It is just a question of time before well-defined, highly purified (possibly produced by recombinant technology) food antigens will be available for skin testing. Availability of standardized antigens will contribute to a more standardized approach to skin testing for food allergy.

Utilizing the presently available commercial extracts the accuracy of prick skin tests for six common food allergens was compared with the clinical outcome of food challenge in children with atopic dermatitis. The spectrum of sensitivity ranged from 73% for eggs to 100% for peanuts and fish. The specificity was significantly lower for all the food extracts tested. In this series the negative predictive accuracy was excellent, but the positive predictive value was poor [11]. Skin prick tests are useful only in the diagnosis of IgE-mediated food allergy; they do not have any diagnostic value in non-IgE-mediated disorders, such as gluten-sensitive enteropathy. Negative skin prick test responses are generally useful in the exclusion of a given IgE-mediated food allergy [12].

Gastrointestinal Procedures

Endoscopic and Radiological Studies after Food Challenge

The IgE bearing mast cells of the alimentary tract represent the first level of specific encounter with food antigens. Specific interaction with food antigens and the consequent mediator release lead to clinical features of food allergy. Indeed, intragastric provocation and endoscopic and/or radiological studies have been used to document food allergy [13]. This technique is of value in clinical research but not practical to screen the role of many suspected food allergens in a given patient.

Eosinophil Mediators in Stools

Encounter of food allergens with mucosal mast cells bearing IgE in the gastrointestinal tract leads to the chemotaxis of eosinophils and recruitment of mast cells to the site of inflammation. Presence of eosinophils in stools or intestinal biopsy samples consequent to oral challenge with suspected food allergens has been cited as a diagnostic test [14,15]. Its utility is confined to clinical research.

Intestinal Permeability Studies

The intestinal epithelium is not an absolute physical barrier or homogenous structure between the intestinal lumen and intestinal wall and its vascular channels. Intestinal permeability represents a state of intestinal mucosa that permits molecules or compounds (such as mannitol, insulin, lactose, or polyethylene glycols) to diffuse across the membrane, even though in the normal state these molecules do not cross the intestinal barrier as they have no active transport system.

Derangements of this barrier (secondary to mediators of allergic inflammation in food-induced allergy) have been documented by several investigators using the tracer molecules mentioned previously. Intestinal permeability abnormalities have been described by several investigators, using different markers such as PEG 600 or 4000, [51Cr]ethylene diaminetetraacetic acid (EDTA), rhamnose, and lactulose [16]. In a series of children with atopic dermatitis, analyses of intestinal permeability tests carried out during a food provocation procedure documented that in 14 of 35 subjects the permeability was increased [17]. The value of this test in clinical practice needs to be established and standardized. Nevertheless, it represents a noninvasive approach to understanding mucosal immunity in food allergy.

Rectal Mucosal Imprint/Biopsy

Rectal mucosal imprint/biopsy has been utilized by Japanese investigators to identify the food-induced inflammatory response. They have documented the migration of eosinophils and mast cells in rectal tissue consequent to food challenge and have used it as a marker of food allergy [18]. Again, it is of limited value in clinical practice.

Bronchial Reactivity after Food Challenge

Food allergy manifested by release of mediators of allergic response might alter the state of bronchomotor tone and hence bronchial reactivity to histamine or methacholine. This altered bronchial reactivity is quantitated by the histamine or methacholine provocative test and expressed as that dose of methacholine or histamine that causes a 20% drop in forced expiratory volume (FEV_1) before and after challenge with the offending food. James et al. studied the effects of food allergens on airway hyperresponsiveness in 16 patients with mild to severe asthma and documented food hypersensitivity by DBPCFC [19]. They evaluated the usefulness of spirometry and methacholine challenge performed before and after DBPCFC. There were 22 positive DBPCFC reactions overall, and 12 involved chest symptoms. The symptoms included coughing, chest tightness, and/or wheezing. Methacholine induced airway hyperresponsiveness increased significantly in 7 of these patients, in a patient with a positive DBPCFC result and no chest symptoms, and in a patient with a negative DBPCFC finding. In only 1 patient did the FEV_1 change significantly. This study clearly points out two important practical aspects: First, it endorses the concept that food induced allergic reactions can increase air reactivity in patients with asthma without inducing an acute asthmatic reaction and contribute to clinical deterioration. Second, it indicates the diagnostic value of methacholine induced bronchial hyperreactivity in such subjects when spirometry is not so useful in corroborating a diagnosis of food induced asthma. Similar conclusions have been reported in patients with tartrazine sensitivity [20].

Food Diary and Elimination Diet

A detailed food diary may be helpful in subjects with a history of intermittent episodes of acute urticaria and cutaneous pruritus (with or without oral allergy manifestations). Any suggestion of a causal effect indicated by the timing of the ingestion of a food (or its related antigen) needs to be explored with a detailed history and examination and followed up by skin prick tests. In these situations diagnostic elimination of the food from the diet must be carried out. If the skin test results are positive and the symptoms resolve or remit consequent to elimination of specific food (or antigenically related food), then a pathogenic role for the food in question is clearly implicated [12].

If the finding of the initial evaluation (detailed history, food diary, skin tests, or in vitro tests) is negative, careful removal of the highly allergenic food may be helpful. In subjects with severe symptoms use of an amino acid–based formula (elemental formula) may be necessary [12]. Such a drastic approach must be done with dietary supervision and may be useful in eliminating the symptoms/signs of food allergy. Once the clinical state is stable, an allergist/dietician supervised food challenge may help in the identification of the relevant food allergen.

Elimination diets are time consuming and necessitate careful planning, patient compliance, and thorough chronological data on symptoms/signs. Nevertheless they are rewarding to both patients and clinicians.

Double-Blind Placebo-Controlled Food Challenge

The gold standard in substantiating an adverse reaction to food irrespective of the mechanism is the DBPCFC. Its clinical utility and scientific validity have been extensively documented [21,22]. The "blinding" of both the clinician and the patient eliminates any possibility of an interpretational or subjective bias, respectively. The following is a brief outline of the DBPCFC adapted from the guidelines published by Sampson and Metcalfe [23].

1. The procedure should be done under controlled conditions, such as in a hospital, clinic, or physician's office.
2. The challenge should be performed by personnel (preferably allergists/immunologists) knowledgeable about the manifestations of adverse reaction to food and in the management of anaphylaxis.
3. The patient/family must be fully informed of the objective and procedures involved to relieve any apprehension.
4. The suspected food should be eliminated from the diet 10–14 days prior to challenge.
5. Antihistamines should be discontinued 12 hr prior to challenge.
6. The individual to be challenged should be in a stable cardiovascular, pulmonary, and metabolic condition prior to challenge.
7. The individual to be challenged should be in a fasting state (6–12 hr) when challenged.
8. The challenge should start with a low dose (e.g., 125–500 mg lyophilized food) so as not to provoke symptoms.
9. Gradual increase in dose (suspected food or placebo) should occur by doubling the amount every 15–20 minutes.
10. The maximum dose of food used in the challenge should approximate 10 g of lyophilized food.
11. The minimum recommended observation period after completion of the DBPCFC procedure is as follows:
    a. Suspected anaphylaxis, 2 hr
    b. Isolated gastrointestinal (GI) signs/symptoms, 4–8 hr
    c. Food intolerance reaction, 4–8 hr
12. In follow-up of negative specific food challenge reaction, open feeding with this food is recommended for the subsequent 24–48 hr

DBPCFC is now being coupled with studies of mediators and cellular and/or cytokine responses to enhance the clinicopathological basis of food allergy.

IN VITRO TESTS

Tests for Specific Immunoglobulin E

Tests for specific IgE such as RAST and ELISA are solid-phase immunoassays and are based on a principle similar to that of the indirect Coombs' test. The allergens (food antigens or extracts) are coupled covalently to solid-phase support (such as filter paper disks or cellulose caps or inner walls of microtiter plates) and then incubated with the patient's serum. During incubation the specific antibodies of all immunoglobulin classes bind to the solid-phase allergen. The nonantibody serum components are removed from the solid-phase allergen complex by washing. During the second stage, the solid-phase complex is incubated with radiolabeled (in RAST) or enzyme-linked (in ELISA) affinity purified polyclonal or monoclonal antibody to human IgE. In the case of radiolabeled anti-IgE the allergen solid-phase complex is washed again to remove excess unbound radioactive anti-IgE and counted in a gamma counter. In the case of ELISA, the excess unbound enzyme-labeled anti-IgE is also removed by washing, and the allergen solid-phase complex is incubated with a chromogenic substrate for the enzyme. The enzyme substrate reaction results in a color change (the intensity of which is proportional to allergen-specific IgE) that is measured in a spectrophotometer [24]. Other indicator systems that have been developed incorporate principles of fluorescence. In immunochemiluminescent assays antihuman IgE antibodies are labeled with horseradish peroxidane (HRP) or acridinium ester in the second stage of the assay. After incubation and washing, the light reaction of the samples is detected in a chemiluminometer by addition of enzyme substrate and hydrogen peroxide and the photoemissions are detected. In the FAST system, the second antibody is coupled to a fluorescein dye, and after washing the intensity of fluorescence is quantitated [24]. The advantages of RAST/ELISA testing for food allergies are as follows:

1. It is sensitive and reproducible.
2. It is useful in patients with dermatographism.
3. It is useful in patients on long-acting antihistaminics or those who cannot stop any H_1 blocker.
4. It is useful in patients with severe anaphylaxis to fish or nuts.
5. In infants and toddlers who require tests with multiple allergens these in vitro tests provide an easy, nontraumatic modality of evaluation.
6. It can be ordered by nonallergists (though its accurate interpretation and clinical relevance often require an allergist) when food allergy is a consideration in the diagnosis of the patient's symptoms.

The disadvantages outweigh its uses:

1. RAST and ELISA detect only antigen-specific IgE in serum and do not provide an evaluation of the biological response consequent to antigen interaction with cell bound IgE as is provided by allergy skin tests.
2. It lacks of standardized allergens coupled to the solid phase.
3. Difficulty and variations in coupling allergens to the solid-phase system occur.
4. Nonspecific IgE and IgE complexes trap to the solid phase.

5. Lectin interference of IgE binding occurs, especially with food allergens.
6. It is expensive and requires sophisticated equipment, trained personnel, and greater turnaround time.
7. RAST interference by IgG blocking antibodies is possible. This has been largely overcome by using sorbents with greater allergen-binding capacity.
8. There is a poor correlation between the RAST scores and the severity of the clinical picture.

RAST Inhibition Test

The RAST inhibition test is a radioimmunoassay very similar to the RAST assay except that the soluble antigen identical to or cross-reactive with the antigen on the solid phase is added with the patient's serum. The resultant inhibition of binding of radiolabeled anti-IgE to the antigen on the solid phase reflects the antigenic identity or cross-reactivity of the soluble antigen with antigen bound to the solid phase. RAST inhibition assays are utilized in standardization of allergenic extracts. Though they are not routinely used in clinical practice, they have helped define some of the antigenic determinants in complex food allergies. For example, in a subject with acute urticaria and angioedema after ingestion of soybean products, the RAST inhibition assay was able to pinpoint IgE antibodies specific for the polypeptides of a soybean trypsin inhibitor as the clinically relevant allergen in soybean [25]. Cross-reactivity among birch pollens, apples, and potatoes has been documented by this assay in subjects with documented allergy to these foods [26].

Gel Diffusion Techniques

Gel diffusion techniques are based on the principle that antigen and antibody diffuse through a semisolid medium (e.g., agar), forming precipitins at the zone of equivalence. IgM, IgG, and IgA form precipitins but IgD and IgE do not. In the radiodiffusion techniques, either antigen or antibody is radioactively labeled and the resulting antigen–antibody complex or precipitate is quantitated by autoradiography. Such techniques have been applied in the evaluation of precipitating antibodies to milk proteins in children with milk allergy. Generally fewer than 25% of normal children may have precipitating antibodies to cow's milk protein. In children with milk allergy the incidence of these antibodies is well over 50%. The incidence of positive results increases dramatically in patients with intestinal diseases and antibody deficiency syndromes. In these situations the precipitins may represent an immune response to milk proteins absorbed excessively or processed inappropriately by an altered gastrointestinal mucosal barrier [27]. The technique of immunoblot or Western blot involves separation of the antigenic determinant of food allergens (based on their molecular size) on polyacrylamide gels. These gels are then reacted with patients' serum, and the specific IgE to the various fractions of the food allergen is developed by using anti-IgE antibodies labeled with radioactive isotope. The resulting radioactive bands are then developed by autoradiography. The advantage of this technique is its ability to identify the various immunogenic determinants in complex food antigens. Such a technique has been used to characterize common determinants among diverse foods such as banana, kiwi, or avocado. The clinical value of this technique is that it identifies cross-reactive food antigens and in some instances the interrelationship between food allergy and latex allergy [28,29].

Basophil Histamine Release Tests

Perturbation of the basophil membrane by either IgE dependent pathways or anaphylatoxins can result in histamine release. Histamine release can be measured by bioassay, fluorometry, radioimmunoassay, and radioisotopic enzymatic assays or by evaluation of basophil degranulation. Basophil histamine release testing has become popular and semiautomated methods are being evaluated in clinical practice. The predictive values of allergen induced basophil histamine release and skin prick testing were compared in 57 children admitted for DBPCFC. For milk, egg, and peanuts, the positive predictive value for skin prick tests ranged from 25% to 69% whereas that for basophil histamine release was only 16%–30% [30]. Studies have shown that food allergic children with atopic dermatitis have higher rates of spontaneous basophil histamine release than with those children with atopic dermatitis who do not have food allergies or normal nonatopic children [31]. The basophil histamine release correlates with RAST, skin prick tests, and positive food challenge results in this group of food allergic subjects [30,32]. At the present time, basophil histamine release assay is not available as a routine clinical test even though it has been shown to have limited clinical value in the follow-up evaluation of food allergic children with severe clinical features. In this group, spontaneous basophil releasability was lost after 4 to 6 months of an appropriate food allergen elimination diet. With the description of various chemokines and their role in modulating basophil histamine release, it is just a question of time before a more meaningful cellular test for food allergy will be developed.

Lymphocyte Proliferation Assays

The hallmark of an immunologically committed lymphocyte is its transformation from a small naïve cell into a large blast that proliferates as well as secretes specific cytokines. A number of stimuli such as the lectins—phytohemagglutinin

(PHA) and concanavalin A (ConA)—nonspecifically stimulate resting lymphocytes to proliferate. Food antigens, on the other hand, stimulate only a few specifically sensitized lymphocytes. The standard assay for lymphocyte proliferation in response to mitogens and food antigens measures the incorporation of radiolabeled thymidine into deoxyribonucleic acid (DNA). It is to be noted that such foods as legume and wheat have lectinlike properties that cause false positive results that are due to their lectin activity rather than their action through the T cell receptor. Some studies have reported the value of the proliferative assay in patients with delayed-type symptoms [33]. The limitations of these assays include individual variability, poor standardization, and considerable cost and turnaround time. Future trends include fluorocytometric evaluation as well as production of cytokines after food challenge.

Leukocyte Migration Inhibition Test

The leukocyte migration inhibition (LMI) test measures the lymphokine, leukocyte migration inhibitory factor (LIF), which is produced as a result of antigen recognition by the T cell receptor of sensitized lymphocytes. This cytokine inhibits leukocyte polymorphonuclear-(PMN) migration and provides the rationale for using PMN indicator cells. Many techniques have been utilized for this assay, including the agarose microdroplet technique. In a study all 24 children with cow's milk allergy had significant LIF production after their lymphocytes were stimulated with β-lactoglobulin. In contrast, none of the 10 children with acute gastroenteritis and only 2 of 24 controls had high normal values [34]. This test also is not routinely available for clinical use. It does, however, indicate the importance of T cell responses to food antigens and the role of cytokines in allergic diseases.

Complement Activation

Complement activation results in the production of the anaphylatoxins C3a and C5a via both pathways and of C4a via the classical pathway alone. These anaphylatoxins activate mast cells and basophils and promote the release of mediators of allergic response. Therefore, immune complexes formed between food allergens and IgG or IgM can participate in this mechanism. In milk allergic children C3 has been shown to be activated (as documented by a fall in serum C3 level) 90 minutes after milk challenge. In the controls C3 was not activated on ingestion of milk. These children had positive skin prick test reactions, improved on elimination of milk, and relapsed on reintroduction of milk [35]. Routine evaluation of complement activation (by measuring either CH50 or individual complement proteins) has not been clinically useful and therefore remains an area of research potential.

Cytokine Profiles

Cytokine profiles in subjects with food allergy mirror those of a TH-2 response, as has been established in atopic dermatitis, asthma, and allergic rhinitis [36]. The dichotomy of TH-1 versus TH-2 response is now a paradigm of allergic inflammation, with TH-2 response predominating and resulting in the preferential production of interleukin 4 (IL-4) and IL-5. IL-4 and gamma interferon (γ-IFN) production by stimulated T cells was evaluated in 15 adults with food allergy manifesting as urticaria, rhinitis, and even anaphylaxis, to diverse but common antigens such as peanuts, wheat, soybean, and tomatoes. Compared with the 15 controls these allergic individuals had mononuclear cells that produced more IL-4 and less gamma interferon [37]. This study endorses the concept of TH-1 versus TH-2 imbalance in allergic diseases and their potential for diagnostic evaluation by cytokine assays. It is conceivable that in situ PCR for detecting the mitochondrial ribonucleic acid (mRNA) of TH-1 and TH-2 cytokine gene products might add another dimension to the diagnosis of allergic diseases in general and food allergy in particular.

Food allergy continues to pose a challenge in all aspects. The clinical spectrum ranges from anaphylaxis to delayed nonspecific cutaneous erythema, pruritus, and even enterocolitis; laboratory diagnoses require judicious use of both in vivo and in vitro tests, relating the results to the present "gold standard," the DBPCFC. This heterogeneity necessitates cost-effective and risk-conscious management plans in the care of patients with food allergy.

REFERENCES

1. Bruijnzeei-Koomen C, Ortolani C, Aaas K et al. Adverse reaction to food: position paper. Allergy 1995; 50:623.
2. Sampson HA. Diagnosing food allergy. In: Spector SL, ed. Provocation Testing in Clinical Practice. New York; Marcel Dekker, 1995, 623.
3. Prausnitz C, Kustner H. Studies on supersensitivity. Centrabl Bakteriol 1921; 86:160.
4. Ishizaka K, Ishizaka T. Identification of IgE-antibodies as a carrier of reaginic activity. J Immunol 1967; 99:1187.
5. Vanselow NA. Skin testing and other diagnostic procedures. In: Sheldon JM, Lovell RG, Mathews KP, eds. A Manual of Clinical Allergy. Philadelphia: WB Saunders, 1967.
6. Ovary Z. Passive cutaneous anaphylaxis in the albino rat. Int Arch Allergy 1952; 3:293.
7. Bousquet J, Michel FB. In vivo methods for study of allergy: skin tests, techniques and interpretation. In: Middleton E, Jr., Reed CE, Ellis EF, eds. Allergy: Principles and Practice. St. Louis: Mosby, 1993, p 573.
8. Burks AW, Williams LW, Connaughton C et al. Identification and characterization of a

second major peanut allergen, Ara h II, with the use of the sera of patients with atopic dermatitis and positive peanut challenge. J Allergy Clin Immunol 1992; 90:962.

9. Anderson JA. Food allergy and Intolerance. In: Lieberman P, Anderson JA, eds. Allergic Diseases: Diagnosis and Treatment. Clifton, NJ: Humana Press, 1997, p 255.

13. Reimann HJ, Schmidt U, Zellmar A et al. Intragastric provocation under endoscopic control. In: Ring J, Burg G, eds. New Trends in Allergy II. Vol. 146 Berlin: Springer Verlag, 1986, p 53.

14. Lavo B, Knudson L, Loof L et al. Challenge with gliadin induces eosinophil and mast cell activation in the jejunum of patients with celiac disease. Am J Med 1989; 87:655.

15. Ferguson A, McMowar A, Strobel S et al. T-Cell mediated immunity in food allergy. Ann Allergy 1983; 51:246.

16. Dupont C. Evaluation of intestinal permeability in food hypersensitivity disorders. In: deWeck AL, Sampson HA, eds. Intestinal immunology and food allergy. Nestle Nutrition Workshop series. Volume 34. New York: Raven Press, 1995, p 73.

17. Dupont C, Barau E, Molkhou P et al. Food-induced alterations in intestinal permeability in children with cow's milk sensitive enteropathy and atopic dermatitis. J Pediatr Gastroenterol Nutr 1989; 8:459.

18. Honma K, Kohno Y, Hirano K et al. Diagnosis of food allergy based on rectal mucosal cytology (in Japanese). Aerugi 1992; 41:749.

19. James JM, Eigenmann PA, Eggleston PA et al. Airway reactivity changes in asthmatic patients undergoing blinded food challenges. Am J Respir Crit Care Med 1996; 153:597.

20. Hariprasad D, Wilson N, Dixon C et al. Oral tartarazine challenge in childhood asthma: effect on bronchial reactivity. Clin Allergy 1984; 14:81.

21. Bock SA, Atkins FM. Patterns of food hypersensitivity during sixteen years of double-blind, placebo controlled food challenges. J Pediatr 1990; 117:561.

22. Sampson HA. Immediate hypersensitivity reactions to foods: blinded food challenges in children with atopic dermatitis. Ann Allergy 1986; 57:209.

23. Sampson HA, Metcalfe DD. Food allergies. JAMA 1992; 268:2840.

24. Yunginger JW. Diagnostic testing. skin tests, IgE quantitation. In: Kaplan AP, ed. Allergy-Philadelphia: WB Saunders, 1997, p 326.

25. Moroz LA, Yang WH. Kunitz soybean trypsin inhibitor. A specific allergen in food anaphylaxis. N Engl J Med 1980; 302:1126.

26. Lowenstein H, Ericksson NE. Hypersensitivity to foods among birch pollen allergic patients: immunochemical inhibition studies for evaluation of possible mechanisms. Allergy 1983; 38:577.

27. Cunningham-Rundles C, Brandeis WE, Good RA et al. Bovine antigens and the formation of circulating immune complexes in selective immunoglobulin A deficiency. J Clin Invest 1979; 64:272.

28. Varjonen E, Savolainen J, Mattila L et al. IgE binding components of wheat, rye, barley and oats recognized by immunoblotting analysis with sera from adult atopic dermatitis patients. Clin Exp Allergy 1994; 22:481.

29. Pastorello EA, Pravettoni V, Espano M et al. Identification of the allergic components of kiwi fruit and evaluation of their cross-reactivity with timothy and birch pollens. J Allergy Clin Immunol 1996; 98:601.

30. Sampson HA. In vitro diagnosis and mediator assays for food allergies. Allergy Proc 1993; 14:259.
31. Sampson HA, Broadbent KR, Bernheisel-Broadbent J. Spontaneous release of histamine from basophils and histamine-releasing factor in patients with atopic dermatitis and food hypersensitivity. N Engl J Med 1989; 321:228.
32. Nolte H, Schiotz PO, Kruse A et al. Comparison of intestinal mast cell and basophil histamine release in children with food allergic reactions. Allergy 1989; 44: 554.
33. Van Sickle GJ, Powell GK, McDonald PJ et al. Milk and soy protein induced enterocolitis: evidence for lymphocyte sensitization to specific food proteins. Gastroenterology 1985; 88:1915.
34. Ashkenazi A, Levin S, Idar D et al. In vitro cell-mediated immunological assay for cow's milk allergy. Pediatrics 1980; 66:399.
35. Matthews TS, Soothill JF. Complement activation after milk feeding in children with cow's milk allergy. Lancet 1970; 2:893.
36. Knapik M, Frieri M. Altered cytokine production in atopic dermatitis: a preliminary study, Pediatr Asthma Allergy Immunol 1993; 7:122–133.
37. Andre F, Pene J, Andre C. Interleukin-4 and interferon-gamma production by peripheral blood mononuclear cells from food-allergic patients. Allergy 1996; 51:350. (1996).

20

Unproven Methods of Diagnosis and Treatment of Food Allergy

ABBA I. TERR
Stanford University School of Medicine, Stanford, California

INTRODUCTION

Allergic diseases are illnesses that arise out of the action of the immune system through its ability to recognize foreign substances and to mount an immune response whenever it encounters these substances. Acquired immunity is the critical element in overcoming infections, but the immune response is equally capable of recognizing and reacting to antigens that are not harmful, including essential environmental agents such as foods. Most individuals elicit no detectable immune response to foods, although many healthy people have very low levels of circulating immunoglobulin G (IgG) antibodies to some foods with no clinical deleterious effect [1].

A few atopic persons, however, have sufficient IgE antibodies to certain foods that they experience allergic reactions on ingestion of these foods. Some nonatopic individuals experience IgE-mediated anaphylaxis caused by eating minute amounts of a food; peanuts, shellfish, nuts, and berries are especially likely to induce such a response.

Well-documented cases of food allergy are almost always attributable to IgE antibodies. Although IgG antibodies may also give rise to an allergic response, as in serum sickness and hypersensitivity pneumonitis, bona fide allergy to ingested foods is almost invariably caused by the IgE antibody. Therefore, the reaction is an immediate one displaying objective signs consistent with IgE-triggered, mast cell–derived mediator action on target tissues such as the skin, gastrointestinal mucosa, or blood vessels.

Rare cases of delayed-onset pulmonary disease in infants and small children believed to be caused by IgG antibodies have been reported [2], but this proposed mechanism for the induction of food-related immune disease has not yet been firmly established [3].

The pathophysiology of allergic disease caused by IgE antibody rests on a firm scientific foundation. The clinical manifestations, diagnostic testing methods, and appropriate treatment and prophylaxis of IgE-mediated food allergy are well established. Unfortunately, there are today many physicians, "alternative" health care providers, and patients who adhere to certain controversial and unscientific theories of food "allergy." As a result, there are a number of unproven and unvalidated procedures purported to diagnose and treat a variety of conditions improperly ascribed to food allergy.

Controversial Practices (Alternative and Complementary)

The controversial theories and unproven methods described in this chapter are part of a larger group of pseudomedical practices that are often referred to as "alternative" or "complementary." These terms are misleading, because none of these practices can substitute for or add to the efficacy of medical procedures that are based on scientific evidence. Nevertheless, such modalities as acupuncture, homeopathy, herbalism, and numerous forms of unsubstantiated nutritional advice form a large and pervasive industry [4]. The services and products of this industry appeal to many people because of persuasive advertising and seductive claims. Practitioners who use many of these modalities claim that a single procedure can diagnose and treat a variety of unrelated diseases; allergies, arthritis, cancer, depression, autoimmune diseases, and many others. Food allergy diagnosis and dietary advice are common components of many of these practices.

CONTROVERSIAL THEORIES OF FOOD ALLERGY

Allergic Toxemia

"Allergic toxemia" (also called the allergic tension–fatigue syndrome) is a poorly defined term for a diagnosis applied to certain persons who typically suffer from a sensation of fatigue accompanied by numerous other subjective symptoms [5–7]. The diagnosis of allergic toxemia implies that the illness is caused by multiple food allergies. It is used to explain fatigue and listlessness in children, especially when they complain of generalized bone and joint aches in the absence of any objective signs of physical disease. The recommended treatment is to eliminate milk, wheat, chocolate, corn, and sometimes other foods from the diet. There is, however, no confirmation that these foods are responsible for the symptoms, nor is there evidence that the diet is effective. The symptoms of so-called allergic toxemia are commonly experienced in a transient fashion by most healthy children and adults, and if they become excessive or persistent, the patient should be evaluated for a systemic disease or psychopathological condition. There is no defined mechanism for ascribing fatigue per se to food allergy or toxicity.

Delayed Food Allergy

The concept of delayed food allergy is frequently cited in connection with most of the unproven methods of diagnosis and treatment discussed here. Immediate food allergy is a well-established phenomenon, and IgE antibodies to the food are responsible. The clinical manifestations of these reactions—typically systemic anaphylaxis, acute urticaria/angioedema, or allergic gastroenteropathy—are completely consistent with the pathophysiological properties of the various endogenous mediators released or activated from mast cells or basophils. Because of the rapidity of these events and the prompt effects—typically within minutes—of these mediators on target tissues, the onset of IgE antibody-mediated food allergy occurs shortly after exposure to the food allergen, i.e., within minutes and almost invariably within 2 hr [8]. The immediacy of the reaction is reported by the patient, and it has been confirmed by deliberate experimental challenge.

The concept of delayed food allergy mediated by non-IgE specific immune responses has been the subject of a number of studies, but to date only rare cases of illness associated with IgG antibodies to foods and presumptively ascribed to a serum sickness–like mechanism have been reported. Confirmation is even more rare, although the possibility of such diseases cannot be dismissed. The *concept* of delayed food allergy, however, has been adopted as the explanation for ascribing "allergy" to foods in patients with a variety of unexplained subjective symptoms, psychiatric diseases, or chronic physical diseases of uncertain cause. Many of these patients welcome such an explanation as an alternative to a psychiatric or idiopathic cause. Acceptance of the belief that food allergy is responsible for their illness empowers them to have a meaningful role in management of their disease by dietary manipulation. Since the "delay" in onset of symptoms after ingestion of food may be incorrectly interpreted as a matter of days or even weeks, and since the concept always includes that of multiple food allergies, the patient may be preoccupied with complicated elimination diets for many months or years. Regrettably, this only prolongs the time before effective therapy might be instituted.

To add to the folly of this situation, additional unproven concepts of "spreading" and "masking" [9] are used by some practitioners to "explain" why the anticipated benefits of elimination diets do not materialize. If the patient gets sicker on the diet, it is explained as the spreading of allergy to other unrelated foods than those previously deemed to be responsible for illness. If the patient gets better in spite of eating putative allergy-causing foods, a masking phenomenon is invoked.

Food Additive Allergy/Toxicity

Numerous chemicals are routinely added to the food supply to preserve the food, inhibit microbial growth, add color, enhance taste, prolong shelf life, and change the physical properties and appearence [10]. Of the many thousands of food additives in current use, several have been shown to be potential causes of disease.

Of greatest concern to allergic patients are the sulfites that are added to foods to inhibit certain enzymes such as those that cause browning of fresh fruits and vegetables. Most if not all asthmatics are likely to experience an acute asthma exacerbation as a result of inhalation of sulfur and various sulfur compounds [11]. A small but uncertain percentage of asthmatic patients experience acute asthma caused by ingestion of sulfite-containing foods and beverages [12]. In some cases the reaction is severe and even fatal [13]. The mechanism is not thought to have an allergic cause.

Monosodium glutamate (MSG) produces in some susceptible people a complex of symptoms including headache, burning, and sweating [14]. This is popularly referred to as the Chinese restaurant syndrome [15], since MSG is frequently used as a taste enhancer in some Chinese food. In spite of widespread reports of intolerance to MSG, reproducing these effects in susceptible individuals by using a double-blind controlled protocol has proved to be very difficult.

In addition to these well-defined examples of adverse effects of food additives, there is considerable public concern about the safety of adding "unnatural chemicals" to foods. Along with this concern have appeared complaints from numerous people that many specific and nonspecific symptoms or certain illnesss are caused by food additives. One prominent example is the belief that chronic urticaria is sometimes caused by the yellow food dye tartrazine. In spite of anecdotal reports and uncontrolled studies, no properly controlled experimental study has yet confirmed that this chemical causes urticaria or angioedema.

Allergists periodically uncover rare or unique cases of allergic reactions to an intentional or unintentional chemical food additive, but these cases invariably involve well-defined allergic reactions such as anaphylaxis or acute urticaria. The burgeoning use of genetic engineering techniques in the production of improved foodstuffs will most likely herald the appearance of new allergens in the food supply. Vigilance in searching for a hidden allergen in foods must continue, but this should not involve the use of unproven and unreliable diagnostic methods.

INAPPROPRIATE DIAGNOSTIC PROCEDURES

The Cytotoxic Test

The cytotoxic test for food allergy is predicated on the erroneous concept that allergy to foods may be manifested as leukocyte cytotoxicity. The procedure consists of examining leukocytes in a blood sample for morphological changes such as swelling or crenation when the blood is exposed in vitro to a food extract on a microscope slide. The testing is done without controlling for such factors as pH, temperature, or humidity that might be responsible for the observed changes [16,17]. The test "results" invariably are reported as indicating multiple food allergies, but investigation of these reports shows clearly that there is no correlation with clinical food allergy or intolerance, and the results are not reproducible [18–21].

IgG Antibodies to Foods

Although allergic reactions to foods are mediated exclusively by IgE antibodies, certain commercial clinical laboratories offer tests for specific IgG antibodies to foods. The testing is based on the radioallergosorbent test (RAST) procedure, which can detect minute quantities of these antibodies in serum samples. With the possible exception of very rare cases of pulmonary disease in small children [2,3], disease caused by IgG antibodies to foods is not currently a recognizable clinical phenomenon. Furthermore, healthy individuals may have such antibodies to certain foods at levels detectable by a number of sensitive in vitro methods [22,23]. In patients with IgA deficiency, these antibody levels are higher than in normal individuals, although even in this group of individuals IgG antibodies to foods have no proven pathogenic effects [24–26]. There is thus no current diagnostic implication of the test for IgG food antibodies, and a positive test result should not be used to recommend an elimination diet.

Food Immune Complexes

A method for detecting circulating immune complexes containing food antigen has been devised and sometimes recommended as a diagnostic test for food allergy [27,28]. It is also possible by using the appropriate method to determine whether the antibody in the complex is of the IgG or IgE isotype [29–31]. There is no evidence to date that indicates whether such complexes are pathogenic for a certain disease or simply a normal postprandial event [32]. The test cannot be recommended for clinical use [33].

The Pulse Test

An increase in the pulse rate of greater than 10 beats per minute after eating a food has been claimed to indicate allergy to that food. The rationale behind this suggestion is obscure, and there is no empirical evidence to support such a test [34]. Nevertheless, the test has been recommended, especially in the popular press.

Provocation Neutralization Testing

A modification of the standard intradermal skin testing to elicit subjective symptoms from the patient in addition to (or instead of) the local wheal and erythema response is known as provocation neutralization [35–37]. A known quantity of a food (or other) allergen extract is injected intradermally or subcutaneously; afterward the patient records any and all subjective sensations that arise during the ensuing 10 minutes. Any report of a symptom or sensation is accepted as a positive test result, and this is interpreted as allergy to the tested food. In the event that the patient reports no symptoms, the test is repeated, using different dosages until a "positive" result is obtained. Additional test doses are then given until the patient reports no symptoms, at which time the "reaction" is said to be neutralized, thereby "confirming" the prior positive test result and providing the patient with a suitable dose of the food extract for therapeutic administration.

In spite of the reliance on this test by certain practitioners, there is no scientific basis for relating the coming and going of uncontrolled subjective sensations after such exposures to food allergens to any allergic disease caused by the food. More likely, the patient is simply being made aware under the conditions of the testing procedure of myriad normal bodily sensations or emotions. In fact, when the procedure was evaluated under double-blind, placebo-controlled conditions, it revealed that patients reacted with equal frequency to the placebo control tests as to the active food extracts [38].

Sublingual Testing

The provocation neutralization procedure described previously is also performed using the sublingual route of administration of the test doses of food extract [39,40]. This method is no more reliable than the injection procedure, but it does raise concern for the danger of inducing a severe allergic reaction if the patient happens to be anaphylactically sensitive to the food being tested [41].

Applied Kinesiology

The term "applied kinesiology" refers to a bizarre procedure in which the patient is examined for the loss of muscle strength of an extremity, usually the arm, after being exposed to a food. Incredibly, the test is performed not by feeding the test food allergen, but rather by placing the food extract on the person's body, often without removing the clothing. There is no rational theory to support such a "test," and there have been no clinical trials to support its use [42].

Electrodermal Testing

Another bizarre procedure offered as a means of allergy diagnosis is electrodermal testing, in which a machine is used purportedly to measure the electrical resistance of the skin in the presence and absence of a solution of food extract in the machine's electrical circuit [43,44]. It is claimed that a change in resistance in the presence of the food is diagnostic of allergy to that food. Although the physical appearance of the machine may be imposing to the patient, the theory is untested and scientifically implausible, and the diagnostic efficacy has never been tested.

UNPROVEN THERAPIES

Food Allergy Immunotherapy

The process of allergen immunotherapy has a very long record of clinical use in the management of some patients with allergic rhinitis and/or asthma caused by inhaled allergens such as pollens, fungi, house dust mite, and animal danders. There have been a large number of blinded placebo-controlled clinical trials, which showed in most cases that long-term injections of single antigens favorably affect the symptoms and signs of these diseases [45]. In clinical practice, most patients are allergic to more than one allergen and therefore receive mixtures of multiple allergens. Efficacy has been shown to require repeated injections of high doses of allergens to which the patient is sensitive, and the effect is immunologically specific. Similarly, injections of high doses of *Hymenoptera* venom monthly for 5 years are almost always curative in patients with *Hymenoptera* venom anaphylaxis [46]. Achieving the necessary long-term maintenance dosage to treat respiratory allergy or venom anaphylaxis requires a preliminary series of allergen injections at progressively increasing dosage, beginning at a level that will not cause local or systemic reactions.

It would be desirable if a similar form of immunotherapy were effective in eliminating life-threatening anaphylaxis in those patients with such exquisite sensitivity to a food that trace amounts of the allergen in obscure or hidden form pose a constant hazard. Attempts to use allergen immunotherapy in peanut-sensitive patients have to date been reported in only a handful of cases with questionable results and an unacceptably high rate of systemic reactions [13]. There has been one reported death from a dosage error.

Neutralization Therapy by Injection or Sublingual Administration

The proponents of the provocation neutralization procedure described previously recommend the therapeutic administration of allergen extracts to "neutralize" symptoms on an ongoing basis as a form of treatment of allergic disease caused by foods or other allergens [36,47–50]. Dosages are minute, much less than the amounts shown to be required for allergen immunotherapy. Unlike allergen immunotherapy, which, when effective, prophylactically reduces the signs and symptoms of allergy on a long-term basis, "neutralizing" therapy is used to give immediate symptom relief, a claim for which there is no substantiation [51–53].

There have been no studies of the efficacy of sublingual or subcutaneous "neutralizing therapy" in documented instances of food-induced anaphylaxis. Instead, its use seems to be relegated to a population of people with multiple symptoms that are in most cases psychologically induced and amenable to relief by suggestion.

Elimination Diets

The only certain method of prophylaxis in food allergy is the dietary elimination of the allergen, and this is the standard practice of allergists. Using proper techniques of skin testing or in vitro detection of the food allergen–specific IgE antibody (e.g., RAST) in conjunction with the patient's history and, if necessary, a trial diagnostic elimination diet, the therapeutic elimination diet is rarely restrictive or nutritionally inadequate, because in the majority of cases the individual patient with clinically significant food allergy caused by IgE antibodies has only one or very few food sensitivities.

In sharp contrast, the various unproven diagnostic methods described almost always "diagnose" allergy to multiple foods, so that reliance on these procedures results in the recommendation to eliminate numerous foods from the patient's diet. The result is likely to be an inadequate diet for the purpose of proper nutrition. Furthermore, since the test results are spurious, the patient may at best experience only temporary relief based on suggestion, and ultimately the underlying clinical condition recurs, especially if it is a psychiatric one. This will then trigger elimination of additional foods and delay in uncovering the correct explanation for the patient's symptoms.

The practitioners of these unproven tests for food allergy are aware of the danger of highly restrictive diets, so they often prescribe a so-called rotary diversified diet. This consists of a diet plan in which individual foods are eaten in a rotary schedule so that the same food is not consumed more frequently than once every 4 or 5 days. There are various unsubstantiated theories to support such a schedule. It has been claimed, for example, that the risk of development of food allergy is positively correlated with the frequency of consumption of that food, although there is no evidence for such a statement. Ironically, the adaptation/deadaptation theory (described previously) would predict just the opposite, i.e. avoidance of the food for several days should deadapt and therefore increase the likelihood of enhanced sensitivity. In practice, the majority of patients who attempt to maintain highly restrictive or rigorous rotational diets abandon them in short order because of the practical difficulty in compliance and the lack of clinical benefit.

Dietary Supplements

The recommendation to treat allergic (and many other) diseases with dietary supplements, such as multiple vitamins, minerals, and amino acids, is a widespread practice that is a common feature of many "alternative" therapies [54]. The rationales for this vary, but they generally fall into one of three categories: (a) allergy is caused by a deficiency of nutrients, (b) nutritional supplements "boost" the immune system, and (c) antioxidants such as vitamins C and E correct or prevent the damage caused by the generation of oxidative free radicals in allergic inflammation. There is no scientific basis for the first two statements, and there is no clinical or experimental proof that exogenous antioxidant vitamins mitigate localized tissue oxidative processes in allergy.

These compounds are readily available without prescription, and a large segment of the healthy population uses them to "feel well" and to "stay healthy." Fortunately, most of these supplements can be consumed in supraphysiological doses for long periods with no obvious ill effect, although high-dose supplementation of the fat-soluble vitamins is potentially dangerous. With very rare exceptions (e.g., maternal consumption of folic acid during pregnancy to prevent neural tube defects in the fetus), the only medical indications for these supplements are documented specific deficiencies.

Enzyme-Potentiated Desensitization

Enzyme-potentiated desensitization consists of mixing an aqueous extract of a food or any other allergen with a small quantity of β-glucuronidase, which is then immediately injected intradermally as a form of treatment. The rationale is obscure, but it has been speculated that the enzyme has an immune-suppressant effect, although there is no current proof of this effect [55,56]. The quantity of enzyme injected is a small fraction of the amount normally circulating in the blood, thereby suggesting that a pharmacological effect is unlikely. Various treatment protocols have been recommended on the basis of empirical observations. There are to date no controlled clinical trials to support the use of this procedure, and possible adverse effects are unknown.

SUMMARY

Foods that are required for nutrition may occasionally be responsible for disease, including allergic reactions. Food allergy can vary from a mild annoyance to severe life-threatening anaphylactic shock. Fortunately food allergy is not common. The diagnostic methods for detecting food allergies are the same as those used for diagnosing allergy to inhaled substances. These include the medical and environmental history, physical examination, skin testing, RAST, and occasionally a diagnostic elimination diet. In every case, the physician must consider alternative causes of reaction by using an appropriate differential diagnosis. Management of food allergy can be accomplished only when it is based on an accurate diagnosis.

Unfortunately, there are a significant number of unproven and pseudoscientific procedures advocated for the diagnosis and treatment of food allergy, most of which are based on theories that are neither rational nor scientifically plausible. A false diagnosis of food allergy, particularly of multiple food allergies, based on these procedures will result in an unnecessary if not dangerous diet and ineffective use of drug and nutritional supplements.

Clinicians who encounter patients who have been subjected to these unproven tests and treatments or inquire about them should be knowledgeable about these procedures and their potential adverse effects.

REFERENCES

1. Johansson SGO, Dannaeus A, Lilja G. The relevance of antifood antibodies for the diagnosis of food allergy. Ann Allergy 1984; 53:665–672.
2. Heiner DC, Sears JW. Chronic respiratory disease associated with multiple circulating precipitins to cow's milk. Am J Dis Child 1960; 100:500–502.
3. Lee SK, Kniker WT, Cook CD et al. Cow's milk-induced pulmonary disease in children. Adv Pediatr 1978; 25:39–57.
4. Raso J. The Dictionary of Metaphysical Healthcare, Alternative Medicine, Paranormal Healing, and Related Methods. Loma Linda, CA. The National Council Against Health Fraud, Inc., 1996
5. Rowe AH. Allergic toxemia and fatigue. Ann Allergy 1950; 8:72.
6. Speer F. The allergic tension fatigue syndrome. Pediatr Clin North Am 1954; 1:1029.
7. Crook WG. Nervous-system symptoms, emotional behavior, and learning problems: the allergic tension fatigue syndrome. In Crook WG: Your Allergic Child. New York: MedCom Press, 1973.

8. Bock SA, Lei Y, Remigo LK *et al.* Studies of hypersensitivity reactions to foods in infants and children. J Allergy Clin Immunol 1978; 62:327.
9. Randolph TG. The specific adaptation syndrome. J Lab Clin Med. 1956; 48:934.
10. Furia TE. Handbook of Food Additives. Cleveland: The Chemical Rubber Co., 1968.
11. Schwartz HJ, Chester E. Bronchospastic responese to aerosolized metabisulfite in asthmatic subjects: potential mechanisms and clinical implications. J Allergy Clin Immunol 1984; 74:511.
12. Lee RJ, Braman SS, Settipane GA. Reproducibility of metabisulfite sensitivity in patients with asthma. Am J Respir Dis 1984; 130:1027.
13. Oppenheimer JJ, Nelson HS, Bock SA, Christensen F, Leung DYM. Treatment of peanut allergy with rush immunotherapy. J Allergy Clin Immunol 1992; 90:256–262.
14. Reif-Lehrer L. Adverse reactions in humans thought to be related to ingestion of elevated levels of MSG. Fed Proc 1977; 36:1617.
15. Schaumburg HH, Byck R, Gerstl R et al. Monosodium 1-glutamate: its pharmacology and role in the Chinese-restaurant syndrome. Science 1969; 163:826.
16. Black AP. A new diagnostic method in allergic disease. Pediatrics 1956; 17:716.
17. Bryan WTK, Bryan M. The application of in vitro cytotoxic reactions to clinical diagnosis of food allergy. Laryngoscope 1960; 70:810.
18. Lieberman P, Crawford L. Bjelland J *et al.* Controlled study of the cytotoxic food test. JAMA 1974; 231:728.
19. Benson TE, Arkins JA. Cytotoxic testing for food allergy: evaluations of reproducibility and correlation, J. Allergy Clin. Immunol. 1976; 58:471.
20. Lehman CW. The leukocytotoxic food allergy test: a study of its reliability and reproducibility: effect of diet and sublingual food drops on this test. Ann. Allergy 1980; 45:150.
21. Terr AI. the cytotoxic test (editorial). West J Med 1983; 139:702.
22. Rothberg RM, Farr RS. Anti-bovine serum albumin and anti-alphalactalbumin in the serum of children and adults. Pediatrics 1965; 35:571.
23. Cunningham-Rundels C, Brandeis WE, Good RA, Day NK. Milk precipitins, circulating immune complexes and IgA deficiency. Proc. Natl. Acad. Sci. (USA) 1978; 75:3387.
24. Husby S, Oxelius VA, Teisner B, *et al.* Humoral immunity to dietary antigens in healthy adults: occurrence, isotype and IgG subclass distribution of serum antibodies to protein antigens. Int Arch Allergy Appl Immunol 1985; 77:416.
25. Cunningham-Rundels C, Brandeis WE, Good RA, Day NK. Bovine proteins and the formation of circulating immune complexes in selective IgA deficiency. J Clin Invest 1979; 64:272.
26. Cunningham-Rundels C, Brandeis WE, Safai B, *et al.* Selective IgA deficiency and circulating immune complexes containing bovine proteins in a child with chronic graft vs. host disease. Am J Med 1979; 67:883.
27. Leary HL, Halsey JF. An assay to measure antigen-specific immune complexes in food allergy patients. J Allergy Clin Immunol 1984; 74:190.
28. Inganas M, Johansson SGO, Dannaeus A. A method for estimation of circulating immune complexes after oral challenge with ovalbumin. Clin Allergy 1980; 10:293.

29. Djurup R, Kappelgaard E, Stahl Skov P. *et al.* Determination of IgE-containing immune complexes in human sera: evaluation of polyethylene glycol precipitation of nonomeric and complex IgE and of the detectable of IgE in complexes. Allergy 1984; 39:395.

30. Haddad ZH, Vetter M, Friedman J, *et al.* Detection and kinetics of antigen-specific IgE and IgG immune complexes in food allergy. Ann Allergy 1983; 51:255.

31. Brostoff J, Carini C. Production of IgE complexes by allergen challenge in atopic patients and the effect of sodium cromoglycate. Lancet 1979; 1:1268.

32. Paganelli R, Quinti I, D'Offizi GP et al. Immune-complexes in food allergy: a Critical appraisal. Ann Allergy 1987; 58:157–

33. Sheffer AL, Lieberman PL, Aaronson DW et al. Position statement: measurement of circulating IgG and IgE food-immune complexes. J. Allergy Clin. Immunol. 1988; 81:758.

34. Coca AF. The pulse test. Carol Publishing Group, 1982.

35. Willoughby JW. Serial dilution titration skin tests inhalant allergy: a clinical quantitative assessment of biologic skin reactivity to allergenic extracts. Otolaryngol Clin North Am 1974; 7:579.

36. Lee CH, Williams RT, Binkley EL. Provocative testing and treatment for foods. Arch Otolaryngol 1969; 90:87.

37. Willoughby JW. Provocative food test technique. Ann Allergy 1965; 23:543.

38. Jewett DL, Fein G, Greenberg MH. Double blind study of symptoms provocation to determine food sensitivity. N Engl J Med 1990; 323:429.

39. Lehman CW. A double-blind study of sublingual provocation food testing: a study of its efficacy. Ann Allergy 1980; 45:144.

40. Green M. Sublingual provocative testing for food and FD and C dyes. Ann Allergy 1974; 33:274.

41. Breneman JC, Crook WC, Dreamer W *et al.* Report of the food allergy committee on the sublingual method of provocation testing for food allergy, April 12, 1983. Ann Allergy 1973; 31:382.

42. Garrow JS. Kinesiology and food allergy. Br Med J 1988; 296:1573.

43. Voll R. The phenomenon of medicine testing in electroacupuncture according to Voll. Am J Acupuncture 1980; 8:87.

44. Tsuei JJ, Lehman CW, Lam FMK, Zhu DAH. A food allergy study utilizing the EAV acupuncture technique. Am J Acupuncture 1984; 12:105.

45. Van Metre TE, Adkinson NF. Immunotherapy for aeroallergen disease. In: Middleton E et al, eds. Allergy Principles and Practice. 4th ed. St. Louis: Mosby, 1993; pp 1489–1510.

46. Golden DBK, Addison Bl, Gadde J et al. Prospective observations on stopping prolonged venom immunotherapy. J Allergy Clin Immunol 1989; 84:162.

47. Dickey LD, Pfeiffer G. Sublingual therapy in allergy. Trans Am Soc Ophthal Otolaryngol Allergy 1964; 5:37.

48. Kailin EW, Collier R. "Relieving" therapy for antigen exposure. JAMA 1971; 217:78.

49. Lee CH, Williams RT, Binkley EL. Provocative inhalation testing and treatment. Arch Otolaryngol 1969; 90:173.

50. Morris DL. Use of sublingual antigen in diagnosis and treatment of food allergy. Ann Allergy 1971; 27:289.
51. Van Metre TE, Adkinson NF, Lichtenstein LM, *et al.* A controlled study of the effectiveness of the Rinkel method of immunotherapy for ragweed pollen hay fever. J Allergy Clin Immunol 1980; 65:288.
52. Van Metre TE, Adkinson NF, Amodio FJ *et al.* A comparative study of the effectiveness of the Rinkel method and the current standard method of immunotherapy for ragweed pollen hay fever. J Allergy Clin Immunol 1980; 66:500.
53. Hirsch SR, Kalbfleisch JH, Golbert TM, *et al.* Rinkel injection therapy: a multicenter controlled study. J Allergy Clin Immunol 1981; 68:133.
54. Kershner J, Hawke W. Megavitamin therapy, J Nutr 1979; 109:819.
55. McEwen LM, Starr MS. Enzyme potentiated desensitization. I. The effect of pretreatment with glucuronidase, hyaluronidase and antigen on anaphylactic sensitivity of guinea pigs, rats and mice. Int Arch Allergy 1972; 42:153.
56. McEwen LM. Enzyme potentiated hyposensitization. II. Effects of glucose, glucosamine, N-acetylamino-sugars and gelatin on the ability of glucuronidase to block the anamnestic response to antigen in mice. Ann Allergy 1973; 79:

21

The Management and Prevention of Food Allergy

DAVID J. HILL AND CLIFFORD S. HOSKING
Royal Children's Hospital, Melbourne, Australia

FOOD ALLERGY—AN OVERVIEW

Food allergy has been defined as an adverse clinical reaction attributed to the interaction of one or more food proteins with one or more immune mechanisms. These may be immunoglobulin E– (IgE-) or non-IgE-associated. The IgE-associated disorders include immediate hypersensitivity food reactions affecting the skin (urticaria, atopic dermatitis) and gastrointestinal and respiratory tracts, whereas non-IgE disorders predominantly effect the gastrointestinal tract [1].

Food allergy tends to be a problem of early childhood [2] and is often replaced by respiratory allergy, which appears in middle to later childhood as food allergy wanes, i.e., the atopic march. However, allergy to some foods may persist throughout life.

Recent studies of Australian infants and young children have shown that up to the age of 2 years the most common food allergens are cow's milk, egg, peanut, tree nuts, sesame seed, wheat, soy, fish, and crustaceans [3].

Allergy to cow's milk protein, the food allergy studied in most detail, can

TABLE 1   The Incidence of
Food Allergy in Australian
Children

Egg	3.2%
Cow's milk	2.0%
Peanut	1.9%
Sesame seed	0.42%
Cashew nut	0.33%
Hazelnut	0.18%
Walnut	0.16%
Brazil nut	0.07%
Almond	0.02%
Wheat	0.15%
Soy	0.10%
Fish	0.07%

Source: Ref. 3.

have diverse clinical manifestations mainly affecting skin and the respiratory and gastrointestinal tracts with eczema, wheezing, and vomiting [4]. Symptoms may commence within minutes (IgE-associated), hours, or, rarely, a few days (non-IgE-associated) of milk ingestion in the challenge situation. A similar spectrum of reactions to other foods has recently been described [5,6]. It is unclear how much colic [6] or reflux esophagitis of infancy may be due to food hypersensitivity [7,8].

The diagnosis of food allergy on clinical grounds can be difficult because of the diversity and nonspecific nature of many of the symptoms and their delayed onset from the time of ingestion. Although there is an association between the size of the skin prick test response and the probability of a positive food challenge result [9], the response to an appropriately managed challenge with the suspect food is the only completely reliable means of diagnosis [10]. There are no screening tests available for the identification of non-IgE-related food allergy disorders that can allow preventative measures to be implemented on a large-scale basis. These diseases are less severe and remit at a younger age than those of the IgE type. There has been little research on the prevention of non-IgE food disorders, and they are not discussed further in this chapter.

FOOD ALLERGY AND THE EVOLUTION OF ATOPIC DISEASE

As IgE responses to foods often precede the development of IgE responses to inhalant allergens it was hoped the avoidance of IgE-associated food allergy may prevent the subsequent emergence of allergic airway disease.

In 1936 Grulee and Sanford first showed that cow's milk–fed infants had sevenfold more eczema than breast fed infants [11]. This led to speculation that breast milk may be protective against eczema. Subsequent studies have shown conflicting results, some confirming reduction in the prevalence of eczema [12–14], and others showing no benefit [15,16]. Furthermore, Ferguson [17,18] showed the importance of parental atopy and the range of antigens introduced with early solid feeds in promoting eczema. Maternal dietary food allergens are transferred in breast milk [19], and infants may have allergic reactions on their first known contact with a food suggesting prior exposure either via breast milk or before birth [20]. Although recent studies have demonstrated specific IgE antibodies against cow's milk in cord blood from newborn infants with and without an atopic predisposition [21], there is no evidence that restricting maternal diet in the last trimester of pregnancy influences the subsequent development of allergic disease. Such diets may compromise foetal growth [22].

In the last decade a number of large-scale studies have reexamined the value of food allergen avoidance by lactating mothers, use of hypoallergenic infant milk substitutes, and regulation of the introduction of solid foods in an attempt to prevent the development of food allergy–related disorders.

PREVENTION OF FOOD ALLERGY

It is useful to consider the options for preventative management of IgE- mediated food hypersensitivity from an epidemiological viewpoint.

1. Primary prevention: prevention of IgE sensitization
2. Secondary prevention: prevention of disease despite prior IgE sensitization
3. Tertiary prevention: suppression of symptoms after disease manifestation

Primary Prevention

Within the last decade a number of studies have been undertaken in an attempt to demonstrate the benefit of dietary manipulation in the prevention of food related atopic disorders. These diets variably excluded high-allergen foods from the diet of breast feeding mothers, used partially or extensively hydrolyzed infant formula in those unable to breast feed fully, and introduced low-allergen solids only after 4 to 6 months and other foods beyond 12 months of age. It was hoped these diet modifications would prevent the development of food allergy–related disorders and arrest the "atopic march" from hypersensitivity to ingested allergens to hypersensitivity to inhaled allergens, thus preventing asthma. In an excellent review of the value of dietary modification in the primary prevention of atopic disease, Zeiger has compared the results of several prospective randomized control studies performed in the last decade [23]. The details of the dietary modification and their effects are shown in Table 2, prepared by Zeiger [23].

A detailed review of the data in Zeiger's own study [23], which in our view the most scientifically rigorous of those performed to date, shows that at the age of 12 months, 16% (period prevalence) of infants at risk for atopy manifest food allergy–related disorders compared with 4% in those whose mothers were able to follow a restricted low-allergen diet program ($p = 0.006$). At 2 year follow-up evaluation only 10% and 4% (p = n.s.) of these same groups still showed disease. Thus, if these measures were introduced on a widespread basis for infants at risk for atopy, only 12 of every 100 such infants at 1 year and 6 at 2 years would benefit. It would at this stage seem hard to justify such stringent dietary measures at a general community level in a country like Australia where the incidence of potentially atopic infants is only 19.3% [3]. In addition there is a scarcity of reliable data on the long-term effects of dietary restriction on maternal and child health.

Because of different methods of analysis, it is not possible to compare the results of the Isle of Wight study with Zeiger's data. However, a Danish group led by Halken and Host have suggested that dietary restrictions, less stringent than those examined by Zeiger, can reduce food related atopic disease [24]. They reported that moderate diet restriction, breast feeding (without modification of maternal diet), and use of extensively hydrolyzed infant formula as supplements when necessary, together with the avoidance of solids for the first 6 months of life, significantly reduces the prevalence of food allergy–related diseases and prevents the development of cow's milk allergy [24]. They showed the cumulative incidence of atopic dermatitis at 18 months in infants who followed the moderate-allergen avoidance program was 14% compared with 31% in a control group of infants who had participated in an earlier study. The significance of these findings is obscured because the control and treatment groups were not contemporaneous. However, it should be noted that this incidence of atopic dermatitis of 14% in the Danish diet-restricted infants is similar to the 13% that Zeiger documented in his "control" infants, who were also encouraged to breast feed and avoid solids until 4 to 6 months (they followed the routine recommendations for infant feeding of the American Academy of Pediatrics).

Halken also emphasised the importance of such at-risk infants' *totally* avoiding cow's milk in the first 6 months and particularly during the first days of life as breast feeding is being established [24]. Host had previously noted in a large study a significantly lower incidence of cow's milk allergy (CMA) in "exclusively" breast fed infants (0.5%) compared to infants supplemented with cow's milk formula (2.2%) [25]. In a review of the feeding history of the so-called exclusively breast fed infants in whom CMA developed Host noted that they had ingested up to 4 ounces of cow's milk formula in the first few days after delivery and suggested that this exposure may have been responsible for cow's

TABLE 2 Prospective Randomized Controlled Studies of the Effect of Food Allergen Avoidance on the Development of Atopic Disease in Infants of Atopic Parents

Study [reference]	Subjects (n)	Maternal pregnancy diet	Mom lactation diet	Infant diet	Follow-up	SPT/RAST	DBPCFC	Atopic disease
Magnusson et al. [39–41]	197	Third trimester (no egg, CM) vs. no restriction	None	Breast +/or casein hydrolysate (3 Mo), Solids (>4 Mo), CM (>6 Mo); egg/fish (>9 Mo)	5 Yr	Not significant	No	Not significant
Lifja et al. [42, 43]	162	Third trimester (no egg, CM) vs. no restrictions	None	Exclusive breast (5–6 Mo) vs. no restrictions	1.5 Yr	Not significant	No	Not significant
Chandra et al. [44]	71	Entire pregnancy (No egg. CM, fish, peanut, beef) vs. no restrictions	Entire lactation (same as pregnancy) vs. no restrictions	Exclusive breast (5–6 Mo) vs. no restrictions	1 Yr	Not determined	No	Reduced AD severity by [a] 1 Yr
Zeiger et al. [8, 37]	288	Third trimester (no egg, CM, peanut) vs. no restrictions	Entire lactation (same as pregnancy)	Breast and/or casein hydrolysate (12 mo). solids (>6 Mo), CM, soy, corn (>12), egg, fish, peanut (>24 mo) vs. AAP guidelines	7 Yr	Reduced CM IgE prevalence at 1[a] and 2 Yr[b]	Yes; half consented, 80% positive challenges	Reduced current prevalence of AD[a] and food allergy[b] at 1 yr asthma and AR unaffected by 7 Yr
Hattevig et al. [45–47]	115	None	First 3 Mg, of lactation (no egg, CM, fish) vs. no restrictions	Breast +/or casein hydrolysate (6 mo) CM/solids (>6 mo). egg/fish, (>9 Mo)	4 Yr	Reduced no. of CM and/or egg IgE tests at 3 MO[b]	No	Reduced AD at 3[b], 6[a], and 48[b] Mo

TABLE 2 Continued

Study [reference]	Subjects (n)	Maternal pregnancy diet	Mom lactation diet	Infant diet	Follow-up	SPT/ RAST	DBPCFC	Atopic disease
Chandra et al. [48]	97	None	Entire lactation (no egg, CM, peanuts, soy, fish) vs. no restrictions	Exclusive breast (~6 Mo). solids (~6 Mo)	15 Yr	Not determined	No	Reduced AD by 1.5 Yr[a]
Chandra et al. [48]	124 (3 group)	None	None	Exclusive casein hydrolysate vs CM or soy. No breast feeding	1.5 Yr	Not determined	No	Reduced AD[a] by 1.5 Yr with casein hydrolysate
Chandra et al. [49,50]	288 (4 group)	None	None	Exclusive partial whey hydrolysate (6 Mo) vs CM, soy, or breast feeding × 6 Mo	1.5 Yr	No difference in CM IgE at 2 and 6 Mo	No	Reduced 6 and 12 Mo AD cumulative prevalence[a]
Lucas et al. [51]	75 [Preterm]	None	None	Human milk vs preterm formula ×1.5 mo	1.5 Yr	Not determined	No	Reduced AD by 1.5 yr[a]

Arshad et al. [53,54]	120	None	Entire lactation (no egg, CM, fish, nuts) vs no restrictions	Breast +/or soy hydrolysate (9 mo); CM/soy (9 mo); egg (11 mo). all others (12 mo) plus mite avoidance (acaricide and encasing) vs no restrictions	2 Yr	Not significant at 1 yr, significantly reduced at 2 Yr	No	Reduced AD[a] and asthma[a] by 1 yr, any atopy at 2 yr
Mallet/Henocq [55]	165	None	None	Pregetimil vs CM formula = breast milk + no solids × 4 Mo	4 Yr	Not determined	No	Reduced eczema at 4 mo ($p = 0.07$). 2 & 4 Yr ($p = 0.01$)
Hatken et al. [56]	141	None	None	Breast ($n = 20$) Nutramigen ($n = 59$) vs Profylac ($n = 62$) and delayed solids and CM for 6 mo	1.5 Yr	CM IgE in 4/5 with CMPA/CMPI	Open challenge	CMPA/CMPI = 1/20 vs 1/59 vs 3/62, in grps, respectively

CM, cow's milk; AD, atopic dermatitis; CMA, CM allergy; CMPI, CM protein intolerance; AR, allergic rhinitis; DBPCFC, double-blind, placebo-controlled food challenge; mo, month; yr, year.

[a] $p < 0.05$.
[b] $p < 0.01$.
Source: Ref. 55.

milk sensitization. He calculated the quantity of β-lactoglobulin in this volume of cow's milk (1–3 g) is the same amount that the infant would obtain by ingesting 1 liter of breast milk per day for 17 years [26].

Host and Halken's studies imply that there is a critical period during the first days of life during which sensitisation to cow's milk may occur and that late exposure, i.e., beyond the first 6 months of life, apparently is more readily tolerated. However, if early postnatal feeding is hypothesized as the major mechanism by which infants become sensitized to foods, it is difficult to account for the development of sensitivity to egg and peanut reported in allergen avoidance studies when these foods are introduced after the age of 12 months. The possibility that increased mucosal permeability primarily induced by intestinal cow's milk allergy [27] may facilitate absorption of egg, peanut, and other food allergens in breast milk, thereby enhancing their allergenicity, cannot be excluded. A similar effect may be induced in bottle fed infants fed solids prematurely. However, data by Linfors suggest that cow's milk feeds given repeatedly and in large amounts before breast milk was available were associated with a reduced risk of allergic disease in infants with a family history of allergic disease [28].

We are not aware of any controlled study whose primary hypothesis is that the delayed introduction of solid foods beyond the age of 4 or 6 months reduces the development of food related atopic diseases has been tested. However, Ferguson et al. have shown that the early introduction of solids (before 4 months) is a risk factor for the development of recurrent or chronic atopic dermatitis at the age of 2 years (1.6 times) [29] and at the age of 10 years (2.5 times) [30].

There is evidence that delayed introduction of solids for 4 to 6 months would be an acceptable public health measure to reduce food allergy–related disease. In an ongoing study of 620 Australian infants at risk for the development of atopic disease (Melbourne Atopy Cohort Study [MACS]) it was recommended that low-allergen solids be introduced into the diet after 4 months of age; 80% of parents readily complied with this direction [31]. In addition, in a recent Italian study by Marini et al. more than 90% of 279 parents complied with advice not to introduce solids before 4 months. Marini et al. noted in the 80 control infants given no specific dietary advice that >90% had solids before four months [32].

In summary, restrictive diets for breast feeding mothers cannot be recommended as broad measures to reduce the incidence of food allergy–related diseases in the community at large because of the high incidence of noncompliance, the transient and limited benefits, and the lack of reliable data related to their effect on maternal health and infant development. Delayed introduction of solids would appear to be one method of prevention acceptable to the general community.

When the family wish to pursue primary prevention methods, it seems reasonable to encourage breast feeding (without maternal diet restriction), avoid cow's milk formula ingestion in the perinatal period, and delay the introduction of low-allergen solids till 4 to 6 months. High-allergen foods (including milk, egg, nuts, fish) are introduced after 12 months of age according to the results of allergen skin prick testing. For mothers unable to breast feed the data are far from clear but favor the use of extensively hydrolyzed formula till 6 months of age [24,31], followed by cow's milk formula and the introduction of solids as outlined.

Secondary Prevention—Prevention of Food Allergy Diseases Despite Prior IgE Sensitization

Secondary prevention entails identifying patients IgE-sensitized to various foods, who are to avoid these foods until remission of the sensitivity. To be cost-effective, secondary prevention must

1. Identify high-risk groups
2. Screen for the development of food sensitivity by inexpensive methods, prior to deliberate ingestion
3. Avoid foods to which IgE sensitization has developed before clinical allergic disease occurs

Identification of Infants at High Risk

Kjellman reported that 13% of children with food hypersensitivity have no parental history of atopic disease, 25% of young children exhibit food hypersensitivity when there is a unilateral family history of atopic disease, and 58% experience food hypersensitivity when there is a bilateral family history of atopic disease [34].

If one sibling has cow's milk allergy there is a 1 in 3 chance that other siblings may be affected [35,36].

Dean, in an elegant review of factors predicting food sensitivity, summarized some of the recent data from the Isle of Wight studies [37]. Twelve hundred and eighteen infants were followed from birth to 4 years in a population-based prospective study to assess the natural history of allergic disorders. Children were regarded as having a positive family history of atopy if either parent or a sibling suffered from one or more atopic disorders. In Table 3, the association of food intolerance and family history is shown. Table 3 indicates that a higher proportion of children with any food allergy have a family history of respiratory allergic disease ($p < 0.01$), atopy (p < 0.01), and food allergy.

Dean performed a multivariate regression analysis of confounding factors to obtain adjusted odds ratios for a number of factors investigated (Table 4). Milk, egg, and peanut allergies were analyzed (as independent variables) in relation to all risk factors of interest. In Table 4 the adjusted odds ratios for these factors related to food intolerance are shown. As indicated in Table 4, if there is a

TABLE 3 The Association of Food Intolerance and Family History on the Isle of Wight

		Milk	Egg	Wheat	Peanut	Any food
Family history of	Yes	6.2	2.9	1.0	1.7[a]	10.0[b]
atopy	No	3.6	1.6	0.8	0.2	4.8
Family history of	Yes	11.6[c]	5.4[a]	0.6	3.9[b]	18.16[a]
food intolerance	No	4.3	2.0	0.8	0.7	6.5
Family history of	Yes	6.2	3.1	0.7	1.6	10.0[a]
respiratory	No	4.2	1.8	1.0	0.6	6.0
allergic disease						

All figures in percentages.
[a] $p < 0.05$.
[b] $p < 0.01$.
[c] $p < 0.001$.
Source: Ref. 34.

family history of food intolerance the overall risk for any food allergy is increased 3.6-fold.

Dean also reviewed the value of cord blood IgE levels in predicting food allergy. Although the initial studies using preselected infants looked promising, the Isle of Wight study, using a random birth cohort, showed cord blood IgE was a poor predictor for food allergy at the 4 year follow-up evaluation. (see Table 5). There was no difference in the incidence of allergy to milk, egg, wheat, and nuts in infants whose cord blood IgE was >0.5 KU/liter compared to those whose levels were lower.

In summary the groups of infants at highest risk for food allergy are (a) those with a bilateral family history of atopic disease [34]. and (b) those with an immediate family history of food allergy [37].

If secondary prevention is to be economically viable, it is important to know the likely incidence of such at-risk groups in the general community. Recently the incidence of these high-risk groups in the first year of life in the general community has been reported. Bergman [38], in the German Multi-Centre Atopy Study (MAS-90), reported that 7.4% of the general German population have two atopic family members and approximately 8% of Australian infants will have a sibling with food allergy [3].

Screening Methods to Identify Food Allergy Prior to Deliberate Exposure

Our recent studies have defined the sensitivity and specificity for SPT weal diameters to diagnose IgE hypersensitivity to cow's milk, egg, and peanut [3]. We have preliminary data that similar methods may be used in the diagnosis of clin-

TABLE 4 Adjusted Odds Ratios (95% Confidence Limits) for Factors Related to Food Intolerance on the Isle of Wight

	Milk	Egg	Peanut	Any food
Family history of atopy	—	—	—	2.2 (1.0–4.9)
Family history of food intolerance	2.5 (1.2–9.7)	—	—	3.6 (1.6–9.6)
Infantile eczema	3.1 (1.4–10.0)	7.1 (2.5–21.0)	—	2.8 (1.3–6.7)
Eczema at 4 years	—	—	7.3 (2.1–26.1)	2.1 (1.1–4.1)
Wheeze in infancy	3.7 (1.3–10.5)	—	—	3.7 (1.5.–9.2)
Aeroallergen sensitization	-	4.3 (1.1–17.4)	—	3.1 (1.4–6.6)

Source: Ref. 34.

ical hypersensitivity to tree nuts, fish, and sesame seed but not to soy preparations or wheat. In our experience SPTs are simpler to perform and are of more clinical value than In vitro measurements of IgE antibodies to foods for the diagnosis of food allergy in the first 2 years of life [9]. In older children (median age 4 years) Sampson has performed an in vitro assay of IgE binding to allergens (CAP). He determined the cut-off points for 95% PPV and 95% NPV for serum IgE antibodies for cow's milk, egg, fish, peanut, wheat, and soy and suggested they were useful for the diagnosis of food allergy but not wheat and soy allergy [39]. The value of these in vitro antibody measurements in the diagnosis of food allergy in the first 2 years of life requires further evaluation.

Development of Prevention Strategies

Not all children who have IgE skin sensitivity or IgE antibodies to common foods have clinical food allergy. Only those children with very large SPT weal diameters to foods or very high IgE antibody levels to foods will have a positive food challenge outcome predicted [9] by these tests. On the basis of our studies of cow's milk allergy and other investigations we predict that about 30% of children with IgE food hypersensitivity to milk, egg, peanut, tree nut, and fish can be diagnosed by SPT alone [3,9]. The remaining children with lower levels of SPTs and IgE antifood antibodies should be challenged in a safe environment.

In summary, if secondary prevention is to be practiced, then children need to be screened by SPT at 6 and/or 12 months before symptoms have developed. If those tests are diagnostic of food sensitization, avoidance of the food will be undertaken and treatment implemented. If the SPT finding is negative or only weakly positive, sequential introduction of initially low-allergen

TABLE 5   Cord IgE Predictor of Food Allergy in Isle of Wight Birth Cohort Study

		Milk	Egg	Wheat	Peanut	Any food
Cord IgE	Yes	5.8	3.6	1.4	2.2	12.2
≥0.5 KU/liter	No	5.1	2.3	0.9	0.9	7.4

foods (as discussed under Primary Prevention) is undertaken. If an adverse reaction occurs the food is avoided, as discussed in the Treatment section.

It is our current clinical experience that increasing numbers of parents with an affected child will present their next child for screening by SPT at 6 and 12 months of age.

Tertiary "Prevention" of Food Allergy

Tertiary prevention is the suppression of symptoms once the diagnosis of food allergy has been established. It is effective in the management of children with food hypersensitivity. A period of food avoidance is associated with the remission of disease in the majority of children.

However, we believe tertiary prevention should include more than the simple treatment of established food allergy. To us, it entails

1. Recognition of the different symptoms of food allergy at a primary care giver level
2. Rapid referral of patients with suspected food allergy to trained allergy specialists for immediate detailed investigations and implementation of effective treatment programs

This active intervention is to be contrasted with current treatment approaches, in which many children with food allergy receive treatment up to 12 months [1] to 4 years [40] after symptoms develop. By contrast, prospective studies of infants who have food allergy show symptoms invariably develop within 1 to 4 weeks of commencing a food in full amounts [25]. This means most IgE food allergy can be diagnosed in the first 12 months of life, and in particular nut allergy may be diagnosed by SPT in early infancy prior to direct exposure.

Thus the key to successful tertiary prevention is better diagnostic skill at the primary care giver level among nurse practitioners, family practitioners, and pediatricians.

At the primary care giver level, two key points are emphasized for the early diagnosis of IgE food allergy:

1. If an infant has atopic dermatitis the chance of food allergy is three to seven times greater than if a child does not have atopic dermatitis [37]; i.e., it would be appropriate to refer infants with significant atopic dermatitis for detailed evaluation of food allergy.
2. If an infant has an immediate hypersensitivity reaction to one food, there is a 50% to 75% chance of an immediate hypersensitivity reaction to another food [5]. That is, this group of infants needs to be screened for other potential food allergens by immediate referral. Many infants with cow's milk allergy or egg allergy have peanut and nut allergy, which can be diagnosed by SPT prior to direct peanut or other nut exposure.

At the specialist level it is important that the broad spectrum of food allergy in infancy and early childhood particularly be appreciated as it is in this period that it has its greatest impact. We have recently approached this problem from a clinical viewpoint, attempting to quantify the probability of a child's having food allergy (diagnosed on food challenge) exemplified by cow's milk allergy on the basis of the features at clinical presentation [4].

At a clinical level it is possible to recognize the following groups of potentially food allergic children.

A. High probability
    i. Anaphylaxis, urticaria, angioedema, eczema; vomiting and diarrhea

These reactions develop within minutes or hours of ingestion of small volumes of food.

B. Moderate probability
    i. Eczema
    ii. Abdominal cramping with or without vomiting
    iii. Failure to thrive with gastrointestinal symptoms with or without atopic disease
    iv. Inflammatory bowel disease symptoms:
        a. Colitis
        b. Eosinophilic enteropathy
        c. Breast milk colitis

Reactions develop slowly hours or days after ingestion of moderate amounts of food.

C. Low probability:
    i. Recurrent rhinorrhea, nasal obstruction
    ii. Recurrent middle ear disease
    iii. Recurrent cough including asthma

Symptoms usually affect single systems and develop in the second or third year of life; i.e., these symptoms are likely to be due to vital infections.

D. Other confusing entities
   i. Munchhausen by proxy syndrome

These infants are placed on restricted diets as a form of food deprivation; i.e., this is a form of child abuse associated with parental psychosis.

Tertiary prevention attempts to improve the outcome of diseases associated with food allergy by their early recognition, rapid referral to a specialist facility for confirmation, diagnosis, and implementation of effective treatment programs. These measures will improve the rate of morbidity and are likely to be highly cost-effective.

Specific management issues relating to food allergy are discussed in the Treatment section.

TREATMENT OF FOOD ALLERGY

It is important to realize that there is a broad spectrum of manifestations of food allergy, ranging from trivial and transient skin rashes and intestinal upsets to life-threatening anaphylaxis. Therefore, the nature of the investigations and treatment regimens needs to be in proportion to the severity of the disease.

It is useful to consider treatment under general issues and those related to the management of specific clinical problems associated with food allergy.

General Issues

General Medical Care

Treatment of symptoms associated with food allergy is relatively nonspecific, i.e., topical steroids for atopic dermatitis, possible use of prokinetic agents and H_2 antagonists for management of gastrointestinal symptoms unresponsive to dietary management, and beta-agonists and preventative medications for asthma.

Availability of Epinephrine for Children with Immediate IgE Food Hypersensitivity

A decision should be made as to whether or not parents are to be issued epinephrine kits. We advise all parents of patients who have anaphylactic life-threatening reactions to a food to have access to Epi-Pen or Epi-Pen Junior at all times. In addition we encourage children who have asthma and IgE food hypersensitivity—irrespective of the severity of the latter problem—to have access to epinephrine because of the increased risk of severe reactions in such patients [41]. Where the manifestations of food allergy are less severe, i.e., perioral or generalized cutaneous eruptions or exacerbations of atopic dermatitis, availability of oral antihistamines in the home is recommended.

Specific Issues

Management of food allergy entails identification of the relevant food allergen and its exclusion from the diet until remission of the disorder. When food allergy develops in infancy such exclusions may compromise nutrition and growth. Therefore, during this period specific formulas and supplements may be required to ensure optimal nutrition, and the assistance of a nutritionist should be considered.

By contrast, in adolescents and adults in whom the oral allergy syndrome (OAS) develops, such nutritional considerations are usually not necessary, but practical dietary advice to optimize care may be required.

The following topics are relevant to this discussion:

1. Selection of formula for infants and young children with cow's milk allergy
2. Management of infants with multiple food allergy
3. Peanut and nut hypersensitivity
4. Oral allergy syndrome

Management of Cow's Milk Allergy

The mainstays of treatment of cow's milk allergy are complete avoidance of cow's milk proteins and use of a replacement formula. Elimination of cow's milk antigens responsible for the disorder alleviates symptoms and helps preserve intestinal integrity [42].

Between 70% and 90% of infants with cow's milk allergy are tolerant of soy formula [5,43]. Those intolerant of soy formula will require extensively hydrolyzed casein or whey preparations or occasionally an amino acid–based complete infant formula. Hydrolyzed soy preparations are currently being evaluated in the management of cow's milk allergy.

There is evidence that infant formulas with molecular weight <1200 Da are suitable for infants with nonanaphylactic CMA. Most of these formulas are prepared by varying degrees of hydrolysis, which may not render the formula hypoallergenic. This may be in part due to the variability of the degree of hydrolysis so that the molecular weight of peptides is not uniformly <1200 Da. Isolauri has compared the concentration of β-lactoglobulin detected in partially and extensively hydrolyzed casein and whey formulas as well as two preparations of complete infant formulas made up of individual amino acids [44] (see Table 6).

Table 6 indicates that the β-lactoglobulin content of the extensively hydrolyzed preparations was much less than that of partially hydrolyzed preparations

TABLE 6   Mean β-Lactoglobulin Concentrations (µg/g)in Different Infant Formulas

Batch	W_p	C_{42}	W_{42}	A	AA
1	82	0.020	0.017	0.032	0.0017
2	86	0.007	0.005	0.030	0.0015
Mean	84	0.014	0.011	0.031	0.0016

W_p, partially hydrolyzed whey; C_{42}, extensively hydrolyzed casein; W_{42}, extensively hydrolyzed whey; A and AA, amino acid–derived formulas.
Source: Ref. 41.

and similar to that in human breast milk. Interestingly one of the amino acid complete infant formula preparations contained greater concentrations of β-lactoglobulin than the extensively hydrolyzed casein and whey preparations. Presumably this amino acid product became contaminated with milk protein during manufacture despite standard precautions.

Infants with Hypersensitivity to Multiple Foods

There are two clinical situations to consider. oligo food allergy in infants multiple food protein intolerance (MFPI) of infancy.

Oligo Food Allergy

Oligo food allergy is characterized by hypersensitivity reactions in a group of infants and young children not only to cow's milk but to two or three other foods. Host reported that in 54% of infants with cow's milk allergy in a community based study other food intolerances, including hypersensitivity to egg and nuts, developed [45]. In a hospital referred population the incidence of these associated food hypersensitivities is higher [5]. The relatively benign nature of this clinical problem of allergy to a few foods needs to be contrasted with multiple food protein intolerance (MFPI), in which the spectrum of adverse reactions and foods is much wider and consequently dietary restriction is more severe and nutritional requirements are more difficult to meet without specific dietary supplements [43].

Multiple Food Protein Intolerance of Infancy [43]

In Table 7, the incidence of hypersensitivity to soy milk, extensively hydrolyzed casein formula, wheat, eggs, nuts, fish, and meats in the first 100 young children we studied with cow's milk allergy proved by cow's milk challenge is shown. This study identified a small group of infants who showed hypersensitivity to a wide range of foods. In the last decade at the Children's Allergy Centre, Melbourne, more than 60 infants who demonstrated hypersensitivity to all the hy-

TABLE 7 The Percentage of CMA Children Studied over 5 Years with an Adverse Reaction to Other Foods: Total Number of Children Reported to React to Each Food Compared to the Total Number Exposed

Egg	56/97	58%
Wheat	16/97	16%
Soy milk	37/78	47%
Casein hydrolysate	13/58	22%
Banana	17/93	18%
Apple	5/97	5%
Pear	8/96	8%
Orange	33/93	35%
Strawberry	10/90	11%
Tomato	11/90	12%
Fish	12/95	13%
Peanut	34/97	34%
Lamb	7/97	7%
Beef	14/96	14.5%
Chicken	9/96	9%

Source: Ref. 5.

poallergenic formula available and several other foods have been identified. In order to achieve symptomatic control nutrition was compromised. Because these infants and young children were characterized by intolerance to multiple food proteins we called the disorder multiple food protein intolerance (MFPI) of infancy. Three years ago Neocate (SHS—Liverpool), a nutritionally complete amino acid–based formula for infant use became available; it was well tolerated by young patients with this disorder.

In the initial cohort of 18 infants with MFPI the typical clinical features were a history of immediate or slowly evolving reactions to common foods with persistent protracted diarrhea, vomiting, and distressed behavior (attributed and often demonstrated to be due to reflux esophagitis), and/or severe atopic dermatitis unresponsive to standard dermatological treatment and low-allergen formula preparations. The persistence of symptoms despite the use of low-allergen formulas and dietary restriction suggested hypersensitivity to those low-allergen formulas and dietary components. Symptoms remitted within 2 weeks of commencing Neocate and relapsed when extensively hydrolyzed casein and whey formula as well as soy formula were used in double-blind placebo-controlled procedures. Once the patients' conditions were stabilized and low-allergen foods were introduced, it was found that on average each patient had a relapse of symptoms after the ingestion of 6 of the following 10 relatively low-allergen foods: rice, wheat, potato, pumpkin, broccoli, zucchini, apple, pear, chicken, and lamb. The patients with failure to thrive regained normal growth when they commenced Neocate.

The natural history of this disease is similar to that of other forms of food allergy. Our preliminary analysis suggests that in most cases tolerance to vegetables, fruits, and meats was achieved by the age of 2 years, and to most other foods by the age of 5 years. Occasionally hypersensitivity to milk, egg, peanut, and nuts persisted beyond this age if very high levels of IgE sensitization to foods were evident at the outset. In many of these young children both non-IgE and IgE adverse reactions to different foods ware seen in the same patient [46].

Most infants with MFPI will require assessment by a qualified nutritionist to ensure they have adequate caloric, calcium, and vitamin intake. Once a stable and nutritionally adequate diet has been achieved, it is our practice for all patients with food allergy to review growth on a 6 month basis and challenge them every 12 months until remission of their disease. It is our practice when a child with food allergy is first seen to skin test a wide range of common dietary and inhalant allergens. This may allow the identification of potential food allergens to which a child has not yet been exposed and may serve to identify inhalant allergens that may become releyant to the subsequent development of allergic airway disease.

HYPERSENSITIVITY TO PEANUT AND TREE NUTS

In the United States 80% of infants are exposed to peanut in the first 12 months of life and all have encountered it by the age of 2 years. There is increasing concern regarding fatal anaphylactic reactions, particularly in adolescents, because of peanut hypersensitivity [47]. In Australian infants 1.9% of the population is peanut allergic [3], whereas in the United Kingdom the incidence is reported as 0.5% at the age of 4 years [48]. Peanut, together with cow's milk, is the second most common food allergen after egg in Australian children. A recent review of the rate of sensitization to tree nuts and sesame seed in consecutive children attending the Children's Allergy Centre, Melbourne, as a result of possible peanut hypersensitivity is summarized in Table 8 [49].

Table 8 shows how frequently sensitization to botanically unrelated tree nuts occurs in children with peanut hypersensitivity and indicates the relatively high incidence of sensitization to sesame seed in Australian children. In our experience more than 85% of infants and young children with a very high skin test score on SPT to peanut, nuts, or sesame seed will demonstrate immediate hypersensitivity on challenge [49].

TABLE 8 Skin Test Sensitivity to Peanut, Nuts, and Sesame Seed in Children with Suspected Food Allergy (Children's Allergy Centre, Melbourne, 1990–1996)

	Sensitization[a]					
	0	1+	2+	3+	4+	5+
Peanut	2,175	36	222	525	127	949
Almond	236	6	22	58	7	7
Brazil	440	8	46	80	16	25
Cashew	1,394	19	126	188	34	153
Hazelnut	838	24	92	144	24	77
Walnut	515	16	54	84	20	68
Sesame seed	2,071	23	164	294	61	176

[a]Sensitization to nut extracts (Hollister-Stier USA) was scored by comparing the skin wheal diameter to a histamine control (1 mg/ml) (on average 3 mm): 1+ if less than half the diameter of the histamine control, 2+ if equal to half the diameter, 3+ if equal to the diameter, 4+ if equal to twice the diameter, and 5+ if greater than twice the diameter of the histamine control.

Three key points characterize peanut and nut hypersensitivity:

1. The reactions can be extremely violent and life-threatening with minimal exposure [48].
2. Peanut hypersensitivity is likely to persist through childhood and probably throughout life [50].
3. Peanut (legume) hypersensitivity is frequently associated with other nonlegume and seed hypersensitivity [49].

It is critical that when a patient has a history of anaphylaxis or a severe immediate hypersensitivity reaction to a nut the precise diagnosis be established with certainty. This may require a formal challenge in a safe environment with different nut preparations. Only when a definite adverse reaction can be attributed to the ingestion of a specific nut or nuts should the final diagnosis be made and specific advice regarding avoidance of the relevant substance be given. Not infrequently patients who have experienced nut anaphylaxis may be told they have peanut allergy, whereas the true cause of the anaphylaxis may be an unrelated tree nut, or alternatively anaphylactic hypersensitivity to other nuts may coexist in patients with peanut hypersensitivity.

The wide distribution of peanut and nut preparations in food outside the domestic environment is not generally appreciated. In particular these allergens are often present in reworked ice cream or chocolate preparations without being identified. In addition foods may be contaminated with peanut protein from pressed or extruded peanut oils, or oils or utensils used to cook foods containing peanuts. There is a need for better labeling of peanut and nut products in food substances. Prevention of cross-contamination in packaging is essential [47].

ORAL ALLERGY SYNDROME

Oral allergy syndrome (OAS) is a complex of clinical symptoms including oral itching, angioedema of the lips, and occasionally glottic edema after ingestion of various fruits and vegetables. Approximately 2% to 4% of European adults experience this syndrome [51,52], and in Israel hypersensitivity to fruits and vegetables is believed to be the most common cause of food allergy in patients above the age of 10 years [53]. It is caused by an IgE immediate reaction to predominantly heat-labile allergens in various foods. Symptoms are unpleasant but usually not dangerous unless associated with a nut hypersensitivity, when anaphylaxis after nut ingestion may occur. The syndrome is due to hypersensitivity to cross-reactive determinants shared by the different fruits and vegetables. In some instances this extends to cross-reactivity with various pollens. The full spectrum of the syndrome and the shared allergenic determinants in the different substances is under continuing investigation.

For a clinical viewpoint it is useful to consider these syndromes with respect to pollenosis associated versus non–pollen associated OAS.

1. Pollenosis associated OAS: Approximately 35% of patients with the following types of pollenosis show hypersensitivity to antigenically related fruits and vegetables:
   a. Birch pollen—apple, hazelnut, carrot, potato, celery, kiwi fruit
   b. Mugwort/birch pollen—celery, carrot, spices
   c. Rye grass—melon, tomato, peanut, watermelon
   d. Ragweed pollen—melon, watermelon, banana, zucchini, cucumber
2. Non–pollen associated OAS. These symptoms have been attributed to the following:
   a. Cross-reactivity to carbohydrate determinants on different substances: grass pollen, buckwheat, potato, bee venom
   b. Fruits of the Prunoideae genera: peach, plum, apricot, cherry
   c. Latex-fruit-cluster hypersensitivity: latex, banana, kiwi fruit, avocado

Because of the heat lability of many of the allergens, skin prick testing needs to be performed with the fresh food product: i.e., uncooked food must be used to detect skin test reactivity. Many of the syndromes associated with pollenosis may be restricted to the period of such pollen exposure. Although the full spectrum of OAS associated with pollenosis (because pollenosis does not usually develop until late childhood) is not usually seen in infants and young children, some of the fruits and vegetables associated with this disorder can elicit perioral urticaria and occasionally anaphylaxis. Such severe reactions are most commonly associated with the ingestion of banana and kiwi fruit.

Treatment consists of avoidance of the relevant foods. The effect of pollen desensitization on pollenosis associated OAS is not clear.

TREATMENT FAILURES IN FOOD ALLERGY

There are a small number of patients who fail to respond to what appear to be appropriate food allergen exclusion diets. These treatment failures can be considered in (a) infants and young children and (b) older children, adolescents, and adults.

Infants and Young Children

Maternally Ingested Food Antigens in Breast Milk

Cow's milk, egg, and wheat antigens have been identified in breast milk [39]. In a significant number of infants who are totally breast fed, uncontrolled atopic dermatitis; recurrent urticaria; some distressed behavior, i.e., colic or reflux esophagitis; and breast milk colitis may be due to hypersensitivity to maternally ingested dietary antigens. Many of these symptoms respond to modification of the maternal diet. Occasionally this is not effective, and when the mother is losing weight, cessation of breast feeding and implementation of hypoallergenic formula feeding may be required.

Failure to Follow a Strict Allergen-Free Diet

Noncompliance with a strict diet is usually seen in infants and young children with cow's milk allergy when care givers are not aware of the distribution of milk antigens in bread, butter, chocolate, and commercially available infant food preparations and the significance of ingredients such as "whey protein," "casein solids," and "milk solids." Small amounts of cow's milk protein in these foods are sufficient to exacerbate symptoms of CMA in highly sensitized infants [41]. Children in child care facilities may inadvertently be given milk-containing products that cause exacerbations and continuing symptoms of CMA, particularly the more subtle forms of the disease.

Multiple Food Allergies

As has been discussed, between 50% and 75% of children with cow's milk allergy have hypersensitivity to other foods, and failure to recognize that hypersensitivity may lead to treatment failure [5]. In Table 7 the incidence of reported adverse reactions to other foods in the first 100 children with CMA we studied is shown. These data emphasize the frequency with which hypersensitivity to multiple foods can occur in children with apparent hypersensitivity to a single food.

Older Children, Adolescents, and Young Adults

Peanut and Nut Hypersensitivity

There is increasing concern about an apparent rise in the incidence of peanut and nut hypersensitivity [47]. This has been associated with an apparent increase in mortality due to food hypersensitivity of adolescence. Two factors that appear to be contributing to this increase in morbidity and mortality in adolescent food allergy are (a) that the nut responsible for the adverse reaction has not been correctly identified, and that (b) unlabeled peanut and nut products are widely used in foods.

The Oral Allergy Syndrome

The OAS is a relatively new entity and treatment failures arise because of the incompleteness of our knowledge of cross-reactive antigens between different food substances. Exciting research that is currently under way should allow precise dietary advice to be given to sufferers of this condition.

CONCLUDING REMARKS

This discussion has been largely confined to the treatment and prevention of food allergy disorders in infancy and early childhood because it is at this age that IgE food hypersensitivity has its greatest impact. Studies that have attempted to modify the development of these food allergy disorders have been reviewed. We are not convinced that current food allergy primary preventative measures are sufficiently effective at a community level to recommend their widespread use. Secondary prevention may well be useful in particular families in which a high probability of an infant's having food allergic diseases exists. At present we believe major emphasis should be given to education of primary care givers about the very high incidence of food hypersensitivity in infants and the importance of their having appropriate treatment strategies ready, i.e., tertiary prevention.

In order to assist patients with established food allergy there is a need for regulatory authorities to insist on accurate labeling of food products and for manufacturers to prevent contamination of food products with highly allergenic food substances [54].

ACKNOWLEDGMENTS

The assistance with preparation of this chapter of Dr. Ian Humphrey and Mrs. Joan Sedmak is gratefully acknowledged.

REFERENCES

1. Hill DJ, Firer MA, Shelton MA, Hosking CS. Manifestations of milk allergy in infancy: clinical and immunological findings. *J Pediatr 1986; 109:*270.
2. Hill DJ, Bannister DG, Hosking CS, Kemp AS. Cow milk allergy within the spectrum of atopic disorders. *Clin Exp Allergy 1994; 24:*1137.
3. Hill DJ, Hosking CS, Chen YZ et al. The frequency of food allergy in Australia and Asia. *Toxicol Lett* in press.
4. Hill DJ, Hosking CS. The cow milk allergy complex: overlapping disease profiles in infancy. *Eur J Clin Nutr 1995; 48*(suppl 1):S1.
5. Bishop JM, Hill DJ, Hosking CS. Natural history of cow milk allergy: clinical outcome. *J Pediatr 1990; 116:*862.
6. Hill DJ, Hudson IL, Sheffield LJ et al. A low allergen diet is a significant intervention in infantile colic: results of a community based study. *J Allergy Clin Immunol 1995; 96:*886.
7. Iacono G, Carroccio A, Cavatio F et al. Gastroesophageal reflux in cow's milk allergy in infants: a prospective study. *J Allergy Clin Immunol 1996; 97:*822.
8. Hill DJ, Catto-Smith ACS, Cameron DJS et al. Is multiple food protein intolerance (MFPI) the cause of "reflux oesophagitis" in distressed infants. *J Allergy Clin Immunol* 1997; 336
9. Hill DJ, Duke AM, Hosking CS, Hudson IL. Clinical manifestations of cow's milk allergy in childhood. II. The diagnostic value of skin test and RAST. *Clin Allergy 1988; 18:*481.
10. Bock SA, Sampson HA, Atkins FM et al. Double-blind placebo-controlled food challenges as an office procedure: a manual. *J Allergy Clin Immunol 1988; 88:*986.
11. Grulee C, Sandford H. The influence of breast feeding and artificial feeding in infantile eczema. *J Pediatr 1936; 9:*223.
12. Sarrinen UM, Kajossari M, Backman A, Siimes MA. Prolonged breast feeding as prophylaxis for atopic disease. *Lancet 1979; 2:*163.
13. Matthew DJ, Taylor B, Norman AP, et al. Prevention of eczema. *Lancet 1997; 1:*321.
14. Chandra RK, Pun S, Suraiya C et al. Influence of maternal food antigen avoidance during pregnancy and lactation on incidence of atopic eczema in infants. *Clin Allergy 1986; 16:*565.
15. Halpem SR, Sellars WA, Johnson RB et al. Development of childhood allergy in infants fed breast, soy or cow milk. *Allergy Clin Immunol 1973; 51:*139.
16. Golding J, Butler NR, Taylor B. Breast feeding and eczema/asthma (letter). *Lancet 1982; 1:*623.
17. Ferguson DM, Horwood LJ, Beutrais AL. et al. Eczema and infant diet. *Clin Allergy 1981; 11:*325.
18. Ferguson DM, Horwood LJ. Early solid food and eczema in childhood: a 10 year longitudinal study. *Pediatr Allergy Immunol 1994; (suppl 1):*44.
19. Gerrard JW. Allergies in breast fed babies to foods ingested by the mother. *Clin Rev Allergy 1984; 2:*143.
20. Van Asperen PP, Kemp AS, Mellis CM. Immediate food hypersensitivity reactions on the first known exposure to the food. *Arch Dis Child 1983; 58:*253.

21. Jacobsen SP, Halken S, Host A, Bender L. Specific IgE antibodies against cow milk protein in cord blood from newborn infants with or without atopic disposition. *Pediar Allergy Immunol Suppl 1995; 8:*98.

22. Falth-Magnusson K, Kjellman NIM. Development of atopic disease in babies whose mothers were receiving exclusion diet during pregnancy: a randomised study. *J Allergy Clin Immunol 1987; 80:*868.

23. Zeiger RS. Secondary prevention of allergic disease: an adjunct to primary prevention. *Pediatr Allergy Immunol 1995; 6:*127.

24. Halken S, Jacobsen HP, Host A, Holmenwund D. The effect of hypoallergenic formulas in infants at risk of allergic disease. *Eur J Clin Nutr 1995; 49:*(suppl 1):77.

25. Host A, Husbe S, Osterballe O. A prospective study of cow's milk allergy in exclusively breast fed infants. Acta Pediatr Scand 1988; 77:663.

26. Host A. Cow's milk protein allergy and intolerance in infancy. *Paediatr Allergy Immunol 1994; (suppl 5):*5.

27. Heyman M, Darmon N, Dupont C, Dugas B, Hirribaren A, Blaton M, Desjeux JF. Mononuclear cells from infants allergic to cow's milk secrete tumour necrosis factor Alpha altering intestinal function. *Gastroenterology 1994; 106:*1516.

28. Lindfors A, Enocksson E. Development of atopic disease after early administration of cow milk formula. *Allergy 1988; 43:*11.

29. Fergusson D, Horwood L Shannon F. Asthma and infant diet. *Arch Dis Child 1983; 58:*48.

30. Fergusson DM, Horwood LJ, Shannon FT. Early solid feeding in recurrent eczema: a 10-year longitudinal study. *Pediatrics 1990; 86:*541.

31. Hill DJ, Hosking CS. The Melbourne Atopy Cohort Study.

32. Marini A, Agosti M, Motta G, Mosca F. Affects of a dietary and environmental prevention program on the incidence of allergic symptoms in high atopic risk infants: a 3-years follow-up. *Acta Pediatr Scand Suppl 1996; 414:*1.

33. Bruijnzell-Koomen C, Ortolani C, Aas K, Bindslev-Jensen C, Bjorksten B, Moneret-Vautrin D, Wuthrich B. Adverse reactions to foods. *Allergy 1955; 50:*623–635.

34. Kjellmann NIM. Natural history and prevention of food hypersensitivity. In: Metcalfe DD, Sampson HI, Simon RA, eds. *Food Allergy: At Risk Reactions to Foods and Food Additives.* Boston: Blackwell Scientific, 1991, p 319.

35. Gerrard JW, McKenzie JWA, Goluboff N, Garson JZ, Maningas CS. Cow's milk allergy: prevalence and manifestations in an unselected series of newborns. *Acta Pediatr Scand 1973; 273*(suppl 1):273.

36. Gerrard JW, Lubos MC, Hardy LW, Holmlund BA, Webster VA. Milk allergy: clinical picture and familial incidence. Can Med Assoc J 1967; 97:780–785. (1967).

37. Dean T. Factors predicting food allergy. *Toxicol Lett*

38. Bergman RL. The allergy march: from food to pollen. *Toxicol Lett*

39. Sampson HA, Ho DG. The utility of the Pharmacia CAP system (RAST. FEIA/TM CAP) in diagnosing IgE-mediated food hypersensitivity. *J Allergy Clin Immunol 1995; 1 (p 2):*329

40. Sampson HA. Mast cell involvement in food allergy. In: Kaliner MA, Metcalfe DD, eds. *The Mast Cell in Health and Disease.* New York: Marcel Dekker, 1993, p 609.

41. Sampson HA, Mendelson LM, Rose JP. Fatal and near fatal anaphylactic reactions to food in children and adolescents. *N Engl J Med 1992; 327:*380.
42. Heyman M, Grasset E, Ducroc R, Desjeux JF. Antigen absorption by jejunal epithelium of children with cow's milk allergy. *Pediatr Resp 1988; 24:*197.
43. Businco L, Bruno G, Giampietro PG, Cantani A, Allergenicity and nutrititional adequacy of soy protein formulas. *J Pediatr 1992; 121:*S21.
44. Isolauri E, Sutas Y, Makinen-Kiljunen S, Oja SS, Isosomppi R, Turjanmaa K. Efficacy and safety of hydrolysed cow milk and amino acid-derived formulas in infants with cow milk allergy. J Pediatr 1995; 127:550.
45. Host A. Cow's milk protein allergy and intolerance in infancy: some clinical epidemiological and immunological aspects. *Pediatr Allergy Immunol 1994; 5 (suppl S5):*5.
46. Hill DJ, Cameron DJS, Francis DEM, Gonzales-Andaya A, Hosking CS. Challenge confirmation of late onset reactions to extensively hydrolysed formulas in infants with multiple food protein intolerance. *J Allergy Clin Immunol 1995; 96:*386.
47. Sampson H. The management of peanut allergy. *Br Med J 1996; 312:*1050.
48. Tariq SM, Stevens M, Matthews S, Ridaut S, Twiselton R, Hide DW. Cohort study of peanut and tree nut sensitisation by the age of 4 years. *Br Med J 1996; 313:*514.
49. Sporik R, Hill DJ. Allergy to peanuts, nuts and sesame seed in Australian children. *Br Med J 1996; 313:*147.
50. Bock SA, Atkins FM. The natural history of peanut allergy. *J Allergy Clin Immunol 1996; 83:*900.
51. Vieths S. Allergenic cross-reactivity food allergy and pollen. *Toxicol Lett*
52. Pastorelo EA, Ortolani C. Oral allergy syndrome. In Metcalf DD, Sampson HA, Simon RA, eds. *Food Allergy: Adverse Reactions to Foods and Food Additives.* 2nd ed. Cambridge, MA: Blackwell Scientific, 1997, p 221.
53. Kivity S, Dunnel K, Marian Y. The pattern of food hypersensitivity in patients with onset after 10 years of age. *Clin Exp Allergy 1994; 24:*19.
54. Steinman HA. "Hidden" allergies in foods. *J Allergy Clin Immunol 1996; 98:*241.
55. Zeiger RS. Pediatr Allergy Immunol 1994; 5(suppl2): 33–43.

22

Food Allergies and Their Implications in Diets and Nutrition

SUSAN C. STURGESS
Winthrop-University Hospital, Mineola, New York

As health care providers involved with food, nutrition, or medical nutrition therapy, we are responsible for ensuring that our clients or patients consume optimal calories, protein, and micronutrients to meet their nutritional needs. It is equally, if not more, important that we provide this nutrition in a diet that is safe for and well tolerated by each individual. In the United States today, researchers estimate that approximately 7% of adults and 13% of children have some type of allergic reaction to food [1]. The typical manifestations of food allergies may be asthma, exacerbation of eczema, gastrointestinal symptoms, and, in the most severe cases, anaphylaxis [2]. When encountering a patient with a reported history of "food allergy," we must first determine the type of reaction that exists.

An adverse reaction to food is defined as any clinically abnormal response caused by the ingestion of a food substance [3]. The offending agent may be the food itself or an ingredient added in processing. Sulfites, monosodium glutamate, tartrazine, and aspartame are among the most common food additives implicated in adverse reactions [2]. Although the Food and Drug Administration

(FDA) has banned the use of sulfites in raw fruits and vegetables, it allows their use in packaged foods, such as dried fruits, beer, and wine [1]. People sensitive to sulfites may exhibit hives, vomiting, or wheezing, and in the most severe cases, a fatal asthma attack. Monosodium glutamate (MSG) is used as a flavor enhancer in certain foods, such as Chinese dishes. Many people attribute headache, dizziness, palpitations, or wheezing to the ingestion of MSG, but the relationship is still widely debated among scientists [3]. Tartrazine is more commonly known as FDC yellow dye number 5. It is used as a food coloring in ice cream and other desserts, beverages, and salad dressings and in some medications, such as enteric coated tablets. Tartrazine has been suggested to cause hives and wheezing in some cases, but the mechanism of its action remains unclear [4]. Aspartame is an artificial sweetener made from the amino acids phenylalanine and aspartic acid. It is widely used in dietetic products, such as sugar-free desserts and calorie-free soft drinks, and people have attributed hives and migraine headaches to its ingestion, but these claims remain unsubstantiated [2]. Artificial flavoring and coloring, and preservatives have also been suggested to exacerbate symptoms in children with attention deficit hyperactivity disorders, although further study is needed to confirm these suspicions [6].

A food allergy is an immunological reaction to the exposure to a food antigen [7]. This reaction must be reproducible with repeat exposure to the allergen. The majority of recognized food allergies are the Immunoglobulin E–(IgE) mediated degranulation of the mast cells in response to a food allergen, primarily glycoprotein. This response is the body's immune system's reaction to the presence of a foreign antigen in a food consumed through an IgE-mediated immune reaction and is the classic food allergy response [3]. The most severe of the food hypersensitivities may result in anaphylaxsis and can often end in death if not attended to quickly. One source states that in the United States more children and adolescents die annually of food-induced anaphylaxis than of insect stings [2]. The most common IgE-mediated food allergy reactions in the United States are caused by cow's milk, fish, eggs, bananas, melon, peanuts, nuts, shellfish, soy, and wheat [1].

Another type of adverse reaction to food is a food intolerance: an abnormal, nonimmunological response to a food ingested, which is the most common food-related adverse reaction [3]. Food intolerances can include toxic reaction, such as food poisoning, or reaction to a contaminant in a food, such as aflatoxin, mercury, penicillin, or pesticides; pharmacological reactions, such as shakiness from caffeine, alkaloids in mushrooms, goitrogens in cabbage, or pressor amines in bananas; and metabolic reactions, such as diarrhea caused by lactose consumption in a lactose-intolerant individual. A metabolic food intolerance may have a primary cause, such as a congenital lactase deficiency, or may be secondary to another disease process, such as transient lactose intolerance after an acute viral enteritis. Such food intolerances are commonly mislabeled food allergies by patients.

It is important to determine which component of the offending food is responsible for the adverse reaction. For example, if a mother tells you her child is allergic to milk, does she mean it is the milk protein (the casein or lactalbumin) that causes a hypersensitive immune response, or is the child's diarrhea caused by the inability to digest the milk sugar lactose? Symptoms such as anaphylaxsis and eczema are most likely IgE-mediated responses to a food's glycoprotein, whereas symptoms such as diarrhea, wheezing, and migraines may be adverse reactions to a starch, fat, amino acid, or preservative in the food implicated [2]. Symptoms of insomnia, fatigue, and hyperactivity due to food ingestion are still debated by many physicians and remain controversial. It is of the utmost importance to ensure that the patient does not consume a food that causes him or her to have a severe or harmful reaction, but it is important not to overrestrict a person's dietary intake, especially if he or she is a growing child or is suffering from malnutrition.

Adverse symptoms to food ingestion may be acute and caused by a single exposure, or they may be dose related. In my own experience and in the assessment of patients, I have observed certain people who are able to eat small quantities of their allergy-causing food without any negative effects. If they exceed a certain amount of that food over a short time, however, symptoms may develop. Keep in mind that a symptomatic response to a specific food may not occur with each ingestion because the quantity may be insufficient to cause the adverse effect. Varying the method by which the food is prepared may also alter the response if the offending antigen is denatured in the preparation. Severity of symptoms or reaction may also be exacerbated by alcohol or certain medications. The most notable example of such a reaction is the occurrence of a hypertensive crisis that results from ingesting tyramine-containing foods or beverages, such as aged cheese or red wine, while on a drug containing a monoamine oxidase inhibitor, found in some antidepressants [1].

Elimination diets can be useful in helping to determine which foods in the diet are causing an adverse reaction. In the most simple of the elimination diets, a single food is eliminated and reintroduced while symptoms are monitored. The reintroduction of a suspected allergenic food is referred to as a food challenge. If the symptoms disappear with the elimination of the food and reappear with its reintroduction, it is presumed that the individual is allergic to this food. A challenge should only be used in cases of mild to moderate adverse reaction and not with those foods that are known to cause anaphylaxis in an individual. In a multiple elimination diet, foods that are commonly known to cause allergic reactions are simultaneously omitted from the diet for 2–3 weeks and then introduced one at a time [4].

There is continuing debate about which foods to eliminate from the baseline test diet. The strictest of the elimination diets excludes eggs, milk, fish, poultry, and all meats except lamb; allows white and sweet potatoes and tapioca; does not allow wheat, oats, corn, millet, barley, or rye; includes all fruits except citrus, strawberries, and tomatoes; allows all vegetables except corn and peas; limits fats to olive oil, coconut oil, sesame oil, and safflower oil; and limits sweeteners to cane sugar, beet sugar, and maple syrup [3]. It is recommended that this restrictive a diet be used for as short a time as possible and that a multivitamin/mineral supplement be given during this time to prevent micronutrient deficiencies [4].

Before imposing a strict or minimal elimination diet, as outlined here, many experts recommend a trial of a wheat-, egg-, and milk-free diet, with the additional elimination of specific foods suspected of causing adverse reaction [9]. Others suggest keeping food diaries and recording the occurrence of allergy symptoms to identify foods most likely responsible before eliminating any foods from the diet [2].

A food may be reintroduced into the diet in a number of ways. An *open challenge* is a reintroduction in which both the person eating the food and the person observing the symptoms are aware of the food being tested. This is probably the most feasible method for patients to make use of in their own homes. In a single-blind challenge, only the patient is unaware of the food being tested. In this type of test, the antigen could be provided in a form other than the original food, such as in a capsule or mixed into another, stronger tasting, nonoffending food. Using this method would help to eliminate reactions brought on by food aversions that may be seen when presenting the patient with the food in its original form. A single-blind test is still subject to observer bias but can be useful in many situations. The optimal test for definitively diagnosing a food sensitivity is the double-blind food challenge, in which neither the patient nor the observer is aware of the food being given.

Although many clinicians have varying protocols on administering a food challenge, a fairly common regimen may include the following steps:

1. Patient is observed to have food allergy symptoms.
2. Diet history is recorded and implicates specific food.
3. Patient follows diet, eliminating this suspect food for approximately 14 days.
4. If symptoms persist, further elimination is imposed, to be followed by reintroduction:
   a. Continue food diary, identifying additional suspect foods and eliminating them as well.
   b. Try diet excluding wheat, milk, and egg foods as well as suspected allergens.
   c. Try strict or minimal elimination diet plus avoidance of suspect foods.
   d. If symptoms persist at this point of elimination, reevaluate for non-food causes of the symptoms, such as the environment or medication.

5. If 14 day diet free of offending food causes a disappearance of symptoms, provide an oral challenge with a small amount of a single suspect food every 4 hr.

6. If the patient remains symptom-free for approximately 48 hr, repeat the challenge, increasing the quantity of food given gradually to a full portion.

7. If the patient continues to be symptom-free, he or she now consumes the food in question for 3 consecutive days in the amount typically eaten.

8. If the patient is still symptom-free at this point, the food is allowed in the diet as desired by the patient.

9. The next food is then reintroduced 7 days after this challenge is completed.

One of the most important steps in diagnosing and managing a food allergy is the patient's keeping an accurate and detailed food diary. The patient or care giver should be instructed to record everything the patient eats or drinks for several consecutive days, usually at least 2 weekdays and 1 weekend day. The food listing should specify time of day consumed, brand name if applicable, methods of preparation, serving size and quantity consumed, and location where the food is eaten. The preparation and serving of the food should include, but not be limited to, noting whether the food is raw; washed or unwashed; cooked in liquid, shortening, wine, or extracts; broiled, and, if so, on what surface; smoked; fermented; contains mold, artificial coloring, flavoring, or preservatives. The symptoms should also be recorded, each time they appear, including the time of day of onset, the interval after eating when they occur, the severity of the reaction, and a description of the symptoms [8]. A trained registered dietitian can then evaluate these diaries, along with the physician, to determine patterns relating the consumption of certain foods to adverse reactions. The dietitian and physician will look for trends in the time frame between the ingestion of the food and the symptoms, the quantity of the food needed to produce a reaction, the frequency of the reaction, the effect of food preparation on the reaction, and the environmental conditions under which the food is eaten. It is those foods identified by the dietitian and physician that will be eliminated and challenged in the patient's diet.

Whole foods, such as raw fruits and vegetables and unprocessed meats, are often easier for the patient and the health care professionals to identify than processed or combination foods. It is crucial that the dietitian educate the patient and his or her care givers about the importance of reading labels and understanding what ingredients combination foods contain. For example, the following ingredients indicate the presence of a food substance:

Ingredient listed	Origin
Casein, caseinate, sodium caseinate, calcium caseinate, whey, lactalbumin, lactose	All indicate milk
Albumin	Eggs
Wheat bran, gum, or starch; gluten, food starch, enriched flour, vegetable starch/gum	All may indicate wheat
Shortening, lard, gelatin	Beef or pork
Vegetable oil, starch, or gum	May also indicate corn or soy
Margarine, corn syrup, or food starch	May also indicate corn
Textured vegetable protein	May indicate soy

In addition to being integral components of the combination food, many allergenic food substances can be added to a food during processing for flavor, texture, preservative, or emusification purposes or as fillers, For example:

If patient reacts to	Watch out for
Citrus fruits	Citric acid preservative in foods, lime juice in tortilla chips
Lactose	Processed nonkosher meats (i.e., hot dogs)
Sulfites	Frozen potatoes and frozen shrimp, tea mixes, beet sugar, vinegars, wines
Egg whites	Instant coffee, bouillon, marshmallows
Corn	Jellies and ketchup made with corn syrup
Wheat	Salad dressing, whiskey, vinegar
Soy	Some canned green beans

Patients are able to discover these additives or ingredients when they read labels of foods they are preparing for themselves, but they must be even more careful to ask specific questions about ingredients and preparation when eating out at restaurants. Many experts believe that people with multiple anaphylactic food allergies should not take the chance of eating in a restaurant. There have been documented cases in which people with anaphylactic reactions to shrimp have died because a person at a nearby table in a restaurant was served sizzling shrimp fajitas and there was enough shrimp glycoprotein aerosolized in the steam to kill them [3].

Even at a friend's house, patients must be sure that the cook understands the severity of their allergy and considers any exposure, even in food preparation. If a patient with severe food allergies orders a grilled hamburger or chicken breast at a restaurant or a neighbor's barbecue, it is extremely important that he or she find out what other foods have been cooked recently on the same grill. There may be enough residue left from previously grilled foods to cause an adverse reaction. Again, shrimp can be a likely offender, especially now that many people, in their efforts to be calorie conscious, have started grilling seafood instead of just meat and poultry. Another case recently reported in the media was one in which a girl died of chick-pea anaphylaxis because her friend's mother was cooking a dish containing chick-peas near where the children were playing. Again the culprit was aerosolized glycoprotein, this time from the chick-peas [10].

When eating out, persons with food allergies must be familiar with menu terms in order to be aware of the ingredients used in making various dishes. For example:

When the menu says	The dish probably contains
Français or soufflé	Eggs
Bolognaise	Meat (usually beef or pork)
Provençale	Tomatoes
Hollandaise	Egg and butter
Deviled	Mayonnaise (eggs)
Au gratin	Cheese (milk)
Scallopini	Mushrooms
Ceviche or carpaccio	Raw fish/seafood
Bisque	Cream (milk)
Florentine	Spinach

One ingredient that seems omnipresent in a wide range of foods is gluten. This ingredient poses a particular challenge for individuals who are gluten-intolerant, a condition also known as celiac sprue or gluten-sensitive enteropathy. Gluten, commonly known as wheat protein, is a major component of wheat endosperm, but similar proteins called prolamins are also found in barley, oats, and rye. (A mnemonic for gluten-containing foods is BROW, for barley, rye, oats, and wheat.) Gliadin is one of the proteins found in gluten and is also thought to contribute to adverse symptoms in people with gluten intolerance [9]. Symptoms are primarily diarrhea and/or vomiting, which is reflective of malabsorption caused by damage to the intestinal mucosa. The exact cause of celiac disease remains unclear, but the diagnosis can be confirmed with an intestinal biopsy. The biopsy of the small bowel of a person with celiac disease shows a flattened intestinal mucosa, loss of villi, and an increased presence of immune cells in the gastrointestinal (GI) tract [4]. Management of celiac disease involves strict compliance with a gluten-free diet. Compliance can be evaluated by a rebiopsy of the small bowel and subsequent assessment of further damage versus improved histological findings. One problem a patient with celiac disease faces when he or she is noncompliant with a gluten-free diet is that the diarrhea and intestinal damage caused by the ingestion of gluten can lead to malabsorption of other nutrients, such as vitamins and minerals.

Although it may not be difficult to identify gluten-containing foods whose main ingredients are wheat flour, such as bread and pasta, it is the foods that contain hidden sources of gluten that may present a problem to gluten-intolerant individuals. Literally thousands of the foods that Americans include in their daily diets are made with some form of wheat protein or related compound. Most soups, gravies, sauces, salad dressings, soy sauce, and some seasonings are made with some form of gluten or gliadin used in their processing. Other foods that contain gluten and/or gliadin include most ice creams, frozen yogurts, and puddings; malted milk products, distilled vinegars, horseradish, and some chewing gums; whiskey, gin, vodka, beer, and ale; many hot dogs, cold cuts, and some sausages; those cheeses that contain oat gum; thickened fruit products, such as pie filling; baked beans, creamed vegetables, and frozen or canned vegetables that are prepared in a sauce [2].

Patients with gluten intolerance must substitute products made from rice, corn, soy, tapioca, or potato flour for those foods that contain gluten. Several specialty food companies (such as Ener-G Foods in Seattle, Washington) make breads, pastas, and breakfast cereals of non-gluten-containing flours, such as those mentioned. Many of these gluten-free starch foods are fortified with the same vitamins and minerals as standard fortified or enriched wheat-based products, but patients must read labels to ensure that they are not missing essential micronutrients. Specific vitamin and mineral levels that should be monitored in a patient with celiac sprue include iron, vitamin B_{12}, folate, calcium, and vitamin D. Clotting time (PT/PTT) should be monitored for the need of vitamin K supplementation, and fluid status and electrolytes should be monitored and replaced as needed in celiac patients with active diarrhea. There are several organizations that provide information and support for gluten-intolerant individuals, which are listed at the end of this chapter.

When eliminating offending foods from the diet, one must take care not to cause insufficient intake of micronutrients. It is important to determine what nutrients the eliminated foods would have contributed to the diet and to substitute those foods with suitable replacements.

For example:

Eliminated food	Possible deficiency	Try to use
Milk/dairy	Calcium	Calcium fortified soy milk, spinach, salmon canned with bones,
Lactose products	Calcium	Lactose-free milk
Citrus fruit	Vitamin C	Broccoli, green peppers
Meats and nuts	Thiamine	Barley, brewers' yeast
Beef	Iron	Prunes, spinach, kidney beans, molasses
Wheat (gluten)	Thiamine, riboflavin, niacin, iron	Fortified gluten-free products (must read labels)

It is important that patients eliminating many foods from their diets keep food diaries that a registered dietitian can analyze. Using a computerized diet analysis program, a dietitian can determine which nutrients are deficient in the patient's restricted diet and can then recommend increases in appropriate alternate foods based on the patient's food preferences.

In the age of genetic engineering, people with severe food allergies must also be careful of encountering allergens in foods that have been engineered from other foods. There was recently a case cited in the literature in which soybeans were biogenetically combined with Brazil nuts to enrich the soybeans with the amino acid they lack naturally, methionine. Analysis showed that the new supersoybeans contained 2S albumin, the major allergen from Brazil nuts, and that people allergic to Brazil nuts also reacted to the 2S albumin from the new soybeans when tested. The researchers suggested that the FDA should require companies that sell transgenic foods to label the source of the donor food for the purpose of averting potential allergic reactions [5].

Cross-reactivity between antigens may also occur in some patients with food allergies, but not in all. People allergic to one food in a biological class may also be allergic to other foods in that class [4]. For example:

If one is allergic to	He or she may also be allergic to [4]
Gourds (squash)	Cucumber, melon, cantaloupe
Plums	Sloe (gin)
Laurel	Bay leaf, cinnamon, avocado
Peas (beans)	Peanuts, licorice
Lily	Asparagus, onion, garlic
Grass	Barley, rye, oats, wheat, corn, rice

Patients with a ragweed allergy may also be allergic to banana, melon, and chamomile tea, because of the presence of a like glycoprotein [2]. Similarly, patients with a strong allergy to birch tree pollen may have a sensitivity to apples [8]. An allergy to aspirin may also include sensitivity to salicylate-containing foods, including avocado, berries, cucumbers, melon, root beer, quick breads, potatoes, tomatoes, red and green peppers, pickles, olives, almonds, peanuts, wintergreen flavoring, and foods or drugs containing tartrazine dye [4]. The increasing use of latex products in our society has led to an increased incidence of latex allergies in recent years. Health care workers must be extremely cautious not to use latex-containing examination gloves, intravenous (IV) tubing, breathing tubes, or other latex based supplies near a patient who suffers from severe latex sensitivity, to prevent an anaphylactic reaction. Patients with such sensitivity should be sure to wear medical alert tags indicating this allergy at all times. These patients should also be made aware that eating certain foods, such as avocado, bananas, chestnuts, kiwi, or mango, may increase their sensitivity to latex.

Patients and health care workers alike should also be aware of the potential presence of food allergy–related antigens in other medical treatments. Egg phospholipid is commonly used as an emulsifier in intravenous vaccines, such as flu shots; therefore, people with a severe food allergy to eggs are not able to receive inoculation in IV format. Similarly, patients with anaphylaxis to eggs should not be given IV lipid preparation when receiving parenteral nutrition solutions, because of the use of egg phospholipid for emulsification in these mixtures as well.

A causative agent for food intolerance, lactose, can also be found in many medications, such as tablet forms of antibiotics, pain relievers, and even vitamin and mineral supplements. Although lactose may be present in small amounts, it must be taken into consideration when a patient is extremely sensitive or when a patient with a moderate intolerance is taking multiple lactose-containing medications. In addition, many medications are prescribed to be taken on an empty stomach. Although some individuals may be able to tolerate small amounts of lactose with a meal of non-lactose-containing foods, they may experience gastrointestinal distress when consuming a lactose source, such as a pill, on an empty stomach.

Many health care providers are also involved in recommending, prescribing, or administering oral or enteral calorie/protein supplements, such as "instant breakfast" drinks or milk shakes; other nutritive beverages, such as Sustacal, Resource, or Ensure; and tube feedings. Many of the powdered mixes and refrigerated shakes are milk based and therefore contain lactose. Several nutritional supplement companies, such as Nutrabalance, however, do make lactose-free "milk shakes." It is important that nutritionists and physicians become familiar with the variety of products on the market and that they make their patients aware of their availability. Most of the canned and brick-pack, or "juice box," forms of oral nutritional supplements (Sustacal, Resource, Ensure), are lactose-free and gluten-free, but health care providers should read labels to ensure they are dispensing appropriate formulas.

Like oral supplements, most of the tube feeding formulas on the market today are both gluten-free and lactose-free, and ingredients are listed on the labels of all cans or packets. Representatives of the pharmaceutical companies that manufacture the various tube feedings can provide information that details the special features of each product and lists cautions for use in patients with certain medical conditions or food allergies. Nutritionists, physicians, and patients should all be aware that lactose-free does not mean milk-free. Many of the lactose-free tube feedings and oral supplements use casein, or milk protein, as a protein source. Therefore, anyone with a severe food allergy to milk protein would have to use a product that is also casein-free, with the protein provided from another source, such as beef or egg. Once again label reading is a most important tool in preventing adverse reactions to food or nutrition support products.

I have included at the end of this chapter a list of organizations that provide information about food allergies. Be aware as well that food manufacturers are also a resource for patients and health care professionals and can provide detailed information on ingredients, preservatives, or processing agents used in the foods they produce. Most have written information they will mail or fax consumers, by request, and many of the larger food companies also have toll-free phone numbers you can call to speak to a representative, who will answer your questions about the company's products over the phone.

It is the responsibility of health care professionals to educate patients with food allergies about the dangers and solutions in choosing foods. Anyone with severe food allergies must thoroughly investigate any new food, whether it is from a store, a restaurant, a friend's kitchen, or his or her garden, before incorporating it into the diet.

REFERENCES

1. American Academy of Allergy and Immunology. Understanding Food Allergy. Washington, DC: International Food Information Council Foundation, 1993.
2. Beaudette T. Adverse Reactions to Food. Chicago: American Dietetic Association, 1991.
3. Sampson HA. Food hypersensitivity: manifestations, diagnosis and natural history. Food Technol 1992; 46:141–144.
4. Krause, Mahan. Food, Nutrition and Diet Therapy. 7th ed. Philadelphia: WB Saunders, 1984.
5. Nordlee JA, Taylor SL, Townsend JA, Thomas LA, Bush RK. Allergen in transgenic soybeans. N Engl J Med 1996; 334:688–692.
6. Boris M, Mandel FS. Foods and additives are common causes of the attention deficit hyperactivity disorder in children. Ann Allergy 1994; 72(5):462–468.

7.   Hensyl WR. Stedman's Medical Dictionary. 24th ed. Baltimore: Williams & Wilkins, 1982.
8.   Zeman FJ, Ney DM. Applications of Clinical Nutrition. 1st ed. Englewood Cliffs, NJ: Prentice Hall, 1988.
9.   Zeman FJ. Clinical Nutrition and Dietetics. 2nd ed. Englewood Cliffs, NJ: Prentice Hall, 1993.
10. Associated Press. Cooking Fumes Kill Girl Allergic to Beans. Newsday, Feb 11, 1994.

ORGANIZATIONS THAT PROVIDE INFORMATION ON FOOD ALLERGIES

Allergy and Asthma Network/Mothers of Asthmatics, Inc.
3554 Chain Bridge Road
Suite 200
Fairfax. VA 22030-2709
(800) 878-4403

American Academy of Allergy, Asthma & Immunology
611 East Wells Street
Milwaukee, WI 53202
(414) 272-6071

The American Dietetic Association
216 West Jackson Boulevard
Suite 800
Chicago. IL 60607
(800) 366-1655

The Asthma and Allergy Foundation of America
Information line: (800) 727-8462

Celiac Sprue Association
P.O. Box 31700
Omaha, NE 68131-0700
(402) 558-0600

The Food Allergy Network
17400 Eaton Place
Suite 107
Fairfax, VA 22030-2208
(703) 691-3179
(800) 929-4040

Food and Drug Administration
FDA, HFE-88
5600 Fishers Lane
Rockville, MD 20857
Consumer inquiries information line: (301) 443-3170
(FDA Consumer Special Report: Focus on Food Labeling)

The Gluten Intolerance Group of North America
P.O. Box 23053
Seattle, WA 98102-0353
(206) 325-6980
(Leave message on answering machine for introductory package)

Hotline Printing & Publishing
Allergy Hotline (newsletter)
5329 Diplomat Place
Orlando, FL 32810
(407) 628-1377

International Food Information Council Foundation
1100 Connecticut Avenue, N.W.
Suite 430
Washington, DC 20036
(202) 296-6540

National Digestive Diseases Information Clearinghouse
2 Information Way
Bethesda, MD 20892-3570
(publications include Lactose Intolerance Information Packet)

National Institute of Allergy and Infectious Diseases
31 Center Drive
MSC 2520
Bethesda, MD 20892
(301) 496-5717

23

Milk-Free, Egg-Free, Corn-Free, and Wheat-Free Diets

STEFANIE TORRENS
Massapequa Park, New York

Food allergies are generally treated by the dietary elimination of the offending foods [1–4]. When eliminating certain foods, individual diets should provide variation by using allowed foods and should be nutritionally balanced with carbohydrates, protein, fat, vitamins, and minerals. A qualified dietitian experienced in managing food allergic patients should be consulted to assist the allergist with treatment, in order to provide a complete nutritional assessment, education, dietary planning, and evaluation of individual dietary compliance. Avoidance measures should be outlined for each patient. The individual's age, atopic history, symptoms, and number of suspect allergens are among the items that must be considered for appropriate dietary planning. Energy and nutrient intake of individuals with multiple food allergies or allergies to a staple food such as milk, wheat, corn, or egg should be monitored closely to ensure nutritional adequacy. The potential for nutritional inadequacies increases if several foods must be eliminated or if the food is a major source of nutrients in the diet. Nutritional deficiencies resulting from use of elimination diets have been reported [5–8]. In addition, an evaluation of nutrient and food intake in individuals with reported food allergies was presented at the New York State Dietetic Association meeting in April 1995. Results of this study showed that subjects reporting an allergy to milk had low intakes of calcium and vitamin D. Several other subjects also had low intakes of various nutrients [9]. Nutritional evaluation and education should be considered for all individuals reporting food allergies in order to provide advice on the consumption of a nutritionally adequate diet.

MILK-FREE DIET

Food Selection Guidelines

Treatment of cow's milk allergy consists of eliminating all food sources of this allergen from the individual's diet. Food selection guidelines for a milk-free diet are outlined in Table 1.

When milk is restricted in the diet, many excellent sources of nutrients are eliminated. Milk is a major source of calcium and an important source of protein, riboflavin, vitamin A, and vitamin D. A calcium supplement with vitamin D may be necessary if intake of these nutrients through other food sources is not adequate. Intake of calcium and vitamin D should be closely monitored and supplemented as needed to meet the RDAs (Recommended Dietary Allowances) for these nutrients (see Table 2). Alternative nondairy calcium sources include fortified tofu or soybean curd, calcium fortified orange juice, broccoli, kale, collard greens, salmon, and sardines (canned fish with bones), dried peas and beans, dried fruits, and nuts. Other major nutrients found in milk can be obtained from alternative sources such as meats, whole grain breads and cereals, enriched grain products, and dark green leafy vegetables. In addition, vitamin D can be synthesized by the body from sunlight.

Label Reading

Labels should be read carefully and any foods that contain the following words should be avoided.

Milk	Casein	Cheese
Instant nonfat dry milk	Casein hydrosylate	Cheese food
Nonfat milk	Sodium caseinate	Cottage cheese
Milk solids	Calcium caseinate	Custard
Curds	Lactalbumin	Cream
Whey	Lactoglobulin	Ice cream
Whey solids	Butter	Sour cream
Ghee	Buttermilk	
Chocolate (products may use milk solids)		
Simplesse (fat substitute containing milk protein)		

Sources: Adapted from Ref. 12; Ref. 13.

TABLE 1 Food Selection Guidelines for Milk-Free Diet

Food group	Avoid	Acceptable substitutes
Milk/beverages	Fluid milk (whole, 2%, 1%, skim, evaporated, condensed), buttermilk, nonfat dry milk, yogurt, Ovaltine, all cheeses, cream, hot chocolate or cocoa mixes, goat's milk, eggnog, malted milk, milk shakes, cow's milk–based infant formulas	Milk protein hydrolyzed cow's formulas, soy and soy milk formulas
Meat, egg, cheese, fish, poultry	Any prepared with milk or milk products, some hot dogs and luncheon meats, sausage, any meat/fish seared in butter or margarine, breaded or creamed meat, all cheeses, egg, fish, poultry, or egg substitutes made with milk products	Plain meats/fish and those that do not contain milk or milk products, kosher prepared meats and products labeled *parve* or *pareve*, soy cheese, and tofu
Breads/cereals	Any prepared with or served with milk, milk solids, butter or margarine; pancakes, waffles, many baking mixes	Any made without milk/milk products, most French and Italian bread, bagels, saltines or soda crackers, bread labeled *parve*
Potatoes and substitutes	Any potato, rice, or pasta prepared with milk, butter, margarine, cheese, cream (e.g., au gratin, scalloped, mashed, creamed, macaroni and cheese)	All pasta, macaroni, potatoes, and rice prepared without milk or milk products
Soups	Any prepared with milk, cream, butter or margarine (e.g., bisques, cream soups, chowders)	Any prepared without milk products
Fruits/vegetables	Any prepared or served with milk or milk products	Any prepared without milk
Desserts/sweets	Any prepared with milk products ice cream, sherbet, whipped toppings, custard, pudding mixes, cake, cookies, pastries, cream pies, candies containing milk, (e.g., caramels, milk chocolate, nougats, fudge)	Any made without milk products, milk-free sherbets, ices, sorbets, gelatin, angel food cake, frozen tofu desserts
Fats	Butter, many margarines, salad dressing containing milk products, many coffee creamers, cream, sour cream	Milk-free margarine and salad dressing, oil, nuts, peanut butter, nondairy creamers without milk protein
Miscellaneous	White and cheese sauces, creamed foods, Hollandaise sauce, imitation chocolate chips	

Sources: Adapted from Ref. 13; Ref. 10.

TABLE 2   Recommended Dietary Allowances for Calcium and Vitamin D

	Age (years)	Calcium (mg)	Vitamin D (μg)
Infants	0–0.5	400	7.5
	0.5–1.0	600	10
Children	1–10	800	10
Males	11–24	1200	10
	25–50	800	5
	51+	800	5
Females	11–24	1200	10
	25–50	800	5
	51+	800	5
Pregnant/lactating		1200	10

Source: Ref. 14.

Substitutions in Cooking

In recipes calling for milk, fruit juice, or herbal tea can be used as a substitute, provided there is no cross-reactivity to fruit and herbal ingredients. They add a spicy fragrance to bread, cakes, and cookies. Soy or cashew milk can be used as a milk replacement, provided there is no allergy to these items. Combine 1 cup soy powder or ground cashews with 3 cups water in a large saucepan. Whisk until well dissolved. Bring to boil over high heat, stirring constantly. Lower heat and simmer for 3 minutes. Makes 3 cups and may be served hot or cold [10].

EGG-FREE DIET

Food Selection Guidelines

Treatment of egg allergy consists of eliminating all food sources of this allergen from the individual's diet. Food selection guidelines for an egg-free diet are outlined in Table 3.

Eggs are good dietary sources of many nutrients, including protein and iron. These nutrients, however, can be provided readily from a variety of other food sources in the diet. Since egg or egg derivatives are found in many prepared foods, especially grain products, care must be taken so that foods that contain important nutrients such as B vitamins and iron are not unnecessarily restricted.

TABLE 3 Food Selection Guidelines for Egg-Free Diet

Food group	Avoid	Acceptable substitutes
Beverages	Eggnog, some malted drinks, Ovaltine, Ovomalt (wine, root beer, coffee may be clarified with egg; read labels or contact manufacturer regarding these items)	Milk, tea, carbonated beverages, fruit drinks, pure cocoa
Meat, egg, cheese, fish, poultry	Eggs, in any form; many egg substitutes such as Egg Beaters Scramblers, any meat or cheese mixture prepared with or containing egg (meatloaf, meatballs, breaded meats, patties, croquettes), casseroles, gefiltefish, many prepared meats (luncheon meats, imitation seafood)	Plain, fresh meats, poultry, fish, cheese; fish canned in oil, brine, or water; prepared meats and imitation seafood without eggs
Breads/cereals	Any containing egg as an ingredient, challah, egg rolls, or any brushed with egg white glaze; prepared mixtures for pancakes, waffles	Egg-free baked goods, pita bread, rice cakes, potato chips, ready to eat or hot breakfast cereals
Breads/cereals	Biscuits, muffins; French toast, quick breads, pretzels; egg bagels, batters, bread crumbs	
Potatoes and substitutes	Any prepared with egg (duchess potatoes, potato puffs) egg noodles; all pastas unless egg-free	White or sweet potatoes, rice, pasta (egg-free), spaghetti, macaroni
Soups	Bouillons, consommé or other stock soup cleared with egg, noodle soups, egg drop	
Fruits/vegetables	Fruit whips; any served with custard, creamed vegetables, batter fried fruit or vegetables; any served with egg sauces (Hollandaise), vegetable soufflés	All fresh, canned, frozen or dried fruits/vegetables, nectars; all pure fruit or vegetable juices
Desserts/sweets	Meringues, macaroons, custards, angel food cake, puddings or gelatin desserts made with egg, frostings, marshmallows; cakes, cookies, and pastries made with egg or egg products; fruit whips, sherbet, ice cream, doughnuts, candy such as chocolate, fondants, or nougats	Egg-free baked goods, cornstarch puddings made without eggs, Popsicles, fruit ices, gelatin, jellies, jams, pure chocolate and cocoa, fruit pies

TABLE 3   Continued

Food group	Avoid	Acceptable substitutes
Fats	Mayonnaise, some salad dressings, tartar sauce, hollandaise sauce, fat substitute; Simplesse contains egg protein	Butter, margarine, vegetable oils, shortening, olives, gravy and sauces made without
Miscellaneous	Food made with batter or coated with batter, breaded foods; baking powder may contain egg derivatives (check ingredients carefully)	Salt, pepper, spices, herbs, extracts, catsup, mustard, food colorings, lemon juice, vinegar, cornstarch, cream of tartar, yeast

Sources: Adapted from Ref. 10; Ref. 11; Ref. 13.

Label Reading

Labels should be read carefully and any foods that contain the following words should be avoided:

Egg powder or dried egg	Albumin	Ovovitellin
Egg yolk	Ovalbumin	Livetin
Egg white	Ovomucin	Globulin
Egg white solids	Ovomucoid	Ovoglobulin egg albumin
Yolks	Vitellin	

Sources: Adapted from Ref. 12; Ref. 13.

Substitutions in Cooking

In baking, replace one egg by combining 2 tablespoons whole wheat flour, $1/2$ tsp oil, $1/2$ tsp baking powder, and 2 tablespoons liquid (milk, water, or fruit juice). Egg-free substitutes can also be used; however, to prevent problems with consistency, 1 tsp of baking powder can be used for each egg omitted. Some baking powders may contain egg derivatives and ingredients should be checked prior to use [10].

CORN-FREE DIET

Food Selection Guidelines

Treatment of corn allergy consists of eliminating all food items containing this allergen from the individual's diet. Food selection guidelines for the corn-free diet are outlined in Table 4.

TABLE 4 Food Selection Guidelines for Corn-Free Diet

Food group	Avoid	Acceptable substitutes
Beverages	Carbonated beverages, sweetened fruit juice, powdered fruit drinks, milk in paper cartons, instant breakfast, milk shakes, instant coffee or tea, fermented beverages made with corn (bourbon, gin, vodka, whiskey, ale, beer, scotch), many liqueurs, soybean milks and yogurts, nondairy creamers	Milk, buttermilk, pure fruit juice, flavored seltzer, home-made shakes, rum (must be made from cane sugar)
Meat, poultry, fish, egg, cheese	Ham (cured or tenderized), processed meats (i.e., cold cuts or luncheon meats, frankfurters, bacon—unless corn free), sausages, self-basting turkey with hydrolyzed vegetable protein, meat, fish, poultry breaded with corn flour or meal, commercial entrées unless corn free, imitation seafood, cheese spreads unless corn-free	Processed meats made without corn products, fresh meats, poultry, fish, eggs, fish canned in water
Breads/cereals	Bread made with corn products including corn bread, corn muffins, corn chips, tortillas, English muffins, graham crackers, biscuits, waffles, pancake flour and other prepared mixes containing corn products, baking powder with corn derivatives All cereals made with corn (i.e., (Cornflakes, Rice Krispies, Kix, Cheerios, Corn Toasties), hominy grits, some presweetened cereals	Breads, crackers, and cereals made from rice, wheat, rye, oats, barley, bran without corn or corn products, wheat tortillas
Potatoes and substitutes	Any prepared mixes made with corn containing ingredients (i.e., au gratin), canned spaghetti and sauces, potato or macaroni with sauces thickened with cornstarch	Plain white and sweet potatoes, yams, macaroni, noodles, spaghetti, rice
Soups	Vegetable soup, creamed soup, commercial soups unless corn-free, any thickened with cornstarch	Soups made without corn products

TABLE 4 Continued

Food group	Avoid	Acceptable substitutes
Fruits and vegetables	Canned and frozen fruits and juices with added corn sugars, dates and dried fruits, canned baked beans, canned peas, canned vegetables, frozen vegetables in waxed containers, corn, succotash, hominy, Harvard beets, vegetables with sauces containing corn ingredients	Fresh fruits and vegetables, unsweetened fruit juices, pure vegetable juices
Desserts/sweets	Any prepared with corn products, including commercially prepared cakes, candies, cookies, pastries, puddings, cream pies, ices, sherbet, ice cream, gelatin desserts, cake frosting, powdered sugar, corn syrup, jams, jellies, or preserves, Karo syrup, commercial fructose, candied fruits, pancake syrup, chewing gum	Homemade baked goods without corn products, granulated cane or beet sugar, honey, pure maple syrup, molasses, brown sugar, sorghum syrup, artificially sweetened gelatin, sugarless gums, frozen desserts without added corn sweeteners
Fats	Some salad dressings, gravies and sauces thickened with cornstarch, commercial nondairy creamers, some mayonnaise, corn oil or vegetable oil,[a] corn oil margarine[a]	Butter, shortening, vegetable oils (i.e. safflower, peanut, soybean), sour cream, cream cheese
Miscellaneous	Popcorn, catsup, BBQ sauce, peanut butter (unless corn-free), monosodium glutamate, distilled vinegar, chewing gum, Equal, cornstarch, vanillin, maraschino cherries, sweet pickles and sweet peppers, some baking powders, caramel coloring, many vitamins, medicines, tablets capsules, and liquids	Sea salt, baking soda, tapioca, dextrins, herbs and spices, pure extracts without added corn ingredients

[a]Tolerated by most people with corn allergy; advise caution for those with history of anaphylaxis.
Sources: Adapted from Ref. 10; Ref. 11; Ref. 13.

Although corn in itself does not contribute any specific nutrients, it is widely used in a variety of food products, usually in the form of corn sweeteners or cornstarch. It is possible that nutrient intake could be affected if food items that contain corn products are eliminated and not replaced with alternative nutrient sources.

In addition to its widespread use in food products, cornstarch is used in many paper or cardboard products, including milk cartons and paper cups. Foods packaged in these types of containers may need to be avoided. Other items that also contain corn products include breath sprays, drops, many chewing gums, and the glue on stamps, stickers, envelopes, and labels. Contact with these products should be avoided. In addition, products such as vitamins and drugs in tablet, capsule, or liquid form; toothpaste; and cough medicine may also contain corn derivatives. Caution should also be used with other nonfood products that may contain corn, including baby powders, hairsprays, and laundry starch.

Label Reading

Labels should be read carefully and any foods that contain the following words should be avoided:

Corn: fresh, canned, or creamed	Baking powder (unless corn-free)	Alcohol
		Lactic acid
Corn syrup	Dextrins	Popcorn
Cornstarch	Maltodextrins	Sorbitol
Corn flour	Dextrose	Corn solids
Corn sugar or sweetener	Fructose	Hydrolyzed vegetable
Vegetable starch	Vegetable gum	protein
Modified food starch	Vinegar	Vegetable oil[a]
Maize		Corn oil[a]
Cornmeal		

[a] Tolerated by most people with corn allergy. Caution is advised for those with history of anaphylaxis.
Sources: Adapted from Ref. 12; Ref. 13.

Substitutions in Cooking

In place of cornstarch, use equal amounts of arrowroot or potato starch or double the amount of whole wheat, soy, or barley flour. Since most baking powders contain cornstarch, a corn-free baking powder can be made by combining $1/4$ tsp baking soda with $1/2$ tsp cream of tartar. This is equivalent to 1 tsp baking powder and may be used for a leavening agent [10].

WHEAT-FREE DIET

Food Selection Guidelines

Treatment of wheat allergy consists of eliminating all food items containing this allergen from the individual's diet. Food selection guidelines for a wheat-free diet are outlined in Table 5.

Wheat is an important source of thiamine, riboflavin, niacin, and iron in the diet and in addition provides other important vitamins and minerals. Alternative food sources that contain these nutrients must be provided to ensure nutritional adequacy of a wheat-free diet.

Label Reading

Food labels and grain products should be checked carefully for the following ingredients, which indicate the presence of wheat protein:

Wheat	Graham flour	Farina
Wheat bran	All-purpose flour	Modified food starch
Bran	Cake flour	Malt or cereal extract
Wheat germ	Durum flour	Vegetable gums
Gluten	Pastry flour	Vegetable starches
Semolina	Whole wheat flour	

Sources: Adapted from Ref. 12; Ref. 13.

Substitutions in Cooking

Any of the following may be used as a thickening substitute for 1 tablespoon wheat flour:

$1\frac{1}{2}$ teaspoons cornstarch	$1\frac{1}{2}$ teaspoons white, brown, or sweet rice flour
$1\frac{1}{2}$ teaspoons potato starch	2 teaspoons quick-cooking tapioca
$1\frac{1}{2}$ teaspoons arrowroot starch	

Any of the following may be used as a baking substitute for 1 cup wheat flour:

1 cup barley flour	$\frac{3}{4}$ cup rice flour
1 cup corn flour	$1\frac{1}{4}$ cup rye flour
$\frac{3}{4}$ cup plain cornmeal, coarse	1 cup rye meal
1 scant cup plain cornmeal, fine	$1\frac{1}{2}$ cup ground rolled oats
$\frac{5}{8}$ cup potato starch flour	

Source: Ref. 12.
It should be noted that use of substitutes for wheat flour may alter food products' texture or flavor. Experimentation with alternate flours and recipes may be necessary to create an acceptable product.

TABLE 5   Food Selection Guidelines for Wheat-Free Diet

Food group	Avoid	Acceptable substitutes
Beverages	Malted milk, instant Breakfast, Postum, Ovaltine; gin, malt beer, ale, whiskey; flavor syrups that contain malt or wheat products	Plain milk, ground coffee, tea, fruit drinks, unfortified wines, rums; pure cocoa powder
Meat, egg, cheese, poultry, fish	Processed meat products (luncheon meats, cold cuts, hotdogs, sausage); meats prepared with flour, cracker crumbs, or other wheat products casseroles, croquettes, timbales, meatloaf, meatballs, some hamburgers, Swiss steak) breaded meat, fish, chicken	Meat products without added wheat; all fresh meat, fish, poultry, eggs, and cheese
Breads/cereals	All breads, rolls, crackers made with wheat flour, bran, graham flour, wheat germ, wheat gluten, cracker meal; muffins, biscuits, waffles, pancakes, and othe r prepared mixes containing wheat; bread crumbs and breaded foods; all ready to eat and cooked cereals containing wheat products, malted cereals, wheat germ	Wheat-free breads and baked goods; wheat-free cereals, Rice Chex, Cream of Rice, rice cakes/crackers, corn tortillas
Potatoes and substitutes	Any potatoes prepared with wheat products (scalloped, creamed, au gratin); wheat tortillas, some packaged rice mixes; pasta, spaghetti, noodles, macaroni made with wheat products	Rice, plain potatoes, sweet potatoes, yams, hominy, wheat-free pastas
Soups	Bouillon cubes, all creamed soups thickened with wheat flour; soups with macaroni, noodles, etc.	Creamed soups thickened with potato flour, cream, or cornstarch
Fruits/vegetables	Strained fruits with added cereal fruits prepared or thickened with wheat products (i.e., pie fillings), breaded or creamed vegetables served with wheat thickened sauce, some canned peas, beans, corn	All fresh fruits and vegetables and pure juices; canned plain fruits and vegetables

TABLE 5 Continued

Food group	Avoid	Acceptable substitutes
Desserts/sweets	Any prepared with flour as an ingredient: cakes, cookies, pies, pastries, doughnuts, bread pudding, prepared mixes, pudding thickened with wheat flour; ice cream cones some ice creams (use wheat products as thickening agents), some syrups and chocolate candies	Homemade baked goods and puddings made without wheat, gelatin, sherbet, or ices; ice creams made without wheat products
Fats	Commercial prepared salad dressings, gravies and sauces thickened with wheat products	Butter, margarine, vegetable oils, shortening; gravies and sauces made with acceptable thickening agents (cornstarch, potato starch, etc.)
Miscellaneous	Breaded foods, soy sauce, some yeasts, some powdered seasoning mixes	

Sources: Adapted from Ref. 10; Ref. 13.

DIETARY SUGGESTIONS FOR MANAGEMENT OF FOOD ALLERGIES

Label reading is perhaps the most important skill for the individual with food allergies. Being well informed about what foods are acceptable and carefully reading labels continuously are of utmost importance. Food manufacturers may change ingredients over time, without warning, and food labels must be carefully scrutinized prior to purchase or consumption. Grocery shopping and food preparation will probably take extra time. Specialty food stores, health food stores, and larger supermarkets may be checked for suitable alternatives.

Individuals with food allergies can safely eat out at restaurants and away from home, if they keep the following guidelines in mind:

1. Order plain food products and avoid mixed foods or processed foods, which may be prepared with a potential allergen that may cause distress.
2. Call in advance, state your specific allergies, and see whether food can be specially prepared.
3. Ask what specific ingredients are in the foods.
4. Take "safe" foods to substitute for foods that may contain an allergen.
5. Arrangements must be made for children when they eat outside the home. Other care givers and schools should be notified of the child's

allergy and given proper instructions concerning the child's diet. Effective communication between parents and school/care givers regarding the child's allergy is extremely imporsafe foods.

6. Individuals should be alerted to the possibility that the allergen may be a hidden ingredient or cross-contaminant and may need to carry epinephrine in case of accidental ingestion.

In treating the patient with food allergies, it is important that the diet provide variation using allowed foods and be nutritionally balanced, while restricting the offending allergen. A qualified dietitian can be of assistance to the physician with the assessment, education, and dietary planning of affected individuals. In addition, recipes, references, and sources of specialty products are helpful, allowing the individual to maintain variety in the diet. With the proper education and counseling, the food-allergic individual can learn to understand the food allergy, plan an adequate diet, and maintain a comfortable life-style.

RECIPE REFERENCES AND PATIENT RESOURCES

Allergy Information Association: The Food Allergy Cookbook (Diets Unlimited for Limited Diets). New York: St. Martin's Press, 1983.

American Academy of Allergy and Immunology, 611 East Wells Street, Milwaukee, WI 53202.

Asthma and Allergy Foundation of America, 1125 15th Street NW, Suite 502, Washington, DC 20005.

Dobler ML. Food Allergies. Chicago: American Dietetic Association, 1991.

Dong FM. All about Food Allergy. Philadelphia: George Stickley, 1984.

Ener-G-Foods, Inc, P.O. Box 24723, Seattle, WA 98124. This company sells specialty foods for wheat,- corn,- soy,- and egg-free diets.

The Food Allergy Network, 4744 Holly Avenue, Fairfax, VA 22030-5647.

Moyer J. Cooking for the Allergic Child. Bellefonte, PA: Grove Printing, 1987.

Roth J. The Allergic Gourmet. Chicago: Contemporary Books, 1983.

Williams ML. Cooking Without: Recipes for the Allergic Child (and FamYoder ER. Allergy-Free Cooking. Reading, PA: Addison-Wesley, 1987.

REFERENCES

1. American Academy of Allergy and Immunology, Committee on Adverse Reactions to Food and National Institute of Allergy and Infectious Diseases. Adverse Reactions to foods. NIH Publication No. 84-2442, July 1984.
2. Rao Y, Bahna SL. Dietary Management of Food Allergies. In: Chiaramonte LT, Schneider AT, Lifshitz F, eds. Food Allergy: A Practical Approach to Diagnosis and Management. New York: Marcel Dekker, 1988, pp 351–363.

3. Sampson HA, Metcalfe DD. Food allergy. JAMA 1992; 268:2840–2844.
4. Koerner CB, Sampson HA. Diets and Nutrition. In: Metcalfe DD, Sampson HA, Simon RA, eds. Food Allergy: Adverse Reactions to Food and Food Additives. Boston: Blackwell Scientific Publication, 1991.
5. Bierman CW, Shapiro CG, Christies DL VanArsdel, Jr., P.O., Furukawa, CT, and Ward BH. Allergy Grand Rounds: Eczema, Rickets and Food Allergy. J Allergy Clin Immunol 1978; 61:119–127.
6. David TJ, Waddington E, Stanton RHJ. Nutritional hazards of elimination diets in children with atopic eczema. Arch Dis Child 1984; 59:323–325.
7. Lloyd-Still JD. Chronic diarrhea of childhood and the misuse of elimination diets. J Pediatr 1979; 95:10–13.
8. Davidovits M, Levy Y, Avramovitz. Calcium deficiency rickets in a four-year-old boy with milk allergy. J Pediatr 1993; 122:249–251.
9. Torrens S, Gizis F, Frieri M. Evaluation of nutrient and food intake in individuals with reported food allergies. Abstract presented at New York State Dietetic Association 65th Annual Meeting, April 27, 1995.
10. Adams EJ. Nutritional care in food allergy and food intolerance. In: Mahan LK, Arlin M, eds. Krause's Food Nutrition and Diet Therapy. Philadelphia: WB Saunders, 1992:653–669.
11. Greenberg LE, Moses NS. Egg-free and corn-free diets. In: Chiaramonte LT, Schneider AT, Lifshitz F. Food Allergy: A Practical Approach to Diagnosis and Management. New York: Marcel Dekker, 1988, pp 441–452.
12. Dobler ML. Food Allergies. Chicago: The American Dietetic Association, 1991.
13. Kendall PA, Gloeckner JW. Allergies and adverse reactions: managing food allergies and sensitivities. Top Clin Nutr 1994; 9(3):4–6.
14. National Academy of Sciences. Recommended Dietary Allowances. 10th ed. Washington DC: National Academy Press, 1989.

24

Hypoallergenic Formulas

JAYA M. THERATTIL
Nassau County Medical Center, East Meadow, New York

SAMI L. BAHNA
University of South Florida, All Children's Hospital, St. Petersburg, Florida

Hypoallergenic formulas were developed as substitute diets for children with cow's milk allergy or intolerance. Depending on the protein source as well as on the method of preparation there are a wide variety of these formulas with different degrees of immunogenicities. Immunogenicity is the capacity of molecules or immunogens to elicit an immune response. The factors that contribute to immunogenicity include the molecular weight, "foreignness" of the immunogen, chemical complexity, dose, route of exposure, and method of sensitization.

Several studies have investigated the antigen content and allergenicity of hypoallergenic formulas. The allergenic potential of a protein can be reduced by enzymatic hydrolysis and heat treatment. On the basis of the degree of such hydrolysis, formulas can be classified as partially or extensively hydrolyzed. Several studies have shown that in the partial hydrolysate formulas the quantity of intact antigen is significant and the immunogenicity can be high, whereas in the extensively hydrolyzed formulas, the antigen content is greatly reduced [1–5].

RECOMMENDED STANDARDS FOR HYPOALLERGENIC FORMULAS

The American Academy of Pediatrics Subcommittee on Nutrition and Allergic Disease has proposed the following criteria for hypoallergenic formula [6].

- Nutritional adequacy to promote growth in healthy infants
- Preclinical testing in vitro and in vivo for allergenicity
- Clinical testing in allergic infants for allergenicity
- Clinical testing in infants at high risk of allergy for allergenicity

The objectives of preclinical testing are to

1. Characterize the molecular properties of the protein or peptides to assess residual antigenicity
2. Estimate the actual reduction in antigenicity of the starting protein
3. Develop methods that ensure batch-to-batch consistency of the hydrolyzed protein

After the appropriate preclinical studies are conducted, double-blind placebo-controlled trials should be performed in infants with symptoms caused by documented hypersensitivity to cow's milk or cow's milk–based infant formula and/or when given to similar subjects with documented hypersensitivity to the protein from which the hydrolysate is derived. After the double-blind placebo-controlled trial, an open challenge should be performed. The number of infants or children studied should be sufficient to project with 95% confidence that at least 90% of milk-allergic infants will not react to the formula.

ALLERGIC REACTIONS TO HYDROLYSATE FORMULAS

Hydrolysate formulas, particularly the extensively hydrolyzed ones, contain significantly less allergen than the regular formulas and are tolerated by the majority of milk-sensitive patients. Certain subjects with exquisite sensitivity may react to these formulas, and the reactions can be severe [7–14]. Hence, in such subjects it would be prudent before prescribing any milk formula to try it cautiously under supervision.

Elemental Formulas

The elemental formulas consist of synthesized amino acids and therefore have the least immunogenicity. Several preparations are available (Tables 1 and 2).

TABLE 1 Types and Preparations of Hypoallergenic Formulas

	Manufacturer
A. Extensively hydrolyzed bovine casein	
1. Nutramigen	Mead Johnson
2. Pregestemil	Mead Johnson
3. Alimentum	Ross
B. Extensively hydrolyzed bovine whey	
1. Alfa-Re	Nestle
2. Ultra	Nestle
3. Profylac	ALK
4. Almiron Pepti	Nucticia/Loma Linda
5. Nutrilon Pepti	Nutricia
6. Nutrilon Pepti Plus	Nutricia
7. Pepti Junior	Nutricia
8. Peptamen	Clintec Nutrition
9. Peptamen Junior	Clintec Nutrition
10. Peptidi-Tutteli	Valio
C. Extensively hydrolyzed bovine casein and whey	
1. Damira	Wander
D. Extensively hydrolyzed soy plus bovine collagen	
1. Pregomin, Hydrolac	Milupa
E. Elemental diet	
1. Vivonex	Sandoz Nutrition
2. Tolerex	Sandoz Nutrition
3. Vivasorb	Phrimer A/S
4. Neocate	Scientific Hospital Supplies
5. Neocate One Plus	Scientific Hospital Supplies
6. Nutri-Junior	Nutricia
F. Partially hydrolyzed bovine whey	
1. Beba HA, Nan HA, Nidina HA	Nestle
2. Good Start	Carnation Nestle
3. Vivena HA	Dieterba
G. Partially hydrolyzed bovine casein and whey	
1. Aptamil	Milupa

Vivonex is available in three forms, Vivonex pediatric, Vivonex plus, and Vivonex T.E.N. Neocate [15–17] is one of the newest elemental formulas and is available in two forms, Neocate for infants under 1 year of age and Neocate One+ for older children.

Table 1 contains the types and preparations of various formulas that are considered "hypoallergenic" in various countries. Table 2 shows the nutritional constituents of some of these formulas.

TABLE 2 Nutritional Constituents of Some Hypoallergenic Formulas per 100 kcal of Product

	Neocate[c]	Pregestimil[a]	Nutramigen[a]	Alimentum[b]
Form	Powder	Powder	Powder	Liquid
Flavor	Unflavored	Unflavored	Unflavored	Unflavored
Energy kcal/ml	0.67	0.67	0.67	0.67
Protein equivalent	3.1	2.8	2.8	2.75
Protein source	Limoteic acids	Hydrolyzed casein	Hydrolyzed casein	Hydrolyzed casein
Fat g	4.5	5.6	2.0	1.6
L-amino acid g	.67	.94	2.0	1.6
MCT	5%	55%	0%	50%
LCT	95%	45%	100%	50%
Carbohydrate g	11.7	10.3	13.4	10.2
Minerals				
Calcium, mg	123	94	94	105
Phosphorus, mg	93.1	63	63	75
Magnesium, mg	12.4	10.9	10.9	7.5
Iron, mg	1.85	1.88	1.88	1.8
Zinc, mg	1.66	.94	.78	.75
Manganese, mg	0.09	0.03	0.03	0.03
Copper, mg	.124	0.09	0.09	0.075
Iodine, mcg	15.4	7.0	7	15
Sodium, mg	37.3	39	47	44
Potassium, mg	155.1	109	109	118
Chloride, mg	77.2	86	86	80
Selenium, µg	3.73	2.3	2.3	Not stated
Chromium, µg	3.38	Not stated	Not stated	Not stated
Molybdenum, µg	4.75	Not stated	Not stated	Not stated
Vitamins				
Vitamin A, µg RE	122.7	114	93	90
Vitamin D, µg	2.175	1.88	1.58	1.13
Vitamin E, mg a-TE	.765	2.55	2.1	2.01
Vitamin K, µg	8.79	18.8	15.6	15
Vitamin C, mg	9.26	11.7	8.1	9
Thiamine, mg	.0926	0.08	0.08	0.06
Riboflavin, mg	.1378	0.09	0.09	0.09
Vitamin B_4, mg	.1235	0.06	0.06	0.06
Vitamin B_{12}, µg	.170	.31	.31	.45
Niacin, mg	1.5440	1.25	1.25	1.35
Folic acid, µg	10.2	15.6	15.6	15
Panthothenic acid, mg	.62	.47	.47	.75
Biotin, µg	3.1	7.8	7.8	4.5
Choline, mg	13.1	13.3	13.3	8.0

TABLE 2 Continued

	Neocate[c]	Pregestimil[a]	Nutramigen[a]	Alimentum[b]
Inositol, mg	23.3	4.7	4.7	5.0
Osmolality at standards dilution (m Osm/kg H_2O)	342	320	320	370

	Neocate[c] One	Vivonex[d] Pediatric	Vivonex[d] T.E.N.	Vivonex[d] Plus	Tolerex	Peptamen[e] Oral
Form	Liquid and powder	Powder	Powder	Powder	Powder	Liquid
Flavor	Liquid: Orange Pineapple Powder: Unflavored	Unflavored	Unflavored	Unflavored	Unflavored	Vanilla
Energy (Kcal/m)	1.0	.8	1.0	1.0	1.0	1.0
Protein Equivalent g	2.5	3	3.8	4.5	2.1	4
Protein Source	L-amino acids	L-amino acids	L-amino acids	L-amino acids	L-amino acids	Hydrolyzed whey
Fat, g	3.5	2.94	.28	.67	.15	4
Linoleic Acid, g	.38	.49	.22	.1	.12	.06
% MCT	35%	68%	0%	0%	0%	70%
% LCT	65%	32%	100%	100%	100%	30%
Carbohydrate, g	14.6	15.75	21	19	23	12.7
Minerals						
Calcium, mg	62	121.5	50	55.7	56	80
Phosphorus, mg	62	100	50	55.7	56	70
Magnesium, mg	9	25	20	22	22	40
Iron, mg	.77	1.25	.9	.1	.1	1.2
Zinc, mg	.77	1.5	1	1.3	.83	1.4
Magnesnese, mg	.1	.25	.09	.17	.16	.27
Copper, mg	.1	.15	.1	.11	.11	.14
Iodine, µg	6	15	7.5	8.3	8.30	10
Sodium, mg	20	50	46	61	47	50
Potassium, mg	93	150	78	110	120	125
Chloride, mg	35	125	82	94	95	100
Selenium, µg	1.54	3.75	5	5.6	8.3	4
Chromium, µg	3	5.65	1.7	8.3	2.78	4
Molybdenum, µg	3.5	9.4	5	14	8.3	12

TABLE 2 Continued

	Neocate[c] One	Vivonex[d] Pediatric	Vivonex[d] T.E.N.	Vivonex[d] Plus	Tolerex	Peptamen[e] Oral
Vitamins						
Vitamin A,						
mcg RE	35	93.8	75	126	84	120
Vitamin D, μg	.78	1.56	.5	.83	.55	.7
Vitamin E, mg						
α-TE	.55	2.52	.1	1.7	1.14	1.88
Vitamin K, μg	1.5	5	2.2	4.4	3.7	8
Vitamin C, mg	3.08	12.5	6	6.7	3.3	14
Thiamine, mg	.054	.19	.15	.17	.08	.2
Riboflavin, mg	.065	.225	.17	.19	.09	.24
Vitamin B_6, mg	.08	.25	.2	.22	11	.4
Vitamin B_{12}, μg	.07	.375	.6	.67	.33	.8
Niacin, mg	.9	2.5	2	2.2	1.11	2.8
Folic acid, μg	6	25	40	44.3	22	54
Pantothenic acid,						
mg	.24	.625	1	1.11	.56	1.4
Biotin, μg	2	12.5	30	33	17	40
Choline, mg	18.3	25	7.4	22	4.1	45
Inositol, mg	1.8	7.5	not stated	not stated	not stated	not stated
Osmolality at						
standard	Liquid: 835					
dilution		360	630	650	550	380
(mOsm/kg	Powder: 610					
H_2O**)**						

[a]Mead Johnson Pediatrics, Pediatric Products Handbook, Evansville, IN: Mead Johnson & Co. 1993
[b]Ross Products Handbook, Columbus, OH: Ross Products Division, Abbott Laboratories, 1994
[c]Scientific Hospital Supplies
[d]Vivonex Pediatric, Minneapolis, MS: Clinical Products Division, Sandoz Nutrition Corporation, 1994
[e]Clintec Enteral Product Guide, Deerfield, IL: Clintec Nutrition Company, 1994.

REFERENCES

1. Leary LH: Non-clinical testing of formulas containing hydrolysed milk protein. J Pediatr 121:545, 1992.
2. Makinen-Kiljunen S, Sorva R: Bovine B-lactoglobulin levels in hydrolysed protein formulas for infant feeding. Clin exp Allergy 23:287, 1993.
3. McLaughlan P, Anderson KJ, Widdowson EM, et al: Effect of heat on the anaphy-

lactic-sensitizing capacity of cows milk, goats milk, and various infant formulae fed to guinea-pigs. Arch Dis Child 56:165, 1981.

4. Oldaeus G, Bjorksten B, Einarsson R, et al: Antigenicity and allergenicity of cow milk hydrolysates intended for infant feeding. Pediatr Allergy Immunol 4:156, 1991.

5. Oldaeus G, Bradley CK, Bjorksten B, et al: Allergenicity screening of "hypoallergenic milk-based formulas". J Allergy Clin Immunol 90:133, 1992.

6. Kleinman RE, Bahna SL, Powell GF, Sampson HA: Use of infant formulas in infants with cow milk allergy: A review and recommendations. Pediatr Allergy Immunol 4:146, 1991.

7. Amonette MS, Schwartz RH, Maltson L, et al: Double-blind placebo-controlled food challenges (DBPCFC) demonstrating acute IgE mediated allergic reactions to Good Start, Untrafiltered Good Start, Alfare, Nutramigen and Alimentum in a seven-year-old. Pediatr Asthma Allergy Immunol 5:245, 1991.

8. Businco L, Cantani A, Longhi MA, et al: Anaphylactic reactions to a cow's milk whey protein hydrolysate (Alfa-Re Nestle) in infants with cow's milk allergy. Ann Allergy 62:333, 1989.

9. Ellis MH, Short JA, Heiner DC: Anaphylaxis after ingestion of a recently introduced hydrolysed whey protein formula. J Pediatr 118:74, 1991.

10. Kelso JM, Sampson HA: Food protein-induced enterocolitis to casein hydrolysate formulas. J Allergy Clin Immunol 92:909, 1993.

11. Rosenthal E, Schliesinger Y, Birnbaum Y, et al: Intolerance to casein hydrolysate formula. Acta Paediatr Scand 80:958, 1991.

12. Rugo E, Wahl R, Wahn U: How allergenic are hypoallergenic infant formulae? Clin exp Allergy 22:635, 1992.

13. Sampson HA, Bernhisel-Broadbent J, Yang E, et al: Safety of casein hydrolysate formula in children with cow milk allergy. J Pediatr 118:520, 1991.

14. Saylor JD, Bahna SL: Anaphylaxis to casein hydrolysate formula. J Pediatr 118:71, 1991.

15. Hill DJ, Cameron DJS, and Francis, DEM, et al. Challenge confirmation of late onset reactions to extensively hydrolyzed formulae in infants with multiple food protein intolerance. J Allergy Clin Immunol, 96:386, 1995.

16. Sampson HA, James JM and Bernhisel-Broadbent J: Safety of an amino acid-derived infant formula in children allergic to cow milk. Pediatrics 90, (3), 463, 1992.

17. Isolauri E and Turjanmaa K: Combined skin prick and patch testing enhances identification of food allergy in infants with atopic dermatitis. J Allergy Clin Immunol 97:9, 1996.

25

Available Patient Resources

ANNE MUÑOZ-FURLONG
The Food Allergy Network, Fairfax, Virginia

The diagnosis of food allergy and recommendation of a strict elimination diet may leave patients feeling overwhelmed at the task ahead. However, learning to incorporate the elimination diet into everyday situations and to always be prepared to handle the unexpected is the cornerstone to managing food allergies.

Following are names and phone numbers for health organizations, support groups, supply companies, and other sources of information created to help patients learn to manage their allergy successfully. Most organizations will send patients free information or provide assistance by phone. Many will send free samples to physicians' offices to facilitate distribution to patients.

Please make this list available to patients as you make your diagnosis so that the patient can immediately become connected to a support system and begin to learn that it is possible to live a normal life in spite of a food allergy.

Health Professionals: For a List of Local Doctors Patients Can Call

American Academy of Allergy Asthma & Immunology
611 East Wells Street
Milwaukee, WI 53202
Toll Free: (800) 822-2762
Phone: (414) 272-6071
Web Site: http://www.aaaai.org

American College of Asthma, Allergy and Immunology
1645 Oakton Street
Des Plaines, IL 60018
Toll Free: (800) 842-7777
Web Site: http://www.allergy.mcg.edu

American Dietetic Association
216 West Jackson Boulevard
Chicago, IL 60606-6995
Toll Free: (800) 366-1655
Web Site: http:/www.eatright.org

National Jewish Medical and Research Center
1400 Jackson Street
Denver, CO 80206
Toll Free: (800) 222-LUNG
Web Site: http://www.njc.org

Patient Educational Sources

Allergy and Asthma Network/Mothers of Asthmatics, Inc.
2751 Prosperity Avenue, Suite 150
Fairfax, VA 22031-4397
Toll Free: (800) 878-4403
Phone: (703) 385-4403
Web Site: http://www.aanma.org
Nonprofit organization, provides monthly newsletter and other educational materials for managing asthma and allergies.

Asthma and Allergy Foundation of America
1125 15th Street, NW, Suite 502
Washington, DC 20005
Toll Free: (800)-7-ASTHMA
Phone: (202) 466-7643
Fax: (202) 466-8940
Web Site: http://www.aafa.org

The Asthma and Allergy Foundation of America (AAFA) is a private, not-for-profit organization dedicated to finding a cure for and controlling asthma and allergic diseases. Has a network of chapters and support groups located throughout the nation.

Nancy Carol Sanker, OTR
Coordinator of Support Group Services
Asthma and Allergy Foundation of America
1412 Miramont Drive
Ft. Collins, CO 80524
Phone: (970) 221-9165
Fax: (970) 482-6235
Provides information and guidance for creating local support groups.

Allergy/Asthma Information Association
30 Eglinton Avenue West, Suite 750
Mississauga, Ontario
Canada L5R 3E7
Phone: (905) 712-2242
Fax: (905) 712-2245
Patient education, newsletter, and other materials for managing asthma and allergies. Nonprofit organization.

Celiac Sprue Association/United States of America, Inc.
P.O. Box 31700
Omaha, NE 68131-0700
Phone: (402) 558-0600
National support organization provides information and referral services for persons with celiac sprue. Has published a series of low-cost brochures on the gluten-free diet, gluten-free commercial foods, and gluten-free medications.

Celiac Disease Foundation
13251 Ventura Boulevard, Suite 1
Studio City, CA 91504-1838
Phone: (818) 990-2354
Fax: (818) 990-2379
email: cdefprimenet.com
Web Site: http://www.csaceliacs.org
A California nonprofit public benefit corporation dedicated to providing services and support to persons with celiac disease and dermatitis herpetiformis through programs of awareness, education, advocacy, and research.

Ellie Goldberg Education Rights Specialist
70 Elmore Street
Newton, MA 02159
Phone: (617) 965-9637
Fax: (617) 965-5407

Specializes in issues pertaining to children in the school system. Publishes literature, provides free advice for enforcing children's legal rights.

The Food Allergy Network
10400 Eaton Place, Suite 107
Fairfax, Virginia 22030-2208
Toll Free: (800) 929-4040
Phone: (703) 691-3179
Fax: (703) 691-2713
Web Site: http://www.foodallergy.org
A nonprofit organization devoted solely to patient education about food allergies. Mission is to increase public awareness of food allergies and anaphylaxis
and to provide emotional support and coping strategies to individuals with
food allergies and their families. Provides videos, pamplets, cookbooks,
newsletter, patient conferences, and EpiPen trainers. Free information available to callers.

Immune Deficiency Foundation
25 W. Chesapeake Avenue, Suite 206
Towson, MD 21204
Toll Free: (800) 296-4433
Phone: (410) 321-6647
Fax: (410) 321-9165
Web Site: http://www.primaryimmune.org
A national organization devoted to research and education for the primary im-
mune deficiency diseases.

International Food Information Council Foundation
1100 Connecticut Avenue, NW, Suite 430
Washington, DC 20036
Phone: (202) 296-6540
Fax: (202) 296-6547
Web Site: http://ificinfo.health.org
Provides sound scientific information on food safety and nutrition to journalists,
health professionals, educators, government officials, and consumers. IFIC is a
nonprofit organization based in Washington, DC.

International Glutamate Association
555 13th Street NW, Suite 7W304
Washington, DC 20004
Phone: (202) 783-6135
Web Site: http://www.msgfacts.com
Trade association that provides information and research studies on MSG.

Medic Alert Foundation United States
2323 Colorado Avenue
Turlock, CA 95382
Phone: (209) 668-3333
Fax: (209) 669-2495
Web Site: http://www.medicalert.org
Nonprofit 501 corporation founded to provide quick, accessible, vital personal medical information to protect its members and save lives in emergencies. The trademarked Medic Alert emblem is worn as a bracelet or necklace that bears the internationally recognized insignia of the medical profession with the words "Medic Alert." The emblem specifies medical conditions of the wearer and the telephone number of the Emergency Response Center. Emergency personnel can call this number collect from any phone around the world.

National Center for Nutrition and Dietetics
216 West Jackson Boulevard, Suite 800
Chicago, IL 60606-6995
Toll Free: (800) 366-1655
Public education initiative of the American Dietetic Association (ADA) and its foundation. Dedicated to promoting the nutritional health of Americans. Disseminates objective and timely nutrition information.

National Eczema Association
1221 SW Yamhill, #303
Portland, OR 97205
Phone: (503) 228-4430
A national nonprofit patient-oriented organization dedicated to atopic dermatitis education and research. Provides educational and informational services, working to increase public awareness, support training, and research funding for atopic dermatitis.

RECOMMENDED READING FOR PATIENTS

Bock MD, Allan S. *Food Allergy: A Primer for People.* Vantage Press, 1988.
Muñoz-Furlong A, Goldberg E. *Students with Food Allergies: What Do the Laws Say?* The Food Allergy Network, 1994.
Muñoz-Furlong A. *The School Food Allergy Program.* The Food Allergy Network, 1995.

Index

About the Editors

Marianne Frieri is the Director of Clinical Immunopathology and the Allergy-Immunology Training Program at Nassau County Medical Center, East Meadow, New York (affiliated with North Shore University Hospital), and Associate Professor of Medicine and Pathology, State University of New York at Stony Brook. She is the author or coauthor of more than 120 abstracts, book chapters, and journal articles, and a frequent local, national, and international lecturer on allergy, immunology, and immunopathology. She is a past president of the Long Island Allergy and Asthma Society, a Fellow of the local Arthritis Foundation, and a member of the American Society of Clinical Pathologists, the American Federation of Clinical Research, and the American Academy and College of Allergy, Asthma and Immunology. Dr. Frieri received the B.S. degree (1967) in biology and medical technology from the State University of New York at Buffalo, the M.S. degree (1970) in biology from Canisius College, Buffalo, the Ph.D. degree (1976) in microbiology from the University of Health Sciences, Chicago Medical School, Illinois, and the M.D. degree (1978) from Loyola University, Stritch School of Medicine, Maywood, Illinois.

Brett Kettelhut is currently an Assistant Clinical Professor of Pediatrics at the Children's Hospital Medical Center, Cincinnati, Ohio, and a private practice allergist at the Cincinnati Allergy and Asthma Center. He is a Fellow of the American Academy of Allergy, Asthma and Immunology and the American Academy of Pediatrics, and a member of the American Thoracic Society, Dr. Kettelhut received the B.S. degree (1974) in chemistry from the University of Nebraska, Omaha, and the M.D. degree (1982) from the University of Nebraska College of Medicine, Omaha, and completed his allergy and immunology fellowship at the National Institutes of Health in 1988.

Milton Keynes UK
Ingram Content Group UK Ltd.
UKHW020007071024
449327UK00031B/2691